GROUP HOME COOKBOOK

PART 2

MEAT AND SEAFOOD

Standard Recipes with Food Safety Guidelines, Therapeutic Diet Modifications, Texture Diet Modifications, and Allergy Alert

THIS BOOK IS PART OF A SERIES. THIS COOKBOOK INCLUDE BEEF, HAM, LAMB, PORK SAUSAGE, AND SEAFOOD RECIPES

Managing Editor

Jacqueline Larson M.S., R.D.N.

This publication was developed for and under the direction and supervision of the Jacqueline Larson M.S., R.D.N and Associates. All rights under federal copyright laws are held by Jacqueline Larson M.S. R.D.N. and Associates.

All parts of this publication may not be reproduced in any form of printed or visual medium. Any reproduction of this publication may not be sold for profit or reproduction costs without the exclusive permission of Jacqueline Larson M.S., R.D.N. Any reproduction of this cookbook in whole or part, shall acknowledge Jacqueline Larson M.S., R.D.N. in writing.

Jacqueline Larson, M.S., R.D.N.

Consultant Dietitian

Cookbook Series Coordinator

www.Consultantdietitian.com

Copyright © 2020 Jacqueline Larson M.S., R.D.N.
All rights reserved.
ISBN: 9798648292390

ACKNOWLEDGMENT

"The Group Home Cookbook " was first developed in 1986 by Jacqueline Larson M.S., R.D.N. and Associates. After the overwhelming success of "The Group Home Cookbook" the new version has been converted into a series of cookbooks. This will be the forth version. This new series has even more delicious and nutritious recipes. The collaborative efforts of this group have resulted in a series of recipes designed for use by health care professionals in providing nutrition care to individuals in Long Term Care smaller communities. Ideal for group homes, rehabilitation centers, board and care communities and small schools. The recipes are standardized for 8 servings. Each recipe includes food safety guidelines, therapeutic diet modification guidelines, texture diet modifications guidelines and allergy alerts. This Cookbook is part of a series of cookbooks. Other cookbooks in the series included in the series:

Other cookbooks in the series included in the series:

Group Home Cookbook Part 1 Poultry and Eggs

Group Home Cookbook Part 2 Meats and Seafood

Group Home Cookbook Part 3 Vegan and Vegetarian

Group Home Cookbook Part 4 Soups, Sauces and Appetizers

Group Home Cookbook Part 5 Breads, Starchy Sides, Desserts and Beverages

Group Home Cookbook Part 6 Fruits, Vegetables, Salads and Dressings

Other books of interest:

High Calorie High Protein Supplements

The Diet Manual (coordinates with the cookbook series)

Preparing Puree Meals

On-going revisions will occur as advancements in medical nutritional therapy continue to be made. The information in this manual is current as possible in a continuously changing field.

DISCLAIMER

The information provided here is as up to date, accurate and as practical as possible in a field that moving very quickly and is full of controversy. Any preparations in this manual should be discussed with and managed by your medical physician. The implementation should be supervised by a registered dietitian nutritionist. It is highly recommended individuals with chewing and/or swallowing difficulties consult with a qualified Speech and Language Pathologist and/or qualified Occupational Therapeutics. Great effort has been taken to assure the accuracy of this manual; however, we know that errors do occur, and caution should be used when feeding or preparing meals of individuals with special needs. The author and publisher disclaim any responsibility for any adverse consequences resulting from the use of this manual

IMPORTANT NOTICE

Specialized diets should only be done under the supervision of your medical physician. Always consult your medical physician before starting any type of special diet.

Copyright 2020- Jacqueline Larson M.S., R.D.N. and Associates.   All Rights Reserved

TABLE OF CONTENTS

INTRODUCTION TO MEAT AND SEAFOOD	7
BEEF DINNER RECIPES	9
BEEF LUNCH RECIPES	94
HAM DINNER RECIPES	114
HAM LUNCH RECIPES	141
LAMB DINNER RECIPES	148
PORK DINNER RECIPES	152
PORK LUNCH RECIPES	213
SAUSAGE DINNER RECIPES	221
SAUSAGE LUNCH RECIPES	243
SEAFOOD DINNER RECIPES	249
SEAFOOD LUNCH RECIPES	342
RECIPE INDEX	370

Copyright 2020 Jacqueline Larson M.S., R.D.N. and Associates.   All Rights Reserved

Meats

Meats are defined as domesticated animals raised for their meat. This includes beef, pork, chicken and lamb. Chicken is the most popular meat consumed in the United States. Meats are a high-quality protein foods. A high quality protein is a protein source which meets the protein requirements for humans. Meat composition may include muscle, fat, cartilage and bone. Removing the fat from the meat will decrease the amount of fat and calories. Pay attention when selecting ground meats. Not all ground meats are created equal. Read labels carefully to ground meat because fat is sometimes added. Choose leaner ground meat when cooking. To reduce fat choose the 7% or less fat ground meat. It is leaner and more cost effective.

Purchasing Meat

The Federal Meat Inspection Act of 1906 made inspection of all meat crossing state lines mandatory. The USDA is responsible for meat inspections. Look for the USDA meat inspection stamp on meats to ensure wholesomeness. When purchasing meat for a 3 oz. serving ,purchase a 4 oz. serving to account for losses during cooking. Purchase refrigerated or frozen items after selecting your non-perishables. Never choose meat or poultry in packaging that is torn or leaking. Do not buy food past "Sell-By," "Use-By," or other expiration dates.

Choosing low fat meats

Not all cuts of meats are created equal. Look for beefs labeled "USDA Select" grade. It is lower in fat and calories than choice or prime. Meats with the word "loin" or "round" are usually leaner choices. When cooking meats trim all fats before cooking, and remove fats from stews, soups and casseroles. Avoid frying meats.

Thawing Meat

Freezing meat can protect against bacterial growth. The refrigerator is the best place to thaw meat. NEVER THAW MEAT AT ROOM TEMPERATURE. The larger the meat cut the more time it will take to thaw.

Refrigerator: The refrigerator allows slow, safe thawing. Make sure thawing meat and poultry juices do not drip onto other food.

Cold Water: For faster thawing, place food in a leak-proof plastic bag. Submerge in cold tap water. Change the water every 30 minutes. Cook immediately after thawing.

Preparation of Meat

There are 2 types of cooking methods for meat. Dry heat methods and Moist heat methods. Moist heat methods are usually preferred for tougher cuts of meat. Meats should be prepared properly is tender and juicy. Over cooking meat can cause the flesh to become dry, tough and stringy. Dry Heat Methods include: Roasting, Baking, Broiling, Grilling, Frying. Moist Heat Methods include : Braising, Stewing, Poaching. Meats should always be heated until the minimum temperature to enhance the flavor and to minimize the risk of food borne illness. Doneness must be determined by taking the internal temperature. Avoid over cooking meats.

Minimum internal cooking temperature:165°F (74°C) for <1 second (Instantaneous)
- Poultry—whole or ground chicken, turkey or duck
- Stuffing made with fish, meat, or poultry
- Stuffed meat, seafood, poultry, or pasta
- Dishes that include previously cooked TCS ingredients

Minimum internal cooking temperature: 155°F (68°C) for 17 seconds
- Ground meat—beef, pork, and other meat
- Injected meat—including brined ham and flavor-injected roasts
- Mechanically tenderized meat
- Ground meat from game animals commercially raised and inspected
- Ratites—including ostrich and emu
- Ground seafood—including chopped or minced seafood
- Shell eggs that will be hot-held for service

Minimum internal cooking temperature: 145°F (63°C) for 15 seconds
- Seafood—including fish, shellfish, and crustaceans
- Steaks/chops of pork, beef, veal, and lamb
- Commercially raised game
- Shell eggs that will be served immediately

Minimum internal cooking temperature: 145°F (63°C) for four minutes
- o Roasts of pork, beef, veal, and lamb
- o Alternate cooking times/temperatures

  - 130°F (54°C) 112 minutes
  - 131°F (55°C) 89 minutes
  - 133°F (56°C) 56 minutes
  - 135°F (57°C) 36 minutes
  - 136°F (58°C) 28 minutes
  - 138°F (59°C) 18 minutes
  - 140°F (60°C) 12 minutes
  - 142°F (61°C) 8 minutes
  - 144°F (62°C) 5 minutes

Rinsing or Soaking Meats
Washing raw meat before cooking it is not recommended. Bacteria in raw meat can be spread to other foods, utensils, and surfaces. This is called cross-contamination. Rinsing or soaking meat does not destroy bacteria. Only cooking will destroy any bacteria that might be present on fresh meat.

Safe Meat Handling
Fresh Meats: Meat is kept cold during distribution to retail stores to prevent the growth of bacteria and to increase its shelf life. Meat should feel cold to the touch when purchased. Select fresh meat just before checking out at the register. Put packages of meats in disposable plastic bags (if available) to contain any leakage which could cross-contaminate cooked foods or produce. Make the grocery store your last stop before going home. At home, immediately place meats in a refrigerator that maintains a temperature of 40 °F (4.4 °C) or below. Use it within 1 or 2 days or freeze it at 0 °F (-17.8 °C). If kept frozen continuously, it will be safe indefinitely.

Meats may be frozen in its original packaging or repackaged. If freezing meats longer than 2 months, overwrap the porous store plastic packages with airtight heavy-duty foil, plastic wrap, or freezer paper, or place the package inside a freezer bag. Use these materials or airtight freezer containers to freeze the chicken from opened packages or repackage family packs of chicken into smaller amounts.

Proper wrapping prevents "freezer burn," which appears as grayish-brown leathery spots and is caused by air reaching the surface of food. Cut freezer-burned portions away either before or after cooking the meat. Heavily freezer-burned products may have to be discarded because they may be too dry or tasteless.

Food Safety Tips for Meats
Safe steps in food handling, cooking, and storage are essential to prevent foodborne illness. You can't see, smell, or taste harmful bacteria that may cause illness.

Clean — Wash hands and surfaces often.
Separate — Don't cross-contaminate.
Cook — Cook to the right temperature.
Chill — Refrigerate promptly.

Storage
Always refrigerate perishable food within 2 hours—1 hour when the temperature is above 90 °F (32.2 °C). Check the temperature of your refrigerator and freezer with an appliance thermometer. The refrigerator should be at 40 °F (4.4 °C) or below and the freezer at 0 °F (-17.7 °C) or below. Cook or freeze fresh poultry, fish, ground meats, and variety meats within 2 days; other beef, veal, lamb, or pork, within 3 to 5 days. Perishable food such as meat and poultry should be wrapped securely to maintain quality and to prevent meat juices from getting onto other food. To maintain quality when freezing meat and poultry in its original package, wrap the package again with foil or plastic wrap that is recommended for the freezer. Canned foods are safe indefinitely as long as they are not exposed to freezing temperatures, or temperatures above 90 °F. If the cans look ok, they are safe to use. Discard cans that are dented, rusted, or swollen. High-acid canned food (tomatoes, fruits) will keep their best quality for 12 to 18 months; low-acid canned food (meats, vegetables) for 2 to 5 years.

Preparation
Always wash hands with warm water and soap for 20 seconds before and after handling food.
Don't cross-contaminate. Keep raw meat, poultry, fish, and their juices away from other food. After cutting raw meats, wash cutting board, utensils, and countertops with hot, soapy water.

Cutting boards, utensils, and countertops can be sanitized by using a solution of 1 tablespoon of unscented, liquid chlorine bleach in 1 gallon of water.

Marinate meat and poultry in a covered dish in the refrigerator.

When slicing meat, slice meat across the grain.

Refrigerator: The refrigerator allows slow, safe thawing. Make sure thawing meat and poultry juices do not drip onto other food.

Cold Water: For faster thawing, place food in a leak-proof plastic bag. Submerge in cold tap water. Change the water every 30 minutes. Cook immediately after thawing.

Microwave: Cook meat and poultry immediately after microwave thawing.

Serving

Hot food should be held at 140 °F (60 °C) or warmer.

Cold food should be held at 40 °F (4.4 °C) or colder.

When serving food at a buffet, keep food hot with chafing dishes, slow cookers, and warming trays. Keep food cold by nesting dishes in bowls of ice or use small serving trays and replace them often.

Perishable food should not be left out more than 2 hours at room temperature—1 hour when the temperature is above 90 °F (32.2 °C).

Always wear gloves when handling ready to eat foods.

Leftovers

Discard any food left out at room temperature for more than 2 hours—1 hour if the temperature was above 90 °F (32.2 °C).

Place food into shallow covered containers and immediately put in the refrigerator or freezer for rapid cooling.

Label and date leftovers.

Use cooked leftovers within 2 days.

Reheat leftovers to 165 °F (73.9 °C).

Portion sizes:

The recipes in this cookbook are standardized. Dinner recipes yield 3 oz. or more edible portion of protein and lunch recipes yield 2 oz. or more edible portion of protein.

For texture modified diets measuring cups may be used for portion size. *

Breakfast 1 oz. = ¼ cup

Lunch 2 oz. = 1/3 cup

Dinner 3 oz. = ½ cup

*Each community may have different standards. Check with the dietitian if you are not sure.

Seafood

In the United States there are over 20,000 known species of edible fish and sea mammals. Approximately 250 species are harvested to be consumed by humans and animals. Shellfish and Fish are often classified in three different ways: Vertebrate and Invertebrate; Salt Water or Fresh Water; or Lean or Fatty. Vertebrate fish have fins and internal skeletons. Invertebrate fish or shellfish have external skeletons and do not have backbones. Examples of invertebrate fish include: crab, crayfish, lobster, shrimp, clams, mussel, oysters, scallop. Examples of Vertebrate fin fish include: tuna, cod, salmon, catfish, and sole.

Fish Classification

Fish in general is not very fatty but fish is sometimes classified as lean versus fatty. A 3 oz. portion of a lean fish is usually less than 2.5 g. of fat. Some fish like salmon, mackerel and tuna can have 5-10 g. fat per 3 oz. serving. The fat in fish is polyunsaturated and depending on the type of fish may be high in Omega-3 fatty acids. Good seafood sources of omega-3 fatty acids include: Barramundi, Mediterranean seabass, Herring, Oyster, Salmon, Swordfish, Scallops, Shrimp, Sole, Halibut, Perch, Cod, Grouper, Mahi-mahi, and Tuna.

Purchasing Seafood

Unlike inspection of meat and poultry, inspection of seafood is voluntary. When inspection does occur it is based on wholesomeness and the sanitary conditions of the processing plant. Grading is also voluntary. Only finfish can be graded. The grading is based on quality of appearance, texture, uniformity, good flavor, fresh odor, and absence of defects. Fish can be purchased fresh, frozen or canned.

FISH SELECTION:	WHAT TO LOOK FOR:	DO NOT PURCHASE IF:
Fresh Fish	- Color: bright red gills;, bright shiny skin - Texture: firm flesh that springs back when touched - Odor: mild ocean or seaweed smell - Eyes: bright, clear, full - Packaging: product surround by crushed self-draining ice	- Color: dull gray gills; dull dry skin - Texture: Soft flesh that leaves an imprint when touched - Odor: strong fishy or ammonia smell - Eyes: cloud, red-rimmed, sunken - Product: tumors, abscesses or cysts on the skin
Shell Fish	- Odor: mild ocean or seaweed smell - Shells: closed unbroken, indicating that the shellfish are alive - Condition: if fresh, they must be received alive	- Texture: slimy, sticky or dry - Odor: strong fishy smell - Shells: excessively muddy or broken shells - Condition: dead on arrival (open shells that do not close when tapped)
Crustaceans	- Odor: mild ocean or seaweed smell - Condition: shipped alive, packed in seaweed, and kept moist	- Odor: strong fishy smell - Condition: dead on arrival

Preparation of Fish and Shellfish

Overcooking is the most common mistake made when preparing fish. Overcooked fish has excessive flakiness, dryness and flavor loss. Avoid cooking the fish too long or at too high of a temperature. Fish cooks quickly and is done when the bone is no longer pink and the flesh turns from translucent to an opaque color, is firm to the touch and separates easily from the bone. The fish should be moist and flake easily without falling apart. Using the thermometer to test for done is key to prevent food borne illness.

Storage of Fish

Fresh fish is best consumed within a day or two of purchase. If fish is purchased in butcher paper, it should be rewrapped with plastic wrap and aluminum foil. Prepackaged fish and shell fish can in the original package. Fish should be frozen at 0 degree F. or below. Fish should never be refrozen once it is thawed. Canned fish can stay on the shelf for up to 12 months. Frozen fish should be used within 30 days from purchase for optimal quality. Most shell fish must be kept alive prior to preparation.

BEEF DINNER RECIPES

Recipe Name: Asian Skirt Steak
Recipe Category: Dinner Entrée
Portion Size: 3 oz. boneless meat
Ingredients: Yields: 8 servings

Ingredients	Notes:
2 beef Skirt Steak (about 2-1/2 pounds), cut into 4 to 6-inch portions	Trim all visible fat.
1/2 cup reduced-sodium or regular soy sauce	
½ cup dark brown barbecue sauce	
¼ cup creamy peanut butter	
2 teaspoons garlic powder	
8 green onions, cut crosswise in half	Wash thoroughly before cutting

Directions:

Steps:	Directions:	Critical Control Point /Quality Assurance
1	Combine soy sauce, barbecue sauce, peanut butter and garlic powder in small bowl; stir to combine thoroughly. Place beef steaks and soy sauce mixture in sealable container; turn to coat steaks. Close the container and marinate in refrigerator 1 hours or as long as overnight, turning occasionally	Store in refrigerator at less than 40 degrees F while marinating
2	Remove steaks from marinade; discard marinade. Place steaks on rack of broiler pan so surface of beef is 2 to 3 inches from heat. Broil 10 to 13 minutes for medium rare (145°F) to medium (160°F) doneness, turning once. During last 3 minutes of broiling top steaks with green onions.	Discard marinade. Minimum Temperature 145°F for 15 seconds
3	Carve steaks diagonally across grain into thin slices. Serve with green onions.	

Time Temperature Sensitive food. *Food safety Standards: hold food for service at an internal temperature above 140° F. Do not mix old product with new. Cool leftover product quickly (within 4 hours) to below 41° F. Follow proper cooling procedures. Store leftovers in a tightly sealed, labeled and dated container. Use leftover within 72 hours if stored in refrigerator or 30 days if stored in the freezer. Reheat leftover product quickly (within 2 hours) to 165 degrees F for 15 seconds. Reheat left over product only once; discard if not used. Cold holding at 41°F or colder or using time alone (less than four hours).*

Texture Modified Diets:
Soft & Bite Size: (aka Bite size) **Food particle size ½ inch (~width of standard fork)** Food must be moist. Cut foods with a knife to a ½" particle size prior to mixing. Moisten with broth as needed. Foods that do not process well should be omitted. Omit: green onions.
Chopped: Food particle size ¼ inch (~ ½ width of standard fork) Food must be moist. Chop foods with a knife to 1/4" particle size prior to mixing. Moisten with broth as needed. Foods that do not process well should be omitted. Omit: green onions.
Minced and Moist:(aka Minced/Mechanical Soft/Ground) **Food particle size 1/8 inch (fits through prongs of standard fork)** Food must be moist. Use a food processor to grind food particles into 1/8 inch prior to mixing. Moisten with broth as needed. Foods that do not process well should be omitted. Omit: green onions.
Pureed: Smooth and cohesive. Use a food processor to puree to a smooth consistency. Foods are processed by grinding and then pureeing them. May add broth or sauce to puree. Do not add to much liquid. Puree should still hold its shape. Must not be firm or sticky. Puree foods while still hot. Appearance should be smooth like pudding. Foods that do not process well should be omitted. Omit: green onions.

Therapeutic Modified Diets:
Lowfat: No changes needed
Diabetic/No added Sugar/No Conc. Sweets/Calorie Controlled: No changes needed
Bland: omit barbecue sauce, garlic powder and onion
Liberal House Renal: Omit soy sauce, barbeque sauce, peanut butter, season with no salt herbs
No Added Salt: Omit soy sauce
2 Gram Sodium: omit soy sauce, barbecue sauce, peanut butter, season with no salt herbs
Gluten Free: Use GF soy sauce and BBQ sauce. Prepare foods separately to prevent cross contamination.

Allergy Alerts: When an "X" is present, this indicates the allergen is present. Always read all food labels to ensure allergens are not present.

Wheat	Milk	Eggs	Fish Shellfish	Soy	Peanuts/Nuts	Other
X				X	X	

Key: SF= Salt Free D= Diet or Sugarfree LF = Lowfat FF = Fat Free GF = Gluten Free

Copyright 2020 Jacqueline Larson M.S., R.D.N. and Associates.   All Rights Reserved

Recipe Name: Baked Rigatoni with Beef
Recipe Category: Dinner Entrée
Portion Size: ½ cup Meat Sauce and ½ cup Pasta Total 1 cup
Ingredients: Yields: 8 servings

Ingredients	Notes:
32 oz. jar Spaghetti sauce	
2 lbs. lean ground beef	
1 lb. rigatoni pasta	
2 cups shredded low fat mozzarella cheese	
½ c. Parmesan cheese	

Directions:

Steps:	Directions:	Critical Control Point / Quality Assurance
1	Preheat oven to 350 degrees.	
2	Brown ground beef in large skillet. Drain.	Minimum Temperature 165°F for 15 seconds
3	Add spaghetti sauce to beef in large skillet. Cook for 10 minutes until hot.	
4	Cook pasta according to directions on package. Drain.	
5	Combine pasta with meat mixture.	
6	In a large baking dish spread pasta and meat mixture.	
7	Top with mozzarella cheese.	
8	Bake for 30 minutes or until hot.	Temperature check to 165 degrees F.
9	Garnish with Parmesan cheese.	

Time Temperature Sensitive food. *Food safety Standards: hold food for service at an internal temperature above 140°F. Do not mix old product with new. Cool leftover product quickly (within 4 hours) to below 41°F. Follow proper cooling procedures. Store leftovers in a tightly sealed, labeled and dated container. Use leftover within 72 hours if stored in refrigerator or 30 days if stored in the freezer. Reheat leftover product quickly (within 2 hours) to 165 degrees F for 15 seconds. Reheat left over product only once; discard if not used. Cold holding at 41°F or colder or using time alone (less than four hours). Always wash hands and wash and sanitize counter tops utensils and containers between steps when working with raw meat.*

Texture Modified Diets: TIP ; use pasta that is correct particle size.
Soft & Bite Size: (aka Bite size) **Food particle size ½ inch (~width of standard fork)** Food must be moist. Cut foods with a knife to a ½" particle size prior to mixing. Moisten with broth as needed.
Chopped: Food particle size ¼ inch (~ ½ width of standard fork) Food must be moist. Chop foods with a knife to 1/4" particle size prior to mixing. Moisten with broth as needed.
Minced and Moist: (aka Minced/Mechanical Soft/Ground) **Food particle size 1/8 inch (fits through prongs of standard fork)** Food must be moist. Use a food processor to grind food particles into 1/8 inch prior to mixing. Moisten with broth as needed.
Pureed: Smooth and cohesive. Use a food processor to puree to a smooth consistency. Foods are processed by grinding and then pureeing them. May add broth or sauce to puree. Do not add to much liquid. Puree should still hold its shape. Must not be firm or sticky. Puree foods while still hot. Appearance should be smooth like pudding. Puree Pasta while hot for best results. Serve ½ c. meat sauce serving and ½ cup pasta separately

Therapeutic Modified Diets:
Lowfat: No changes needed
Diabetic/No added Sugar/No Conc. Sweets/Calorie Controlled: No changes needed
Bland: omit spaghetti sauce, serve hamburger patty plain and plain pasta
Liberal House Renal: Omit spaghetti sauce Mozzarella cheese, and Parmesan cheese. Serve hamburger patty plain and SF plain pasta. May toss pasta with salt free herbs/spices.
No Added Salt: No changes
2 Gram Sodium: Omit spaghetti sauce. Serve hamburger patty plain and plain SF pasta. May toss pasta with salt free herbs/spices, and fresh tomatoes
Gluten Free: Use GF spaghetti sauce and GF pasta. Prepare foods separately to prevent cross contamination.

Allergy Alerts: When an "X" is present, this indicates the allergen is present. Always read all food labels to ensure allergens are not present.

Wheat	Milk	Eggs	Fish Shellfish	Soy	Peanuts/Nuts	Other
X	X	X				

Key: SF= Salt Free D= Diet or Sugarfree LF = Lowfat FF = Fat Free GF = Gluten Free

Recipe Name: Beef and Broccoli
Recipe Category: Dinner Entrée
Portion Size: Approx. 1 1/3 cups (1/2 cup rice(starch), ½ cup broccoli (vegetable),1/3 cup beef (3 oz. Protein)
Ingredients: Yields: 8 servings

Ingredients	Notes:
2 1/2 Pounds beef top or bottom sirloin, cut into thin strips	Trim all visible fat..
1 cup low sodium beef broth	
¼ cup lite soy sauce	
3 tablespoons cornstarch	
2 teaspoons sugar	
1 teaspoon garlic powder	
1 teaspoon ground ginger	
Nonstick cooking spray	
4 cups broccoli flowerets.	Washed, trimmed and cut up
2 medium carrots	Washed, peeled and sliced thin
2 tablespoons cooking oil	
4 cups hot cooked brown rice	See recipe for brown rice

Directions:

Steps:	Directions:	Critical Control Point /Quality Assurance
1	Heat oil in a large skillet or wok.	
2	Add beef and garlic. Sauté until beef is no longer pink. Remove from skillet.	Temperature check 145 degrees for 15 seconds. Minimum Temperature 145°F for 15 seconds
3	In a small bowl combine beef broth, soy sauce, cornstarch, sugar and ginger; set aside.	
4	Lightly coat a wok or large skillet with cooking spray. Heat to medium- high heat. Add carrots and broccoli. Stir fry for 3 to 4 minutes or until vegetables are crisp-tender. Remove from wok or skillet.	
5	Add beef to wok or skillet and push to sides. .	
6	In the center add the sauce and heat until bubbly.	
7	Add vegetable to beef in wok or skillet.	
8	Stir all ingredients together to coat with sauce. Heat thoroughly. Serve hot over rice.	

Time Temperature Sensitive food. *Food safety Standards: hold food for service at an internal temperature above 140° F. Do not mix old product with new. Cool leftover product quickly (within 4 hours) to below 41° F. Follow proper cooling procedures. Store leftovers in a tightly sealed, labeled and dated container. Use leftover within 72 hours if stored in refrigerator or 30 days if stored in the freezer. Reheat leftover product quickly (within 2 hours) to 165 degrees F for 15 seconds. Reheat left over product only once; discard if not used. Cold holding at 41°F or colder or using time alone (less than four hours). Always wash hands and wash and sanitize counter tops utensils and containers between steps when working with raw meat.*

Texture Modified Diets:

Soft & Bite Size: (aka Bite size) **Food particle size ½ inch (~width of standard fork)** Food must be moist. Cut foods with a knife to a ½" particle size after cooking. Moisten with broth as needed. Serve ½ c. meat serving ½ cup rice and ½ vegetables separately. Moisten with broth/sauce if needed

Chopped: Food particle size ¼ inch (~ ½ width of standard fork) Food must be moist. Chop foods with a knife to 1/4" particle size after cooking. Moisten with broth as needed. Serve ½ c. meat serving ½ cup rice and ½ vegetables separately. Moisten with broth/sauce if needed

Minced and Moist:(aka Minced/Mechanical Soft/Ground) **Food particle size 1/8 inch (fits through prongs of standard fork)** Food must be moist. Use a food processor to grind food particles into 1/8 inch after cooking. Serve ½ c. meat serving ½ cup rice and ½ vegetables separately. Moisten with broth/sauce if needed.

Pureed: Smooth and cohesive. Use a food processor to puree to a smooth consistency. Foods are processed by grinding and then pureeing them. May add broth or sauce to puree. Do not add to much liquid. Puree should still hold its shape. Must not be firm or sticky. Puree foods while still hot. Appearance should be smooth like pudding. Serve ½ c. meat serving ½ cup rice and ½ vegetables separately. Moisten with broth/sauce if needed

Therapeutic Modified Diets:
Lowfat: No changes needed

Diabetic/No added Sugar/No Conc. Sweets/Calorie Controlled: No changes needed
Bland: omit broccoli and sub. Green beens, omit garlic and ginger
Liberal House Renal: Omit sauce, no broth or soy sauce. Season with no salt herbs/spices
No Added Salt: Omit sauce, no broth or soy sauce. Season with no salt herbs/spices
2 Gram Sodium: Omit sauce, no broth or soy sauce. Season with no salt herbs/spices
Gluten Free: Use GF soy sauce and GF broth . Prepare foods separately to prevent cross contamination.
Allergy Alerts: When an "X" is present, this indicates the allergen is present.
Always read all food labels to ensure allergens are not present.

Wheat	Milk	Eggs	Fish Shellfish	Soy	Peanuts/Nuts	Other
X				X		

Key: SF= Salt Free D= Diet or Sugarfree LF = Lowfat FF = Fat Free GF = Gluten Free

Recipe Name: Beef and Brown Rice Casserole
Recipe Category: Dinner Entrée
Portion Size: 1 cup (½ cup meat and ½ cup rice)
Ingredients: Yields: 8 servings

Ingredients	Notes:
2 cups light sour cream	
1 cup low sodium beef broth	
1/4 teaspoon pepper	
1 teaspoon garlic powder	
1 teaspoon thyme	
2 1/2 Pounds lean ground beef	
4 cups cooked brown rice	
1 cup sliced mushrooms	Washed, trimmed and sliced
1 small onion diced	Washed, peeled and diced
1 tablespoon olive oil	
2 cups low fat cheese	Suggestion: cheddar for beef or Swiss for Turkey

Directions:

Steps:	Directions:	Critical Control Point /Quality Assurance
1	Preheat oven to 350 degrees.	
2	In a large skillet, heat to medium high heat. Add ground beef and cook until browned. Drain excess fat.	Check temperature. Minimum Temperature 165°F for 15 seconds
3	Place in a large mixing bowl.	
4	In the same large pan, sauté onion and mushrooms in oil until tender. Add onions and mushrooms to ground beef.	
5	Stir in sour cream, broth, pepper, garlic powder, thyme and rice.	
6	Place mixture into a casserole dish. Top with cheese.	
7	Bake in preheated oven for 30 minutes.	Check temperature 165 F degrees

Time Temperature Sensitive food. Food safety Standards: hold food for service at an internal temperature above 140° F. Do not mix old product with new. Cool leftover product quickly (within 4 hours) to below 41° F. Follow proper cooling procedures. Store leftovers in a tightly sealed, labeled and dated container. Use leftover within 72 hours if stored in refrigerator or 30 days if stored in the freezer. Reheat leftover product quickly (within 2 hours) to 165 degrees F for 15 seconds. Reheat left over product only once; discard if not used. Cold holding at 41°F or colder or using time alone (less than four hours). Always wash hands and wash and sanitize counter tops utensils and containers between steps when working with raw meat.

Texture Modified Diets:
Soft & Bite Size: (aka Bite size) **Food particle size ½ inch (~width of standard fork)** Food must be moist. Cut foods with a knife to a ½" particle size prior to mixing. Moisten with broth as needed.
Chopped: Food particle size ¼ inch (~ ½ width of standard fork) Food must be moist. Chop foods with a knife to 1/4" particle size prior to mixing. Moisten with broth as needed.
Minced and Moist: (aka Minced/Mechanical Soft/Ground) **Food particle size 1/8 inch (fits through prongs of standard fork)** Food must be moist. Use a food processor to grind food particles into 1/8 inch prior to mixing. Moisten with broth as needed.
Pureed: Smooth and cohesive. Use a food processor to puree to a smooth consistency. Foods are processed by grinding and then pureeing them. May add broth or sauce to puree. Do not add to much liquid. Puree should still hold its shape. Must not be firm or sticky. Puree foods while still hot. Appearance should be smooth like pudding. Serve ½ c. meat serving and ½ cup rice separately. Separate meat out before baking and puree. Add broth to meat to puree. Add rice, onions, mushroom, sour cream, pepper, garlic powder, and thyme to casserole dish. Bake rice mixture.

Therapeutic Modified Diets:
Lowfat: No changes needed
Diabetic/No added Sugar/No Conc. Sweets/Calorie Controlled: No changes needed
Bland: omit garlic, thyme, mushrooms and onions
Liberal House Renal: Use SF broth or water, omit cheese and sour cream. Season with SF herbs/spices.
No Added Salt: No changes
2 Gram Sodium: Use SF broth or water, omit cheese and sour cream. Season with SF herbs/spices
Gluten Free: Use GF broth. Prepare foods separately to prevent cross contamination.

Allergy Alerts: When an "X" is present, this indicates the allergen is present. Always read all food labels to ensure allergens are not present.

Wheat	Milk	Eggs	Fish Shellfish	Soy	Peanuts/Nuts	Other
X	X					

Key: SF= Salt Free D= Diet or Sugarfree LF = Lowfat FF = Fat Free GF = Gluten Free

Copyright 2020 Jacqueline Larson M.S., R.D.N. and Associates.   All Rights Reserved

Recipe Name: Beef and Brown Rice Salad
Recipe Category: Dinner Entrée
Portion Size: 1 ½ cups (3 oz. meat, ½ cup starch, ½ cup vegetables)
Ingredients: **Yields: 8 servings**

Ingredients	Notes:
2 1/2 lbs. beef Top Round Steak, cut 3/4 inch thick	Trim all visible fat.
2 teaspoons olive oil	
2 cups asparagus pieces (2-inch pieces)	Wash all produce, prior to cutting
2 cups medium yellow squash,	Wash and cut lengthwise in half, then crosswise into 1/4-inch thick slices
4 cups hot cooked brown rice	See recipe for brown rice
1 cup diced, seeded tomatoes	Wash, seeded and diced
1 cup canned garbanzo beans	Rinsed and drained
1/4 cup fresh basil, thinly sliced	Or 2 Tablespoons dried
1/2 teaspoon salt	
Marinade Ingredients ½ cup olive oil ¾ cup soy sauce ½ cup lemon juice ½ cup Worcestershire sauce 2 tablespoons Dijon mustard 1 clove garlic, minced ¼ teaspoon pepper to taste	

Directions:

Steps:	Directions:	Critical Control Point / Quality Assurance
1	Combine marinade ingredients in small bowl. Place beef steak and 1/4 cup marinade in sealable container; turn steak to coat. Close container securely and marinate in refrigerator 1 hour or as long as overnight. Reserve remaining marinade in refrigerator for dressing.	Store marinate and steak in refrigerator at 40F degrees or less.
2	Remove steak from marinade; discard marinade. Place steak on rack in broiler pan so surface of beef is 2 to 3 inches from heat. Broil 12 to 13 minutes for medium rare (145°F) doneness, turning once. Remove; keep warm.	Discard Marinade. Check Temperature. Minimum Temperature 145°F for 15 seconds for beef or pork 165 °F for chicken
3	Heat oil in large nonstick skillet over medium-high heat until hot. Add asparagus and squash; cook and stir 7 to 8 minutes or until tender. Toss with rice, tomatoes, beans, basil, salt and reserved marinade in large bowl. Chill.	
4	Carve steak into thin slices. Serve warm over chilled rice salad.	

Time Temperature Sensitive food. *Food safety Standards: hold food for service at an internal temperature above 140° F. Do not mix old product with new. Cool leftover product quickly (within 4 hours) to below 41° F. Follow proper cooling procedures. Store leftovers in a tightly sealed, labeled and dated container. Use leftover within 72 hours if stored in refrigerator or 30 days if stored in the freezer. Reheat leftover product quickly (within 2 hours) to 165 degrees F for 15 seconds. Reheat left over product only once; discard if not used. Cold holding at 41°F or colder or using time alone (less than four hours). Always wash hands and wash and sanitize counter tops utensils and containers between steps when working with raw meat.*

<u>Texture Modified Diets:</u>

Soft & Bite Size: (aka Bite size) **Food particle size ½ inch (~width of standard fork)** Food must be moist. Cut foods with a knife to a ½" particle size prior to mixing. Moisten with broth as needed.

Chopped: Food particle size ¼ inch (~ ½ width of standard fork) Food must be moist. Chop foods with a knife to 1/4" particle size prior to mixing. Moisten with broth as needed.

Copyright 2020 Jacqueline Larson M.S., R.D.N. and Associates.   All Rights Reserved

Minced and Moist: (aka Minced/Mechanical Soft/Ground) **Food particle size 1/8 inch (fits through prongs of standard fork)** Food must be moist. Use a food processor to grind food particles into 1/8 inch prior to mixing. Moisten with broth as needed.

Pureed: Smooth and cohesive. Use a food processor to puree to a smooth consistency. Foods are processed by grinding and then pureeing them. May add broth or sauce to puree. Do not add to much liquid. Puree should still hold its shape. Must not be firm or sticky. Puree foods while still hot. Appearance should be smooth like pudding. Serve ½ c. meat serving, ½ cup vegetables, and ½ cup rice separately.

<u>Therapeutic Modified Diets:</u>

Lowfat: No changes needed

Diabetic/No added Sugar/No Conc. Sweets/Calorie Controlled: No changes needed

Bland: omit garbanzo beans, basil, tomatoes, lemon juice, Dijon mustard, and pepper

Liberal House Renal: Omit salt, tomatoes, soy sauce, and Worcestershire sauce

No Added Salt: No changes

2 Gram Sodium: omit salt, soy sauce and Worcestershire sauce

Gluten Free: Use gluten free soy sauce. Prepare separately to prevent cross contamination.

Allergy Alerts: When an "X" is present, this indicates the allergen is present.
Always read all food labels to ensure allergens are not present.

Wheat	Milk	Eggs	Fish Shellfish	Soy	Peanuts/Nuts	Other
X			X			

Key: SF= Salt Free D= Diet or Sugarfree LF = Lowfat FF = Fat Free GF = Gluten Free

Recipe Name: Beef and Tater Casserole
Recipe Category: Dinner Entrée
Portion Size: 1 cup
Ingredients: **Yields: 8 servings**

Ingredients	Notes:
1 cup fat free evaporated milk	
1 cup light sour cream	
8 oz. package sliced mushrooms	Wash, trim and slice
2 cups low salt beef broth	
1 (32 oz.) package frozen tater tots	
1/2 Teaspoon pepper	
1 teaspoon ground sage	
2 1/2 Pounds lean ground beef	
1/4 Teaspoon garlic powder	
1 medium onion, chopped	Wash, peel and chop.
2 cups shredded low fat cheddar cheese	

Directions:

Steps:	Directions:	Critical Control Point /Quality Assurance
1	Preheat oven to 350 degrees.	
2	In a large skillet cook ground beef with onion and mushrooms. Drain.	Check temperature. Minimum Temperature 165°F for 15 seconds
3	Add evaporated milk, sour cream, broth, pepper, garlic powder and sage.	
4	Spread in a baking dish.	
5	Top with tater tots and then top with cheddar cheese.	
6	Bake at 350 degree oven for 1 hour and 20 minutes.	Check temperature to 165 F.

Time Temperature Sensitive food. Food safety Standards: hold food for service at an internal temperature above 140° F. Do not mix old product with new. Cool leftover product quickly (within 4 hours) to below 41° F. Follow proper cooling procedures. Store leftovers in a tightly sealed, labeled and dated container. Use leftover within 72 hours if stored in refrigerator or 30 days if stored in the freezer. Reheat leftover product quickly (within 2 hours) to 165 degrees F for 15 seconds. Reheat left over product only once; discard if not used. Cold holding at 41 °F or colder or using time alone (less than four hours). Always wash hands and wash and sanitize counter tops utensils and containers between steps when working with raw meat.

Texture Modified Diets:
Soft & Bite Size: (aka Bite size) **Food particle size ½ inch (~width of standard fork)** Food must be moist. Cut foods with a knife to a ½" particle size prior to mixing. Moisten with broth as needed.
Chopped: Food particle size ¼ inch (~ ½ width of standard fork) Food must be moist. Chop foods with a knife to 1/4" particle size prior to mixing. Moisten with broth as needed.
Minced and Moist:(aka Minced/Mechanical Soft/Ground) **Food particle size 1/8 inch (fits through prongs of standard fork)** Food must be moist. Use a food processor to grind food particles into 1/8 inch prior to mixing. Moisten with broth as needed.
Pureed: Smooth and cohesive. Use a food processor to puree to a smooth consistency. Foods are processed by grinding and then pureeing them. May add broth or sauce to puree. Do not add to much liquid. Puree should still hold its shape. Must not be firm or sticky. Puree foods while still hot. Appearance should be smooth like pudding. Serve ½ c. meat serving.
Serve ½ c. puree meat mixture and ½ cup puree potato cheese mixture separately. Separate after baking. Moisten with broth/milk if needed

Therapeutic Modified Diets:
Lowfat: No changes needed
Diabetic/No added Sugar/No Conc. Sweets/Calorie Controlled: No changes needed
Bland: omit sage, pepper, onion and garlic
Liberal House Renal: Serve plain 3 oz. hamburger patty and ½ cup rice seasoned with herb/spices
No Added Salt: No changes
2 Gram Sodium: Serve plain 3 oz. hamburger patty and ½ cup unsalted tater tots.
Gluten Free: Use GF broth. Prepare foods separately to prevent cross contamination.
Allergy Alerts: When an "X" is present, this indicates the allergen is present.
Always read all food labels to ensure allergens are not present.

Wheat	Milk	Eggs	Fish Shellfish	Soy	Peanuts/Nuts	Other
X	X					

Key: SF= Salt Free D= Diet or Sugarfree LF = Lowfat FF = Fat Free GF = Gluten Free

Copyright 2020 Jacqueline Larson M.S., R.D.N. and Associates.   All Rights Reserved

Recipe Name: Beef Barley Skillet
Recipe Category: Dinner Entrée
Portion Size: 1 cup
Ingredients: **Yields: 8 servings**

Ingredients	Notes:
2 1/2 Pounds beef stew meat	Trim all visible fat. Cut into ½ inch pieces.
1 teaspoon salt	
1/4 teaspoon black pepper.	
1 tablespoon oil	
2 cups low sodium beef broth	
1 8-ounce fresh mushrooms	Wash, trim and slice
2 cups medium pearl barley	
1 onion, chopped	Wash, peel and dice.
1 16-ounce can stewed tomatoes	Undrained
2 cups water	

Directions:

Steps:	Directions:	Critical Control Point /Quality Assurance
1	Season beef with salt and pepper.	
2	Brown stewing beef in oil.	
3	Pour off excess fat and add beef broth. Cover and simmer for 30 minutes.	
4	Add mushrooms, barley, onion, tomatoes, and water.	
5	Cover and bring to boil.	
6	Reduce heat and simmer for 45 minutes or until barley is tender and liquid is absorbed	Temperature check. Minimum Temperature 165°F for 15 seconds.

Time Temperature Sensitive food. *Food safety Standards: hold food for service at an internal temperature above 140° F. Do not mix old product with new. Cool leftover product quickly (within 4 hours) to below 41° F. Follow proper cooling procedures. Store leftovers in a tightly sealed, labeled and dated container. Use leftover within 72 hours if stored in refrigerator or 30 days if stored in the freezer. Reheat leftover product quickly (within 2 hours) to 165 degrees F for 15 seconds. Reheat left over product only once; discard if not used. Cold holding at 41°F or colder or using time alone (less than four hours). Always wash hands and wash and sanitize counter tops utensils and containers between steps when working with raw meat.*

Texture Modified Diets:
Soft & Bite Size: (aka Bite size) **Food particle size ½ inch (~width of standard fork)** Food must be moist. Cut foods with a knife to a ½" particle size prior to mixing. Moisten with broth as needed.
Chopped: Food particle size ¼ inch (~ ½ width of standard fork) Food must be moist. Chop foods with a knife to 1/4" particle size prior to mixing. Moisten with broth as needed.
Minced and Moist:(aka Minced/Mechanical Soft/Ground) **Food particle size 1/8 inch (fits through prongs of standard fork)** Food must be moist. Use a food processor to grind food particles into 1/8 inch prior to mixing. Moisten with broth as needed.
Pureed: Smooth and cohesive. Use a food processor to puree to a smooth consistency. Foods are processed by grinding and then pureeing them. May add broth or sauce to puree. Do not add to much liquid. Puree should still hold its shape. Must not be firm or sticky. Puree foods while still hot. Appearance should be smooth like pudding. Serve ½ c. puree meat ½ c. barley separately. Barley can be cooked in water separately. Cook meat with broth separately and then puree (step 2). For barley do NOT combine with meat. Cook barley then puree.

Therapeutic Modified Diets:
Lowfat: No changes needed
Diabetic/No added Sugar/No Conc. Sweets/Calorie Controlled: No changes needed
Bland: omit black pepper tomatoes, and onions
Liberal House Renal: Omit salt. Use salt free broth or water. Omit tomatoes
No Added Salt: no changes
2 Gram Sodium: omit salt; Use salt free broth or water. Omit canned tomatoes and use fresh diced tomatoes
Gluten Free: Use GF broth. No barley. Substitute rice for barley. Prepare foods separately to prevent cross contamination.

Allergy Alerts: When an "X" is present, this indicates the allergen is present. Always read all food labels to ensure allergens are not present.

Wheat	Milk	Eggs	Fish Shellfish	Soy	Peanuts/Nuts	Other
X						

Key: SF= Salt Free D= Diet or Sugarfree LF = Lowfat FF = Fat Free GF = Gluten Free

Copyright 2020 Jacqueline Larson M.S., R.D.N. and Associates.   All Rights Reserved

Recipe Name: Beef Barley Soup (or Chicken Barley Soup or Turkey Barley Soup)
Recipe Category: Dinner Entrée
Portion Size: 2 cups (3oz. meat, 1 starch, vegetable, plus broth)
Ingredients: Yields: 8 servings

Ingredients	Notes:
2 ½ Pounds lean stew beef, cut into ½ inch pieces	Trim all visible fat (sub. Boneless skinless chicken or turkey cut into ½ inch pieces)
½ teaspoon salt	
¼ teaspoon pepper	
2 tablespoons olive oil	
2 tablespoons flour	
1 cup celery, diced	Washed, trimmed and diced
1 large onion, diced	Washed, peeled and diced
2 cups carrots,	Washed, peeled and sliced
1 cup potatoes	Washed, peeled and diced
1 cup peas, frozen	
1 cup medium pearl barley	
1 Tablespoon basil	
1/4 cup parsley flakes	
1 teaspoon garlic powder	
1 teaspoon cumin	
1 16-ounce can reduced salt diced tomatoes	
8 cups low sodium beef broth	(sub. Chicken if using chicken or turkey)

Directions:

Steps:	Directions:	Critical Control Point /Quality Assurance
1	Season beef with salt and pepper. In a large stock pot, brown beef in oil.	
2	Sprinkle with flour.	
3	Add onion, carrots, potatoes, parsley, basil, parsley, garlic powder, cumin, stewed tomatoes and broth	
4	Heat on medium high to boil, stirring occasionally.	
5	Reduce heat and simmer until meat is tender about 1 hour.	
6	Add peas just before serving simmer 5 minutes.	Check temperature. Minimum 165 degree F.

Time Temperature Sensitive food. *Food safety Standards: hold food for service at an internal temperature above 140° F. Do not mix old product with new. Cool leftover product quickly (within 4 hours) to below 41° F. Follow proper cooling procedures. Store leftovers in a tightly sealed, labeled and dated container. Use leftover within 72 hours if stored in refrigerator or 30 days if stored in the freezer. Reheat leftover product quickly (within 2 hours) to 165 degrees F for 15 seconds. Reheat left over product only once; discard if not used. Cold holding at 41°F or colder or using time alone (less than four hours). Always wash hands and wash and sanitize counter tops utensils and containers between steps when working with raw meat.*

Texture Modified Diets:
Soft & Bite Size: (aka Bite size) **Food particle size ½ inch (~width of standard fork)** Food must be moist. Cut foods with a knife to a ½" particle size prior to mixing. Moisten with broth as needed.
Chopped: Food particle size ¼ inch (~ ½ width of standard fork) Food must be moist. Chop foods with a knife to 1/4" particle size prior to mixing. Moisten with broth as needed.
Minced and Moist:(aka Minced/Mechanical Soft/Ground) **Food particle size 1/8 inch (fits through prongs of standard fork)** Food must be moist. Use a food processor to grind food particles into 1/8 inch prior to mixing. Moisten with broth as needed.
Pureed: Smooth and cohesive. Use a food processor to puree to a smooth consistency. Foods are processed by grinding and then pureeing them. May add broth or sauce to puree. Do not add to much liquid. Puree should still hold its shape. Must not be firm or sticky. Puree foods while still hot. Appearance should be smooth like pudding. Serve separately, ½ cup puree beef, ½ cup puree barley, ½ cup puree carrots.

Therapeutic Modified Diets:
Lowfat: No changes needed
Diabetic/No added Sugar/No Conc. Sweets/Calorie Controlled: No changes needed

Copyright 2020 Jacqueline Larson M.S., R.D.N. and Associates.   All Rights Reserved

Bland: omit basil, parsley, cumin, garlic, onion, tomatoes and celery
Liberal House Renal: Omit tomatoes and salt, Use SF broth or water
No Added Salt: No changes
2 Gram Sodium: Omit salt. Use SF broth and SF tomatoes (or fresh)
Gluten Free: Use GF broth and GF flour. Substitute brown rice for barley. Prepare foods separately to prevent cross contamination.

Allergy Alerts: When an "X" is present, this indicates the allergen is present. Always read all food labels to ensure allergens are not present.

Wheat	Milk	Eggs	Fish Shellfish	Soy	Peanuts/Nuts	Other
X						

Key: SF= Salt Free D= Diet or Sugarfree LF = Lowfat FF = Fat Free GF = Gluten Free

Recipe Name: Beef Carnitas
Recipe Category: Dinner Entrée
Portion Size: 1 Carnitas with 1 ½ Starch (1 whole grain tortilla and potato) 3 oz. Meat
Ingredients: **Yields: 8 servings**

Ingredients	Notes:
2 1/2 Pounds beef flank steak, cut into thin strips	Trim all visible fat.
8 (10 inch) flour tortillas	May use whole grain
2 tablespoons vegetable oil	
3 tablespoons Worcestershire sauce	
1/4 teaspoon hot pepper sauce	(optional)
2 to 3 garlic cloves, minced	
3 medium baking potatoes, cut into 1/2 inch cubes	Wash thoroughly and peel before cubing
1 pound fresh mushrooms, sliced	Washed, trimmed and sliced
1 medium onion, chopped	Washed, peeled and chopped
1 cup shredded low fat cheddar cheese	
1/2 cup salsa	

Directions:

Steps:	Directions:	Critical Control Point /Quality Assurance
1	In medium bowl, combine steak strips, Worcestershire sauce, hot pepper sauce and garlic. Mix well.	
2	Heat oil in a large skillet over medium high heat until hot.	
3	Add meat mixture and cook until browned. Add potatoes, mushrooms, and onion. Cook 1 minute. Reduce heat and simmer 12 to 14 minutes or until potatoes are tender.	Minimum Temperature 145°F for 15 seconds for beef
4	Heat tortilla according to package directions.	
5	To serve, spoon mixture evenly down center of each warm tortilla. Sprinkle with cheese and roll up. Serve with salsa	

Time Temperature Sensitive food. *Food safety Standards: hold food for service at an internal temperature above 140° F. Do not mix old product with new. Cool leftover product quickly (within 4 hours) to below 41° F. Follow proper cooling procedures. Store leftovers in a tightly sealed, labeled and dated container. Use leftover within 72 hours if stored in refrigerator or 30 days if stored in the freezer. Reheat leftover product quickly (within 2 hours) to 165 degrees F for 15 seconds. Reheat left over product only once; discard if not used. Cold holding at 41°F or colder or using time alone (less than four hours). Always wash hands and wash and sanitize counter tops utensils and containers between steps when working with raw meat.*

Texture Modified Diets:

Soft & Bite Size: (aka Bite size) **Food particle size ½ inch (~width of standard fork)** Food must be moist. Cut foods with a knife to a ½" particle size prior to layering. Moisten with broth as needed.
Chopped: Food particle size ¼ inch (~ ½ width of standard fork) Food must be moist. Chop foods with a knife to 1/4" particle size prior to layering. Moisten with broth as needed.
Minced and Moist:(aka Minced/Mechanical Soft/Ground) **Food particle size 1/8 inch (fits through prongs of standard fork)** Food must be moist. Use a food processor to grind food particles into 1/8 inch prior to layering. Moisten with broth as needed.
Pureed: Smooth and cohesive. Use a food processor to puree to a smooth consistency. Foods are processed by grinding and then pureeing them. May add broth or sauce to puree. Do not add to much liquid. Puree should still hold its shape. Must not be firm or sticky. Puree foods while still hot. Appearance should be smooth like pudding. Serve 3/4 c. puree meat mixture separately. ½ cup puree tortilla separately. May puree salsa and add to top of tortilla to moisten. May melt cheese on meat mixture.

Therapeutic Modified Diets:

Lowfat: No changes needed
Diabetic/No added Sugar/No Conc. Sweets/Calorie Controlled: No changes needed
Bland: omit hot sauce, garlic, onion and salsa
Liberal House Renal: Omit Worchester sauce, pepper sauce, cheese and salsa. Use low sodium tortillas.
No Added Salt: Omit Worchester sauce
2 Gram Sodium: Omit Worchester sauce, pepper sauce, and cheese. Use low sodium tortillas. (see recipe)
Gluten Free: Use GF corn tortillas. Prepare foods separately to prevent cross contamination.
Allergy Alerts: When an "X" is present, this indicates the allergen is present. Always read all food labels to ensure allergens are not present.

Wheat	Milk	Eggs	Fish Shellfish	Soy	Peanuts/Nuts	Other
X	X		X	X		

Key: SF= Salt Free D= Diet or Sugarfree LF = Lowfat FF = Fat Free GF = Gluten Free

Copyright 2020 Jacqueline Larson M.S., R.D.N. and Associates.   All Rights Reserved

Recipe Name: Beef Cube Steaks with Pepper
Recipe Category: Dinner Entrée
Portion Size: 3 oz. meat plus 1 oz. pepper (approx. ½ cup)
Ingredients: Yields: 8 servings

Ingredients	Notes:
2 1/2 Pounds beef cube steaks	Trim all visible fat
2 large green bell peppers	Wash all produce thoroughly before cutting. Core and slice.
1 teaspoon garlic powder	
1/2 teaspoon salt	
1/4 teaspoon black pepper.	
1 tablespoon oil	
1 cup low sodium beef broth	
1 tablespoon cornstarch	
1/4 cup water	

Directions:

Steps:	Directions:	Critical Control Point /Quality Assurance
1	Season beef with salt, garlic powder and pepper.	
2	Spray skillet with cooking spray. Heat skillet over medium high heat until hot.	
	Add steaks. Cook 3 to 4 minutes on each side or to doneness.	Temperature check. Minimum Temperature 145°F for 15 seconds
3	Remove steaks from skillet. Keep warm. .	
4	Sauté peppers in skillet until tender crisp.	
5	Remove from skillet. .	
6	In same skillet, combine broth, water and cornstarch. Cook until thickened and bubbly, stirring constantly.	
7	Add steaks and peppers. Heat and serve	

Time Temperature Sensitive food. Food safety Standards: hold food for service at an internal temperature above 140° F. Do not mix old product with new. Cool leftover product quickly (within 4 hours) to below 41° F. Follow proper cooling procedures. Store leftovers in a tightly sealed, labeled and dated container. Use leftover within 72 hours if stored in refrigerator or 30 days if stored in the freezer. Reheat leftover product quickly (within 2 hours) to 165 degrees F for 15 seconds. Reheat left over product only once; discard if not used. Cold holding at 41°F or colder or using time alone (less than four hours). Always wash hands and wash and sanitize counter tops utensils and containers between steps when working with raw meat.

Texture Modified Diets:
Soft & Bite Size: (aka Bite size) **Food particle size ½ inch (~width of standard fork)** Food must be moist. Cut foods with a knife to a ½" particle size prior to mixing. Moisten with broth as needed.
Chopped: Food particle size ¼ inch (~ ½ width of standard fork) Food must be moist. Chop foods with a knife to 1/4" particle size prior to mixing. Moisten with broth as needed.
Minced and Moist:(aka Minced/Mechanical Soft/Ground) **Food particle size 1/8 inch (fits through prongs of standard fork)** Food must be moist. Use a food processor to grind food particles into 1/8 inch prior to mixing. Moisten with broth as needed.
Pureed: Smooth and cohesive. Use a food processor to puree to a smooth consistency. Foods are processed by grinding and then pureeing them. May add broth or sauce to puree. Do not add to much liquid. Puree should still hold its shape. Must not be firm or sticky. Puree foods while still hot. Appearance should be smooth like pudding. Serve ½ c. puree meat serving Cook meat with broth separately and then puree (step 2). For pepper do NOT combine with meat. Cook peppers then puree and top with 1 Tablespoon on top of meat. (step 3)

Therapeutic Modified Diets:
Lowfat: No changes needed
Diabetic/No added Sugar/No Conc. Sweets/Calorie Controlled: No changes needed
Bland: omit black pepper, garlic, and peppers
Liberal House Renal: Omit salt and peppers. Use salt free broth or water.
No Added Salt: Omit salt.
2 Gram Sodium: omit salt; Use salt free broth or water.
Gluten Free: Use GF broth. Prepare foods separately to prevent cross contamination.
Allergy Alerts: When an "X" is present, this indicates the allergen is present .Always read all food labels to ensure allergens are not present.

Wheat	Milk	Eggs	Fish Shellfish	Soy	Peanuts/Nuts	Other
X						

Key: SF= Salt Free D= Diet or Sugarfree LF = Lowfat FF = Fat Free GF = Gluten Free

Copyright 2020 Jacqueline Larson M.S., R.D.N. and Associates.   All Rights Reserved

Recipe Name: Beef Fajitas (or Shrimp Fajitas or Chicken Fajitas)
Recipe Category: Dinner Entrée
Portion Size: 2 fajitas with 1 (1 whole grain tortilla) plus 1 1/2 oz. Meat for a total of 2 tortillas and 3 oz. meat.
Ingredients: Yields: 8 servings

Ingredients	Notes:
2 1/2 pounds beef flank steak, cut into thin strips	Trim all visible fat.
16 (6 inch) flour tortillas	May use whole grain
2 teaspoons vegetable oil	
3 green bell peppers	Wash, trim and slice into strips
1 tablespoon cornstarch	
2 teaspoons chili powder	
1 teaspoon salt	
1 teaspoon sugar	
½ teaspoon onion powder	
½ teaspoon garlic powder	
¼ teaspoon cayenne pepper	
½ teaspoon ground cumin	
2/3 cup water	
1 cup tomato, diced	Wash, trim and dice
1 cup shredded low fat cheddar cheese	
½ cup light sour cream	
avocado	(optional)

Directions:

Steps:	Directions:	Critical Control Point /Quality Assurance
1	Sauté onions and peppers in 1 teaspoon oil in a large pan until tender crisp on medium high heat. Remove from pan.	
2	In the same pan on medium high heat, sauté beef in 1 teaspoon oil until browned.	
3	In a small bowl combine cornstarch, chili powder, salt, paprika, sugar, onion powder, garlic powder, cayenne pepper, cumin and water.	
4	Combine seasoning mix with cooked beef.	
5	Simmer 10 to 15 minutes.	Minimum Temperature 145°F for 15 seconds
6	Heat tortilla according to package directions.	
7	To serve, spoon meat mixture evenly down center of each warm tortilla. Top with green peppers and onions.	
8	Sprinkle with cheese and roll up. Serve with s cheddar cheese, sour cream, and tomato	

Time Temperature Sensitive food. *Food safety Standards: hold food for service at an internal temperature above 140°F. Do not mix old product with new. Cool leftover product quickly (within 4 hours) to below 41°F. Follow proper cooling procedures. Store leftovers in a tightly sealed, labeled and dated container. Use leftover within 72 hours if stored in refrigerator or 30 days if stored in the freezer. Reheat leftover product quickly (within 2 hours) to 165 degrees F for 15 seconds. Reheat left over product only once; discard if not used. Cold holding at 41°F or colder or using time alone (less than four hours). Always wash hands and wash and sanitize counter tops utensils and containers between steps when working with raw meat.*

<u>*Texture Modified Diets:*</u>
Soft & Bite Size: (aka Bite size) **Food particle size ½ inch (~width of standard fork)** Food must be moist. Cut foods with a knife to a ½" particle size prior to layering. Moisten with broth as needed.
Chopped: Food particle size ¼ inch (~ ½ width of standard fork) Food must be moist. Chop foods with a knife to 1/4" particle size prior to layering. Moisten with broth as needed.
Minced and Moist:(aka Minced/Mechanical Soft/Ground) **Food particle size 1/8 inch (fits through prongs of standard fork)** Food must be moist. Use a food processor to grind food particles into 1/8 inch prior to layering. Moisten with broth as needed.

Pureed: Smooth and cohesive. Use a food processor to puree to a smooth consistency. Foods are processed by grinding and then pureeing them. May add broth or sauce to puree. Do not add to much liquid. Puree should still hold its shape. Must not be firm or sticky. Puree foods while still hot. Appearance should be smooth like pudding. Serve 1/2 c. puree meat mixture separately.1 cup puree tortilla separately. May puree tomato and add to sour cream and tomato top of tortilla to moisten. May melt cheese on meat mixture.

Therapeutic Modified Diets:
Lowfat: No changes needed
Diabetic/No added Sugar/No Conc. Sweets/Calorie Controlled: No changes needed
Bland: omit all seasonings except salt
Liberal House Renal: Omit tomato, salt, cheddar cheese, sour cream and bell pepper, Use low sodium tortillas. (see recipe)
No Added Salt: no changes
2 Gram Sodium: Omit salt, cheddar cheese, sour cream. Use low sodium tortillas. (See recipe)
Gluten Free: Use GF corn tortillas. Prepare foods separately to prevent cross contamination.
Allergy Alerts: When an "X" is present, this indicates the allergen is present.
Always read all food labels to ensure allergens are not present.

Wheat	Milk	Eggs	Fish Shellfish	Soy	Peanuts/Nuts	Other
X	X					

Key: SF= Salt Free D= Diet or Sugarfree LF = Lowfat FF = Fat Free GF = Gluten Free

Recipe Name: Beef Goulash
Recipe Category: Dinner Entrée
Portion Size: 1 cup (1/2 cup pasta ½ cup meat mixture)
Ingredients: Yields: 8 servings

Ingredients	Notes:
2 1/2 Pounds beef stew meat	Trim all visible fat. Cut into ½ inch pieces.
1 teaspoon salt	
1/4 teaspoon black pepper.	
2 tablespoon olive oil	
1 cup onion, chopped	Wash, peel and dice.
1 cup green bell pepper	Wash, trim and slice.
1 cut tomato sauce	
1 cup reduced sodium beef broth	
1 tablespoon paprika	
2 tablespoons flour	
1 lb. pasta	Tip: use whole grain pasta

Directions:

Steps:	Directions:	Critical Control Point /Quality Assurance
1	Heat 1 tablespoon oil. Brown meat on all sides in a large skillet over medium high heat.	
2	Add onions and sauté until transparent.	
3	Add tomato sauce, broth, green pepper, salt, flour and paprika.	
4	Cover the pot and simmer the meat for 1 1/2 hours. In a small sauce pan, melt remaining olive oil and stir in flour. Slowly add flour mixture to sauce. Cook until thickened.	Temperature check. Minimum Temperature 165°F for 15 seconds
5	Prepare pasta according to directions on package.	
6	Serve pasta topped with meat mixture. Serve hot.	

Time Temperature Sensitive food. *Food safety Standards: hold food for service at an internal temperature above 140° F. Do not mix old product with new. Cool leftover product quickly (within 4 hours) to below 41° F. Follow proper cooling procedures. Store leftovers in a tightly sealed, labeled and dated container. Use leftover within 72 hours if stored in refrigerator or 30 days if stored in the freezer. Reheat leftover product quickly (within 2 hours) to 165 degrees F for 15 seconds. Reheat left over product only once; discard if not used. Cold holding at 41 °F or colder or using time alone (less than four hours). Always wash hands and wash and sanitize counter tops utensils and containers between steps when working with raw meat.*

<u>*Texture Modified Diets:*</u> *TIP: use pasta within particle size.*
Soft & Bite Size: (aka Bite size) **Food particle size ½ inch (~width of standard fork)** Food must be moist. Cut foods with a knife to a ½" particle size prior to mixing. Moisten with broth as needed.
Chopped: Food particle size ¼ inch (~ ½ width of standard fork) Food must be moist. Chop foods with a knife to 1/4" particle size prior to mixing. Moisten with broth as needed.
Minced and Moist:(aka Minced/Mechanical Soft/Ground) **Food particle size 1/8 inch (fits through prongs of standard fork)** Food must be moist. Use a food processor to grind food particles into 1/8 inch prior to mixing. Moisten with broth as needed.
Pureed: Smooth and cohesive. Use a food processor to puree to a smooth consistency. Foods are processed by grinding and then pureeing them. May add broth or sauce to puree. Do not add to much liquid. Puree should still hold its shape. Must not be firm or sticky. Puree foods while still hot. Appearance should be smooth like pudding. Serve ½ c. puree meat ½ c. pasta separately.
<u>*Therapeutic Modified Diets:*</u>
Lowfat: No changes needed
Diabetic/No added Sugar/No Conc. Sweets/Calorie Controlled: No changes needed
Bland: omit black pepper, tomato sauce, paprika, green pepper, and onions
Liberal House Renal: Omit salt, flour and green peppers. Use water in place of tomato juice.
No Added Salt: no changes
2 Gram Sodium: omit salt
Gluten Free: Use GF all-purpose flour. Substitute GF pasta. Prepare foods separately to prevent cross contamination.
Allergy Alerts: When an "X" is present, this indicates the allergen is present. Always read all food labels to ensure allergens are not present.

Wheat	Milk	Eggs	Fish Shellfish	Soy	Peanuts/Nuts	Other
X		X				

Copyright 2020 Jacqueline Larson M.S., R.D.N. and Associates.   All Rights Reserved

Recipe Name: Beef Lo Mein
Recipe Category: Dinner Entrée
Portion Size: 3 oz. boneless meat, ½ cup pasta, ½ cup vegetables (approx. 1 ½ cups)
Ingredients: **Yields: 8 servings**

Ingredients	Notes:
2 beef Skirt Steak, Sirloin Steak or flank steak (about 2-1/2 pounds), sliced thin across the grain	Trim all visible fat.
1 lb. spaghetti	May use whole grain
1/2 cup reduced-sodium soy sauce	
1 tablespoon sesame oil	
¼ cup hot water	
1 tablespoon beef bouillon	
¼ cup brown sugar	
2 teaspoons garlic powder or garlic cloves minced	
2 tablespoon oil	
2 cups carrots	Wash thoroughly, peeled, and sliced thin
2 cups broccoli	Wash thoroughly, cut into bite size pieces
1 large onion	Wash thoroughly before cutting, sliced
2 tablespoons sesame seeds, toasted	

Directions:

Steps:	Directions:	Critical Control Point /Quality Assurance
1	In a small bowl, dissolve beef bouillon in hot water. Add soy sauce, brown sugar, sesame oil and garlic in the small bowl. Stir.	
2	Prepare pasta according to directions on package. Drain reserving 1 cup water	
3	In a medium high heated skillet, add oil. Add beef and brown.	
4	Add sauce mixture, cook all together for about 2 minutes and remove from pan.	Minimum Temperature 145°F for 15 seconds for beef
5	In the same pan, sauté onions until golden brown. Remove from heat.	
6	In a separate skillet, stir fry carrot until just tender. Add broccoli and cook until just tender.	
7	In a large pot combine reserved water, pasta, vegetables and beef. Toss to coat.	
8	Top with sesame seeds. Serve hot.	

Time Temperature Sensitive food. *Food safety Standards: hold food for service at an internal temperature above 140° F. Do not mix old product with new. Cool leftover product quickly (within 4 hours) to below 41° F. Follow proper cooling procedures. Store leftovers in a tightly sealed, labeled and dated container. Use leftover within 72 hours if stored in refrigerator or 30 days if stored in the freezer. Reheat leftover product quickly (within 2 hours) to 165 degrees F for 15 seconds. Reheat left over product only once; discard if not used. Cold holding at 41°F or colder or using time alone (less than four hours). Always wash hands and wash and sanitize counter tops utensils and containers between steps when working with raw meat.*

Texture Modified Diets: TIP: use pasta within correct particle size.
Soft & Bite Size: (aka Bite size) **Food particle size ½ inch (~width of standard fork)** Food must be moist. Cut foods with a knife to a ½" particle size prior to mixing. Moisten with broth as needed.
Chopped: Food particle size ¼ inch (~ ½ width of standard fork) Food must be moist. Chop foods with a knife to 1/4" particle size prior to mixing. Moisten with broth as needed.
Minced and Moist: (aka Minced/Mechanical Soft/Ground) **Food particle size 1/8 inch (fits through prongs of standard fork)** Food must be moist. Use a food processor to grind food particles into 1/8 inch prior to mixing. Moisten with broth as needed.
Pureed: Smooth and cohesive. Use a food processor to puree to a smooth consistency. Foods are processed by grinding and then pureeing them. May add broth or sauce to puree. Do not add to much liquid. Puree should still hold its shape. Must not be firm or sticky. Puree foods while still hot. Appearance should be smooth like pudding. Serve ½ c. puree meat serving, ½ cup puree pasta and ½ cup puree vegetables separately. Omit sesame seeds.
Therapeutic Modified Diets:

Copyright 2020 Jacqueline Larson M.S., R.D.N. and Associates.   All Rights Reserved

Lowfat: No changes needed
Diabetic/No added Sugar/No Conc. Sweets/Calorie Controlled: No changes needed
Bland: omit sesame seeds, garlic powder, broccoli and onion
Liberal House Renal: Omit sauce, season with no salt herbs
No Added Salt: Omit sauce
2 Gram Sodium: omit sauce, season with no salt herbs
Gluten Free: Use GF soy sauce. Use gluten free pasta. Prepare foods separately to prevent cross contamination.
Allergy Alerts: When an "X" is present, this indicates the allergen is present.
Always read all food labels to ensure allergens are not present.

Wheat	Milk	Eggs	Fish Shellfish	Soy	Peanuts/Nuts	Other
X		X		X		

Key: SF= Salt Free D= Diet or Sugarfree LF = Lowfat FF = Fat Free GF = Gluten Free

Recipe Name: Beef Pepper Steak
Recipe Category: Dinner Entrée
Portion Size: 3 oz.
Ingredients: **Yields: 8 servings**

Ingredients	Notes:
2-2 1/2 Pounds sirloin, strip or porterhouse steak (boneless)	Trim all visible fat
Marinate:	
12 black peppercorns, coarsely ground	
¼ cup rice vinegar	
2 tablespoons tamari (Japanese Soy Sauce)	
1 clove garlic, minced	
¼ teaspoon white sugar	
¼ teaspoon salt	

Directions:

Steps:	Directions:	Critical Control Point /Quality Assurance
1	In a bowl, combine vinegar, peppercorns, tamari, garlic, sugar and salt. Marinate meat in a sealable container and refrigerate for 1 hour or more.	
2	Put steak on a cold grid or on a greased hot grids over a shallow greased pan, the top surface of the meat 3 inches from the heat source for a 1 1/2 inch steak.	
3	Brown the meat on one side, then turn once and brown the other side, allowing about 7 minutes per side for rare and about 8 minutes for medium.	Cook until internal temperature reaches 145 F degrees for 15 seconds
4	For a 2 inch steak, place meat 4 inches from heat source; turn more frequently, allowing in all about 9 minutes per side for rare and about 10 minutes for medium. Slice thinly across the grain to serve	Cook until internal temperature reaches 145 F degrees for 15 seconds

Time Temperature Sensitive food. *Food safety Standards: hold food for service at an internal temperature above 140°F. Do not mix old product with new. Cool leftover product quickly (within 4 hours) to below 41°F. Follow proper cooling procedures. Store leftovers in a tightly sealed, labeled and dated container. Use leftover within 72 hours if stored in refrigerator or 30 days if stored in the freezer. Reheat leftover product quickly (within 2 hours) to 165 degrees F for 15 seconds. Reheat left over product only once; discard if not used. Cold holding at 41°F or colder or using time alone (less than four hours). Always wash hands and wash and sanitize counter tops utensils and containers between steps when working with raw meat.*

Soft & Bite Size: (aka Bite size) **Food particle size ½ inch (~width of standard fork)** Food must be moist. Cut foods with a knife to a ½" particle size prior to mixing. Moisten with broth as needed. Foods that do not process well should be omitted. Omit: peppercorns

Chopped: Food particle size ¼ inch (~ ½ width of standard fork) Food must be moist. Chop foods with a knife to 1/4" particle size prior to mixing. Moisten with broth as needed. Foods that do not process well should be omitted. Omit: peppercorns

Minced and Moist:(aka Minced/Mechanical Soft/Ground) **Food particle size 1/8 inch (fits through prongs of standard fork)** Food must be moist. Use a food processor to grind food particles into 1/8 inch prior to mixing. Moisten with broth as needed. Foods that do not process well should be omitted. Omit: peppercorns

Pureed: Smooth and cohesive. Use a food processor to puree to a smooth consistency. Foods are processed by grinding and then pureeing them. May add broth or sauce to puree. Do not add to much liquid. Puree should still hold its shape. Must not be firm or sticky. Puree foods while still hot. Appearance should be smooth like pudding. Foods that do not process well should be omitted. Omit: peppercorns

Therapeutic Modified Diets:
Lowfat: No changes needed
Diabetic/No added Sugar/No Conc. Sweets/Calorie Controlled: No changes needed
Bland/Anti Reflux: omit pepper and garlic powder
Liberal House Renal: Omit salt and tamari
No Added Salt: No changes
2 Gram Sodium: Omit salt and tamari
Gluten Free: Use GF tamari. Prepare separately to prevent cross contamination.
Allergy Alerts: When an "X" is present, this indicates the allergen is present.
Always read all food labels to ensure allergens are not present.

Wheat	Milk	Eggs	Fish Shellfish	Soy	Peanuts/Nuts	Other
X				X		

Key: SF= Salt Free D= Diet or Sugarfree LF = Lowfat FF = Fat Free GF = Gluten Free

Recipe Name: Beef Pizza
Recipe Category: Lunch Entrée
Portion Size: 1 Slice (1/8 pizza)
Ingredients: Yields: 8 servings

Ingredients	Notes:
1 pound lean ground beef	
½ teaspoon garlic powder	
1 (1 pound) loaf frozen bread dough	Thawed
1 small jar pizza sauce	
2 cups shredded lowfat mozzarella cheese	

Directions:

Steps:	Directions:	Critical Control Point /Quality Assurance
1	In a skillet, cook beef over medium heat until no longer pink; drain.	Internal temperature of beef should reach 165 degree F
2	Add garlic powder	
3	On a floured surface, roll dough into a 13-inch circle	
4	Press onto the bottom and up the sides of a greased 12-inch pizza pan.	
5	Spread sauce over crust to within 1/2 inch of edge	
6	Top with beef and then cheese.	
7	Bake at 350 degrees F for 20-25 minutes or until crust is golden and cheese is melted	

Time Temperature Sensitive food. Food safety Standards: hold food for service at an internal temperature above 140° F. Do not mix old product with new. Cool leftover product quickly (within 4 hours) to below 41° F. Follow proper cooling procedures. Store leftovers in a tightly sealed, labeled and dated container. Use leftover within 72 hours if stored in refrigerator or 30 days if stored in the freezer. Reheat leftover product quickly (within 2 hours) to 165 degrees F for 15 seconds. Reheat left over product only once; discard if not used. Cold holding at 41 °F or colder or using time alone (less than four hours). Always wash hands and wash and sanitize counter tops utensils and containers between steps when working with raw meat.

Texture Modified Diets:
Soft & Bite Size: (aka Bite size) **Food particle size ½ inch (~width of standard fork)** Food must be moist. Bake crust until soft. If crust is hard, it must be processed to 1/8 inch and moistened before adding the toppings. Cut foods with a knife to a ½" particle size prior to layering. Moisten with broth as needed.
Chopped: Food particle size ¼ inch (~ ½ width of standard fork) Food must be moist. Bake crust until soft. If crust is hard, it must be processed to 1/8 inch and moistened before adding the toppings Chop foods with a knife to 1/4" particle size prior to layering. Moisten with broth as needed.
Minced and Moist: (aka Minced/Mechanical Soft/Ground) **Food particle size 1/8 inch (fits through prongs of standard fork)** Food must be moist. Bake crust until soft. Use a food processor to grind food particles into 1/8 inch prior to layering. Moisten with broth as needed.
Pureed: Smooth and cohesive. Use a food processor to puree to a smooth consistency. Foods are processed by grinding and then pureeing them. May add broth or sauce to puree. Do not add to much liquid. Puree should still hold its shape. Must not be firm or sticky. Puree foods while still hot. Appearance should be smooth like pudding.

Therapeutic Modified Diets:
Lowfat: No changes
Diabetic/No added Sugar/No Conc. Sweets/Calorie Controlled: No changes needed
Bland/Anti Reflux: omit garlic and pizza sauce.
Liberal House Renal: Use alternate menu item
No Added Salt: No changes
2 Gram Sodium: Use alternate menu item
Gluten Free: Use gluten free sauce and gluten free dough. Prepare foods separately to prevent cross contamination.
Allergy Alerts: When an "X" is present, this indicates the allergen is present. Always read all food labels to ensure allergens are not present.

Wheat	Milk	Eggs	Fish Shellfish	Soy	Peanuts/Nuts	Other
X	x					

Key: SF= Salt Free D= Diet or Sugarfree LF = Lowfat FF = Fat Free GF = Gluten Free

Recipe Name: Beef Pot Roast
Recipe Category: Dinner Entrée
Portion Size: 3 oz. beef, ½ c. carrots, ½ c. potatoes
Ingredients: **Yields: 8 servings**

Ingredients	Notes:
3 to 4 pounds chuck, shoulder, top or bottom round, brisket, blade or rump roast	Trim all visible fat
1/4 teaspoon garlic powder	
1 teaspoon salt	
1/4 teaspoon pepper	
1/4 cup flour	
1 tablespoon vegetable oil	
2 cups diced carrots	Washed, peeled and diced
3 cups diced potatoes	Washed, peeled and diced
1/2 cup diced onion	Washed, peeled and diced
1/2 cup diced celery	Washed, trimmed and diced
2 cups low sodium beef stock, low sodium vegetable stock, or water	
1 bay leaf	

Directions:

Steps:	Directions:	Critical Control Point /Quality Assurance
1	Combine garlic powder, salt, pepper, and flour.	
2	Dredge meat in flour mixture.	Discard excess flour
3	Heat oil in a heavy pan.	
4	Brown the meat on all sides in the oil.	
5	Drain excess fat.	
6	Add carrot, onions, potatoes, celery, stock, and bay leaf.	
7	Cover and bake in 300 degree oven for 3 to 4 hours.	
8	During this time turn the meat several times and, if necessary, add additional stock.	Cook until internal temperature reaches 165 degrees F for 4 minutes
9	Discard bay leaf and serve.	
***	***This may also be cooked in a crock pot for 8 to 10 hours on low heat or 6 to 8 hours on high heat.	Cook until internal temperature reaches 165 degrees F for 4 minutes

Time Temperature Sensitive food. *Food safety Standards: hold food for service at an internal temperature above 140° F. Do not mix old product with new. Cool leftover product quickly (within 4 hours) to below 41° F. Follow proper cooling procedures. Store leftovers in a tightly sealed, labeled and dated container. Use leftover within 72 hours if stored in refrigerator or 30 days if stored in the freezer. Reheat leftover product quickly (within 2 hours) to 165 degrees F for 15 seconds. Reheat left over product only once; discard if not used. Cold holding at 41°F or colder or using time alone (less than four hours). Always wash hands and wash and sanitize counter tops utensils and containers between steps when working with raw meat.*

<u>**Texture Modified Diets:**</u>
Soft & Bite Size: (aka Bite size) **Food particle size ½ inch (~width of standard fork)** Food must be moist. Cut foods with a knife to a ½" particle size after cooking. Moisten with broth as needed. Serve ½ c. meat, carrot and potato serving separately. Moisten with broth if needed

Chopped: Food particle size ¼ inch (~ ½ width of standard fork) Food must be moist. Chop foods with a knife to 1/4" particle size after cooking. Moisten with broth as needed. Serve ½ c. meat, carrot and potato serving separately. Moisten with broth if needed

Minced and Moist: (aka Minced/Mechanical Soft/Ground) **Food particle size 1/8 inch (fits through prongs of standard fork)** Food must be moist. Use a food processor to grind food particles into 1/8 inch after cooking. Moisten with broth as needed. Serve ½ c. meat, carrot, and potato serving separately.

Pureed: Smooth and cohesive. Use a food processor to puree to a smooth consistency. Foods are processed by grinding and then pureeing them. May add broth or sauce to puree. Do not add to much liquid. Puree should still hold its shape. Must not be firm or sticky. Puree foods while still hot. Appearance should be smooth like pudding. Serve ½ c. puree meat , carrot and potato serving separately .

<u>**Therapeutic Modified Diets:**</u>
Lowfat: No changes needed
Diabetic/No added Sugar/No Conc. Sweets/Calorie Controlled: No changes needed
Bland/Anti Reflux: omit garlic, pepper, onion, celery and bay leaf
Liberal House Renal: Omit salt, use SF broth or water. Sub. ½ rice for potatoes
No Added Salt: No changes needed
2 Gram Sodium: Omit salt, Use SF broth or water.
Gluten Free: Use gluten free broth and gluten free flour. Prepare foods separately to prevent cross contamination.

Allergy Alerts: When an "X" is present, this indicates the allergen is present. Always read all food labels to ensure allergens are not present.

Wheat	Milk	Eggs	Fish Shellfish	Soy	Peanuts/Nuts	Other
X						

Key: SF= Salt Free D= Diet or Sugarfree LF = Lowfat FF = Fat Free GF = Gluten Free

Copyright 2020 Jacqueline Larson M.S., R.D.N. and Associates.   All Rights Reserved

Recipe Name: Beef Sesame Stir Fry
Recipe Category: Dinner Entrée
Portion Size: ¾ cup
Ingredients: **Yields: 8 servings**

Ingredients	Notes:
2 1/2 pounds boneless tender beef steak (sirloin, rib eye, or top loin)	Trim all visible fat, slice thinly across the grain
1/3 cup Lite Soy Sauce	
¼ cup sugar	
2 cloves garlic, minced	
¼ cup vegetable oil	
4 green onions, sliced	Washed, trimmed, and sliced thin
3 tablespoons sesame seeds	

Directions:

Steps:	Directions:	Critical Control Point / Quality Assurance
1	Cut beef across grain into strips, then into 1 1/2 inch squares.	
2	Mix soy sauce, sugar, oil, and garlic in a large bowl. Add beef and add to bowl. Cover.	
3	Chill in the refrigerator for 30 minutes to 24 hours.	
4	Heat 1 tablespoon oil in hot wok or skillet over high heat.	
5	Add beef and stir fry 1 minute; remove.	Cook until internal temperature reaches 145 F degrees for 15 seconds
6	Add sesame seeds and serve immediately. Garnish green onions.	

Time Temperature Sensitive food. *Food safety Standards: hold food for service at an internal temperature above 140° F. Do not mix old product with new. Cool leftover product quickly (within 4 hours) to below 41° F. Follow proper cooling procedures. Store leftovers in a tightly sealed, labeled and dated container. Use leftover within 72 hours if stored in refrigerator or 30 days if stored in the freezer. Reheat leftover product quickly (within 2 hours) to 165 degrees F for 15 seconds. Reheat left over product only once; discard if not used. Cold holding at 41°F or colder or using time alone (less than four hours). Always wash hands and wash and sanitize counter tops utensils and containers between steps when working with raw meat.*

<u>**Texture Modified Diets:**</u>

Soft & Bite Size: (aka Bite size) **Food particle size ½ inch (~width of standard fork)** Food must be moist. Cut foods with a knife to a ½" particle size prior to mixing. Moisten with broth as needed.

Chopped: Food particle size ¼ inch (~ ½ width of standard fork) Food must be moist. Chop foods with a knife to 1/4" particle size prior to mixing. Moisten with broth as needed.

Minced and Moist:(aka Minced/Mechanical Soft/Ground) **Food particle size 1/8 inch (fits through prongs of standard fork)** Food must be moist. Use a food processor to grind food particles into 1/8 inch prior to mixing. Moisten with broth as needed.

Pureed: Smooth and cohesive. Use a food processor to puree to a smooth consistency. Foods are processed by grinding and then pureeing them. May add broth or sauce to puree. Do not add to much liquid. Puree should still hold its shape. Must not be firm or sticky. Puree foods while still hot. Appearance should be smooth like pudding. Serve ½ c. puree meat. Omit sesame seeds.

<u>**Therapeutic Modified Diets:**</u>
Lowfat: No changes needed
Diabetic/No added Sugar/No Conc. Sweets/Calorie Controlled: No changes needed
Bland/Anti Reflux: omit garlic, vinegar, red pepper, onions and green peppers
Liberal House Renal: Omit soy sauce and sugar
No Added Salt: Omit soy sauce and sugar
2 Gram Sodium: Omit soy sauce and sugar
Gluten Free: Use gluten free soy sauce. Prepare foods separately to prevent cross contamination.
**Allergy Alerts: When an "X" is present, this indicates the allergen is present.
Always read all food labels to ensure allergens are not present.**

Wheat	Milk	Eggs	Fish Shellfish	Soy	Peanuts/Nuts	Other
X				X		

Key: SF= Salt Free D= Diet or Sugarfree LF = Lowfat FF = Fat Free GF = Gluten Free

Recipe Name: Beef Stew
Recipe Category: Dinner Entrée
Portion Size: 1 cup
Ingredients: **Yields: 8 servings**

Ingredients	Notes:
2 1/2 Pounds of lean beef stew meat cut into ½ inch cubes	Trim all visible fat
¼ cup all purpose flour	
2 tablespoons cooking oil	
4 cups cubed potatoes	
4 cups mixed (frozen peas, carrots, corn and green bean variety) vegetables	
2 onions, cut into wedges	Wash, peel and cut into wedges
3 teaspoons low sodium instant beef bouillon granules	
¼ cup Worcestershire sauce	
2 teaspoons oregano	
1 teaspoon basil	
½ teaspoon pepper	
2 bay leaves	
4 cups low salt tomato sauce	

Directions:

Steps:	Directions:	Critical Control Point /Quality Assurance
1	Place flour in a deep dish.	
2	Dredge meat cubes and roll until meat is coated with flour. Shake off excess flour.	
3	In a large skillet, heat oil and brown meat. Turning to brown evenly. Drain off fat.	
4	In a large pot or crock pot layer potatoes, vegetables, and onion. Add meat.	
5	Add bouillon, Worcestershire sauce, oregano, basil, pepper and bay leaf.	
6	If using a crock pot cook on low heat for 10 to 12 hours or on high heat for 5 to 6 hours.	Cook until internal temperature reaches 145 degrees F for 15 seconds
7	If using a large pot on the stove top, bring mixture to boil. Reduce heat and simmer for 1 ½ hour or until meat is tender. Discard bay leaves.	Cook until internal temperature reaches 145 degrees F for 15 seconds

Time Temperature Sensitive food. Food safety Standards: hold food for service at an internal temperature above 140° F. Do not mix old product with new. Cool leftover product quickly (within 4 hours) to below 41° F. Follow proper cooling procedures. Store leftovers in a tightly sealed, labeled and dated container. Use leftover within 72 hours if stored in refrigerator or 30 days if stored in the freezer. Reheat leftover product quickly (within 2 hours) to 165 degrees F for 15 seconds. Reheat left over product only once; discard if not used. Cold holding at 41°F or colder or using time alone (less than four hours). Always wash hands and wash and sanitize counter tops utensils and containers between steps when working with raw meat.

Texture Modified Diets:
Soft & Bite Size: (aka Bite size) **Food particle size ½ inch (~width of standard fork)** Food must be moist. Cut foods with a knife to a ½" particle size prior to mixing. Moisten with broth as needed.
Chopped: Food particle size ¼ inch (~ ½ width of standard fork) Food must be moist. Chop foods with a knife to 1/4" particle size prior to mixing. Moisten with broth as needed.
Minced and Moist: (aka Minced/Mechanical Soft/Ground) **Food particle size 1/8 inch (fits through prongs of standard fork)** Food must be moist. Use a food processor to grind food particles into 1/8 inch prior to mixing. Moisten with broth as needed.
Pureed: Smooth and cohesive. Use a food processor to puree to a smooth consistency. Foods are processed by grinding and then pureeing them. May add broth or sauce to puree. Do not add to much liquid. Puree should still hold its shape. Must not be firm or sticky. Puree foods while still hot. Appearance should be smooth like pudding. Serve ½ c. puree meat, ½ c. puree vegetables and ½ c. puree potatoes separately. serving.

Therapeutic Modified Diets:
Lowfat: No changes needed
Diabetic/No added Sugar/No Conc. Sweets/Calorie Controlled: No changes needed
Bland/Anti Reflux: Use peas and carrots for the vegetable. Omit onion, Worchester sauce, pepper, oregano, basil, bay leaves and tomato sauce.
Liberal House Renal: Use SF broth or water. Omit potatoes, Worcestershire sauce and tomato sauce
No Added Salt: No changes needed
2 Gram Sodium: Use SF broth or water. Use SF tomato sauce or Fresh tomatoes. Omit Worcestershire sauce.
Gluten Free: Use gluten free flour and gluten free bouillon granules.   Prepare foods separately to prevent cross contamination.
Allergy Alerts: When an "X" is present, this indicates the allergen is present. Always read all food labels to ensure allergens are not present.

Wheat	Milk	Eggs	Fish Shellfish	Soy	Peanuts/Nuts	Other
X			X	X		

Key: SF= Salt Free D= Diet or Sugarfree LF = Lowfat FF = Fat Free GF = Gluten Free

Recipe Name: Beef Stroganoff
Recipe Category: Dinner Entrée
Portion Size: ½ cup stroganoff and ½ cup noodles
Ingredients: **Yields: 8 servings**

Ingredients	Notes:
2 1/2 pounds lean fillet of beef	Trim all visible fat,
1 tablespoon olive oil	
1 tablespoon grated onion	Washed, peeled and grated
1 pound sliced mushrooms	Washed, trimmed and sliced
1/2 teaspoon salt	
1/4 teaspoon pepper	
1/2 teaspoon basil	
1 cup light sour cream	
4 Cups cooked noodles or rice	May use whole grain

Directions:

Steps:	Directions:	Critical Control Point /Quality Assurance
1	Cut beef into 1/2 inch slices across the grain.	
2	Pound them until thin. Cut into strips about 1 inch wide.	
3	Heat oil in a pan. Sauté onion in oil.	
4	Add beef and sauté quickly about 5 minutes, until browned. Remove and keep warm.	
5	Add mushrooms to the pan and sauté.	
6	Drain and add the beef, salt, pepper, and basil. Heat through. Stir in sour cream.	Cook until internal temperature reaches 165 degrees F for 15 seconds
7	Serve over noodles or rice.	

Time Temperature Sensitive food. Food safety Standards: hold food for service at an internal temperature above 140° F. Do not mix old product with new. Cool leftover product quickly (within 4 hours) to below 41° F. Follow proper cooling procedures. Store leftovers in a tightly sealed, labeled and dated container. Use leftover within 72 hours if stored in refrigerator or 30 days if stored in the freezer. Reheat leftover product quickly (within 2 hours) to 165 degrees F for 15 seconds. Reheat left over product only once; discard if not used. Cold holding at 41 °F or colder or using time alone (less than four hours). Always wash hands and wash and sanitize counter tops utensils and containers between steps when working with raw meat.

Texture Modified Diets: Tip: use pasta that is the correct particle size.

Soft & Bite Size: (aka Bite size) **Food particle size ½ inch (~width of standard fork)** Food must be moist. Cut foods with a knife to a ½" particle size prior to mixing. Moisten with broth as needed.

Chopped: Food particle size ¼ inch (~ ½ width of standard fork) Food must be moist. Chop foods with a knife to 1/4" particle size prior to mixing. Moisten with broth as needed.

Minced and Moist: (aka Minced/Mechanical Soft/Ground) **Food particle size 1/8 inch (fits through prongs of standard fork)** Food must be moist. Use a food processor to grind food particles into 1/8 inch prior to mixing. Moisten with broth as needed.

Pureed: Smooth and cohesive. Use a food processor to puree to a smooth consistency. Foods are processed by grinding and then pureeing them. May add broth or sauce to puree. Do not add to much liquid. Puree should still hold its shape. Must not be firm or sticky. Puree foods while still hot. Appearance should be smooth like pudding. Serve ½ c. meat and pasta serving separately. Tip: puree pasta while still hot.

Therapeutic Modified Diets:
Lowfat: No changes needed
Diabetic/No added Sugar/No Conc. Sweets/Calorie Controlled: No changes needed
Bland/Anti Reflux: omit onion, pepper and basil.
Liberal House Renal: Omit salt and sour cream
No Added Salt: No changes needed
2 Gram Sodium: Omit salt and sour cream
Gluten Free: Use gluten free pasta. Prepare foods separately to prevent cross contamination.

Allergy Alerts: When an "X" is present, this indicates the allergen is present. Always read all food labels to ensure allergens are not present.

Wheat	Milk	Eggs	Fish Shellfish	Soy	Peanuts/Nuts	Other
X	X	X				

Key: SF= Salt Free D= Diet or Sugarfree LF = Lowfat FF = Fat Free GF = Gluten Free

Recipe Name: Beef Tacos
Recipe Category: Dinner Entrée
Portion Size: 2 small tacos
Ingredients: Yields: 8 servings

Ingredients	Notes:
2 Pounds lean ground beef	
1 tablespoon chili powder	
1/2 teaspoon garlic powder	
1/4 teaspoon onion powder	
1/4 teaspoon dried oregano	
1/2 teaspoon paprika	
1 teaspoon ground cumin	
1/2 teaspoon salt	
1/4 teaspoon ground black pepper	
1/2 teaspoon sugar	
1 16-ounce can low sodium tomato sauce	
2 Cups shredded low fat cheddar cheese	
1 Cups tomatoes, chopped	Wash, trim and chop
3 Cups shredded lettuce	Wash, trim and chop
16 Flour small tortillas	May use whole grain
1/2 Cup light sour cream	
Taco sauce (optional)	

Directions:

Steps:	Directions:	Critical Control Point /Quality Assurance
1	In a large sauce pan, brown ground beef. Drain fat.	
2	In a small bowl combine, chili powder, garlic powder, onion powder, oregano, paprika, cumin, salt, pepper and sugar.	
3	Add seasoning mix and tomato sauce to ground beef. Heat through.	Cook until internal temperature reaches 165 F degrees for 15 seconds.
4	Wrap tortillas in foil and 350 warm in oven for 20 minutes.	
5	Top each with meat and then cheese.	
6	Top with chopped tomatoes, sour cream, and lettuce.	
7	Sprinkle with taco sauce.	

Time Temperature Sensitive food. *Food safety Standards: hold food for service at an internal temperature above 140° F. Do not mix old product with new. Cool leftover product quickly (within 4 hours) to below 41° F. Follow proper cooling procedures. Store leftovers in a tightly sealed, labeled and dated container. Use leftover within 72 hours if stored in refrigerator or 30 days if stored in the freezer. Reheat leftover product quickly (within 2 hours) to 165 degrees F for 15 seconds. Reheat left over product only once; discard if not used. Cold holding at 41°F or colder or using time alone (less than four hours). Always wash hands and wash and sanitize counter tops utensils and containers between steps when working with raw meat.*

Texture Modified Diets:

Soft & Bite Size: (aka Bite size) **Food particle size ½ inch (~width of standard fork)** Food must be moist. Cut foods with a knife to a ½" particle size prior to layering. Moisten with broth as needed. Serve chopped meat mixture, tomatoes, lettuce, cheese and sour cream on top of chopped tortillas.

Chopped: Food particle size ¼ inch (~ ½ width of standard fork) Food must be moist. Chop foods with a knife to 1/4" particle size prior to layering. Serve chopped meat mixture, tomatoes, lettuce, cheese and sour cream on top of chopped tortillas. Moisten with broth as needed.

Minced and Moist:(aka Minced/Mechanical Soft/Ground) **Food particle size 1/8 inch (fits through prongs of standard fork)** Food must be moist. Use a food processor to grind food particles into 1/8 inch prior to layering. Serve ½ c. ground meat mixture, tomatoes, lettuce, cheese, and sour cream on top of ground tortillas. Do not mix. Moisten with broth if needed Moisten with broth as needed.

Pureed: Smooth and cohesive. Use a food processor to puree to a smooth consistency. Foods are processed by grinding and then pureeing them. May add broth or sauce to puree. Do not add to much liquid. Puree should still hold its shape. Must not be firm or sticky. Puree foods while still hot. Appearance should be smooth like pudding. Serve ½ c. puree meat on top of ½ c. puree tortillas serving. Melt cheese on top of meat. Top with1 T. puree tomato and 1 T. puree lettuce and 1 t. sour cream.

Therapeutic Modified Diets:
Lowfat: No changes needed
Diabetic/No added Sugar/No Conc. Sweets/Calorie Controlled: No changes needed
Bland/Anti Reflux: omit chili powder, garlic powder, onion powder, oregano, paprika, cumin, black pepper, sugar, tomato sauce, tomatoes, and taco sauce. (plain ground beef on tortilla topped with cheese, finely chopped lettuce, and sour cream)

Liberal House Renal: Omit salt, tomato sauce, cheese, tomatoes, sour cream and Taco sauce. Use low sodium tortillas. (See recipe.)
No Added Salt: No changes needed
2 Gram Sodium: Omit salt, cheese, sour cream and Taco sauce. Use SF tomato sauce or fresh tomatoes. Use low sodium tortillas. (See recipe)
Gluten Free: Omit flour whole grain tortillas for gluten free corn tortillas. Prepare foods separately to prevent cross contamination.

Allergy Alerts: When an "X" is present, this indicates the allergen is present.
Always read all food labels to ensure allergens are not present.

Wheat	Milk	Eggs	Fish Shellfish	Soy	Peanuts/Nuts	Other
X	X					

Key: SF= Salt Free D= Diet or Sugarfree LF = Lowfat FF = Fat Free GF = Gluten Free

Recipe Name: Beef Tenderloin
Recipe Category: Dinner Entrée
Portion Size: 3 oz.
Ingredients: Yields: 8 servings

Ingredients	Notes:
2-2 1/2 Pounds beef tenderloin roast	Trim all visible fat
½ cup olive oil	
¾ cup light soy sauce	
Seasonings to taste: salt, pepper, rosemary, sherry, or garlic powder	(optional)

Directions:

Steps:	Directions:	Critical Control Point /Quality Assurance
1	Preheat oven to 350 F degrees	
2	Place roast in a shallow baking dish. Pour soy sauce and oil over the tenderloin.	
3	Bake in preheated oven for 10 minutes, then turn the roast over, and continue cooking 35 to 40 minutes, basting occasionally until the internal temperature of the roast is reached. Let meat rest for 10 to 15 minutes before slicing. Slice thinly across the grain to serve	Cook until internal temperature reaches 145 F degrees for 15 seconds

Time Temperature Sensitive food. Food safety Standards: hold food for service at an internal temperature above 140° F. Do not mix old product with new. Cool leftover product quickly (within 4 hours) to below 41° F. Follow proper cooling procedures. Store leftovers in a tightly sealed, labeled and dated container. Use leftover within 72 hours if stored in refrigerator or 30 days if stored in the freezer. Reheat leftover product quickly (within 2 hours) to 165 degrees F for 15 seconds. Reheat left over product only once; discard if not used. Cold holding at 41°F or colder or using time alone (less than four hours). Always wash hands and wash and sanitize counter tops utensils and containers between steps when working with raw meat.

Texture Modified Diets:

Soft & Bite Size: (aka Bite size) **Food particle size ½ inch (~width of standard fork)** Food must be moist. Cut foods with a knife to a ½" particle size after cooking. Moisten with broth as needed.

Chopped: Food particle size ¼ inch (~ ½ width of standard fork) Food must be moist. Chop foods with a knife to 1/4" particle size after cooking. Moisten with broth as needed.

Minced and Moist: (aka Minced/Mechanical Soft/Ground) **Food particle size 1/8 inch (fits through prongs of standard fork)** Food must be moist. Use a food processor to grind food particles into 1/8 inch after cooking. Moisten with broth as needed.

Pureed: Smooth and cohesive. Use a food processor to puree to a smooth consistency. Foods are processed by grinding and then pureeing them. May add broth or sauce to puree. Do not add to much liquid. Puree should still hold its shape. Must not be firm or sticky. Puree foods while still hot. Appearance should be smooth like pudding. Serve ½ c. meat serving.

Therapeutic Modified Diets:

Lowfat: No changes needed
Diabetic/No added Sugar/No Conc. Sweets/Calorie Controlled: No changes needed
Bland/Anti Reflux: omit pepper and garlic powder
Liberal House Renal: Omit salt
No Added Salt: No changes
2 Gram Sodium: omit salt
Gluten Free: No changes needed.
Allergy Alerts: When an "X" is present, this indicates the allergen is present.
Always read all food labels to ensure allergens are not present.

Wheat	Milk	Eggs	Fish Shellfish	Soy	Peanuts/Nuts	Other

Key: SF= Salt Free D= Diet or Sugarfree LF = Lowfat FF = Fat Free GF = Gluten Free

Recipe Name: Beef Tenderloin Medallions
Recipe Category: Dinner Entrée
Portion Size: 3 oz. boneless
Ingredients: Yields: 8 servings

Ingredients	Notes:
2 lbs. boneless beef tenderloin	Trim all visible fat, Thinly slice into thin slices across the grain.
1/4 cup olive oil	Or vegetable oil
1 teaspoon garlic salt	
1 teaspoon pepper	
Optional additional herbs to rub: dried thyme, minced rosemary, fresh minced garlic.	

Directions:

Steps:	Directions:	Critical Control Point /Quality Assurance
1	Season Meat with garlic salt and pepper	
2	Heat oil to medium high heat.	
3	Add beef slices	
4	Cook for 2 minutes until slightly brown	
5	Turn slices and cook until brown	Heat to at least 145 degree with 4 minute rest
6	Serve immediately.	

Time Temperature Sensitive food. *Food safety Standards: hold food for service at an internal temperature above 140° F. Do not mix old product with new. Cool leftover product quickly (within 4 hours) to below 41° F. Follow proper cooling procedures. Store leftovers in a tightly sealed, labeled and dated container. Use leftover within 72 hours if stored in refrigerator or 30 days if stored in the freezer. Reheat leftover product quickly (within 2 hours) to 165 degrees F for 15 seconds. Reheat left over product only once; discard if not used. Cold holding at 41°F or colder or using time alone (less than four hours). Always wash hands and wash and sanitize counter tops utensils and containers between steps when working with raw meat.*

Texture Modified Diets:

Soft & Bite Size: (aka Bite size) **Food particle size ½ inch (~width of standard fork)** Food must be moist. Cut foods with a knife to a ½" particle size after cooking. Moisten with broth as needed.

Chopped: Food particle size ¼ inch (~ ½ width of standard fork) Food must be moist. Chop foods with a knife to 1/4" particle size after cooking. Moisten with broth as needed.

Minced and Moist: (aka Minced/Mechanical Soft/Ground) **Food particle size 1/8 inch (fits through prongs of standard fork)** Food must be moist. Use a food processor to grind food particles into 1/8 inch after cooking. Moisten with broth as needed.

Pureed: Smooth and cohesive. Use a food processor to puree to a smooth consistency. Foods are processed by grinding and then pureeing them. May add broth or sauce to puree. Do not add to much liquid. Puree should still hold its shape. Must not be firm or sticky. Puree foods while still hot. Appearance should be smooth like pudding.

Therapeutic Modified Diets:

Lowfat: No changes needed
Diabetic/No added Sugar/No Conc. Sweets/Calorie Controlled: No changes needed
Bland/Anti Reflux: omit pepper and garlic salt
Liberal House Renal: omit garlic salt and use garlic powder
No Added Salt: No changes needed
2 Gram Sodium: omit garlic salt and use garlic powder
Gluten Free: No changes. Prepare foods separately to prevent cross contamination.
Allergy Alerts: When an "X" is present, this indicates the allergen is present.
Always read all food labels to ensure allergens are not present.

Wheat	Milk	Eggs	Fish Shellfish	Soy	Peanuts/Nuts	Other

Key: SF= Salt Free D= Diet or Sugarfree LF = Lowfat FF = Fat Free GF = Gluten Free

Copyright 2020 Jacqueline Larson M.S., R.D.N. and Associates. All Rights Reserved

Recipe Name: Beef Tips and Noodles
Recipe Category: Dinner Entrée
Portion Size: ½ cup beef tips and ½ cup noodles
Ingredients: **Yields: 8 servings**

Ingredients	Notes:
16 oz. package of whole grain noodles	
2 1/2 lb. sirloin tips, cubed	Trim all visible fat
1 can evaporated fat free milk	
2 tablespoons all purpose flour	
1 onion, chopped	Wash, peel and chop
2 gloves garlic, minced	Wash, peel and mince
1 (8oz) package fresh sliced mushrooms	Wash, trim and slice
2 cups reduced sodium beef broth	
1/2 teaspoon ground black pepper	

Directions:

Steps:	Directions:	Critical Control Point / Quality Assurance
1	Preheat oven to 400 degrees.	
2	In a baking inch pan, combine the milk, beef broth, garlic, mushrooms, flour and onion.	
3	Mix thoroughly with beef tips.	
4	Bake covered in oven for 1 1/2 hours.	Cook until internal temperature reaches 165 F degrees for 15 seconds
5	Cook pasta according to directions on package. Drain.	
6	Serve beef tips and sauce over noodles	

Time Temperature Sensitive food. *Food safety Standards: hold food for service at an internal temperature above 140° F. Do not mix old product with new. Cool leftover product quickly (within 4 hours) to below 41° F. Follow proper cooling procedures. Store leftovers in a tightly sealed, labeled and dated container. Use leftover within 72 hours if stored in refrigerator or 30 days if stored in the freezer. Reheat leftover product quickly (within 2 hours) to 165 degrees F for 15 seconds. Reheat left over product only once; discard if not used. Cold holding at 41 °F or colder or using time alone (less than four hours). Always wash hands and wash and sanitize counter tops utensils and containers between steps when working with raw meat.*

Texture Modified Diets: TIP: Use pasta with correct particle size.

Soft & Bite Size: (aka Bite size) **Food particle size ½ inch (~width of standard fork)** Food must be moist. Cut foods with a knife to a ½" particle size prior to mixing. Moisten with broth as needed.

Chopped: Food particle size ¼ inch (~ ½ width of standard fork) Food must be moist. Chop foods with a knife to 1/4" particle size prior to mixing. Moisten with broth as needed.

Minced and Moist:(aka Minced/Mechanical Soft/Ground) **Food particle size 1/8 inch (fits through prongs of standard fork)** Food must be moist. Use a food processor to grind food particles into 1/8 inch prior to mixing. Moisten with broth as needed.

Pureed: Smooth and cohesive. Use a food processor to puree to a smooth consistency. Foods are processed by grinding and then pureeing them. May add broth or sauce to puree. Do not add to much liquid. Puree should still hold its shape. Must not be firm or sticky. Puree foods while still hot. Appearance should be smooth like pudding. Serve ½ c. meat serving and ½ c. puree noodles separately. Tip: puree noodles while still hot.

Therapeutic Modified Diets:
Lowfat: No changes needed
Diabetic/No added Sugar/No Conc. Sweets/Calorie Controlled: No changes needed
Bland/Anti Reflux: omit garlic and pepper
Liberal House Renal: Use SF broth or water.
No Added Salt: No changes needed
2 Gram Sodium: Use SF broth or water
Gluten Free: Omit flour for gluten free flour. Use gluten free broth. Serve with GF noodles Prepare foods separately to prevent cross contamination.
Allergy Alerts: When an "X" is present, this indicates the allergen is present.
Always read all food labels to ensure allergens are not present.

Wheat	Milk	Eggs	Fish Shellfish	Soy	Peanuts/Nuts	Other
X	X	X				

Key: SF= Salt Free D= Diet or Sugarfree LF = Lowfat FF = Fat Free GF = Gluten Free

Copyright 2020 Jacqueline Larson M.S., R.D.N. and Associates.   All Rights Reserved

Recipe Name: Beef Tostada
Recipe Category: Dinner Entrée
Portion Size: 1/3 c. ground meat, 1/4 c. refried beans, 1 tortilla, ¼ cup tomatoes and, ½ cup lettuce each.
Ingredients: Yields: 8 servings

Ingredients	Notes:
1 pounds lean ground beef	
2 cans fat free refried beans	
1 small can Ortega chili peppers, drained	
2 cups shredded low fat cheddar cheese	
2 cups tomatoes, chopped	
4 cups shredded lettuce	
8 flour tortillas	May use whole grain
Taco sauce (optional)	

Directions:

Steps:	Directions:	Critical Control Point /Quality Assurance
1	Prepare flour tortillas by frying them in hot oil until crisp tender, turning once.	
2	Drain on a paper towel.	
3	In a large sauce pan, brown ground beef. Drain fat.	Cook until internal temperature reaches 165 F degrees for 15 seconds
4	Mix canned refried beans with Ortega chili peppers, heat through.	
5	Place bean mixture on prepared tortillas.	
6	Top each with meat and then cheese.	
7	Top with chopped lettuce and tomatoes.	
8	Sprinkle with taco sauce.	

Time Temperature Sensitive food. *Food safety Standards: hold food for service at an internal temperature above 140° F. Do not mix old product with new. Cool leftover product quickly (within 4 hours) to below 41° F. Follow proper cooling procedures. Store leftovers in a tightly sealed, labeled and dated container. Use leftover within 72 hours if stored in refrigerator or 30 days if stored in the freezer. Reheat leftover product quickly (within 2 hours) to 165 degrees F for 15 seconds. Reheat left over product only once; discard if not used. Cold holding at 41°F or colder or using time alone (less than four hours). Always wash hands and wash and sanitize counter tops utensils and containers between steps when working with raw meat.*

Texture Modified Diets:

Soft & Bite Size: (aka Bite size) **Food particle size ½ inch (~width of standard fork)** Food must be moist. Cut foods with a knife to a ½" particle size prior to layering Do not fry tortilla.. Order: tortillas, beef, beans, cheese, lettuce and tomato. Sprinkle with taco sauce. Moisten with broth if needed

Chopped: Food particle size ¼ inch (~ ½ width of standard fork) Do not fry tortilla. Food must be moist. Chop foods with a knife to 1/4" particle size prior to layering. Order: tortillas, beef, beans, cheese, lettuce and tomato. Sprinkle with taco sauce. Moisten with broth if needed

Minced and Moist:(aka Minced/Mechanical Soft/Ground) **Food particle size 1/8 inch (fits through prongs of standard fork)** Do not fry tortilla. Food must be moist. Use a food processor to grind food particles into 1/8 inch prior to layering. Order: tortillas, beef, beans, cheese, lettuce and tomato. Sprinkle with taco sauce. Moisten with broth if needed

Pureed: Smooth and cohesive. Do not fry tortilla. Use a food processor to puree to a smooth consistency. Foods are processed by grinding and then pureeing them. May add broth or sauce to puree. Do not add to much liquid. Puree should still hold its shape. Must not be firm or sticky. Puree foods while still hot. Appearance should be smooth like pudding. Puree each item separately and layer each puree item on top of each other. (do not mix). May drizzle with taco sauce.

Therapeutic Modified Diets:

Lowfat: Do not fry tortilla
Diabetic/No added Sugar/No Conc. Sweets/Calorie Controlled: No changes needed
Bland/Anti Reflux: Do not fry tortilla, omit beans, chili peppers, tomatoes and taco sauce
Liberal House Renal: Omit refried beans, cheese, tomatoes and taco sauce. Use low sodium tortillas. (see recipe)
No Added Salt: No changes needed
2 Gram Sodium: omit cheese, refried beans and taco sauce. Use low sodium tortillas. (Use low sodium tortillas. (see recipe)
Gluten Free: Omit flour whole grain tortillas and use gluten free corn tortillas. Use GF taco sauce. Prepare foods separately to prevent cross contamination.
Allergy Alerts: When an "X" is present, this indicates the allergen is present.
Always read all food labels to ensure allergens are not present.

Wheat	Milk	Eggs	Fish Shellfish	Soy	Peanuts/Nuts	Other
X	X					

Key: SF= Salt Free D= Diet or Sugarfree LF = Lowfat FF = Fat Free GF = Gluten Free

Recipe Name: Broiled Steak
Recipe Category: Dinner Entrée
Portion Size: 3 oz.
Ingredients: **Yields: 8 servings**

Ingredients	Notes:
2-2 1/2 Pounds sirloin, strip or porterhouse steak (boneless)	Trim all visible fat
Seasonings to taste: salt, pepper, or garlic powder	

Directions:

Steps:	Directions:	Critical Control Point / Quality Assurance
1	Put steak on a cold grid or on a greased hot grids over a shallow greased pan, the top surface of the meat 3 inches from the heat source for a 1 1/2 inch steak.	
2	Brown the meat on one side, then turn once and brown the other side, allowing about 7 minutes per side for rare and about 8 minutes for medium.	Cook until internal temperature reaches 145 F degrees for 15 seconds
3	For a 2 inch steak, place meat 4 inches from heat source; turn more frequently, allowing in all about 9 minutes per side for rare and about 10 minutes for medium. Slice thinly across the grain to serve	Cook until internal temperature reaches 145 F degrees for 15 seconds

Time Temperature Sensitive food. Food safety Standards: hold food for service at an internal temperature above 140° F. Do not mix old product with new. Cool leftover product quickly (within 4 hours) to below 41° F. Follow proper cooling procedures. Store leftovers in a tightly sealed, labeled and dated container. Use leftover within 72 hours if stored in refrigerator or 30 days if stored in the freezer. Reheat leftover product quickly (within 2 hours) to 165 degrees F for 15 seconds. Reheat left over product only once; discard if not used. Cold holding at 41°F or colder or using time alone (less than four hours). Always wash hands and wash and sanitize counter tops utensils and containers between steps when working with raw meat.

Texture Modified Diets:

Soft & Bite Size: (aka Bite size) **Food particle size ½ inch (~width of standard fork)** Food must be moist. Cut foods with a knife to a ½" particle size after cooking. Moisten with broth as needed.

Chopped: Food particle size ¼ inch (~ ½ width of standard fork) Food must be moist. Chop foods with a knife to 1/4" particle size after cooking. Moisten with broth as needed.

Minced and Moist: (aka Minced/Mechanical Soft/Ground) **Food particle size 1/8 inch (fits through prongs of standard fork)** Food must be moist. Use a food processor to grind food particles into 1/8 inch after cooking. Moisten with broth as needed.

Pureed: Smooth and cohesive. Use a food processor to puree to a smooth consistency. Foods are processed by grinding and then pureeing them. May add broth or sauce to puree. Do not add to much liquid. Puree should still hold its shape. Must not be firm or sticky. Puree foods while still hot. Appearance should be smooth like pudding. Serve ½ c. meat serving.

Therapeutic Modified Diets:

Lowfat: No changes needed
Diabetic/No added Sugar/No Conc. Sweets/Calorie Controlled: No changes needed
Bland/Anti Reflux: omit pepper and garlic powder
Liberal House Renal: Omit salt
No Added Salt: No changes
2 Gram Sodium: omit salt
Gluten Free: No changes needed.
Allergy Alerts: When an "X" is present, this indicates the allergen is present.
Always read all food labels to ensure allergens are not present.

Wheat	Milk	Eggs	Fish Shellfish	Soy	Peanuts/Nuts	Other

Key: SF= Salt Free D= Diet or Sugarfree LF = Lowfat FF = Fat Free GF = Gluten Free

Recipe Name: Cabbage Roll Casserole
Recipe Category: Dinner Entrée
Portion Size: 1 ½ cup
Ingredients: **Yields: 8 servings**

Ingredients	Notes:
2 1/2 pounds lean ground beef	
1 cup chopped onion	Wash, peel and chop
1 (29 oz.) can low sodium tomato sauce	
3 ½ pounds chopped cabbage	Wash, trim and chop
1 cup uncooked brown white rice	
1 teaspoon. salt	
2 (14 ounce) cans low salt beef broth	

Directions:

Steps:	Directions:	Critical Control Point /Quality Assurance
1	Preheat oven to 350 degrees.	
2	In a large skillet brown beef over medium high heat until redness is gone	
3	Drain off fat.	
4	In a large mixing bowl combine the onion, tomato sauce, cabbage salt and rice.	
5	Add meat and mix all together.	
6	Pour mixture into large baking dish	
7	Cover and bake for 1 hour.	
8	Remove from oven.	
9	Uncover and stir.	
10	Bake uncovered for 30 additional minutes.	Cook until internal temperature reaches 165 F degrees for 15 seconds

Time Temperature Sensitive food. Food safety Standards: hold food for service at an internal temperature above 140° F. Do not mix old product with new. Cool leftover product quickly (within 4 hours) to below 41° F. Follow proper cooling procedures. Store leftovers in a tightly sealed, labeled and dated container. Use leftover within 72 hours if stored in refrigerator or 30 days if stored in the freezer. Reheat leftover product quickly (within 2 hours) to 165 degrees F for 15 seconds. Reheat left over product only once; discard if not used. Cold holding at 41 °F or colder or using time alone (less than four hours). Always wash hands and wash and sanitize counter tops utensils and containers between steps when working with raw meat.

Texture Modified Diets:

Soft & Bite Size: (aka Bite size) **Food particle size ½ inch (~width of standard fork)** Food must be moist. Cut foods with a knife to a ½" particle size prior to mixing. Moisten with broth as needed.

Chopped: Food particle size ¼ inch (~ ½ width of standard fork) Food must be moist. Chop foods with a knife to 1/4" particle size prior to mixing. Moisten with broth as needed.

Minced and Moist: (aka Minced/Mechanical Soft/Ground) **Food particle size 1/8 inch (fits through prongs of standard fork)** Food must be moist. Use a food processor to grind food particles into 1/8 inch prior to mixing. Moisten with broth as needed.

Pureed: Smooth and cohesive. Use a food processor to puree to a smooth consistency. Foods are processed by grinding and then pureeing them. May add broth or sauce to puree. Do not add to much liquid. Puree should still hold its shape. Must not be firm or sticky. Puree foods while still hot. Appearance should be smooth like pudding. Serve ½ c. puree meat , puree cooked cabbage, and ½ cup puree rice serving separately.

Therapeutic Modified Diets:

Lowfat: No changes needed
Diabetic/No added Sugar/No Conc. Sweets/Calorie Controlled: No changes needed
Bland/Anti Reflux: plain hamburger patty, ½ c. plain rice and ½ c. cooked peas or carrots
Liberal House Renal: Serve plain hamburger patty, ½ c. plain rice and ½ c. SF cabbage
No Added Salt: No changes needed
2 Gram Sodium: Serve SF hamburger patty, ½ c. plain rice and ½ c. SF cabbage.
Gluten Free: Use gluten free broth. Prepare foods separately to prevent cross contamination.
**Allergy Alerts: When an "X" is present, this indicates the allergen is present.
Always read all food labels to ensure allergens are not present.**

Wheat	Milk	Eggs	Fish Shellfish	Soy	Peanuts/Nuts	Other
X						

Key: SF= Salt Free D= Diet or Sugarfree LF = Lowfat FF = Fat Free GF = Gluten Free

Recipe Name: Cheesy Hamburger Casserole
Recipe Category: Dinner Entrée
Portion Size: 1 cup
Ingredients: Yields: 8 servings

Ingredients	Notes:
2 1/2 Pounds lean ground beef	
2 tablespoons yellow mustard	
1-16 oz. pasta	Prepare according directions
1 Small onion, chopped	Wash, peel and chop
1 cup fat free milk	
1 cup light cream cheese	
2 Cans (14 oz.) of low sodium tomato sauce	
2 Cup shredded low fat cheddar cheese	

Directions:

Steps:	Directions:	Critical Control Point / Quality Assurance
1	Brown ground beef with onion. Drain excess fat.	
2	Prepare pasta according to directions on package. Drain.	
3	Combine ground beef, pasta, milk, mustard cream cheese, and tomato sauce.	
4	Pour mixture into a baking dish.	
5	Sprinkle cheese on top.	
6	Bake in a 325 degree oven for about 30-35 minutes.	Cook until internal temperature reaches 165 F degrees for 15 seconds

Time Temperature Sensitive food. Food safety Standards: hold food for service at an internal temperature above 140°F. Do not mix old product with new. Cool leftover product quickly (within 4 hours) to below 41°F. Follow proper cooling procedures. Store leftovers in a tightly sealed, labeled and dated container. Use leftover within 72 hours if stored in refrigerator or 30 days if stored in the freezer. Reheat leftover product quickly (within 2 hours) to 165 degrees F for 15 seconds. Reheat left over product only once; discard if not used. Cold holding at 41°F or colder or using time alone (less than four hours). Always wash hands and wash and sanitize counter tops utensils and containers between steps when working with raw meat.

Texture Modified Diets: Tip: Use pasta that is the correct particle size.

Soft & Bite Size: (aka Bite size) **Food particle size ½ inch (~width of standard fork)** Food must be moist. Cut foods with a knife to a ½" particle size prior to mixing. Moisten with broth as needed.

Chopped: Food particle size ¼ inch (~ ½ width of standard fork) Food must be moist. Chop foods with a knife to 1/4" particle size prior to mixing. Moisten with broth as needed.

Minced and Moist: (aka Minced/Mechanical Soft/Ground) **Food particle size 1/8 inch (fits through prongs of standard fork)** Food must be moist. Use a food processor to grind food particles into 1/8 inch prior to mixing. Moisten with broth as needed.

Pureed: Smooth and cohesive. Use a food processor to puree to a smooth consistency. Foods are processed by grinding and then pureeing them. May add broth or sauce to puree. Do not add to much liquid. Puree should still hold its shape. Must not be firm or sticky. Puree foods while still hot. Appearance should be smooth like pudding. Foods that do not process well should be omitted. Serve 1 c. meat/ bean serving.

Therapeutic Modified Diets:

Lowfat: No changes needed
Diabetic/No added Sugar/No Conc. Sweets/Calorie Controlled: No changes needed
Bland/Anti Reflux: Serve plain hamburger patty and ½ c. plain pasta.
Liberal House Renal: Serve plain hamburger patty and ½ c. SF pasta. May season pasta with SF herbs and spices.
No Added Salt: No changes needed
2 Gram Sodium: Serve plain hamburger patty and ½ c. SF pasta. May season rice with SF herbs and spices
Gluten Free: Use GF pasta. Prepare foods separately to prevent cross contamination.
Allergy Alerts: When an "X" is present, this indicates the allergen is present.
Always read all food labels to ensure allergens are not present.

Wheat	Milk	Eggs	Fish Shellfish	Soy	Peanuts/Nuts	Other
X	X					

Key: SF= Salt Free D= Diet or Sugarfree LF = Lowfat FF = Fat Free GF = Gluten Free

Recipe Name: Chili
Recipe Category: Dinner Entrée
Portion Size: 1 cup
Ingredients: Yields: 8 servings

Ingredients	Notes:
2 Pounds lean ground beef or ground turkey	
1 Small onion, minced	Wash, peel and mince
1 Small green pepper, diced	Wash, trim and dice
1 (14 1/2 oz.) can low sodium red cut tomatoes	
2 (14 1/2 oz.) cans low sodium tomato sauce	
1 (6 oz.) can low sodium tomato paste	
2 (16 oz.) low sodium cans of pinto or kidney beans	Drained and rinsed
1 Tablespoons chili powder	
1 Teaspoon ground cumin	

Directions:

Steps:	Directions:	Critical Control Point /Quality Assurance
1	Sauté onion and ground beef in a nonstick skillet until beef is no longer pink.	
2	Drain fat	
3	Add rest of ingredients.	
4	Stir and bring to boil. Reduce heat simmer for 30 minutes.	Cook until internal temperature reaches 165 F degrees for 15 seconds

Time Temperature Sensitive food. *Food safety Standards: hold food for service at an internal temperature above 140° F. Do not mix old product with new. Cool leftover product quickly (within 4 hours) to below 41° F. Follow proper cooling procedures. Store leftovers in a tightly sealed, labeled and dated container. Use leftover within 72 hours if stored in refrigerator or 30 days if stored in the freezer. Reheat leftover product quickly (within 2 hours) to 165 degrees F for 15 seconds. Reheat left over product only once; discard if not used. Cold holding at 41°F or colder or using time alone (less than four hours). Always wash hands and wash and sanitize counter tops utensils and containers between steps when working with raw meat.*

Texture Modified Diets:

Soft & Bite Size: (aka Bite size) **Food particle size ½ inch (~width of standard fork)** Food must be moist. Cut foods with a knife to a ½" particle size prior to mixing. Moisten with broth as needed.

Chopped: Food particle size ¼ inch (~ ½ width of standard fork) Food must be moist. Chop foods with a knife to 1/4" particle size prior to mixing. Moisten with broth as needed.

Minced and Moist: (aka Minced/Mechanical Soft/Ground) **Food particle size 1/8 inch (fits through prongs of standard fork)** Food must be moist. Use a food processor to grind food particles into 1/8 inch prior to mixing. Moisten with broth as needed.

Pureed: Smooth and cohesive. Use a food processor to puree to a smooth consistency. Foods are processed by grinding and then pureeing them. May add broth or sauce to puree. Do not add to much liquid. Puree should still hold its shape. Must not be firm or sticky. Puree foods while still hot. Appearance should be smooth like pudding. Serve 1 c puree chili mixture

Therapeutic Modified Diets:

Lowfat: No changes needed
Diabetic/No added Sugar/No Conc. Sweets/Calorie Controlled: No changes needed
Bland/Anti Reflux: Serve plain hamburger patty and rice or pasta.
Liberal House Renal: Serve plain hamburger patty with rice or pasta. May season hamburger patty with onion and green pepper. May season pasta or rice with SF herbs/spices
No Added Salt: No changes needed
2 Gram Sodium: Serve plain hamburger patty with rice or pasta. May season hamburger patty with onion and green pepper. May season rice or pasta with SF herbs/spices
Gluten Free: No changes needed. Prepare foods separately to prevent cross contamination.
Allergy Alerts: When an "X" is present, this indicates the allergen is present.
Always read all food labels to ensure allergens are not present.

Wheat	Milk	Eggs	Fish Shellfish	Soy	Peanuts/Nuts	Other

Key: SF= Salt Free D= Diet or Sugarfree LF = Lowfat FF = Fat Free GF = Gluten Free

Recipe Name: Chili and Macaroni
Recipe Category: Dinner Entrée
Portion Size: 1 cup
Ingredients: Yields: 8 servings

Ingredients	Notes:
1/2 Pound macaroni	May use whole grain
2 1/2 Pounds lean ground beef	
1 Medium onion, diced	Washed, peeled and diced
2 Cans (16 ounce) low sodium tomatoes	
2 Cups frozen corn	
1/2 Teaspoon salt	
1/4 Teaspoon pepper	
1/2 Teaspoon cumin	
1 Tablespoon chili powder	

Directions:

Steps:	Directions:	Critical Control Point / Quality Assurance
1	Cook macaroni as directed on package.	
2	Drain.	
3	Brown ground beef and diced onion in a stock pot.	Cook until internal temperature reaches 165 F degrees for 15 seconds
4	Drain fat.	
5	Add tomatoes, corn, macaroni, salt, pepper, cumin, and chili powder to meat.	
6	Cook 20 minutes or until heated through over low heat, stirring occasionally. Add macaroni just before serving.	

Time Temperature Sensitive food. Food safety Standards: hold food for service at an internal temperature above 140° F. Do not mix old product with new. Cool leftover product quickly (within 4 hours) to below 41° F. Follow proper cooling procedures. Store leftovers in a tightly sealed, labeled and dated container. Use leftover within 72 hours if stored in refrigerator or 30 days if stored in the freezer. Reheat leftover product quickly (within 2 hours) to 165 degrees F for 15 seconds. Reheat left over product only once; discard if not used. Cold holding at 41°F or colder or using time alone (less than four hours). Always wash hands and wash and sanitize counter tops utensils and containers between steps when working with raw meat.

Special Diets:

Texture Modified Diets: Tip : Use pasta with correct particle size.

Soft & Bite Size: (aka Bite size) **Food particle size ½ inch (~width of standard fork)** Food must be moist. Cut foods with a knife to a ½" particle size prior to mixing. Moisten with broth as needed. Foods that do not process well should be omitted. Omit: corn

Chopped: Food particle size ¼ inch (~ ½ width of standard fork) Food must be moist. Chop foods with a knife to 1/4" particle size prior to mixing. Moisten with broth as needed. Foods that do not process well should be omitted. Omit: corn

Minced and Moist: (aka Minced/Mechanical Soft/Ground) **Food particle size 1/8 inch (fits through prongs of standard fork)** Food must be moist. Use a food processor to grind food particles into 1/8 inch prior to mixing. Moisten with broth as needed. Foods that do not process well should be omitted. Omit: corn

Pureed: Smooth and cohesive. Use a food processor to puree to a smooth consistency. Foods are processed by grinding and then pureeing them. May add broth or sauce to puree. Do not add to much liquid. Puree should still hold its shape. Must not be firm or sticky. Puree foods while still hot. Appearance should be smooth like pudding. Foods that do not process well should be omitted. Omit: corn. Serve ½ c. puree meat and ½ c. puree pasta serving separately. Tip: Puree pasta while hot. Before adding meat to pasta puree separately.

Therapeutic Modified Diets:

Lowfat: No changes needed
Diabetic/No added Sugar/No Conc. Sweets/Calorie Controlled: No changes needed
Bland/Anti Reflux: Serve plain hamburger patty and pasta
Liberal House Renal: Omit tomatoes and salt. Use SF broth or water.
No Added Salt: No changes needed
2 Gram Sodium: Omit salt and use SF broth or water. Use fresh tomatoes for canned.
Gluten Free: Omit whole grain macaroni for gluten free macaroni. Prepare foods separately to prevent cross contamination.

Allergy Alerts: When an "X" is present, this indicates the allergen is present.
Always read all food labels to ensure allergens are not present.

Wheat	Milk	Eggs	Fish Shellfish	Soy	Peanuts/Nuts	Other
X		X				

Key: SF= Salt Free D= Diet or Sugarfree LF = Lowfat FF = Fat Free GF = Gluten Free

Copyright 2020 Jacqueline Larson M.S., R.D.N. and Associates.   All Rights Reserved

Recipe Name: Corned Beef and Cabbage
Recipe Category: Dinner Entrée
Portion Size: 3 oz., 1/4 c. cabbage, 1/4 c. carrots and ½ c. potatoes
Ingredients: Yields: 8 servings

Ingredients	Notes:
4 pounds corned beef, marinated	Trim all visible fat
1 small head of cabbage,	Washed, trimmed and cut into wedges
8 medium potatoes, pared	Washed, peeled and cut up
4 carrots, peeled	Washed, peeled and cut up
1/2 Cup diced onion	Washed, peeled and diced

Directions:

Steps:	Directions:	Critical Control Point /Quality Assurance
1	In a large pot cover corned beef with water.	
2	Bring to boil.	
3	Cover and simmer for 2 to 3 hours.	
4	Add potatoes, carrots, onions, and cabbage.	
5	Simmer 30 minutes more or until vegetables are tender.	Cook until internal temperature reaches 165 F degrees for 15 seconds
6	Cut corned beef very thin diagonally across the grain.	
	*** This may also be cooked in a crock pot 8 to 10 hours on low or 6 to 8 hour on high heat	

Time Temperature Sensitive food. Food safety Standards: hold food for service at an internal temperature above 140° F. Do not mix old product with new. Cool leftover product quickly (within 4 hours) to below 41° F. Follow proper cooling procedures. Store leftovers in a tightly sealed, labeled and dated container. Use leftover within 72 hours if stored in refrigerator or 30 days if stored in the freezer. Reheat leftover product quickly (within 2 hours) to 165 degrees F for 15 seconds. Reheat left over product only once; discard if not used. Cold holding at 41°F or colder or using time alone (less than four hours). Always wash hands and wash and sanitize counter tops utensils and containers between steps when working with raw meat.

Texture Modified Diets:

Soft & Bite Size: (aka Bite size) **Food particle size ½ inch (~width of standard fork)** Food must be moist. Cut foods with a knife to a ½" particle size after cooking. Serve ½ c. meat serving ½ cup vegetables and ½ cup potatoes. Moisten with broth as needed.

Chopped: Food particle size ¼ inch (~ ½ width of standard fork) Food must be moist. Chop foods with a knife to 1/4" particle size after cooking. Serve ½ c. meat serving ½ cup vegetables and ½ cup potatoes. Moisten with broth as needed.

Minced and Moist: (aka Minced/Mechanical Soft/Ground) **Food particle size 1/8 inch (fits through prongs of standard fork)** Food must be moist. Use a food processor to grind food particles into 1/8 inch after cooking. Serve ½ c. meat serving ½ cup vegetables and ½ cup potatoes. Moisten with broth as needed.

Pureed: Smooth and cohesive. Use a food processor to puree to a smooth consistency. Foods are processed by grinding and then pureeing them. May add broth or sauce to puree. Do not add to much liquid. Puree should still hold its shape. Must not be firm or sticky. Puree foods while still hot. Appearance should be smooth like pudding. Serve ½ c. puree meat serving, 1/4 cup puree carrots, ¼ cup puree cabbage, ½ cup puree potatoes all separately.

Therapeutic Modified Diets:

Lowfat: No corned beef. Serve slice roast beef with potatoes, carrots and cabbage.
Diabetic/No added Sugar/No Conc. Sweets/Calorie Controlled: No changes needed
Bland/Anti Reflux: No corned beef. Serve slice roast beef, potatoes and carrots
Liberal House Renal: No corned beef. Serve slice roast beef, rice or pasta and carrots
No Added Salt: No corned beef. Served slice roast beef, potatoes, cabbage and carrots
2 Gram Sodium: No corned beef. Serve slice roast beef, potatoes, cabbage and carrots.
Gluten Free: No changes. (read label to be sure on corned beef)
Allergy Alerts: When an "X" is present, this indicates the allergen is present.
Always read all food labels to ensure allergens are not present.

Wheat	Milk	Eggs	Fish Shellfish	Soy	Peanuts/Nuts	Other

Key: SF= Salt Free D= Diet or Sugarfree LF = Lowfat FF = Fat Free GF = Gluten Free

Recipe Name: Corn Bread Tamale Bake
Recipe Category: Dinner Entrée
Portion Size: 1 cup
Ingredients: Yields: 8 servings

Ingredients	Notes:
2 1/2 Pounds lean ground beef	
1 diced onion	Washed, peeled and diced
2 cup of low sodium tomato sauce	
2 tablespoons sugar	
1 teaspoon oregano	
1 cup of water	
1/4 teaspoon pepper	
1 teaspoon salt	
1 tablespoon chili powder	
1 cup drained low sodium whole kernel corn	
1 1/2 cup cornmeal	
2 tablespoon flour	
2 tablespoon sugar	
1 teaspoon salt	
3 teaspoons double acting baking powder	
2 eggs, beaten	
2/3 cup nonfat milk	
2 tablespoon vegetable oil	

Directions:

Steps:	Directions:	Critical Control Point / Quality Assurance
1	Sauté the ground beef and onion in a skillet.	
2	When the meat is highly browned and the onion is translucent, drain.	
3	Add tomato sauce, water, pepper, salt, chili powder, oregano, 2 tablespoons sugar, corn, and pepper.	
4	Simmer for 15 minutes.	
5	Preheat oven to 425 degrees.	
6	Meanwhile, sift and mix together cornmeal, flour, 2 tablespoons sugar, salt, and baking powder.	
7	Moisten with egg, milk, and oil.	
8	Place meat mixture in a non stick vegetable sprayed baking dish and cover with the corn bread topping.	
9	The topping will disappear into the meat mixture, but will rise during baking and to form a layer of corn bread.	
10	Bake about 20 to 25 minutes or until cornbread is brown.	Cook until internal temperature reaches 165 F degrees for 15 seconds.

Time Temperature Sensitive food. *Food safety Standards: hold food for service at an internal temperature above 140°F. Do not mix old product with new. Cool leftover product quickly (within 4 hours) to below 41°F. Follow proper cooling procedures. Store leftovers in a tightly sealed, labeled and dated container. Use leftover within 72 hours if stored in refrigerator or 30 days if stored in the freezer. Reheat leftover product quickly (within 2 hours) to 165 degrees F for 15 seconds. Reheat left over product only once; discard if not used. Cold holding at 41°F or colder or using time alone (less than four hours). Always wash hands and wash and sanitize counter tops utensils and containers between steps when working with raw meat.*

Texture Modified Diets:

Soft & Bite Size: (aka Bite size) **Food particle size ½ inch (~width of standard fork)** Food must be moist. Cut foods with a knife to a ½" particle size after cooking. Moisten with broth as needed.

Chopped: Food particle size ¼ inch (~ ½ width of standard fork) Food must be moist. Chop foods with a knife to 1/4" particle size after cooking. Moisten with broth as needed.

Minced and Moist:(aka Minced/Mechanical Soft/Ground) **Food particle size 1/8 inch (fits through prongs of standard fork)** Food must be moist. Use a food processor to grind food particles into 1/8 inch after cooking. Moisten with broth as needed.

Pureed: Smooth and cohesive. Use a food processor to puree to a smooth consistency. Foods are processed by grinding and then pureeing them. May add broth or sauce to puree. Do not add to much liquid. Puree should still hold its shape. Must not be firm or sticky. Puree foods while still hot. Appearance should be smooth like pudding. Puree with broth if needed. Serve 1 c. serving.

Copyright 2020 Jacqueline Larson M.S., R.D.N. and Associates.   All Rights Reserved

Therapeutic Modified Diets:

Lowfat: No changes needed
Diabetic/No added Sugar/No Conc. Sweets/Calorie Controlled: No changes needed
Bland/Anti Reflux: Serve 3 oz. ground beef patty and ½ cup rice or pasta
Liberal House Renal: Serve 3 oz. ground beef patty and ½ cup rice or pasta
No Added Salt: No changes needed
2 Gram Sodium: Serve 3 oz. ground beef patty and ½ cup rice or pasta
Gluten Free: Omit flour for gluten free flour and baking powder. Prepare foods separately to prevent cross contamination.
Allergy Alerts: When an "X" is present, this indicates the allergen is present.
Always read all food labels to ensure allergens are not present.

Wheat	Milk	Eggs	Fish Shellfish	Soy	Peanuts/Nuts	Other
X	X	X				

Key: SF= Salt Free D= Diet or Sugarfree LF = Lowfat FF = Fat Free GF = Gluten Free

Recipe Name: Corn Bread Tamale Pie
Recipe Category: Dinner Entrée
Portion Size: 1 cup
Ingredients: Yields: 8 servings

Ingredients	Notes:
2 1/2 Pounds lean ground beef	
1 diced onion	Washed, peeled and diced
2 cup of low sodium tomato sauce	
2 tablespoons sugar	
1 teaspoon oregano	
1 cup of water	
1/4 teaspoon pepper	
1 teaspoon salt	
1 tablespoon chili powder	
1 cup drained low sodium whole kernel corn	
1 1/2 cup cornmeal	
2 tablespoon flour	
2 tablespoon sugar	
1 teaspoon salt	
3 teaspoons double acting baking powder	
2 eggs, beaten	
2/3 cup nonfat milk	
2 tablespoon vegetable oil	

Directions:

Steps:	Directions:	Critical Control Point / Quality Assurance
1	Sauté the ground beef and onion in a skillet.	
2	When the meat is highly browned and the onion is translucent, drain.	
3	Add tomato sauce, water, pepper, salt, chili powder, oregano, sugar, corn, and pepper.	
4	Simmer for 15 minutes.	
5	Preheat oven to 425 degrees.	
6	Meanwhile, sift and mix together cornmeal, flour, sugar, salt, and baking powder.	
7	Moisten with egg, milk, and oil.	
8	Place meat mixture in a non stick vegetable sprayed baking dish and cover with the corn bread topping.	
9	The topping will disappear into the meat mixture, but will rise during baking and to form a layer of corn bread.	
10	Bake about 20 to 25 minutes or until cornbread is brown.	Cook until internal temperature reaches 165 F degrees for 15 seconds.

Time Temperature Sensitive food. *Food safety Standards: hold food for service at an internal temperature above 140° F. Do not mix old product with new. Cool leftover product quickly (within 4 hours) to below 41° F. Follow proper cooling procedures. Store leftovers in a tightly sealed, labeled and dated container. Use leftover within 72 hours if stored in refrigerator or 30 days if stored in the freezer. Reheat leftover product quickly (within 2 hours) to 165 degrees F for 15 seconds. Reheat left over product only once; discard if not used. Cold holding at 41°F or colder or using time alone (less than four hours). Always wash hands and wash and sanitize counter tops utensils and containers between steps when working with raw meat.*

<u>**Texture Modified Diets:**</u>

Soft & Bite Size: (aka Bite size) **Food particle size ½ inch (~width of standard fork)** Food must be moist. Cut foods with a knife to a ½" particle size after baking. Moisten with broth as needed. Foods that do not process well should be omitted. Omit: corn

Chopped: Food particle size ¼ inch (~ ½ width of standard fork) Food must be moist. Chop foods with a knife to 1/4" particle size after baking. Moisten with broth as needed. Foods that do not process well should be omitted. Omit: corn

Minced and Moist: (aka Minced/Mechanical Soft/Ground) **Food particle size 1/8 inch (fits through prongs of standard fork)** Food must be moist. Use a food processor to grind food particles into 1/8 inch after baking. . Moisten with broth as needed. Foods that do not process well should be omitted. Omit: corn

Pureed: Smooth and cohesive. Use a food processor to puree to a smooth consistency. Foods are processed by grinding and then pureeing them. May add broth or sauce to puree. Do not add to much liquid. Puree should still hold its shape. Must not be firm or sticky. Puree foods while still hot. Appearance should be smooth like pudding. Foods that do not process well should be omitted. Omit: corn Serve 1 c. serving.

Therapeutic Modified Diets:
Lowfat: No changes needed
Diabetic/No added Sugar/No Conc. Sweets/Calorie Controlled: No changes needed
Bland/Anti Reflux: Serve 3 oz. ground beef patty and ½ cup rice or pasta
Liberal House Renal: Serve 3 oz. ground beef patty and ½ cup rice or pasta
No Added Salt: No changes needed
2 Gram Sodium: Serve 3 oz. ground beef patty and ½ cup rice or pasta
Gluten Free: Omit flour for gluten free flour and baking powder. Prepare foods separately to prevent cross contamination.
Allergy Alerts: When an "X" is present, this indicates the allergen is present.
Always read all food labels to ensure allergens are not present.

Wheat	Milk	Eggs	Fish Shellfish	Soy	Peanuts/Nuts	Other
X	X	X				

Key: SF= Salt Free D= Diet or Sugarfree LF = Lowfat FF = Fat Free GF = Gluten Free

Recipe Name: Curried Beef
Recipe Category: Dinner Entrée
Portion Size: ½ cup curried beef and ½ cup rice
Ingredients: **Yields: 8 servings**

Ingredients	Notes:
2 tablespoons cooking oil	
2 1/2 pounds beef round, cut in 1 inch cubes	Trim all visible fat
2 medium onions, sliced	Wash, peel and slice
1 clove garlic	Wash, peel and mince
1 tablespoon curry powder	
1 tablespoon all purpose flour	
1 teaspoon salt	
1 low sodium Beef bouillon cube, crumbled	
1 1/2 cup water	
1/4 cup vinegar	
1/2 cup raisins	
4 cups cooked rice	
1/2 pint low fat plain yogurt	

Directions:

Steps:	Directions:	Critical Control Point /Quality Assurance
1	In skillet brown meat in the cooking oil.	
2	Add onions and garlic and cook until slightly clear.	
3	Add curry powder.	
4	Stir and cook 2 to 3 minutes, being careful curry powder does not burn.	
5	Stir in flour and salt.	
6	Add bouillon cube, water, vinegar and raisins; stir.	
7	Cover and cook over low heat until meat is tender, 2 to 2 1/2 hours, stirring several times.	Cook until internal temperature reaches 165 F degrees for 15 seconds
8	If mixture becomes too dry, an additional half cup of water may be added.	
9	Cook rice according to package directions.	
10	Serve with beef and top with yogurt.	

Time Temperature Sensitive food. *Food safety Standards: hold food for service at an internal temperature above 140° F. Do not mix old product with new. Cool leftover product quickly (within 4 hours) to below 41° F. Follow proper cooling procedures. Store leftovers in a tightly sealed, labeled and dated container. Use leftover within 72 hours if stored in refrigerator or 30 days if stored in the freezer. Reheat leftover product quickly (within 2 hours) to 165 degrees F for 15 seconds. Reheat left over product only once; discard if not used. Cold holding at 41°F or colder or using time alone (less than four hours). Always wash hands and wash and sanitize counter tops utensils and containers between steps when working with raw meat.*

Texture Modified Diets:
Soft & Bite Size: (aka Bite size) **Food particle size ½ inch (~width of standard fork)** Food must be moist. Cut foods with a knife to a ½" particle size prior to mixing. Moisten with broth as needed. Foods that do not process well should be omitted. Omit: raisins
Chopped: Food particle size ¼ inch (~ ½ width of standard fork) Food must be moist. Chop foods with a knife to 1/4" particle size prior to mixing. Moisten with broth as needed. Foods that do not process well should be omitted. Omit: raisins
Minced and Moist:(aka Minced/Mechanical Soft/Ground) **Food particle size 1/8 inch (fits through prongs of standard fork)** Food must be moist. Use a food processor to grind food particles into 1/8 inch prior to mixing. Moisten with broth as needed. Foods that do not process well should be omitted. Omit: raisins
Pureed: Smooth and cohesive. Use a food processor to puree to a smooth consistency. Foods are processed by grinding and then pureeing them. May add broth or sauce to puree. Do not add to much liquid. Puree should still hold its shape. Must not be firm or sticky. Puree foods while still hot. Appearance should be smooth like pudding. Foods that do not process well should be omitted. Omit: raisins Serve ½ c. meat serving and puree rice separately.

Therapeutic Modified Diets:
Lowfat: No changes needed
Diabetic/No added Sugar/No Conc. Sweets/Calorie Controlled: No changes needed
Bland/Anti Reflux: omit onions, garlic, curry powder, vinegar, and raisins
Liberal House Renal: Omit salt, Use SF bouillon or omit. Omit yogurt
No Added Salt: No changes
2 Gram Sodium: omit salt. Use SF bouillon or omit
Gluten Free: Use gluten free flour and gluten free Beef bouillon cube. Prepare foods separately to prevent cross contamination.
Allergy Alerts: When an "X" is present, this indicates the allergen is present. Always read all food labels to ensure allergens are not present.

Wheat	Milk	Eggs	Fish Shellfish	Soy	Peanuts/Nuts	Other
X	X					

Key: SF= Salt Free D= Diet or Sugarfree LF = Lowfat FF = Fat Free GF = Gluten Free

Copyright 2020 Jacqueline Larson M.S., R.D.N. and Associates.   All Rights Reserved

Recipe Name: Curried Beef with Apple Couscous
Recipe Category: Dinner Entrée
Portion Size: 3 oz. meat over ½ c. couscous
Ingredients: Yields: 8 servings

Ingredients	Notes:
2 1/2 pounds boneless beef top sirloin steak, cut into thin slices across the grain	Trim all visible fat
½ teaspoon salt	
½ teaspoon black pepper	
1 tablespoon oil	
1 large red pepper seeded and cut into thin strips	Wash, trim and cut
1 large green pepper, seeded and cut into thin strips	Wash, trim and cut
1 cup water	
1 cup apple juice	
2 teaspoons low sodium instant beef bouillon granules	
1 ½ cups couscous	May use whole wheat
2 apples	Wash, core and coarsely chop
½ cup chopped unsalted peanuts	

Directions:

Steps:	Directions:	Critical Control Point /Quality Assurance
1	Sprinkle steak with salt and pepper.	
2	Grill beef over medium coals or sauté in large skillet.	Cook until internal temperature reaches 145 F degrees for 15 seconds
3	In a large skillet, heat oil over medium heat.	
4	Add peppers and onions. Cook for 5 minutes.	
5	Add curry powder. Cook and stir for 1 minute.	
6	Add the water, apple juice, and bouillon granules.	
7	Bring to boil. Stir in couscous and apple.	
8	Cover and let stand about 5 minutes or until liquid is absorbed.	
9	To serve, fluff couscous mixture with fork. Thinly slice steak across the grain.	
10	Serve steak slices over couscous mixture. Sprinkle with peanuts.	

Time Temperature Sensitive food. *Food safety Standards: hold food for service at an internal temperature above 140° F. Do not mix old product with new. Cool leftover product quickly (within 4 hours) to below 41° F. Follow proper cooling procedures. Store leftovers in a tightly sealed, labeled and dated container. Use leftover within 72 hours if stored in refrigerator or 30 days if stored in the freezer. Reheat leftover product quickly (within 2 hours) to 165 degrees F for 15 seconds. Reheat left over product only once; discard if not used. Cold holding at 41°F or colder or using time alone (less than four hours). Always wash hands and wash and sanitize counter tops utensils and containers between steps when working with raw meat.*

<u>Texture Modified Diets:</u>
Soft & Bite Size: (aka Bite size) **Food particle size ½ inch (~width of standard fork)** Food must be moist. Cut foods with a knife to a ½" particle size prior to mixing. Moisten with broth as needed. Foods that do not process well should be omitted. Omit: nuts. Peel apple.
Chopped: Food particle size ¼ inch (~ ½ width of standard fork) Food must be moist. Chop foods with a knife to 1/4" particle size prior to mixing. Moisten with broth as needed. Foods that do not process well should be omitted. Omit: nuts. Peel Apple.
Minced and Moist:(aka Minced/Mechanical Soft/Ground) **Food particle size 1/8 inch (fits through prongs of standard fork)** Food must be moist. Use a food processor to grind food particles into 1/8 inch prior to mixing. Moisten with broth as needed. Foods that do not process well should be omitted. Omit: nuts. Peel Apple.
Pureed: Smooth and cohesive. Use a food processor to puree to a smooth consistency. Foods are processed by grinding and then pureeing them. May add broth or sauce to puree. Do not add to much liquid. Puree should still hold its shape. Must not be firm or sticky. Puree foods while still hot. Appearance should be smooth like pudding. Foods that do not process well should be omitted. Omit: nuts. Peel apple. Serve ½ c. meat serving

<u>Therapeutic Modified Diets:</u>
Lowfat: Omit nuts
Diabetic/No added Sugar/No Conc. Sweets/Calorie Controlled: No changes needed
Bland/Anti Reflux: omit black pepper, red and green peppers, peel apple, and omit nuts
Liberal House Renal: Omit salt and use SF bouillon or omit
No Added Salt: No changes needed
2 Gram Sodium: omit salt and use SF bouillon or omit
Gluten Free: Use Gluten free instant beef bouillon granules. Use gluten free couscous or pasta. Prepare foods separately to prevent cross contamination.

Allergy Alerts: When an "X" is present, this indicates the allergen is present. Always read all food labels to ensure allergens are not present.

Wheat	Milk	Eggs	Fish Shellfish	Soy	Peanuts/Nuts	Other
X		X			X	

Key: SF= Salt Free D= Diet or Sugarfree LF = Lowfat FF = Fat Free GF = Gluten Free

Recipe Name: English Muffin Pizzas
Recipe Category: Dinner Entrée
Portion Size: 2 halves with toppings
Ingredients: Yields: 8 servings

Ingredients	Notes:
8 whole wheat English muffins	
2 pounds lean Ground beef	
12 oz. low fat Mozzarella cheese	
1 large jar low sodium pizza sauce	
1 teaspoon Garlic Powder	
1 teaspoon Oregano	

Directions:

Steps:	Directions:	Critical Control Point / Quality Assurance
1	Cook ground beef until slightly browned in a pan. Drain fat.	Cook until internal temperature reaches 165 F degrees for 15 seconds
2	Spilt English muffin and toast English muffins.	
3	Combine ground beef and pizza sauce.	
4	Season with garlic powder and oregano.	
5	Put some of the meat mixture on top of each muffin.	
6	Top each with Mozzarella cheese.	
7	Bake 15 minutes at 350 degrees.	

Time Temperature Sensitive food. Food safety Standards: hold food for service at an internal temperature above 140° F. Do not mix old product with new. Cool leftover product quickly (within 4 hours) to below 41° F. Follow proper cooling procedures. Store leftovers in a tightly sealed, labeled and dated container. Use leftover within 72 hours if stored in refrigerator or 30 days if stored in the freezer. Reheat leftover product quickly (within 2 hours) to 165 degrees F for 15 seconds. Reheat left over product only once; discard if not used. Cold holding at 41 °F or colder or using time alone (less than four hours). Always wash hands and wash and sanitize counter tops utensils and containers between steps when working with raw meat.

Texture Modified Diets:

Soft & Bite Size: (aka Bite size) **Food particle size ½ inch (~width of standard fork)** Food must be moist. Cut foods with a knife to a ½" particle size after cooking. Moisten with broth as needed.

Chopped: Food particle size ¼ inch (~ ½ width of standard fork) Food must be moist. Chop foods with a knife to 1/4" particle size after cooking. Moisten with broth as needed.

Minced and Moist: (aka Minced/Mechanical Soft/Ground) **Food particle size 1/8 inch (fits through prongs of standard fork)** Food must be moist. Use a food processor to grind food particles into 1/8 inch after cooking. Moisten with broth as needed.

Pureed: Smooth and cohesive. Use a food processor to puree to a smooth consistency. Foods are processed by grinding and then pureeing them. May add broth or sauce to puree. Do not add to much liquid. Puree should still hold its shape. Must not be firm or sticky. Puree foods while still hot. Appearance should be smooth like pudding. Serve 1 cup puree pizzas.

Therapeutic Modified Diets:

Lowfat: No changes needed
Diabetic/No added Sugar/No Conc. Sweets/Calorie Controlled: No changes needed
Bland/Anti Reflux: omit pizza sauce, garlic and oregano.
Liberal House Renal: Serve plain hamburger patty and ½ cup SF rice or pasta.
No Added Salt: No changes needed
2 Gram Sodium: Serve plain hamburger patty and ½ cup SF rice or pasta
Gluten Free: Use gluten free English muffins or bread. Prepare foods separately to prevent cross contamination.
Allergy Alerts: When an "X" is present, this indicates the allergen is present.
Always read all food labels to ensure allergens are not present.

Wheat	Milk	Eggs	Fish Shellfish	Soy	Peanuts/Nuts	Other
X	X	X				

Key: SF= Salt Free D= Diet or Sugarfree LF = Lowfat FF = Fat Free GF = Gluten Free

Copyright 2020 Jacqueline Larson M.S., R.D.N. and Associates.   All Rights Reserved

Recipe Name: Greek Salad with Steak
Recipe Category: Dinner Entrée
Portion Size: 3 oz. and 1 cup salad
Ingredients: Yields: 8 servings

Ingredients	Notes:
2 1/2 pound boneless beef Top Sirloin or Top Round Steak, or Flank Steak (thinly sliced across the grain)	Trim all visible fat.
8 cups torn romaine lettuce	Wash, trim and tear into bite size pieces.
1 large cucumber	Wash, trim and thinly slice.
1/2 small red onion	Wash, peel and thinly slice.
1/4 cup low fat crumbled feta cheese	
8 Greek or black olives	
2 whole wheat pita breads, toasted, cut into wedges	(optional)
Marinade:	
¼ cup lemon juice	
¼ cup olive oil	
1 teaspoon garlic powder	
½ teaspoon black pepper	
1 teaspoon oregano	
½ teaspoon salt	

Directions:

Steps:	Directions:	Critical Control Point /Quality Assurance
1	Whisk marinade ingredients in small bowl.	
2	Place beef Steak and 1/2 of marinade in sealable container; turn to coat. Close close securely and marinate in refrigerator 30 minutes or as long as overnight, turning occasionally. Reserve remaining marinade.	
3	Remove Steak; discard marinade.	
4	Place Steak on rack in broiler pan so surface of beef is 2 to 3 inches from heat. Broil 10 to 12 minutes for medium rare (145°F) doneness, turning once. Do not overcook. Remove; let stand 10 minutes.	
5	Combine beef, lettuce, cucumber and onion in large bowl.	
6	Add reserved marinade; toss.	
7	Sprinkle with cheese and olives. Serve with pita wedges..	

Time Temperature Sensitive food. *Food safety Standards: hold food for service at an internal temperature above 140° F. Do not mix old product with new. Cool leftover product quickly (within 4 hours) to below 41° F. Follow proper cooling procedures. Store leftovers in a tightly sealed, labeled and dated container. Use leftover within 72 hours if stored in refrigerator or 30 days if stored in the freezer. Reheat leftover product quickly (within 2 hours) to 165 degrees F for 15 seconds. Reheat left over product only once; discard if not used. Cold holding at 41°F or colder or using time alone (less than four hours). Always wash hands and wash and sanitize counter tops utensils and containers between steps when working with raw meat.*

Texture Modified Diets:
Soft & Bite Size: (aka Bite size) **Food particle size ½ inch (~width of standard fork)** Food must be moist. Cut foods with a knife to a ½" particle size prior to mixing. Moisten with broth as needed.
Chopped: Food particle size ¼ inch (~ ½ width of standard fork) Food must be moist. Chop foods with a knife to 1/4" particle size prior to mixing. Moisten with broth as needed.
Minced and Moist: (aka Minced/Mechanical Soft/Ground) **Food particle size 1/8 inch (fits through prongs of standard fork)** Food must be moist. Use a food processor to grind food particles into 1/8 inch prior to mixing. Moisten with broth as needed.
Pureed: Smooth and cohesive. Use a food processor to puree to a smooth consistency. Foods are processed by grinding and then pureeing them. May add broth or sauce to puree. Do not add to much liquid. Puree should still hold its shape. Must not be firm or sticky. Puree foods while still hot. Appearance should be smooth like pudding. Serve ½ c. puree meat and 1 c. puree salad separately. May add pita bread to lettuce for correct consistency.

Therapeutic Modified Diets:
Lowfat: No changes needed
Diabetic/No added Sugar/No Conc. Sweets/Calorie Controlled: No changes needed
Bland/Anti Reflux: omit cucumber and red onion. Finely chop lettuce. Omit lemon juice
Liberal House Renal: Omit salt, feta cheese, olives, pita bread and tomatoes.
No Added Salt: Omit olives
2 Gram Sodium: omit salt, feta cheese, pita bread and olives.
Gluten Free: Use gluten free pita bread. Prepare foods separately to prevent cross contamination.
Allergy Alerts: When an "X" is present, this indicates the allergen is present. Always read all food labels to ensure allergens are not present.

Wheat	Milk	Eggs	Fish Shellfish	Soy	Peanuts/Nuts	Other
X	X					

Key: SF= Salt Free D= Diet or Sugarfree LF = Lowfat FF = Fat Free GF = Gluten Free

Recipe Name: Hamburgers
Recipe Category: Dinner Entrée
Portion Size: 4 oz. patty on bun
Ingredients: **Yields: 8 servings**

Ingredients	Notes:
2 1/2 Pounds lean ground beef	
8 Hamburger buns	Use whole wheat buns.
Optional ingredients to add to ground beef	
1/2 Cup minced onions or 1 Egg or 1/2 Cup bread crumbs and 1/2 Cup milk or 1 Package dried onion soup mix or garlic powder or Worsestershire sauce or 1/2 Cup sautéed mushrooms or 1/2 Cup Roquefort cheese or 1 Teaspoon parsley flakes Salt and pepper to taste	

Directions:

Steps:	Directions:	Critical Control Point / Quality Assurance
1	Mix ground beef with desired ingredients.	
2	Form beef into eight equal beef patties.	
3	Broil, grill, or sauté until no longer pink inside.	Cook until internal temperature reaches 165 F degrees for 15 seconds
4	Serve on hamburger buns.	

Time Temperature Sensitive food. *Food safety Standards: hold food for service at an internal temperature above 140° F. Do not mix old product with new. Cool leftover product quickly (within 4 hours) to below 41° F. Follow proper cooling procedures. Store leftovers in a tightly sealed, labeled and dated container. Use leftover within 72 hours if stored in refrigerator or 30 days if stored in the freezer. Reheat leftover product quickly (within 2 hours) to 165 degrees F for 15 seconds. Reheat left over product only once; discard if not used. Cold holding at 41°F or colder or using time alone (less than four hours). Always wash hands and wash and sanitize counter tops utensils and containers between steps when working with raw meat.*

Chopped: Food particle size ¼ inch (~ ½ width of standard fork) Food must be moist. Chop foods with a knife to 1/4" particle size prior to layering. Moisten with broth as needed.

Minced and Moist:(aka Minced/Mechanical Soft/Ground) **Food particle size 1/8 inch (fits through prongs of standard fork)** Food must be moist. Use a food processor to grind food particles into 1/8 inch prior to layering. Moisten with broth as needed.

Pureed: Smooth and cohesive. Use a food processor to puree to a smooth consistency. Foods are processed by grinding and then pureeing them. May add broth or sauce to puree. Do not add to much liquid. Puree should still hold its shape. Must not be firm or sticky. Puree foods while still hot. Appearance should be smooth like pudding. Serve ½ c. meat serving and 1 c. with condiments puree separately.

<u>Therapeutic Modified Diets:</u>
Lowfat: No Roquefort cheese
Diabetic/No added Sugar/No Conc. Sweets/Calorie Controlled: No changes needed
Bland/Anti Reflux: No dried onion soup mix, Roquefort cheese, parsley flakes or pepper.
Liberal House Renal: Omit salt. No onion soup mix, milk, bread crumbs, Worcestershire sauce, or Roquefort. Wrap in lettuce instead on a bun.
No Added Salt: No changes needed
2 Gram Sodium: Omit salt No onion soup mix, Worcestershire sauce, bread crumbs or Roquefort. Wrap in lettuce instead on a bun.
Gluten Free: Use gluten free bun. No bread crumbs or onion soup mix Prepare foods separately to prevent cross contamination.
Allergy Alerts: When an "X" is present, this indicates the allergen is present.
Always read all food labels to ensure allergens are not present.

Wheat	Milk	Eggs	Fish Shellfish	Soy	Peanuts/Nuts	Other
X	X		X			

Key: SF= Salt Free D= Diet or Sugarfree LF = Lowfat FF = Fat Free GF = Gluten Free

Recipe Name: Korean Beef
Recipe Category: Dinner Entrée
Portion Size: ¾ cup
Ingredients: **Yields: 8 servings**

Ingredients	Notes:
2 1/2 Pounds boneless tender beef steak (sirloin, rib eye, or top loin)	Trim all visible fat, slice thinly across the grain
1/3 cup light soy sauce	
2 tablespoons sesame oil	
2 tablespoons sesame seeds	
2 cloves garlic, minced	Washed, trimmed and minced
2 teaspoon sugar	
1 teaspoon salt	
½ teaspoon ground bell pepper	
2 Tablespoons oil, divided	
4 Carrots, cut diagonally into thinly slices	Washed, peeled and julienned
2 Onions, chunked and separated	Washed, peeled and sliced
4 Green onions	Washed, trimmed and thinly sliced

Directions:

Steps:	Directions:	Critical Control Point /Quality Assurance
1	Cut beef across grain into strips, then into 1 1/2 inch squares.	
2	Combine soy sauce, sesame oil, sesame seeds, garlic sugar and salt in medium bowl; stir in beef.	
3	Let stand in fridge for 30 minutes or longer.	
4	Dry marinate and discard marinate.	
5	Heat 1 tablespoon oil in hot wok or skillet over high heat.	
6	Add beef and stir fry 1 minute; remove.	
7	Heat remaining oil in the same pan.	
8	Add carrots, onion, and green peppers; stir fry 4 minutes.	
9	Add beef and; cook 2 minutes. Serve and top with green onions.	Cook until internal temperature reaches 145 F degrees for 15 seconds

Time Temperature Sensitive food. *Food safety Standards: hold food for service at an internal temperature above 140° F. Do not mix old product with new. Cool leftover product quickly (within 4 hours) to below 41° F. Follow proper cooling procedures. Store leftovers in a tightly sealed, labeled and dated container. Use leftover within 72 hours if stored in refrigerator or 30 days if stored in the freezer. Reheat leftover product quickly (within 2 hours) to 165 degrees F for 15 seconds. Reheat left over product only once; discard if not used. Cold holding at 41°F or colder or using time alone (less than four hours). Always wash hands and wash and sanitize counter tops utensils and containers between steps when working with raw meat.*

Texture Modified Diets:

Soft & Bite Size: (aka Bite size) **Food particle size ½ inch (~width of standard fork)** Food must be moist. Cut foods with a knife to a ½" particle size prior to mixing. Moisten with broth as needed. Omit green onions.

Chopped: Food particle size ¼ inch (~ ½ width of standard fork) Food must be moist. Chop foods with a knife to 1/4" particle size prior to mixing. Moisten with broth as needed. Omit green onions.

Minced and Moist:(aka Minced/Mechanical Soft/Ground) **Food particle size 1/8 inch (fits through prongs of standard fork)** Food must be moist. Use a food processor to grind food particles into 1/8 inch prior to mixing. Moisten with broth as needed. Omit green onions.

Pureed: Smooth and cohesive. Use a food processor to puree to a smooth consistency. Foods are processed by grinding and then pureeing them. May add broth or sauce to puree. Do not add to much liquid. Puree should still hold its shape. Must not be firm or sticky. Puree foods while still hot. Appearance should be smooth like pudding. Serve ½ c. puree meat, ½ cup puree rice and ½ c. puree vegetable separately. Omit green onions.

Therapeutic Modified Diets:

Lowfat: No changes needed
Diabetic/No added Sugar/No Conc. Sweets/Calorie Controlled: No changes needed
Bland/Anti Reflux: Omit sauce
Liberal House Renal: Omit sauce
No Added Salt: Omit sauce
2 Gram Sodium: Omit sauce
Gluten Free: Use gluten free soy sauce. Prepare foods separately to prevent cross contamination.
Allergy Alerts: When an "X" is present, this indicates the allergen is present. Always read all food labels to ensure allergens are not present.

Wheat	Milk	Eggs	Fish Shellfish	Soy	Peanuts/Nuts	Other
X				X		

Key: SF= Salt Free D= Diet or Sugarfree LF = Lowfat FF = Fat Free GF = Gluten Free

Recipe Name: Lasagna
Recipe Category: Dinner Entrée
Portion Size: 1 cup
Ingredients: Yields: 8 servings

Ingredients	Notes:
2 pounds lean ground beef	
1/2 pound low fat ricotta cheese	
1 pound shredded low fat Mozzarella cheese	
1/4 cup Parmesan cheese	
1 (67 oz.) Jar prepared spaghetti sauce	
1 (16 oz.) package lasagna noodles	May use whole grain

Directions:

Steps:	Directions:	Critical Control Point /Quality Assurance
1	Cook lasagna noodles according to package directions.	
2	Brown ground beef in a large skillet.	
3	Drain fat.	
4	Add spaghetti sauce to meat and heat.	
5	In a greased shallow casserole, arrange a layer of lasagna.	
6	Spread a layer of ricotta over this, then a layer of spaghetti sauce mixture, then a layer of mozzarella, topping with Parmesan cheese.	
7	Repeat layer in this order until all ingredients are used, ending with a layer of sauce and a sprinkle of parmesan cheese.	
8	Bake at 350 degree oven for 50 minutes.	Cook until internal temperature reaches 165 F degrees for 15 seconds.
9	Remove from oven and let stand about 15 minutes so that it will be easy to cut.	

Time Temperature Sensitive food. *Food safety Standards: hold food for service at an internal temperature above 140° F. Do not mix old product with new. Cool leftover product quickly (within 4 hours) to below 41° F. Follow proper cooling procedures. Store leftovers in a tightly sealed, labeled and dated container. Use leftover within 72 hours if stored in refrigerator or 30 days if stored in the freezer. Reheat leftover product quickly (within 2 hours) to 165 degrees F for 15 seconds. Reheat left over product only once; discard if not used. Cold holding at 41°F or colder or using time alone (less than four hours). Always wash hands and wash and sanitize counter tops utensils and containers between steps when working with raw meat.*

Texture Modified Diets: Tip: Use correct particle size for pasta.
Soft & Bite Size: (aka Bite size) **Food particle size ½ inch (~width of standard fork)** Food must be moist. Cut foods with a knife to a ½" particle size prior to mixing. Moisten with broth as needed.
Chopped: Food particle size ¼ inch (~ ½ width of standard fork) Food must be moist. Chop foods with a knife to 1/4" particle size prior to mixing. Moisten with broth as needed.
Minced and Moist: (aka Minced/Mechanical Soft/Ground) **Food particle size 1/8 inch (fits through prongs of standard fork)** Food must be moist. Use a food processor to grind food particles into 1/8 inch prior to mixing. Moisten with broth as needed.
Pureed: Smooth and cohesive. Use a food processor to puree to a smooth consistency. Foods are processed by grinding and then pureeing them. May add broth or sauce to puree. Do not add to much liquid. Puree should still hold its shape. Must not be firm or sticky. Puree foods while still hot. Appearance should be smooth like pudding.
Therapeutic Modified Diets:
Lowfat: No changes needed
Diabetic/No added Sugar/No Conc. Sweets/Calorie Controlled: No changes needed
Bland/Anti Reflux: omit tomato sauce. Serve plain ground beef and pasta topped with melted cheese.
Liberal House Renal: Serve plain ground beef and pasta. No cheese or tomato sauce. May season with SF herbs/spices.
No Added Salt: No changes needed
2 Gram Sodium: Serve plain ground beef and pasta. No Cheese. May add fresh tomatoes. May season with SF herbs/spices.
Gluten Free: Use gluten free lasagna noodles or noodles. Prepare foods separately to prevent cross contamination.
Allergy Alerts: When an "X" is present, this indicates the allergen is present.
Always read all food labels to ensure allergens are not present.

Wheat	Milk	Eggs	Fish Shellfish	Soy	Peanuts/Nuts	Other
X	X	X				

Key: SF= Salt Free D= Diet or Sugarfree LF = Lowfat FF = Fat Free GF = Gluten Free

Recipe Name: Lasagna with Beef and Italian Sausage
Recipe Category: Dinner Entrée
Portion Size: 1 cup
Ingredients: **Yields: 8 servings**

Ingredients	Notes:
1 pound lean Italian sausage	
1 1/2 pound lean ground beef	
1/2 cup minced onion	Wash, peel and mince
4 cloves garlic, minced	Wash, peel and mince
1 (28 ounce) can crushed tomatoes*	*Tip: short on time-use prepared large jar of spaghetti sauce in place of these ingredients
2 (6 ounce) cans tomato paste *	
2 (6.5 ounce) cans canned tomato sauce*	
1 cup water *	
3 tablespoons white sugar *	
2 teaspoons dried basil leaves *	
1/2 teaspoon fennel seeds*	
2 teaspoons Italian seasoning*	
1 tablespoon + 1/2 teaspoon salt *	
1/2 teaspoon ground black pepper*	
4 tablespoons chopped fresh parsley + 2 tablespoon for garnish	Wash, trim and chop
12 lasagna noodles (no bake variety)	May use whole wheat noodles
8 ounces low fat ricotta cheese	
1 egg	
1 pound low fat mozzarella cheese, shredded	
3/4 cup grated Parmesan cheese	

Directions:

Steps:	Directions:	Critical Control Point / Quality Assurance
1	In a large pot, cook sausage, ground beef, onion, and garlic over medium heat until well browned.	
2	Drain.	
3	Stir in crushed tomatoes, tomato paste, tomato sauce, and water.	
4	Season with sugar, basil, fennel seeds, Italian seasoning, 1 tablespoon salt, pepper, and 4 tablespoons parsley.	
5	Simmer, covered, for about 1 1/2 hours, stirring occasionally.	
6	In a mixing bowl, combine ricotta cheese with egg, remaining parsley, and 1/2 teaspoon salt.	
7	Preheat oven to 375 degrees F (190 degrees C).	
8	To assemble, spread thin layer meat sauce in the bottom of a baking dish.	
9	Arrange noodles lengthwise over meat sauce.	
10	Spread with one half of the ricotta cheese mixture.	
11	Top with a third of mozzarella cheese.	
12	Spoon 1/3 meat sauce over mozzarella, and sprinkle with 1/4 cup Parmesan cheese.	
13	Repeat layers, and top with remaining mozzarella and Parmesan cheese.	
14	Cover with foil: to prevent sticking, either spray foil with cooking spray, or make sure the foil does not touch the cheese.	
15	Bake in preheated oven for 25 minutes.	Cook until internal temperature reaches 165 F degrees for 15 seconds.
16	Remove foil, and bake an additional 25 minutes.	
17	Cool for 15 minutes before serving.	
18	Garnish with remaining parsley.	

Time Temperature Sensitive food. *Food safety Standards: hold food for service at an internal temperature above 140°F. Do not mix old product with new. Cool leftover product quickly (within 4 hours) to below 41°F. Follow proper cooling procedures. Store leftovers in a tightly sealed, labeled and dated container. Use leftover within 72 hours if stored in refrigerator or 30 days if stored in the freezer. Reheat leftover product quickly (within 2 hours) to 165 degrees F for 15 seconds. Reheat left over product only once; discard if not used. Cold holding at 41°F or colder or using time alone (less than four hours). Always wash hands and wash and sanitize counter tops utensils and containers between steps when working with raw meat.*

Copyright 2020 Jacqueline Larson M.S., R.D.N. and Associates.   All Rights Reserved

Texture Modified Diets: Tip: use pasta in the correct particle size.
Soft & Bite Size: (aka Bite size) **Food particle size ½ inch (~width of standard fork)** Food must be moist. Cut foods with a knife to a ½" particle size prior to layering. Moisten with broth as needed.
Chopped: Food particle size ¼ inch (~ ½ width of standard fork) Food must be moist. Chop foods with a knife to 1/4" particle size prior to layering. Moisten with broth as needed.
Minced and Moist:(aka Minced/Mechanical Soft/Ground) **Food particle size 1/8 inch (fits through prongs of standard fork)** Food must be moist. Use a food processor to grind food particles into 1/8 inch prior to layering. Moisten with broth as needed.
Pureed: Smooth and cohesive. Use a food processor to puree to a smooth consistency. Foods are processed by grinding and then pureeing them. May add broth or sauce to puree. Do not add to much liquid. Puree should still hold its shape. Must not be firm or sticky. Puree foods while still hot. Appearance should be smooth like pudding. Serve 1 c. meat serving.

Therapeutic Modified Diets:
Lowfat: No changes needed
Diabetic/No added Sugar/No Conc. Sweets/Calorie Controlled: No changes needed
Bland/Anti Reflux: Serve ground beef patty topped cheese and SF pasta. May season with SF herbs/spices.
Liberal House Renal: Serve ground beef patty and plain pasta
No Added Salt: No changes
2 Gram Sodium: Serve ground beef patty and SF pasta. May toss with fresh tomatoes and SF herbs/spices.
Gluten Free: Use gluten free lasagna noodles and Italian Sausage. Prepare foods separately to prevent cross contamination.
Allergy Alerts: When an "X" is present, this indicates the allergen is present.
Always read all food labels to ensure allergens are not present.

Wheat	Milk	Eggs	Fish Shellfish	Soy	Peanuts/Nuts	Other
X	X	X				

Key: SF= Salt Free D= Diet or Sugarfree LF = Lowfat FF = Fat Free GF = Gluten Free

Recipe Name: Meat and Pasta Bake
Recipe Category: Dinner Entrée
Portion Size: 1 cup
Ingredients: Yields: 8 servings

Ingredients	Notes:
2 cups, uncooked pasta	May use whole grain pasta
2 1/2 Pounds lean ground beef	
1 cup chopped onion	Wash, peel and chop
1 (8oz.) fresh mushrooms	Wash, trim and slice
1 can fat free evaporated milk	
1 cup low salt beef broth	
2 cups shredded low fat Swiss cheese	
1 (8 ounce) carton light sour cream	
2 Teaspoons Worcestershire sauce	
2 Teaspoon thyme	
2 (10 ounce) packages frozen mixed vegetables	
1/2 cup bread crumbs	

Directions:

Steps:	Directions:	Critical Control Point / Quality Assurance
1	Preheat oven to 350 degree oven.	
2	Cook pasta according to the directions on the package	
3	Drain; set aside.	
4	In a large skillet cook meat and onion till meat is brown.	
5	Drain fat.	
6	Stir in broth, cheese, sour cream, milk, Worcestershire sauce and thyme.	
7	Stir in vegetables and pasta.	
8	Transfer to a baking dish.	
9	Bake covered, in a 375 degree for 30 minutes.	
10	Stir.	
11	Sprinkle with bread crumbs.	
12	Bake, uncovered, for 5 to 10 minutes more or till heated through.	Cook until internal temperature reaches 165 F degrees for 15 seconds

Time Temperature Sensitive food. *Food safety Standards: hold food for service at an internal temperature above 140° F. Do not mix old product with new. Cool leftover product quickly (within 4 hours) to below 41° F. Follow proper cooling procedures. Store leftovers in a tightly sealed, labeled and dated container. Use leftover within 72 hours if stored in refrigerator or 30 days if stored in the freezer. Reheat leftover product quickly (within 2 hours) to 165 degrees F for 15 seconds. Reheat left over product only once; discard if not used. Cold holding at 41°F or colder or using time alone (less than four hours). Always wash hands and wash and sanitize counter tops utensils and containers between steps when working with raw meat.*

Texture Modified Diets: Tip: use pasta in the correct particle size.

Soft & Bite Size: (aka Bite size) **Food particle size ½ inch (~width of standard fork)** Food must be moist. Cut foods with a knife to a ½" particle size prior to mixing. Moisten with broth as needed.

Chopped: Food particle size ¼ inch (~ ½ width of standard fork) Food must be moist. Chop foods with a knife to 1/4" particle size prior to mixing. Moisten with broth as needed.

Minced and Moist: (aka Minced/Mechanical Soft/Ground) **Food particle size 1/8 inch (fits through prongs of standard fork)** Food must be moist. Use a food processor to grind food particles into 1/8 inch prior to mixing. Moisten with broth as needed.

Pureed: Smooth and cohesive. Use a food processor to puree to a smooth consistency. Foods are processed by grinding and then pureeing them. May add broth or sauce to puree. Do not add to much liquid. Puree should still hold its shape. Must not be firm or sticky. Puree foods while still hot. Appearance should be smooth like pudding.
Serve 1 c. meat serving

Therapeutic Modified Diets:
Lowfat: No changes needed
Diabetic/No added Sugar/No Conc. Sweets/Calorie Controlled: No changes needed
Bland/Anti Reflux: Serve plain ground beef patty, pasta and peas with carrots
Liberal House Renal: Serve plain ground beef patty, pasta and peas with carrots.
No Added Salt: No changes needed
2 Gram Sodium: Serve plain ground beef patty, pasta, and peas with carrots.
Gluten Free: Use gluten free pasta and gluten free bread crumbs or cornflakes. Prepare foods separately to prevent cross contamination.
Allergy Alerts: When an "X" is present, this indicates the allergen is present. Always read all food labels to ensure allergens are not present.

Wheat	Milk	Eggs	Fish Shellfish	Soy	Peanuts/Nuts	Other
X	X	X	X			

Key: SF= Salt Free D= Diet or Sugarfree LF = Lowfat FF = Fat Free GF = Gluten Free

Recipe Name: Meatballs in Dijon Gravy
Recipe Category: Dinner Entrée
Portion Size: 4 oz.
Ingredients: **Yields: 8 servings**

Ingredients	Notes:
2 1/2 Pounds lean ground beef	
1 teaspoon salt	
2 tablespoons minced onion	Wash, peel and mince
1/2 cup cooked bread crumbs	
1/2 teaspoon pepper	
½ teaspoon garlic powder	
2 eggs	
1 ½ cups low sodium beef broth	
2 tablespoons Dijon mustard	
3 tablespoons all purpose flour	
3 tablespoons margarine	
¼ teaspoon ground black pepper	

Directions:

Steps:	Directions:	Critical Control Point /Quality Assurance
1	Combine meat, salt, pepper, eggs, garlic powder and onion. Shape into balls.	
2	Brown in a skillet. Drain fat.	
3	In a sauce pan over medium high heat the margarine until melted. Add flour and stir to coat. Whisk in broth, mustard and pepper. Bring to a boil. Reduce heat to simmer until thick about 10 minutes.	
4	Pour over meat balls. Cook about 30 minutes over low heat.	Cook until internal temperature reaches 165 F degrees for 15 seconds

Time Temperature Sensitive food. *Food safety Standards: hold food for service at an internal temperature above 140° F. Do not mix old product with new. Cool leftover product quickly (within 4 hours) to below 41° F. Follow proper cooling procedures. Store leftovers in a tightly sealed, labeled and dated container. Use leftover within 72 hours if stored in refrigerator or 30 days if stored in the freezer. Reheat leftover product quickly (within 2 hours) to 165 degrees F for 15 seconds. Reheat left over product only once; discard if not used. Cold holding at 41°F or colder or using time alone (less than four hours). Always wash hands and wash and sanitize counter tops utensils and containers between steps when working with raw meat.*

Texture Modified Diets:

Soft & Bite Size: (aka Bite size) **Food particle size ½ inch (~width of standard fork)** Food must be moist. Cut foods with a knife to a ½" particle size after cooking. Moisten with sauce as needed.

Chopped: Food particle size ¼ inch (~ ½ width of standard fork) Food must be moist. Chop foods with a knife to 1/4" particle size after cooking. Moisten with sauce as needed.

Minced and Moist:(aka Minced/Mechanical Soft/Ground) **Food particle size 1/8 inch (fits through prongs of standard fork)** Food must be moist. Use a food processor to grind food particles into 1/8 inch after cooking. Moisten with sauce as needed.

Pureed: Smooth and cohesive. Use a food processor to puree to a smooth consistency. Foods are processed by grinding and then pureeing them. May add broth or sauce to puree. Do not add to much liquid. Puree should still hold its shape. Must not be firm or sticky. Puree foods while still hot. Appearance should be smooth like pudding. Serve ½ c. puree meat topped with sauce.

Therapeutic Modified Diets:
Lowfat: No changes needed
Diabetic/No added Sugar/No Conc. Sweets/Calorie Controlled: No changes needed
Bland/Anti Reflux: omit sauce.
Liberal House Renal: Omit salt, no sauce
No Added Salt: no changes needed
2 Gram Sodium: Omit salt, no sauce
Gluten Free: Use GF bread crumbs or GF oatmeal. Use GF flour and broth. Prepare foods separately to prevent cross contamination.
Allergy Alerts: When an "X" is present, this indicates the allergen is present.
Always read all food labels to ensure allergens are not present.

Wheat	Milk	Eggs	Fish Shellfish	Soy	Peanuts/Nuts	Other
X	X	X				

Key: SF= Salt Free D= Diet or Sugarfree LF = Lowfat FF = Fat Free GF = Gluten Free

Recipe Name: Meatballs in Tomato Sauce
Recipe Category: Dinner Entrée
Portion Size: 4 oz.
Ingredients: Yields: 8 servings

Ingredients	Notes:
2 1/2 pounds lean ground beef	
1 teaspoon salt	
2 tablespoons minced onion	Wash, peel and mince
1/2 cup cooked rice	May use brown rice
1/2 teaspoon pepper	
2 cans low sodium tomato sauce	
1 teaspoon basil	
1 tablespoon sugar	
1 teaspoon garlic powder	
1 teaspoon oregano	

Directions:

Steps:	Directions:	Critical Control Point /Quality Assurance
1	Combine meat, salt, rice, pepper, and onion.	
2	Shape into balls.	
3	Brown in a skillet.	
4	Drain fat.	
5	Combine tomato sauce with basil, sugar, garlic powder and oregano.	
6	Pour over meat balls.	
7	Cook about 30 minutes over low heat.	Cook until internal temperature reaches 165 F degrees for 15 seconds

Time Temperature Sensitive food. Food safety Standards: hold food for service at an internal temperature above 140° F. Do not mix old product with new. Cool leftover product quickly (within 4 hours) to below 41° F. Follow proper cooling procedures. Store leftovers in a tightly sealed, labeled and dated container. Use leftover within 72 hours if stored in refrigerator or 30 days if stored in the freezer. Reheat leftover product quickly (within 2 hours) to 165 degrees F for 15 seconds. Reheat left over product only once; discard if not used. Cold holding at 41°F or colder or using time alone (less than four hours). Always wash hands and wash and sanitize counter tops utensils and containers between steps when working with raw meat.

Texture Modified Diets:

Soft & Bite Size: (aka Bite size) **Food particle size ½ inch (~width of standard fork)** Food must be moist. Cut foods with a knife to a ½" particle size after cooking. Moisten with broth as needed.

Chopped: Food particle size ¼ inch (~ ½ width of standard fork) Food must be moist. Chop foods with a knife to 1/4" particle size after cooking. Moisten with broth as needed.

Minced and Moist: (aka Minced/Mechanical Soft/Ground) **Food particle size 1/8 inch (fits through prongs of standard fork)** Food must be moist. Use a food processor to grind food particles into 1/8 inch after cooking. Moisten with broth as needed.

Pureed: Smooth and cohesive. Use a food processor to puree to a smooth consistency. Foods are processed by grinding and then pureeing them. May add broth or sauce to puree. Do not add to much liquid. Puree should still hold its shape. Must not be firm or sticky. Puree foods while still hot. Appearance should be smooth like pudding. Serve ½ c. puree meat topped with tomato sauce.

Therapeutic Modified Diets:

Lowfat: No changes needed
Diabetic/No added Sugar/No Conc. Sweets/Calorie Controlled: No changes needed
Bland/Anti Reflux: omit onion, pepper, tomato sauce, basil, garlic powder and oregano (so sauce)
Liberal House Renal: Omit salt, no sauce
No Added Salt: no changes needed
2 Gram Sodium: omit salt, no sauce
Gluten Free: No changes needed. Prepare foods separately to prevent cross contamination.
Allergy Alerts: When an "X" is present, this indicates the allergen is present.
Always read all food labels to ensure allergens are not present.

Wheat	Milk	Eggs	Fish Shellfish	Soy	Peanuts/Nuts	Other

Key: SF= Salt Free D= Diet or Sugarfree LF = Lowfat FF = Fat Free GF = Gluten Free

Recipe Name: Meatballs with Cheese Sauce
Recipe Category: Dinner Entrée
Portion Size: 4 oz. meatballs and 2 T. sauce
Ingredients: **Yields: 8 servings**

Ingredients	Notes:
2 1/2 pounds lean ground beef	
1/2 cup bread crumbs	
1/4 cup minced onion	
2 egg, slightly beaten	
1/4 teaspoon salt	
2 1/2 cups nonfat milk	
2 tablespoons cornstarch	
2 cups low fat shredded cheese	
1 teaspoon garlic powder	
3 teaspoons parsley	

Directions:

Steps:	Directions:	Critical Control Point /Quality Assurance
1	Mix, beef, bread crumbs, onions, salt, and eggs.	
2	Shape into meatballs.	
3	Brown meatballs in skillet.	Cook until internal temperature reaches 165 F degrees for 15 seconds
4	Pour off drippings.	
5	In a small bowl combine cornstarch with 1/2 cup milk.	
6	In a small sauce pan heat 2 cups milk and cheese until just starts to boil.	
7	Stir in garlic powder and cornstarch mixture.	
8	Cover and cook over low heat for 10 minutes.	
9	Pour sauce over meatballs just before serving.	
10	Top with parsley.	

Time Temperature Sensitive food. *Food safety Standards: hold food for service at an internal temperature above 140° F. Do not mix old product with new. Cool leftover product quickly (within 4 hours) to below 41° F. Follow proper cooling procedures. Store leftovers in a tightly sealed, labeled and dated container. Use leftover within 72 hours if stored in refrigerator or 30 days if stored in the freezer. Reheat leftover product quickly (within 2 hours) to 165 degrees F for 15 seconds. Reheat left over product only once; discard if not used. Cold holding at 41°F or colder or using time alone (less than four hours). Always wash hands and wash and sanitize counter tops utensils and containers between steps when working with raw meat.*

Texture Modified Diets:
Soft & Bite Size: (aka Bite size) **Food particle size ½ inch (~width of standard fork)** Food must be moist. Cut foods with a knife to a ½" particle size after cooking. Moisten with broth as needed.
Chopped: Food particle size ¼ inch (~ ½ width of standard fork) Food must be moist. Chop foods with a knife to 1/4" particle size after cooking. Moisten with broth as needed.
Minced and Moist:(aka Minced/Mechanical Soft/Ground) **Food particle size 1/8 inch (fits through prongs of standard fork)** Food must be moist. Use a food processor to grind food particles into 1/8 inch after cooking. Moisten with broth as needed.
Pureed: Smooth and cohesive. Use a food processor to puree to a smooth consistency. Foods are processed by grinding and then pureeing them. May add broth or sauce to puree. Do not add to much liquid. Puree should still hold its shape. Must not be firm or sticky. Puree foods while still hot. Appearance should be smooth like pudding. Serve ½ c. meat serving.

Therapeutic Modified Diets:
Lowfat: No changes needed
Diabetic/No added Sugar/No Conc. Sweets/Calorie Controlled: No changes needed
Bland/Anti Reflux: omit onion, garlic salt and parsley
Liberal House Renal: Omit salt, bread crumbs and cheese sauce
No Added Salt: No changes
2 Gram Sodium: omit salt, bread crumbs, and cheese sauce
Gluten Free: Use gluten free bread crumbs or GF oats. Prepare foods separately to prevent cross contamination.
Allergy Alerts: When an "X" is present, this indicates the allergen is present.
Always read all food labels to ensure allergens are not present.

Wheat	Milk	Eggs	Fish Shellfish	Soy	Peanuts/Nuts	Other
X	X	X				

Key: SF= Salt Free D= Diet or Sugarfree LF = Lowfat FF = Fat Free GF = Gluten Free

Copyright 2020 Jacqueline Larson M.S., R.D.N. and Associates.   All Rights Reserved

Recipe Name: Meatloaf
Recipe Category: Dinner Entrée
Portion Size: 4 oz.
Ingredients: **Yields: 8 servings**

Ingredients	Notes:
2 1/2 pounds lean ground beef	
3 eggs	
2 teaspoons salt	
1/4 teaspoon pepper	
1 cup quick cooking oats	
1/2 cup catsup	
1 small chopped onion	
1 tablespoon prepared mustard	

Directions:

Steps:	Directions:	Critical Control Point /Quality Assurance
1	Preheat oven to 350 degrees.	
2	In a bowl mix all ingredients.	
3	Shape into a loaf and place into a loaf pan.	
4	Bake for 1 hour.	Cook until internal temperature reaches 165 F degrees for 15 seconds

Time Temperature Sensitive food. *Food safety Standards: hold food for service at an internal temperature above 140° F. Do not mix old product with new. Cool leftover product quickly (within 4 hours) to below 41° F. Follow proper cooling procedures. Store leftovers in a tightly sealed, labeled and dated container. Use leftover within 72 hours if stored in refrigerator or 30 days if stored in the freezer. Reheat leftover product quickly (within 2 hours) to 165 degrees F for 15 seconds. Reheat left over product only once; discard if not used. Cold holding at 41 °F or colder or using time alone (less than four hours). Always wash hands and wash and sanitize counter tops utensils and containers between steps when working with raw meat.*

Texture Modified Diets:

Soft & Bite Size: (aka Bite size) **Food particle size ½ inch (~width of standard fork)** Food must be moist. Cut foods with a knife to a ½" particle size after cooking. Moisten with broth as needed.

Chopped: Food particle size ¼ inch (~ ½ width of standard fork) Food must be moist. Chop foods with a knife to 1/4" particle size after cooking. Moisten with broth as needed.

Minced and Moist: (aka Minced/Mechanical Soft/Ground) **Food particle size 1/8 inch (fits through prongs of standard fork)** Food must be moist. Use a food processor to grind food particles into 1/8 inch after cooking. Moisten with broth as needed.

Pureed: Smooth and cohesive. Use a food processor to puree to a smooth consistency. Foods are processed by grinding and then pureeing them. May add broth or sauce to puree. Do not add to much liquid. Puree should still hold its shape. Must not be firm or sticky. Puree foods while still hot. Appearance should be smooth like pudding. Serve ½ c. meat serving.

Therapeutic Modified Diets:

Lowfat: No changes needed
Diabetic/No added Sugar/No Conc. Sweets/Calorie Controlled: No changes needed
Bland/Anti Reflux: omit pepper, catsup, onion and mustard
Liberal House Renal: Omit salt and catsup
No Added Salt: No changes needed
2 Gram Sodium: omit salt and catsup
Gluten Free: Use gluten free oats. Prepare foods separately to prevent cross contamination.
Allergy Alerts: When an "X" is present, this indicates the allergen is present.
Always read all food labels to ensure allergens are not present.

Wheat	Milk	Eggs	Fish Shellfish	Soy	Peanuts/Nuts	Other
X		X				

Key: SF= Salt Free D= Diet or Sugarfree LF = Lowfat FF = Fat Free GF = Gluten Free

Recipe Name: Mexican Spaghetti
Recipe Category: Dinner Entrée
Portion Size: 1 cup
Ingredients: **Yields:** 8 servings

Ingredients	Notes:
2 1/2 Pounds lean ground beef or turkey	
1 large chopped onion	Wash, peel and chop
2 cups whole kernel corn	Fresh or frozen
¾ cup low sodium tomato sauce	
1 large jar mild salsa (4 cups)	
1 tablespoon chili powder	
1/2 teaspoon garlic powder	
1/4 teaspoon onion powder	
1/4 teaspoon dried oregano	
1/2 teaspoon paprika	
1 teaspoon ground cumin	
1/2 teaspoon salt	
1/4 teaspoon ground black pepper	
1/2 teaspoon sugar	
1 cup low fat Monterrey Jack cheese	
1 pound spaghetti	May use whole grain

Directions:

Steps:	Directions:	Critical Control Point / Quality Assurance
1	Prepare spaghetti according to directions on the package.	
2	Sauté ground meat and onion in a medium size sauce pan until brown. Drain grease.	Cook until internal temperature reaches 165 F degrees for 15 seconds
3	In a small bowl combine chili powder, garlic powder, onion powder, dried oregano, paprika, cumin and salt.	
4	Stir in salsa, corn, water, tomato sauce and seasoning mix with the ground meat	
5	Simmer over low heat for 20 minutes.	
6	Serve the spaghetti on a hot platter, first a layer of pasta, then a layer of sauce. Sprinkle with cheese.	

Time Temperature Sensitive food. Food safety Standards: hold food for service at an internal temperature above 140° F. Do not mix old product with new. Cool leftover product quickly (within 4 hours) to below 41° F. Follow proper cooling procedures. Store leftovers in a tightly sealed, labeled and dated container. Use leftover within 72 hours if stored in refrigerator or 30 days if stored in the freezer. Reheat leftover product quickly (within 2 hours) to 165 degrees F for 15 seconds. Reheat left over product only once; discard if not used. Cold holding at 41 °F or colder or using time alone (less than four hours). Always wash hands and wash and sanitize counter tops utensils and containers between steps when working with raw meat.

Texture Modified Diets: TIP: Use pasta in correct particle size

Soft & Bite Size: (aka Bite size) **Food particle size ½ inch (~width of standard fork)** Food must be moist. Cut foods with a knife to a ½" particle size prior to layering. Moisten with broth as needed.

Chopped: Food particle size ¼ inch (~ ½ width of standard fork) Food must be moist. Chop foods with a knife to 1/4" particle size prior to layering. Moisten with broth as needed.

Minced and Moist: (aka Minced/Mechanical Soft/Ground) **Food particle size 1/8 inch (fits through prongs of standard fork)** Food must be moist. Use a food processor to grind food particles into 1/8 inch prior to layering. Moisten with broth as needed.

Pureed: Smooth and cohesive. Use a food processor to puree to a smooth consistency. Foods are processed by grinding and then pureeing them. May add broth or sauce to puree. Do not add to much liquid. Puree should still hold its shape. Must not be firm or sticky. Puree foods while still hot. Appearance should be smooth like pudding. Serve ½ c. puree meat serving and ½ puree pasta mixture separately.

Therapeutic Modified Diets:
Lowfat: No changes needed
Diabetic/No added Sugar/No Conc. Sweets/Calorie Controlled: No changes needed
Bland/Anti Reflux: Serve plain ground beef with melted cheese on top of plain spaghetti
Liberal House Renal: Serve ground beef seasoned with onion, corn, chili powder, garlic powder, onion powder, oregano, paprika, cumin, and black pepper with plain spaghetti. No cheese
No Added Salt: No changes needed
2 Gram Sodium: follow renal instructions
Gluten Free: Use gluten free spaghetti. Prepare foods separately to prevent cross contamination.
Allergy Alerts: When an "X" is present, this indicates the allergen is present. Always read all food labels to ensure allergens are not present.

Wheat	Milk	Eggs	Fish Shellfish	Soy	Peanuts/Nuts	Other
X	X	X				

Key: SF= Salt Free D= Diet or Sugarfree LF = Lowfat FF = Fat Free GF = Gluten Free

Copyright 2020 Jacqueline Larson M.S., R.D.N. and Associates.   All Rights Reserved

Recipe Name: Mongolian Beef
Recipe Category: Dinner Entrée
Portion Size: ¾ cup
Ingredients: Yields: 8 servings

Ingredients	Notes:
2 1/2 Pounds boneless tender beef steak (sirloin, rib eye, or top loin)	Trim all visible fat, slice thinly across the grain
1/4 Cup cornstarch	
1/2 Cup Teriyaki sauce, divided	
2 Cloves garlic, minced	
2 Cups water	
2 Teaspoon vinegar	
1/4 to 1/2 Teaspoon crushed red pepper	
2 Tablespoons oil, divided	
4 Carrots, cut diagonally into thinly slices	Washed, peeled and cut
2 Onions, chunked and separated	Washed, peeled and chunked
2 Green peppers, chunked	Washed, peeled and chunked

Directions:

Steps:	Directions:	Critical Control Point /Quality Assurance
1	Cut beef across grain into strips, then into 1 1/2 inch squares.	
2	Combine 2 tablespoons cornstarch, 1 tablespoon teriyaki sauce, and garlic in medium bowl; stir in beef.cover	
3	Let stand in fridge for 30 minutes.	
4	Mean while combine water, remaining cornstarch, teriyaki sauce, vinegar and red pepper; set aside.	
5	Heat 1 tablespoon oil in hot wok or skillet over high heat.	
6	Add beef and stir fry 1 minute; remove.	
7	Heat remaining oil in the same pan.	
8	Add carrots, onion, and green peppers; stir fry 4 minutes.	
9	Add beef and teriyaki sauce mixture; cook and stir until sauce boils and thickens.	Cook until internal temperature reaches 145 F degrees for 15 seconds

Time Temperature Sensitive food. Food safety Standards: hold food for service at an internal temperature above 140° F. Do not mix old product with new. Cool leftover product quickly (within 4 hours) to below 41° F. Follow proper cooling procedures. Store leftovers in a tightly sealed, labeled and dated container. Use leftover within 72 hours if stored in refrigerator or 30 days if stored in the freezer. Reheat leftover product quickly (within 2 hours) to 165 degrees F for 15 seconds. Reheat left over product only once; discard if not used. Cold holding at 41°F or colder or using time alone (less than four hours). Always wash hands and wash and sanitize counter tops utensils and containers between steps when working with raw meat.

Texture Modified Diets:

Soft & Bite Size: (aka Bite size) **Food particle size ½ inch (~width of standard fork)** Food must be moist. Cut foods with a knife to a ½" particle size prior to mixing. Moisten with broth as needed.

Chopped: Food particle size ¼ inch (~ ½ width of standard fork) Food must be moist. Chop foods with a knife to 1/4" particle size prior to mixing. Moisten with broth as needed.

Minced and Moist:(aka Minced/Mechanical Soft/Ground) **Food particle size 1/8 inch (fits through prongs of standard fork)** Food must be moist. Use a food processor to grind food particles into 1/8 inch prior to mixing. Moisten with broth as needed.

Pureed: Smooth and cohesive. Use a food processor to puree to a smooth consistency. Foods are processed by grinding and then pureeing them. May add broth or sauce to puree. Do not add to much liquid. Puree should still hold its shape. Must not be firm or sticky. Puree foods while still hot. Appearance should be smooth like pudding. Serve ½ c. puree meat, ½ cup puree rice and ½ c. puree vegetable separately.

Therapeutic Modified Diets:

Lowfat: No changes needed
Diabetic/No added Sugar/No Conc. Sweets/Calorie Controlled: No changes needed
Bland/Anti Reflux: omit garlic, vinegar, red pepper, onions and green peppers
Liberal House Renal: Omit teriyaki sauce
No Added Salt: Omit teriyaki sauce
2 Gram Sodium: Omit teriyaki sauce
Gluten Free: Use gluten free teriyaki sauce. Prepare foods separately to prevent cross contamination.

Allergy Alerts: When an "X" is present, this indicates the allergen is present. Always read all food labels to ensure allergens are not present.

Wheat	Milk	Eggs	Fish Shellfish	Soy	Peanuts/Nuts	Other
X				X		

Key: SF= Salt Free D= Diet or Sugarfree LF = Lowfat FF = Fat Free GF = Gluten Free

Recipe Name: Open Face Roast Beef Sandwich with Mashed Potatoes and Gravy
Recipe Category: Dinner Entrée
Portion Size: 3 oz. beef with 2 tablespoons gravy
Ingredients: **Yields: 8 servings**

Ingredients	Notes:
3 1/2 to 4 Pounds rib roast, rolled rib roast, sirloin rib roast, eye of round or rolled rib roast (boneless)	Trim all visible fat
Seasonings of choice: salt, pepper, garlic powder, seasoning salt, etc.	
Gravy	
1/4 cup drippings	
3 tablespoons flour	
Salt and pepper to taste	
2 cups low sodium beef stock or water	
8 slices of bread	
4 cups prepared Mashed Potatoes	See recipe in starchy side dishes.

Directions:

Steps:	Directions:	Critical Control Point / Quality Assurance
1	Preheat oven to 550 degrees.	
2	Place roast in a roasting pan and season well.	
3	Do not cover and do not add liquid.	
4	Immediately reduce heat to 350 degrees.	
5	Roast 18 to 20 minutes to the pound for medium rare.	Thermometer reading should be between 140 degrees (rare) and 170 degrees(well done.)
6	A rolled roast requires 5 to 10 minutes longer to the pound.	Thermometer reading should be between 140 degrees (rare) and 170 degrees(well done.)
7	Serve sliced thinly across the grain.	
	Gravy	
1	Remove the meat from the pan.	
2	Place it where it will remain hot.	
3	Pour off all but 1/4 cup of drippings.	
4	Blend flour into drippings.	
5	Stir with a wire whisk until the flour has thickened and until the mixture is well combined and smooth.	
6	Continue to cook slowly stir constantly while adding stock.	
7	Cook until desired consistency.	
8	Season with salt and pepper.	
9	To serve: place bread on serving dish, top with 3 oz. roast beef, ½ cup mashed and ¼ cup gravy	

Time Temperature Sensitive food. *Food safety Standards: hold food for service at an internal temperature above 140°F. Do not mix old product with new. Cool leftover product quickly (within 4 hours) to below 41°F. Follow proper cooling procedures. Store leftovers in a tightly sealed, labeled and dated container. Use leftover within 72 hours if stored in refrigerator or 30 days if stored in the freezer. Reheat leftover product quickly (within 2 hours) to 165 degrees F for 15 seconds. Reheat left over product only once; discard if not used. Cold holding at 41°F or colder or using time alone (less than four hours). Always wash hands and wash and sanitize counter tops utensils and containers between steps when working with raw meat.*

Texture Modified Diets:

Soft & Bite Size: (aka Bite size) **Food particle size ½ inch (~width of standard fork)** Food must be moist. Cut foods with a knife to a ½" particle size prior to layering. Moisten with broth as needed.

Chopped: Food particle size ¼ inch (~ ½ width of standard fork) Food must be moist. Chop foods with a knife to 1/4" particle size prior to layering. Moisten with broth as needed.

Minced and Moist:(aka Minced/Mechanical Soft/Ground) **Food particle size 1/8 inch (fits through prongs of standard fork)** Food must be moist. Use a food processor to grind food particles into 1/8 inch prior to layering. Moisten with broth as needed.

Pureed: Smooth and cohesive. Use a food processor to puree to a smooth consistency. Foods are processed by grinding and then pureeing them. May add broth or sauce to puree. Do not add to much liquid. Puree should still hold its shape. Must not be firm or sticky. Puree foods while still hot. Appearance should be smooth like pudding. Serve ½ c. meat serving, ½ cup puree bread and ½ puree potatoes separately.

Therapeutic Modified Diets:

Lowfat: No changes needed
Diabetic/No added Sugar/No Conc. Sweets/Calorie Controlled: No changes needed
Bland/Anti Reflux: omit seasonings except salt. Omit gravy
Liberal House Renal: Omit salt and gravy. Use SF bread. Use SF rice in place of potatoes.
No Added Salt: No changes needed
2 Gram Sodium: omit salt and gravy. Use SF gravy
Gluten Free: Use GF flour, GF bread and GF broth. Prepare foods separately to prevent cross contamination.
Allergy Alerts: When an "X" is present, this indicates the allergen is present.
Always read all food labels to ensure allergens are not present.

Wheat	Milk	Eggs	Fish Shellfish	Soy	Peanuts/Nuts	Other
X	X	X				

Key: SF= Salt Free D= Diet or Sugarfree LF = Lowfat FF = Fat Free GF = Gluten Free

Recipe Name: Pasta with Creamy Tomato Basil Meat Sauce
Recipe Category: Dinner Entrée
Portion Size: 1 cup
Ingredients: Yields: 8 servings

Ingredients	Notes:
2 1/2 pounds lean ground beef	
1 large chopped onion	Wash, peel and slice
1 teaspoon garlic powder	
1 teaspoon salt	
1/4 teaspoon pepper	
4 cups canned low sodium tomato sauce	
2 (8oz.) light cream cheese.	
1 tablespoon basil	
1 teaspoon oregano	
1 pound pasta	May use whole grain
Grated Parmesan cheese	

Directions:

Steps:	Directions:	Critical Control Point / Quality Assurance
1	Prepare pasta according to directions on the package.	
2	Sauté ground beef and onion in a medium size sauce pan.	
3	Drain grease.	
4	Add garlic powder, salt, pepper, basil, oregano, and tomatoes.	
5	Simmer over low heat for 20 minutes. Stir in cream cheese and heat until heated through.	Cook until internal temperature reaches 165 F degrees for 15 seconds
6	Serve the pasta on a hot platter.	
7	First a layer of pasta, then a layer of sauce.	
8	Sprinkle with parmesan cheese.	

Time Temperature Sensitive food. *Food safety Standards: hold food for service at an internal temperature above 140° F. Do not mix old product with new. Cool leftover product quickly (within 4 hours) to below 41° F. Follow proper cooling procedures. Store leftovers in a tightly sealed, labeled and dated container. Use leftover within 72 hours if stored in refrigerator or 30 days if stored in the freezer. Reheat leftover product quickly (within 2 hours) to 165 degrees F for 15 seconds. Reheat left over product only once; discard if not used. Cold holding at 41°F or colder or using time alone (less than four hours). Always wash hands and wash and sanitize counter tops utensils and containers between steps when working with raw meat.*

Texture Modified Diets: Tip: serve pasta in correct particle size.

Soft & Bite Size: (aka Bite size) **Food particle size ½ inch (~width of standard fork)** Food must be moist. Cut foods with a knife to a ½" particle size prior to layering. Moisten with broth as needed.

Chopped: Food particle size ¼ inch (~ ½ width of standard fork) Food must be moist. Chop foods with a knife to 1/4" particle size prior to layering. Moisten with broth as needed.

Minced and Moist: (aka Minced/Mechanical Soft/Ground) **Food particle size 1/8 inch (fits through prongs of standard fork)** Food must be moist. Use a food processor to grind food particles into 1/8 inch prior to layering. Moisten with broth as needed.

Pureed: Smooth and cohesive. Use a food processor to puree to a smooth consistency. Foods are processed by grinding and then pureeing them. May add broth or sauce to puree. Do not add to much liquid. Puree should still hold its shape. Must not be firm or sticky. Puree foods while still hot. Appearance should be smooth like pudding. Serve ½ c. puree meat sauce and ½ c. puree pasta separately. Tip: puree pasta while still hot.

Therapeutic Modified Diets:
Lowfat: No changes needed
Diabetic/No added Sugar/No Conc. Sweets/Calorie Controlled: No changes needed
Bland/Anti Reflux: omit onion, garlic powder, pepper, tomatoes, basil, and oregano
Liberal House Renal: Omit salt, tomatoes, cream cheese and Parmesan cheese
No Added Salt: No changes needed
2 Gram Sodium: omit salt, tomatoes, cream cheese and Parmesan cheese. Sub. Fresh tomatoes for canned
Gluten Free: Use gluten free pasta. Prepare foods separately to prevent cross contamination.
Allergy Alerts: When an "X" is present, this indicates the allergen is present.
Always read all food labels to ensure allergens are not present.

Wheat	Milk	Eggs	Fish Shellfish	Soy	Peanuts/Nuts	Other
X	X	X				

Key: SF= Salt Free D= Diet or Sugarfree LF = Lowfat FF = Fat Free GF = Gluten Free

Recipe Name: Pasta with Tomato Sauce
Recipe Category: Dinner Entrée
Portion Size: 1 cup
Ingredients: **Yields: 8 servings**

Ingredients	Notes:
2 1/2 Pounds lean ground beef	
1 large chopped onion	Wash, peel and slice
1 teaspoon garlic powder	
1 teaspoon salt	
1/4 teaspoon pepper	
4 cups canned low sodium tomato sauce	
1 tablespoon basil	
1 teaspoon oregano	
1 pound pasta	May use whole grain
Grated Parmesan cheese	

Directions:

Steps:	Directions:	Critical Control Point / Quality Assurance
1	Prepare pasta according to directions on the package.	
2	Sauté ground beef and onion in a medium size sauce pan.	
3	Drain grease.	
4	Add garlic powder, salt, pepper, basil, oregano, and tomatoes.	
5	Simmer over low heat for 20 minutes.	Cook until internal temperature reaches 165 F degrees for 15 seconds
6	Serve the pasta on a hot platter.	
7	First a layer of pasta, then a layer of sauce.	
8	Sprinkle with parmesan cheese.	

Time Temperature Sensitive food. *Food safety Standards: hold food for service at an internal temperature above 140° F. Do not mix old product with new. Cool leftover product quickly (within 4 hours) to below 41° F. Follow proper cooling procedures. Store leftovers in a tightly sealed, labeled and dated container. Use leftover within 72 hours if stored in refrigerator or 30 days if stored in the freezer. Reheat leftover product quickly (within 2 hours) to 165 degrees F for 15 seconds. Reheat left over product only once; discard if not used. Cold holding at 41°F or colder or using time alone (less than four hours). Always wash hands and wash and sanitize counter tops utensils and containers between steps when working with raw meat.*

Texture Modified Diets: Tip: serve pasta in correct particle size.

Soft & Bite Size: (aka Bite size) **Food particle size ½ inch (~width of standard fork)** Food must be moist. Cut foods with a knife to a ½" particle size prior to layering. Moisten with broth as needed.

Chopped: Food particle size ¼ inch (~ ½ width of standard fork) Food must be moist. Chop foods with a knife to 1/4" particle size prior to layering. Moisten with broth as needed.

Minced and Moist: (aka Minced/Mechanical Soft/Ground) **Food particle size 1/8 inch (fits through prongs of standard fork)** Food must be moist. Use a food processor to grind food particles into 1/8 inch prior to layering. Moisten with broth as needed.

Pureed: Smooth and cohesive. Use a food processor to puree to a smooth consistency. Foods are processed by grinding and then pureeing them. May add broth or sauce to puree. Do not add to much liquid. Puree should still hold its shape. Must not be firm or sticky. Puree foods while still hot. Appearance should be smooth like pudding. Serve ½ c. puree meat sauce and ½ c. puree pasta separately. Tip: puree pasta while still hot.

Therapeutic Modified Diets:
Lowfat: No changes needed
Diabetic/No added Sugar/No Conc. Sweets/Calorie Controlled: No changes needed
Bland/Anti Reflux: omit onion, garlic powder, pepper, tomatoes, basil, and oregano
Liberal House Renal: Omit salt, tomatoes, and Parmesan cheese
No Added Salt: No changes needed
2 Gram Sodium: omit salt, tomatoes, and Parmesan cheese. Sub. Fresh tomatoes for canned
Gluten Free: Use gluten free pasta. Prepare foods separately to prevent cross contamination.
**Allergy Alerts: When an "X" is present, this indicates the allergen is present.
Always read all food labels to ensure allergens are not present.**

Wheat	Milk	Eggs	Fish Shellfish	Soy	Peanuts/Nuts	Other
X	X	X				

Key: SF= Salt Free D= Diet or Sugarfree LF = Lowfat FF = Fat Free GF = Gluten Free

Recipe Name: Patty Melts
Recipe Category: Dinner Entrée
Portion Size: 4 oz. patty on 2 slices bread
Ingredients: Yields: 8 servings

Ingredients	Notes:
2 1/2 Pounds lean ground beef	
½ teaspoon garlic powder	
¼ teaspoon ground black pepper	
16 slice rye bread	May use whole wheat.
1 large onion	Washed, peeled and diced.
8 slices cheese	
¼ cup margarine, soften	
2 tablespoons catsup	(optional)
2 tablespoons mustard	(optional)

Directions:

Steps:	Directions:	Critical Control Point /Quality Assurance
1	Mix ground beef with garlic and pepper.	
2	Form beef into eight equal beef patties.	
3	Broil, grill, or sauté until no longer pink inside. Set aside	Cook until internal temperature reaches 165 F degrees for 15 seconds
4	Saute onion until tender. Set aside.	
5	Spread 1 slice of slice of bread with margarine.	
6	Heat pan to medium high heat. Place bread with the side down in pan. Top with hamburger, onions, and cheese. May add mustard or catsup as desired. Top with another slice of bread with the margarine side out. Turn when bread is golden brown,	
7	Serve immediately warm.	

Time Temperature Sensitive food. *Food safety Standards: hold food for service at an internal temperature above 140° F. Do not mix old product with new. Cool leftover product quickly (within 4 hours) to below 41° F. Follow proper cooling procedures. Store leftovers in a tightly sealed, labeled and dated container. Use leftover within 72 hours if stored in refrigerator or 30 days if stored in the freezer. Reheat leftover product quickly (within 2 hours) to 165 degrees F for 15 seconds. Reheat left over product only once; discard if not used. Cold holding at 41 °F or colder or using time alone (less than four hours). Always wash hands and wash and sanitize counter tops utensils and containers between steps when working with raw meat.*

Texture Modified Diets:

Soft & Bite Size: (aka Bite size) **Food particle size ½ inch (~width of standard fork) Do not grill bread.** Food must be moist. Cut foods with a knife to a ½" particle size prior to layering. Moisten with broth as needed.

Chopped: Food particle size ¼ inch (~ ½ width of standard fork) Do not grill bread. Food must be moist. Chop foods with a knife to 1/4" particle size prior to layering. Moisten with broth as needed.

Minced and Moist: (aka Minced/Mechanical Soft/Ground) **Do not grill bread. Food particle size 1/8 inch (fits through prongs of standard fork)** Food must be moist. Use a food processor to grind food particles into 1/8 inch prior to layering. Moisten with broth as needed.

Pureed: Smooth and cohesive. Do not grill bread. Use a food processor to puree to a smooth consistency. Foods are processed by grinding and then pureeing them. May add broth or sauce to puree. Do not add to much liquid. Puree should still hold its shape. Must not be firm or sticky. Puree foods while still hot. Appearance should be smooth like pudding. Serve ½ c. meat serving and 1 c. bread with condiments puree separately.

Therapeutic Modified Diets:

Lowfat: No Roquefort cheese
Diabetic/No added Sugar/No Conc. Sweets/Calorie Controlled: No changes needed
Bland/Anti Reflux: Serve plain hamburger
Liberal House Renal: Omit cheese. Use SF margarine or butter. No bread. Wrap in lettuce instead on a bun. Serve with ½ rice or pasta
No Added Salt: No changes needed
2 Gram Sodium: Omit cheese. Use SF margarine or butter. Roquefort. No bread. Wrap in lettuce instead on a bun. Serve with ½ c. rice or pasta
Gluten Free: Use gluten free bread. mix Prepare foods separately to prevent cross contamination.
Allergy Alerts: When an "X" is present, this indicates the allergen is present.
Always read all food labels to ensure allergens are not present.

Wheat	Milk	Eggs	Fish Shellfish	Soy	Peanuts/Nuts	Other
X	X			X		

Key: SF= Salt Free D= Diet or Sugarfree LF = Lowfat FF = Fat Free GF = Gluten Free

Copyright 2020 Jacqueline Larson M.S., R.D.N. and Associates.   All Rights Reserved

Recipe Name: Pasta with Creamy Tomato Basil Meat Sauce
Recipe Category: Dinner Entrée
Portion Size: 1 cup
Ingredients: Yields: 8 servings

Ingredients	Notes:
2 1/2 pounds lean ground beef	
1 large chopped onion	Wash, peel and slice
1 teaspoon garlic powder	
1 teaspoon salt	
1/4 teaspoon pepper	
4 cups canned low sodium tomato sauce	
2 (8oz.) light cream cheese.	
1 tablespoon basil	
1 teaspoon oregano	
1 pound pasta	May use whole grain
Grated Parmesan cheese	

Directions:

Steps:	Directions:	Critical Control Point / Quality Assurance
1	Prepare pasta according to directions on the package.	
2	Sauté ground beef and onion in a medium size sauce pan.	
3	Drain grease.	
4	Add garlic powder, salt, pepper, basil, oregano, and tomatoes.	
5	Simmer over low heat for 20 minutes. Stir in cream cheese and heat until heated through.	Cook until internal temperature reaches 165 F degrees for 15 seconds
6	Serve the pasta on a hot platter.	
7	First a layer of pasta, then a layer of sauce.	
8	Sprinkle with parmesan cheese.	

Time Temperature Sensitive food. Food safety Standards: hold food for service at an internal temperature above 140° F. Do not mix old product with new. Cool leftover product quickly (within 4 hours) to below 41° F. Follow proper cooling procedures. Store leftovers in a tightly sealed, labeled and dated container. Use leftover within 72 hours if stored in refrigerator or 30 days if stored in the freezer. Reheat leftover product quickly (within 2 hours) to 165 degrees F for 15 seconds. Reheat left over product only once; discard if not used. Cold holding at 41°F or colder or using time alone (less than four hours). Always wash hands and wash and sanitize counter tops utensils and containers between steps when working with raw meat.

Texture Modified Diets: Tip: serve pasta in correct particle size.

Soft & Bite Size: (aka Bite size) **Food particle size ½ inch (~width of standard fork)** Food must be moist. Cut foods with a knife to a ½" particle size prior to layering. Moisten with broth as needed.

Chopped: Food particle size ¼ inch (~ ½ width of standard fork) Food must be moist. Chop foods with a knife to 1/4" particle size prior to layering. Moisten with broth as needed.

Minced and Moist: (aka Minced/Mechanical Soft/Ground) **Food particle size 1/8 inch (fits through prongs of standard fork)** Food must be moist. Use a food processor to grind food particles into 1/8 inch prior to layering. Moisten with broth as needed.

Pureed: Smooth and cohesive. Use a food processor to puree to a smooth consistency. Foods are processed by grinding and then pureeing them. May add broth or sauce to puree. Do not add to much liquid. Puree should still hold its shape. Must not be firm or sticky. Puree foods while still hot. Appearance should be smooth like pudding. Serve ½ c. puree meat sauce and ½ c. puree pasta separately. Tip: puree pasta while still hot.

Therapeutic Modified Diets:
Lowfat: No changes needed
Diabetic/No added Sugar/No Conc. Sweets/Calorie Controlled: No changes needed
Bland/Anti Reflux: omit onion, garlic powder, pepper, tomatoes, basil, and oregano
Liberal House Renal: Omit salt, tomatoes, cream cheese and Parmesan cheese
No Added Salt: No changes needed
2 Gram Sodium: omit salt, tomatoes, cream cheese and Parmesan cheese. Sub. Fresh tomatoes for canned
Gluten Free: Use gluten free pasta. Prepare foods separately to prevent cross contamination.
Allergy Alerts: When an "X" is present, this indicates the allergen is present.
Always read all food labels to ensure allergens are not present.

Wheat	Milk	Eggs	Fish Shellfish	Soy	Peanuts/Nuts	Other
X	X	X				

Key: SF= Salt Free D= Diet or Sugarfree LF = Lowfat FF = Fat Free GF = Gluten Free

Recipe Name: Pizza Casserole
Recipe Category: Dinner Entrée
Portion Size: 1 cup
Ingredients: **Yields: 8 servings**

Ingredients	Notes:
2 pounds lean ground beef	
1-12 oz. Package macaroni	May use whole grain
1/4 cup diced onion	Wash, peel and dice
2 tablespoons olive oil	
2 cups small curd low fat cottage cheese	
1/4 cup grated low fat Parmesan cheese	
1-12 oz. can low sodium pizza sauce	
8 oz fresh mushrooms	
1 teaspoon oregano	
1 1/2 teaspoon salt	
1 cup light sour cream	

Directions:

Steps:	Directions:	Critical Control Point /Quality Assurance
1	Cook macaroni, rinse and drain.	
2	Sauté onion in olive oil until transparent.	
3	Add beef and brown, then combine meat with remaining ingredients and mix with macaroni.	
4	Pour into baking dish.	
5	Sprinkle with additional Parmesan cheese.	
6	Bake at 350 degree for 45 to 60 minutes.	Cook until internal temperature reaches 165 F degrees for 15 seconds

Time Temperature Sensitive food. *Food safety Standards: hold food for service at an internal temperature above 140° F. Do not mix old product with new. Cool leftover product quickly (within 4 hours) to below 41° F. Follow proper cooling procedures. Store leftovers in a tightly sealed, labeled and dated container. Use leftover within 72 hours if stored in refrigerator or 30 days if stored in the freezer. Reheat leftover product quickly (within 2 hours) to 165 degrees F for 15 seconds. Reheat left over product only once; discard if not used. Cold holding at 41 °F or colder or using time alone (less than four hours). Always wash hands and wash and sanitize counter tops utensils and containers between steps when working with raw meat.*

Texture Modified Diets: Tip: use pasta in correct particle size.

Soft & Bite Size: (aka Bite size) **Food particle size ½ inch (~width of standard fork)** Food must be moist. Cut foods with a knife to a ½" particle size prior to mixing. Moisten with broth as needed.

Chopped: Food particle size ¼ inch (~ ½ width of standard fork) Food must be moist. Chop foods with a knife to 1/4" particle size prior to mixing. Moisten with broth as needed.

Minced and Moist: (aka Minced/Mechanical Soft/Ground) **Food particle size 1/8 inch (fits through prongs of standard fork)** Food must be moist. Use a food processor to grind food particles into 1/8 inch prior to mixing. Moisten with broth as needed.

Pureed: Smooth and cohesive. Use a food processor to puree to a smooth consistency. Foods are processed by grinding and then pureeing them. May add broth or sauce to puree. Do not add to much liquid. Puree should still hold its shape. Must not be firm or sticky. Puree foods while still hot. Appearance should be smooth like pudding. Serve 1 c. puree serving.

Therapeutic Modified Diets:
Lowfat: No changes needed
Diabetic/No added Sugar/No Conc. Sweets/Calorie Controlled: No changes needed
Bland/Anti Reflux: omit onion, pizza sauce, and oregano. Add 2 cups beef broth
Liberal House Renal: Serve plain beef patty and plain pasta. May season with SF herbs/spices.
No Added Salt: No changes needed
2 Gram Sodium: Serve plain beef patty and plain pasta. May season with SF herbs/spices.
Gluten Free: Use gluten free macaroni. Prepare foods separately to prevent cross contamination.
Allergy Alerts: When an "X" is present, this indicates the allergen is present.
Always read all food labels to ensure allergens are not present.

Wheat	Milk	Eggs	Fish Shellfish	Soy	Peanuts/Nuts	Other
X	X	X				

Key: SF= Salt Free D= Diet or Sugarfree LF = Lowfat FF = Fat Free GF = Gluten Free

Copyright 2020 Jacqueline Larson M.S., R.D.N. and Associates.   All Rights Reserved

Recipe Name: Porcupine Meat Balls
Recipe Category: Dinner Entrée
Portion Size: 4 oz.
Ingredients: Yields: 8 servings

Ingredients	Notes:
2 1/2 pounds lean ground beef	
1 teaspoon salt	
2 tablespoons minced onion	Wash, peel and mince
1/2 cup cooked rice	May use brown rice
1/2 teaspoon pepper	
2 cans low sodium tomato sauce	
1 teaspoon basil	
1 tablespoon sugar	
1 teaspoon garlic powder	
1 teaspoon oregano	

Directions:

Steps:	Directions:	Critical Control Point /Quality Assurance
1	Combine meat, salt, pepper, and onion.	
2	Shape into balls.	
3	Brown in a skillet.	
4	Drain fat.	
5	Combine tomato sauce with basil, sugar, garlic powder and oregano.	
6	Pour over meat balls.	
7	Cook about 30 minutes over low heat.	Cook until internal temperature reaches 165 F degrees for 15 seconds

Time Temperature Sensitive food. *Food safety Standards: hold food for service at an internal temperature above 140° F. Do not mix old product with new. Cool leftover product quickly (within 4 hours) to below 41° F. Follow proper cooling procedures. Store leftovers in a tightly sealed, labeled and dated container. Use leftover within 72 hours if stored in refrigerator or 30 days if stored in the freezer. Reheat leftover product quickly (within 2 hours) to 165 degrees F for 15 seconds. Reheat left over product only once; discard if not used. Cold holding at 41°F or colder or using time alone (less than four hours). Always wash hands and wash and sanitize counter tops utensils and containers between steps when working with raw meat.*

Texture Modified Diets:

Soft & Bite Size: (aka Bite size) **Food particle size ½ inch (~width of standard fork)** Food must be moist. Cut foods with a knife to a ½" particle size after cooking. Moisten with broth as needed.

Chopped: Food particle size ¼ inch (~ ½ width of standard fork) Food must be moist. Chop foods with a knife to 1/4" particle size after cooking. Moisten with broth as needed.

Minced and Moist:(aka Minced/Mechanical Soft/Ground) **Food particle size 1/8 inch (fits through prongs of standard fork)** Food must be moist. Use a food processor to grind food particles into 1/8 inch after cooking. Moisten with broth as needed.

Pureed: Smooth and cohesive. Use a food processor to puree to a smooth consistency. Foods are processed by grinding and then pureeing them. May add broth or sauce to puree. Do not add to much liquid. Puree should still hold its shape. Must not be firm or sticky. Puree foods while still hot. Appearance should be smooth like pudding. Serve ½ c. puree meat topped with tomato sauce.

Therapeutic Modified Diets:

Lowfat: No changes needed
Diabetic/No added Sugar/No Conc. Sweets/Calorie Controlled: No changes needed
Bland/Anti Reflux: omit onion, pepper, tomato sauce, basil, garlic powder and oregano (so sauce)
Liberal House Renal: Omit salt, no sauce
No Added Salt: no changes needed
2 Gram Sodium: omit salt, no sauce
Gluten Free: No changes needed. Prepare foods separately to prevent cross contamination.
Allergy Alerts: When an "X" is present, this indicates the allergen is present.
Always read all food labels to ensure allergens are not present.

Wheat	Milk	Eggs	Fish Shellfish	Soy	Peanuts/Nuts	Other

Key: SF= Salt Free D= Diet or Sugarfree LF = Lowfat FF = Fat Free GF = Gluten Free

Recipe Name: Pot Roast in Foil
Recipe Category: Dinner Entrée
Portion Size: 3 oz.
Ingredients: **Yields: 8 servings**

Ingredients	Notes:
3 to 4 Pounds chuck roast or 7 bone roast	Trim all visible fat
1 Package dehydrated onion soup mix	Or use 4 teaspoons beef bouillon granules, 3 tablespoons dried onion flakes, 2 teaspoons onion powder, 1 teaspoon garlic powder and ½ teaspoon black pepper.

Directions:

Steps:	Directions:	Critical Control Point / Quality Assurance
1	Preheat oven to 300 degrees.	
2	Place roast in large piece of foil and sprinkle with soup mix.	
3	Wrap the roast carefully with the foil, seaming so that no juices can escape.	
4	Place the package in a pan and bake 3 1/2 to 4 hours.	
**	This may also be cooked in a crock pot for 6 to 8 hours on high heat or 8 to 10 hours on low heat.	Cook until internal temperature reaches 165 F degrees

Time Temperature Sensitive food. *Food safety Standards: hold food for service at an internal temperature above 140° F. Do not mix old product with new. Cool leftover product quickly (within 4 hours) to below 41° F. Follow proper cooling procedures. Store leftovers in a tightly sealed, labeled and dated container. Use leftover within 72 hours if stored in refrigerator or 30 days if stored in the freezer. Reheat leftover product quickly (within 2 hours) to 165 degrees F for 15 seconds. Reheat left over product only once; discard if not used. Cold holding at 41°F or colder or using time alone (less than four hours). Always wash hands and wash and sanitize counter tops utensils and containers between steps when working with raw meat.*

Texture Modified Diets:

Soft & Bite Size: (aka Bite size) **Food particle size ½ inch (~width of standard fork)** Food must be moist. Cut foods with a knife to a ½" particle size after cooking. Moisten with broth as needed.

Chopped: Food particle size ¼ inch (~ ½ width of standard fork) Food must be moist. Chop foods with a knife to 1/4" particle size after cooking. Moisten with broth as needed.

Minced and Moist:(aka Minced/Mechanical Soft/Ground) **Food particle size 1/8 inch (fits through prongs of standard fork)** Food must be moist. Use a food processor to grind food particles into 1/8 inch after cooking. Moisten with broth as needed.

Pureed: Smooth and cohesive. Use a food processor to puree to a smooth consistency. Foods are processed by grinding and then pureeing them. May add broth or sauce to puree. Do not add to much liquid. Puree should still hold its shape. Must not be firm or sticky. Puree foods while still hot. Appearance should be smooth like pudding. Serve ½ c. meat serving.

Therapeutic Modified Diets:

Lowfat: No changes needed
Diabetic/No added Sugar/No Conc. Sweets/Calorie Controlled: No changes needed
Bland/Anti Reflux: omit dehydrated onion mix
Liberal House Renal: Omit dehydrated onion mix. May season with SF herb/spices and a diced onion..
No Added Salt: Omit dehydrated onion mix. May season with SF herb/spices and a diced onion.
2 Gram Sodium: omit dehydrated onion mix. May season with SF herb/spices and a diced onion.
Gluten Free: Omit onion soup mix. Season with salt, diced onion and pepper. Prepare foods separately to prevent cross contamination.
Allergy Alerts: When an "X" is present, this indicates the allergen is present.
Always read all food labels to ensure allergens are not present.

Wheat	Milk	Eggs	Fish Shellfish	Soy	Peanuts/Nuts	Other
X				X		

Key: SF= Salt Free D= Diet or Sugarfree LF = Lowfat FF = Fat Free GF = Gluten Free

Recipe Name: Pot Roast with Potatoes and Carrots
Recipe Category: Dinner Entrée
Portion Size: 3 oz. meat, ½ cup potatoes, ½ cup carrots
Ingredients: **Yields: 8 servings**

Ingredients	Notes:
3 1/2 to 4 Pounds rib roast, rolled rib roast, sirloin rib roast, eye of round or rolled rib roast (boneless)	Trim all visible fat
2 teaspoon paprika	
½ teaspoon dried basil	
½ teaspoon dried oregano	
½ teaspoon thyme	
1 teaspoon garlic powder	
½ cup water	
½ cup red wine vinegar	
1 can (14 oz.) low sodium beef broth	
8 medium Red potatoes (4 cups)	Wash and trim
½ teaspoon salt	
¼ teaspoon black pepper	
8 carrots, cut into 1 ½ inch thick pieces (4 cups)	Wash, trim and peel

Directions:

Steps:	Directions:	Critical Control Point / Quality Assurance
1	Preheat oven to 300 degrees.	
2	Place in a large pot coated with cooking spray over medium-high heat.	
3	Season roast with paprika, basil, oregano, thyme, and garlic.	
4	Add roast to heated pot and brown all sides.	
5	Remove from pan; reduce heat to medium.	
6	Add onion; sauté 10 minutes.	
7	Add water, vinegar, and broth; bring to boil.	
8	Peel a half inch strip around each potato.	
9	Stir in salt, pepper, carrots and potatoes.	
10	Return roast to pan.	
11	Cover and bake at 300 degree for 2 hours.	Thermometer reading should be 165 degrees

Time Temperature Sensitive food. *Food safety Standards: hold food for service at an internal temperature above 140° F. Do not mix old product with new. Cool leftover product quickly (within 4 hours) to below 41° F. Follow proper cooling procedures. Store leftovers in a tightly sealed, labeled and dated container. Use leftover within 72 hours if stored in refrigerator or 30 days if stored in the freezer. Reheat leftover product quickly (within 2 hours) to 165 degrees F for 15 seconds. Reheat left over product only once; discard if not used. Cold holding at 41 °F or colder or using time alone (less than four hours). Always wash hands and wash and sanitize counter tops utensils and containers between steps when working with raw meat.*

Texture Modified Diets:

Soft & Bite Size: (aka Bite size) **Food particle size ½ inch (~width of standard fork)** Food must be moist. Peel potatoes. Cut foods with a knife to a ½" particle size after cooking. Moisten with broth as needed.

Chopped: Food particle size ¼ inch (~ ½ width of standard fork) Food must be moist. Peel potatoes Chop foods with a knife to 1/4" particle size after cooking. Moisten with broth as needed.

Minced and Moist: (aka Minced/Mechanical Soft/Ground) **Food particle size 1/8 inch (fits through prongs of standard fork)** Food must be moist. Peel potatoes Use a food processor to grind food particles into 1/8 inch after cooking. Moisten with broth as needed.

Pureed: Smooth and cohesive. Peel potatoes Use a food processor to puree to a smooth consistency. Foods are processed by grinding and then pureeing them. May add broth or sauce to puree. Do not add to much liquid. Puree should still hold its shape. Must not be firm or sticky. Puree foods while still hot. Appearance should be smooth like pudding.
Serve ½ c. meat, ½ c. puree potatoes and ½ c. puree carrots separately.

Therapeutic Modified Diets:

Lowfat: No changes needed
Diabetic/No added Sugar/No Conc. Sweets/Calorie Controlled: No changes needed
Bland/Anti Reflux: omit paprika, basil, oregano, thyme, garlic powder, red wine vinegar and pepper. Peel potatoes.
Liberal House Renal: Omit salt, Use SF broth or water
No Added Salt: No changes needed
2 Gram Sodium: omit salt, Use SF broth or water
Gluten Free: Use GF broth. Prepare foods separately to prevent cross contamination.

Allergy Alerts: When an "X" is present, this indicates the allergen is present. Always read all food labels to ensure allergens are not present.

Wheat	Milk	Eggs	Fish Shellfish	Soy	Peanuts/Nuts	Other
X						

Key: SF= Salt Free D= Diet or Sugarfree LF = Lowfat FF = Fat Free GF = Gluten Free

Copyright 2020 Jacqueline Larson M.S., R.D.N. and Associates.   All Rights Reserved

Recipe Name: Roast Beef and Gravy
Recipe Category: Dinner Entrée
Portion Size: 3 oz. beef with 2 tablespoons gravy
Ingredients: Yields: 8 servings

Ingredients	Notes:
3 1/2 to 4 Pounds rib roast, rolled rib roast, sirloin rib roast, eye of round or rolled rib roast (boneless)	Trim all visible fat
Seasonings of choice: salt, pepper, garlic powder, seasoning salt, etc.	
Gravy	
1/4 cup drippings	
3 tablespoons flour	
Salt and pepper to taste	
2 cups low sodium beef stock or water	

Directions:

Steps:	Directions:	Critical Control Point /Quality Assurance
1	Preheat oven to 550 degrees.	
2	Place roast in a roasting pan and season well.	
3	Do not cover and do not add liquid.	
4	Immediately reduce heat to 350 degrees.	
5	Roast 18 to 20 minutes to the pound for medium rare.	Thermometer reading should be between 140 degrees (rare) and 170 degrees (well done.)
6	A rolled roast requires 5 to 10 minutes longer to the pound. Serve sliced thinly across the grain.	
	Gravy	
1	Remove the meat from the pan.	
2	Place it where it will remain hot.	
3	Pour off all but 1/4 cup of drippings.	
4	Blend flour into drippings.	
5	Stir with a wire whisk until the flour has thickened and until the mixture is well combined and smooth.	
6	Continue to cook slowly stir constantly while adding stock.	
7	Cook until desired consistency.	
8	Season with salt and pepper.	

Time Temperature Sensitive food. *Food safety Standards: hold food for service at an internal temperature above 140° F. Do not mix old product with new. Cool leftover product quickly (within 4 hours) to below 41°F. Follow proper cooling procedures. Store leftovers in a tightly sealed, labeled and dated container. Use leftover within 72 hours if stored in refrigerator or 30 days if stored in the freezer. Reheat leftover product quickly (within 2 hours) to 165 degrees F for 15 seconds. Reheat left over product only once; discard if not used. Cold holding at 41°F or colder or using time alone (less than four hours). Always wash hands and wash and sanitize counter tops utensils and containers between steps when working with raw meat.*

Texture Modified Diets:
Soft & Bite Size: (aka Bite size) **Food particle size ½ inch (~width of standard fork)** Food must be moist. Cut foods with a knife to a ½" particle size after cooking. Moisten with broth as needed.
Chopped: Food particle size ¼ inch (~ ½ width of standard fork) Food must be moist. Chop foods with a knife to 1/4" particle size after cooking. Moisten with broth as needed.
Minced and Moist: (aka Minced/Mechanical Soft/Ground) **Food particle size 1/8 inch (fits through prongs of standard fork)** Food must be moist. Use a food processor to grind food particles into 1/8 inch after cooking. Moisten with broth as needed.
Pureed: Smooth and cohesive. Use a food processor to puree to a smooth consistency. Foods are processed by grinding and then pureeing them. May add broth or sauce to puree. Do not add to much liquid. Puree should still hold its shape. Must not be firm or sticky. Puree foods while still hot. Appearance should be smooth like pudding.
Serve ½ c. meat serving.

Therapeutic Modified Diets:
Lowfat: No changes needed
Diabetic/No added Sugar/No Conc. Sweets/Calorie Controlled: No changes needed
Bland/Anti Reflux: omit seasonings except salt
Liberal House Renal: Omit salt and gravy
No Added Salt: No changes needed
2 Gram Sodium: omit salt and gravy
Gluten Free: Use GF flour and GF broth. Prepare foods separately to prevent cross contamination.
Allergy Alerts: When an "X" is present, this indicates the allergen is present.
Always read all food labels to ensure allergens are not present.

Wheat	Milk	Eggs	Fish Shellfish	Soy	Peanuts/Nuts	Other
X						

Key: SF= Salt Free D= Diet or Sugarfree LF = Lowfat FF = Fat Free GF = Gluten Free

Recipe Name: Salisbury Steak
Recipe Category: Dinner Entrée
Portion Size: 4 oz.
Ingredients: **Yields: 8 servings**

Ingredients	Notes:
4 slices of bread	May use whole wheat
1/2 cup nonfat milk	
2 1/2 pounds lean ground beef	
1 teaspoon salt	
1/4 teaspoon pepper	
1 teaspoon Worcestershire sauce	
4 strips lean turkey bacon, cooked and crumbled	
2/3 cup bread crumbs	

Directions:

Steps:	Directions:	Critical Control Point / Quality Assurance
1	Remove the crusts from the bread and soak bread in the milk until soft.	
2	Squeeze our excess milk, then lightly mix the moist bread with the ground beef until thoroughly absorbed.	
3	Add the salt, pepper and Worcestershire sauce and shape into a large round about 1 inch thick.	Divide into 8 servings.
4	Preheat the broiler.	
5	Place meat on an oiled broiler rack and cook 4 inches from heat on one side for 5 minutes, then turn and sprinkle the bacon and the bread crumbs over the top and broil another 5-6 minutes until done.	Cook until internal temperature reaches 165 F degrees for 15 seconds

Time Temperature Sensitive food. *Food safety Standards: hold food for service at an internal temperature above 140° F. Do not mix old product with new. Cool leftover product quickly (within 4 hours) to below 41° F. Follow proper cooling procedures. Store leftovers in a tightly sealed, labeled and dated container. Use leftover within 72 hours if stored in refrigerator or 30 days if stored in the freezer. Reheat leftover product quickly (within 2 hours) to 165 degrees F for 15 seconds. Reheat left over product only once; discard if not used. Cold holding at 41°F or colder or using time alone (less than four hours). Always wash hands and wash and sanitize counter tops utensils and containers between steps when working with raw meat.*

Texture Modified Diets:
Soft & Bite Size: (aka Bite size) **Food particle size ½ inch (~width of standard fork)** Food must be moist. Cut foods with a knife to a ½" particle size after cooking. Moisten with broth as needed.

Chopped: Food particle size ¼ inch (~ ½ width of standard fork) Food must be moist. Chop foods with a knife to 1/4" particle size after cooking. Moisten with broth as needed.

Minced and Moist: (aka Minced/Mechanical Soft/Ground) **Food particle size 1/8 inch (fits through prongs of standard fork)** Food must be moist. Use a food processor to grind food particles into 1/8 inch after cooking. Moisten with broth as needed.

Pureed: Smooth and cohesive. Use a food processor to puree to a smooth consistency. Foods are processed by grinding and then pureeing them. May add broth or sauce to puree. Do not add to much liquid. Puree should still hold its shape. Must not be firm or sticky. Puree foods while still hot. Appearance should be smooth like pudding. Serve ½ c. meat serving.

Therapeutic Modified Diets:
Lowfat: No changes needed
Diabetic/No added Sugar/No Conc. Sweets/Calorie Controlled: No changes needed
Bland/Anti Reflux: omit pepper, Worcestershire sauce and bacon
Liberal House Renal: Omit salt, Worcestershire sauce, bread crumbs, bread and bacon
No Added Salt: Omit bacon.
2 Gram Sodium: omit salt, Worcestershire sauce, bread crumbs, bread and bacon.
Gluten Free: Use gluten free bread and omit bread crumbs. Use GF oats in place of bread crumbs Prepare foods separately to prevent cross contamination.
Allergy Alerts: When an "X" is present, this indicates the allergen is present.
Always read all food labels to ensure allergens are not present.

Wheat	Milk	Eggs	Fish Shellfish	Soy	Peanuts/Nuts	Other
X	X	X	X			

Key: SF= Salt Free D= Diet or Sugarfree LF = Lowfat FF = Fat Free GF = Gluten Free

Copyright 2020 Jacqueline Larson M.S., R.D.N. and Associates.   All Rights Reserved

Recipe Name: Sauerbraten
Recipe Category: Dinner Entrée
Portion Size: 3 oz. meat and 2 Tablespoon sauce
Ingredients: **Yields: 8 servings**

Ingredients	Notes:
3 1/2 to 4 Pounds Beef shoulder, chuck, rump or round (boneless)	Trim all visible fat
1 teaspoon salt	
1 teaspoon peppercorn	
1/4 cup sugar	
1 tablespoon vegetable oil	
2 cups vinegar	
1/2 cup diced onion	
2 cups water	
2 Bay leaves	
1/4 cup brown sugar	
1/4 cup cornstarch, mixed with 1/2 cup water	
1 cup low fat cream or low fat sour cream	

Directions:

Steps:	Directions:	Critical Control Point /Quality Assurance
1	Season beef with salt.	
2	Combine vinegar, water, onions, bay leaves, sugar and bay leaves.	
3	Heat marinate but do not boil.	
4	Place meat in a deep crock or glass bowl.	
5	Pour the marinade over beef; more than half should be covered.	
6	Cover with a lid and refrigerate for 1-2 days, turning occasionally.	
7	Heat oil in a heavy pan.	
8	Brown beef on both sides.	
9	Sprinkle meat with brown sugar.	
10	Add marinate and cook until beef is tender. Remove meat. Slowly add cornstarch and water. Heat until thick.	Cook until internal temperature reaches 165 F degrees for 4 minutes
11	Add cream or sour cream and serve immediately.	

Time Temperature Sensitive food. *Food safety Standards: hold food for service at an internal temperature above 140° F. Do not mix old product with new. Cool leftover product quickly (within 4 hours) to below 41° F. Follow proper cooling procedures. Store leftovers in a tightly sealed, labeled and dated container. Use leftover within 72 hours if stored in refrigerator or 30 days if stored in the freezer. Reheat leftover product quickly (within 2 hours) to 165 degrees F for 15 seconds. Reheat left over product only once; discard if not used. Cold holding at 41°F or colder or using time alone (less than four hours). Always wash hands and wash and sanitize counter tops utensils and containers between steps when working with raw meat.*

Texture Modified Diets:

Soft & Bite Size: (aka Bite size) **Food particle size ½ inch (~width of standard fork)** Use ground pepper in place of pepper corns. Food must be moist. Cut foods with a knife to a ½" particle size after cooking. Moisten with broth as needed.

Chopped: Food particle size ¼ inch (~ ½ width of standard fork) Use ground pepper in place of pepper corns. Food must be moist. Chop foods with a knife to 1/4" particle size after cooking. Moisten with broth as needed.

Minced and Moist:(aka Minced/Mechanical Soft/Ground) **Food particle size 1/8 inch (fits through prongs of standard fork)** Use ground pepper in place of pepper corns. Food must be moist. Use a food processor to grind food particles into 1/8 inch after cooking. Moisten with broth as needed.

Pureed: Smooth and cohesive. Use ground pepper in place of pepper corns. Use a food processor to puree to a smooth consistency. Foods are processed by grinding and then pureeing them. May add broth or sauce to puree. Do not add to much liquid. Puree should still hold its shape. Must not be firm or sticky. Puree foods while still hot. Appearance should be smooth like pudding. Serve ½ c. meat serving.

Therapeutic Modified Diets:
Lowfat: No changes needed
Diabetic/No added Sugar/No Conc. Sweets/Calorie Controlled: No changes needed
Bland/Anti Reflux: omit peppercorn, onion, and bay leaves
Liberal House Renal: Omit salt and sour cream
No Added Salt: Omit salt
2 Gram Sodium: omit salt
Gluten Free: No changes needed. Prepare foods separately to prevent cross contamination.
Allergy Alerts: When an "X" is present, this indicates the allergen is present. Always read all food labels to ensure allergens are not present.

Wheat	Milk	Eggs	Fish Shellfish	Soy	Peanuts/Nuts	Other
	X					

Key: SF= Salt Free D= Diet or Sugarfree LF = Lowfat FF = Fat Free GF = Gluten Free

Copyright 2020 Jacqueline Larson M.S., R.D.N. and Associates.   All Rights Reserved

Recipe Name: Sauté Beef Liver and Onions
Recipe Category: Dinner Entrée
Portion Size: 4 oz.
Ingredients: **Yields: 8 servings**

Ingredients	Notes:
2 pounds beef liver	
Flour	
1 tablespoon olive oil	
Salt and pepper	
1 large onion sliced	

Directions:

Steps:	Directions:	Critical Control Point / Quality Assurance
1	Coat liver on both sides with flour, salt, and pepper.	
2	Heat olive oil in a large skillet.	
3	Brown liver on both sides.	
4	Add onions and sauté.	

Time Temperature Sensitive food. *Food safety Standards: hold food for service at an internal temperature above 140° F. Do not mix old product with new. Cool leftover product quickly (within 4 hours) to below 41° F. Follow proper cooling procedures. Store leftovers in a tightly sealed, labeled and dated container. Use leftover within 72 hours if stored in refrigerator or 30 days if stored in the freezer. Reheat leftover product quickly (within 2 hours) to 165 degrees F for 15 seconds. Reheat left over product only once; discard if not used. Cold holding at 41 °F or colder or using time alone (less than four hours). Always wash hands and wash and sanitize counter tops utensils and containers between steps when working with raw meat.*

Texture Modified Diets:

Soft & Bite Size: (aka Bite size) **Food particle size ½ inch (~width of standard fork)** Food must be moist. Cut foods with a knife to a ½" particle size after cooking. Moisten with broth as needed.

Chopped: Food particle size ¼ inch (~ ½ width of standard fork) Food must be moist. Chop foods with a knife to 1/4" particle size after cooking. Moisten with broth as needed.

Minced and Moist: (aka Minced/Mechanical Soft/Ground) **Food particle size 1/8 inch (fits through prongs of standard fork)** Food must be moist. Use a food processor to grind food particles into 1/8 inch after cooking. Moisten with broth as needed.

Pureed: Smooth and cohesive. Use a food processor to puree to a smooth consistency. Foods are processed by grinding and then pureeing them. May add broth or sauce to puree. Do not add to much liquid. Puree should still hold its shape. Must not be firm or sticky. Puree foods while still hot. Appearance should be smooth like pudding. Serve ½ c. meat serving.

Therapeutic Modified Diets:
Lowfat: Use alternate menu item
Diabetic/No added Sugar/No Conc. Sweets/Calorie Controlled: No changes needed
Bland/Anti Reflux: use alternate menu item
Liberal House Renal: Omit salt
No Added Salt: No changes needed
2 Gram Sodium: omit salt
Gluten Free: Use gluten free flour. Prepare foods separately to prevent cross contamination.
Allergy Alerts: When an "X" is present, this indicates the allergen is present.
Always read all food labels to ensure allergens are not present.

Wheat	Milk	Eggs	Fish Shellfish	Soy	Peanuts/Nuts	Other
X	X					

Key: SF= Salt Free D= Diet or Sugarfree LF = Lowfat FF = Fat Free GF = Gluten Free

Recipe Name: Shepherds Pie
Recipe Category: Dinner Entrée
Portion Size: 1 cup
Ingredients: **Yields: 8 servings**

Ingredients	Notes:
1 can evaporated fat free milk	
1/2 cup light sour cream	
2 tablespoon flour	
2 1/2 lbs. lean ground beef	
1/2 teaspoon basil or thyme	
1/2 teaspoon salt	
1/4 teaspoon pepper	
1 tablespoon chopped parsley	
4 cups mashed potatoes	See recipe in cookbook
4 cups mixed vegetables	Fresh or frozen
1 tablespoon margarine	

Directions:

Steps:	Directions:	Critical Control Point /Quality Assurance
1	In a large skillet brown ground beef.	
2	Drain excess fat.	
3	Heat and stir sour cream, flour and milk over low heat until thickened in a sauce pan.	
4	Add ground beef basil or thyme, salt, pepper, and parsley.	
5	Preheat oven to 400 degrees.	
6	Spread ground beef in a large baking dish.	
7	Top with mixed vegetables and cover with mashed potatoes.	
8	Brush with margarine.	
9	Bake until potatoes are browned. (about 15 minutes)	Cook until internal temperature reaches 165 F degrees for 15 seconds

Time Temperature Sensitive food. *Food safety Standards: hold food for service at an internal temperature above 140° F. Do not mix old product with new. Cool leftover product quickly (within 4 hours) to below 41° F. Follow proper cooling procedures. Store leftovers in a tightly sealed, labeled and dated container. Use leftover within 72 hours if stored in refrigerator or 30 days if stored in the freezer. Reheat leftover product quickly (within 2 hours) to 165 degrees F for 15 seconds. Reheat left over product only once; discard if not used. Cold holding at 41°F or colder or using time alone (less than four hours). Always wash hands and wash and sanitize counter tops utensils and containers between steps when working with raw meat.*

Texture Modified Diets:

Soft & Bite Size: (aka Bite size) **Food particle size ½ inch (~width of standard fork)** Food must be moist. Cut foods with a knife to a ½" particle size prior to layering. Moisten with broth as needed.

Chopped: Food particle size ¼ inch (~ ½ width of standard fork) Food must be moist. Chop foods with a knife to 1/4" particle size prior to layering. Moisten with broth as needed.

Minced and Moist: (aka Minced/Mechanical Soft/Ground) **Food particle size 1/8 inch (fits through prongs of standard fork)** Food must be moist. Use a food processor to grind food particles into 1/8 inch prior to layering. Moisten with broth as needed.

Pureed: Smooth and cohesive. Use a food processor to puree to a smooth consistency. Foods are processed by grinding and then pureeing them. May add broth or sauce to puree. Do not add to much liquid. Puree should still hold its shape. Must not be firm or sticky. Puree foods while still hot. Appearance should be smooth like pudding. Serve ½ c. meat, ½ cup potatoes and ½ cup vegetables separately.

Therapeutic Modified Diets:

Lowfat: No changes needed
Diabetic/No added Sugar/No Conc. Sweets/Calorie Controlled: No changes needed
Bland/Anti Reflux: omit basil, thyme, pepper, parsley. Use peas and carrots
Liberal House Renal: Serve 3 oz. SF ground beef and rice or pasta
No Added Salt: No changes needed
2 Gram Sodium: Serve 3 oz. SF ground beef patty and SF mashed potatoes
Gluten Free: Use gluten free flour. Prepare foods separately to prevent cross contamination.
Allergy Alerts: When an "X" is present, this indicates the allergen is present.
Always read all food labels to ensure allergens are not present.

Wheat	Milk	Eggs	Fish Shellfish	Soy	Peanuts/Nuts	Other
X	X			X		

Key: SF= Salt Free D= Diet or Sugarfree LF = Lowfat FF = Fat Free GF = Gluten Free

Copyright 2020 Jacqueline Larson M.S., R.D.N. and Associates.   All Rights Reserved

Recipe Name: Sloppy Joe on Bun
Recipe Category: Dinner Entrée
Portion Size: ½ c. on 1 small bun
Ingredients: **Yields: 8 servings**

Ingredients	Notes:
2 1/2 pounds lean ground beef	
1/2 cup minced onion	Wash, peel and mince
1/2 cup celery	Wash, trim and chop fine
1/2 cup green pepper	Wash, trim and chop fine
1 (6 oz.) tomato paste	
¼ cup light corn syrup	
¼ cup white vinegar	
1 teaspoon chili powder	
1 teaspoon Worcestershire sauce	
¼ teaspoon all spice	
¼ teaspoon garlic powder	
¼ teaspoon black pepper	
1/2 cup water	
1/2 teaspoon salt	
8 Small Hamburger buns	May use whole grain

Directions:

Steps:	Directions:	Critical Control Point /Quality Assurance
1	Heat ground beef, onion, celery, and green peppers in a skillet.	
2	Cook until ground beef is no longer pink. Drain fat.	
3	Add tomato paste, corn syrup, vinegar, chili powder, Worcestershire sauce, all spice, garlic powder, black pepper, water, and salt.	
4	Simmer uncover over low heat about 20 minutes until thickened enough to spoon onto buns.	Cook until internal temperature reaches 165 F degrees for 15 seconds

Time Temperature Sensitive food. Food safety Standards: hold food for service at an internal temperature above 140° F. Do not mix old product with new. Cool leftover product quickly (within 4 hours) to below 41° F. Follow proper cooling procedures. Store leftovers in a tightly sealed, labeled and dated container. Use leftover within 72 hours if stored in refrigerator or 30 days if stored in the freezer. Reheat leftover product quickly (within 2 hours) to 165 degrees F for 15 seconds. Reheat left over product only once; discard if not used. Cold holding at 41°F or colder or using time alone (less than four hours). Always wash hands and wash and sanitize counter tops utensils and containers between steps when working with raw meat.

Texture Modified Diets:

Soft & Bite Size: (aka Bite size) **Food particle size ½ inch (~width of standard fork)** Food must be moist. Cut foods with a knife to a ½" particle size prior to layering. Moisten with broth as needed.

Chopped: Food particle size ¼ inch (~ ½ width of standard fork) Food must be moist. Chop foods with a knife to 1/4" particle size prior to layering. Moisten with broth as needed.

Minced and Moist: (aka Minced/Mechanical Soft/Ground) **Food particle size 1/8 inch (fits through prongs of standard fork)** Food must be moist. Use a food processor to grind food particles into 1/8 inch prior to layering. Moisten with broth as needed.

Pureed: Smooth and cohesive. Use a food processor to puree to a smooth consistency. Foods are processed by grinding and then pureeing them. May add broth or sauce to puree. Do not add to much liquid. Puree should still hold its shape. Must not be firm or sticky. Puree foods while still hot. Appearance should be smooth like pudding. Serve ½ c. meat serving separate from 1 cup puree bun.

Therapeutic Modified Diets:

Lowfat: No changes needed
Diabetic/No added Sugar/No Conc. Sweets/Calorie Controlled: No changes needed
Bland/Anti Reflux: Serve plain ground beef on bun. May season with salt
Liberal House Renal: Omit salt, tomato paste, bun and Worcester sauce. Serve ½ cup pasta or rice.
No Added Salt: No changes needed
2 Gram Sodium: omit salt, bun and Worcester sauce. Serve over ½ cup pasta or rice.
Gluten Free: Use gluten free hamburger buns. Prepare foods separately to prevent cross contamination.
Allergy Alerts: When an "X" is present, this indicates the allergen is present.
Always read all food labels to ensure allergens are not present.

Wheat	Milk	Eggs	Fish Shellfish	Soy	Peanuts/Nuts	Other
X	X	X	X			

Key: SF= Salt Free D= Diet or Sugarfree LF = Lowfat FF = Fat Free GF = Gluten Free

Recipe Name: Spaghetti and Meat Sauce
Recipe Category: Dinner Entrée
Portion Size: ½ cup sauce and ½ c. pasta
Ingredients: **Yields: 8 servings**

Ingredients	Notes:
2 1/2 pounds lean ground beef	
1/2 pound fresh mushrooms (optional)	Wash, trim and slice
1 large chopped onion	Wash, peel and chop
1 teaspoon garlic powder	
3/4 teaspoon salt	
1/8 teaspoon pepper	
2 1/2 cups low sodium tomato sauce	
1/2 teaspoon basil	
1/2 teaspoon oregano	
1 pound spaghetti	May use whole wheat spaghetti
¼ cup Grated Parmesan cheese	

Directions:

Steps:	Directions:	Critical Control Point /Quality Assurance
1	Prepare spaghetti according to directions on the package.	
2	Sauté ground beef, onion, and mushroom in a medium size sauce pan.	
3	Drain grease.	
4	Add garlic powder, salt, pepper, basil, oregano, and tomato sauce.	
5	Simmer over low heat for 20 minutes.	Cook until internal temperature reaches 165 F degrees for 15 seconds
6	Serve the spaghetti on a hot platter.	
7	First a layer of pasta, then a layer of sauce.	
8	Sprinkle with parmesan cheese.	

Time Temperature Sensitive food. *Food safety Standards: hold food for service at an internal temperature above 140° F. Do not mix old product with new. Cool leftover product quickly (within 4 hours) to below 41° F. Follow proper cooling procedures. Store leftovers in a tightly sealed, labeled and dated container. Use leftover within 72 hours if stored in refrigerator or 30 days if stored in the freezer. Reheat leftover product quickly (within 2 hours) to 165 degrees F for 15 seconds. Reheat left over product only once; discard if not used. Cold holding at 41°F or colder or using time alone (less than four hours). Always wash hands and wash and sanitize counter tops utensils and containers between steps when working with raw meat.*

Texture Modified Diets: Tip: Use pasta in correct particle size.

Soft & Bite Size: (aka Bite size) **Food particle size ½ inch (~width of standard fork)** Food must be moist. Cut foods with a knife to a ½" particle size prior to layering. Moisten with broth as needed.

Chopped: Food particle size ¼ inch (~ ½ width of standard fork) Food must be moist. Chop foods with a knife to 1/4" particle size prior to layering. Moisten with broth as needed.

Minced and Moist: (aka Minced/Mechanical Soft/Ground) **Food particle size 1/8 inch (fits through prongs of standard fork)** Food must be moist. Use a food processor to grind food particles into 1/8 inch prior to layering. Moisten with broth as needed.

Pureed: Smooth and cohesive. Use a food processor to puree to a smooth consistency. Foods are processed by grinding and then pureeing them. May add broth or sauce to puree. Do not add to much liquid. Puree should still hold its shape. Must not be firm or sticky. Puree foods while still hot. Appearance should be smooth like pudding. Serve ½ c. meat serving and ½ cup puree pasta separately.

Therapeutic Modified Diets:

Lowfat: No changes needed
Diabetic/No added Sugar/No Conc. Sweets/Calorie Controlled: No changes needed
Bland/Anti Reflux: omit onion, garlic powder, pepper, tomato sauce, basil, oregano
Liberal House Renal: Omit salt, tomato sauce and Parmesan cheese
No Added Salt: No changes needed
2 Gram Sodium: omit salt and Parmesan cheese.
Gluten Free: Use gluten free spaghetti. Prepare foods separately to prevent cross contamination.
Allergy Alerts: When an "X" is present, this indicates the allergen is present.
Always read all food labels to ensure allergens are not present.

Wheat	Milk	Eggs	Fish Shellfish	Soy	Peanuts/Nuts	Other
X	X	X				

Key: SF= Salt Free D= Diet or Sugarfree LF = Lowfat FF = Fat Free GF = Gluten Free

Recipe Name: Steak with Barley and Kale Salad
Recipe Category: Dinner Entrée
Portion Size: 3 oz. meat and 1 cup Kale salad
Ingredients: **Yields: 8 servings**

Ingredients	Notes:
8 beef Tenderloin Steaks, cut 1 inch thick (about 4 ounces each)	Trim all visible fat
1/4 plus 1/8 teaspoon cracked black pepper, divided	
Salt	
3 cloves garlic, minced, divided	Wash, peel and mine
4 cup reduced-sodium beef broth	
2 cup pearlized barley	
4 cups thinly sliced kale	Wash, trim, and slice thin. Remove tough stems
1/2 cup dried sweetened cranberries or cherries	
3 tablespoons sliced almonds	
3 teaspoons fresh lemon juice	

Directions:

Steps:	Directions:	Critical Control Point /Quality Assurance
1	Combine 1 clove garlic and 1/4 teaspoon pepper; press evenly onto beef steaks.	
2	Combine beef broth, barley, remaining 2 cloves garlic and remaining 1/8 teaspoon pepper in small saucepan.	
3	Bring to a boil; reduce heat to low.	
4	Cover and simmer 35 to 45 minutes or until most broth has been absorbed and barley is tender.	May need to add more water.
5	Remove from heat.	
6	Stir in kale and cranberries.	
7	Cover; let stand 5 minutes.	
8	Stir in almonds and lemon juice.	
9	Season with salt, as desired.	
10	Meanwhile, place steaks on rack in broiler pan so surface of steaks is 2 to 3 inches from heat, turning once.	Broil 13 to 16 minutes for medium rare (145°F) to medium (160°F) doneness,
11	Season steaks with salt. Slice thinly across the grain	
12	Serve with barley mixture.	

Time Temperature Sensitive food. *Food safety Standards: hold food for service at an internal temperature above 140° F. Do not mix old product with new. Cool leftover product quickly (within 4 hours) to below 41° F. Follow proper cooling procedures. Reheat leftover product quickly (within 2 hours) to 165 degrees F for 15 seconds. Cold holding at 41°F or colder or using time alone (less than four hours).*

Texture Modified Diets:

Soft & Bite Size: (aka Bite size) **Food particle size ½ inch (~width of standard fork)** Food must be moist. Cut foods with a knife to a ½" particle size prior to mixing. Moisten with broth as needed. Foods that do not process well should be omitted. Omit: almond and dried cranberries or cherries

Chopped: Food particle size ¼ inch (~ ½ width of standard fork) Food must be moist. Chop foods with a knife to 1/4" particle size prior to mixing. Moisten with broth as needed. Foods that do not process well should be omitted. Omit: almond and dried cranberries or cherries

Minced and Moist: (aka Minced/Mechanical Soft/Ground) **Food particle size 1/8 inch (fits through prongs of standard fork)** Food must be moist. Use a food processor to grind food particles into 1/8 inch prior to mixing. Moisten with broth as needed. Foods that do not process well should be omitted. Omit: almond and dried cranberries or cherries

Pureed: Smooth and cohesive. Use a food processor to puree to a smooth consistency. Foods are processed by grinding and then pureeing them. May add broth or sauce to puree. Do not add to much liquid. Puree should still hold its shape. Must not be firm or sticky. Puree foods while still hot. Appearance should be smooth like pudding. Foods that do not process well should be omitted. Omit: almond and dried cranberries or cherries. Serve ½ c. meat and 1 cup puree barley mixture separately..

Therapeutic Modified Diets:
Lowfat: No changes needed
Diabetic/No added Sugar/No Conc. Sweets/Calorie Controlled: No changes needed
Bland/Anti Reflux: omit black pepper, garlic and almonds. Cook kale.
Liberal House Renal: Omit salt. Use SF broth or water.
No Added Salt: no changes
2 Gram Sodium: omit salt. Use SF broth or water
Gluten Free: Substitute rice or quinoa for barley.

Allergy Alerts: When an "X" is present, this indicates the allergen is present. Always read all food labels to ensure allergens are not present.

Wheat	Milk	Eggs	Fish Shellfish	Soy	Peanuts/Nuts	Other
X						

Key: SF= Salt Free D= Diet or Sugarfree LF = Lowfat FF = Fat Free GF = Gluten Free

Recipe Name: Stuffed Peppers
Recipe Category: Dinner Entrée
Portion Size: 4 oz. meat
Ingredients: **Yields: 8 servings**

Ingredients	Notes:
2 1/2 pounds lean ground beef	
8 medium green peppers	Wash, , remove stem and seeds, leave whole to stuff
1/2 cup chopped onion	Wash, peel and chop
1 cup whole kernel corn	Use frozen and low salt canned
2 cans low sodium tomato sauce	
1 cup cooked rice	May use brown rice
1 teaspoon salt	
1/4 teaspoon pepper	

Directions:

Steps:	Directions:	Critical Control Point /Quality Assurance
1	In a large kettle over medium high heat, blanch peppers in boiling salted water for 3 to 5 minutes.	
2	Drain and rinse in cold water; set aside.	
3	In a skillet over medium heat brown beef and onion; drain.	
4	Add onion, corn, salt, pepper and rice. Mix well.	
5	Loosely stuff into peppers.	
6	Place in a baking pan. Pour tomato sauce over peppers.	
7	Bake, uncovered, at 350 degrees for 30 to 35 minutes or until peppers are done and filling is hot.	Cook until internal temperature reaches 165 F degrees for 15 seconds

Time Temperature Sensitive food. *Food safety Standards: hold food for service at an internal temperature above 140° F. Do not mix old product with new. Cool leftover product quickly (within 4 hours) to below 41° F. Follow proper cooling procedures. Store leftovers in a tightly sealed, labeled and dated container. Use leftover within 72 hours if stored in refrigerator or 30 days if stored in the freezer. Reheat leftover product quickly (within 2 hours) to 165 degrees F for 15 seconds. Reheat left over product only once; discard if not used. Cold holding at 41°F or colder or using time alone (less than four hours). Always wash hands and wash and sanitize counter tops utensils and containers between steps when working with raw meat.*

<u>*Texture Modified Diets:*</u>

Soft & Bite Size: (aka Bite size) **Food particle size ½ inch (~width of standard fork)** Food must be moist. Cut foods with a knife to a ½" particle size prior to mixing. Peppers can be mixed with tomato sauce and poured over meat. Moisten with broth as needed. Foods that do not process well should be omitted. Omit: corn

Chopped: Food particle size ¼ inch (~ ½ width of standard fork) Food must be moist. Chop foods with a knife to 1/4" particle size prior to mixing. Peppers can be mixed with tomato sauce and poured over meat. Moisten with broth as needed. Foods that do not process well should be omitted. Omit: corn

Minced and Moist: (aka Minced/Mechanical Soft/Ground) **Food particle size 1/8 inch (fits through prongs of standard fork)** Food must be moist. Use a food processor to grind food particles into 1/8 inch prior to mixing. Peppers can be mixed with tomato sauce and poured over meat. Moisten with broth as needed. Foods that do not process well should be omitted. Omit: corn

Pureed: Smooth and cohesive. Use a food processor to puree to a smooth consistency. Foods are processed by grinding and then pureeing them. May add broth or sauce to puree. Do not add to much liquid. Puree should still hold its shape. Must not be firm or sticky. Puree foods while still hot. Appearance should be smooth like pudding. Foods that do not process well should be omitted. Omit: corn. Serve. ½ c. puree meat and ½ c. puree pepper/tomato mixture separately.

<u>*Therapeutic Modified Diets:*</u>

Lowfat: No changes needed
Diabetic/No added Sugar/No Conc. Sweets/Calorie Controlled: No changes needed
Bland/Anti Reflux: omit peppers, onion, corn, tomato sauce and pepper
Liberal House Renal: Omit salt and tomato sauce
No Added Salt: no changes needed
2 Gram Sodium: omit salt and tomato sauce. May top with fresh tomatoes
Gluten Free: No changes needed. Prepare foods separately to prevent cross contamination.
Allergy Alerts: When an "X" is present, this indicates the allergen is present.
Always read all food labels to ensure allergens are not present.

Wheat	Milk	Eggs	FishShellfish	Soy	Peanuts/Nuts	Other

Key: SF= Salt Free D= Diet or Sugarfree LF = Lowfat FF = Fat Free GF = Gluten Free

Recipe Name: Stuffed Potatoes with Chili
Recipe Category: Dinner Entrée
Portion Size: ½ cup chili, 1 small potato
Ingredients: Yields: 8 servings

Ingredients	Notes:
1 tablespoon chili powder	
1 teaspoon garlic powder,	
2 tablespoons minced onion	Wash, peel and mince
1 teaspoon sugar	
1 teaspoon ground cumin	
1 teaspoon salt	
1/2 teaspoon paprika	
1 1/2 Pound lean ground beef or turkey	
1 can (15 1/4 ounce) low sodium kidney beans,	Drained and rinsed
1 can (14 1/2 ounce) low sodium whole peeled tomatoes, undrained and cut up	
1 cup water	
8 Medium potatoes, washed and pierced with fork	
2 cups (8 ounces) grated low fat cheddar cheese	
1/2 cup thinly sliced green onions	

Directions:

Steps:	Directions:	Critical Control Point /Quality Assurance
1	In a large skillet brown ground beef or turkey. Drain excess fat.	Cook until internal temperature reaches 165 F degrees for 15 seconds
2	Stir in chili powder, onion, garlic, sugar, cumin, salt and paprika.	
3	Add kidney beans, water and tomatoes. Bring to boil. Reduce heat simmer 20 minutes.	
4	Microwave potatoes on high 25 minutes, turning over after 12 minutes	Or follow recipe for baked potatoes
5	Slit potatoes lengthwise and pull back skin.	
6	Fluff with a fork. Top each potatoes with prepared chili, cheese, and onions.	

Time Temperature Sensitive food. *Food safety Standards: hold food for service at an internal temperature above 140° F. Do not mix old product with new. Cool leftover product quickly (within 4 hours) to below 41° F. Follow proper cooling procedures. Store leftovers in a tightly sealed, labeled and dated container. Use leftover within 72 hours if stored in refrigerator or 30 days if stored in the freezer. Reheat leftover product quickly (within 2 hours) to 165 degrees F for 15 seconds. Reheat left over product only once; discard if not used. Cold holding at 41°F or colder or using time alone (less than four hours). Always wash hands and wash and sanitize counter tops utensils and containers between steps when working with raw meat.*

Texture Modified Diets:

Soft & Bite Size: (aka Bite size) **Food particle size ½ inch (~width of standard fork)** Food must be moist. Cut foods with a knife to a ½" particle size prior to mixing. Moisten with broth as needed. Foods that do not process well should be omitted. Omit: green onion

Chopped: Food particle size ¼ inch (~ ½ width of standard fork) Food must be moist. Chop foods with a knife to 1/4" particle size prior to mixing. Moisten with broth as needed. Foods that do not process well should be omitted. Omit: Omit: green onion

Minced and Moist:(aka Minced/Mechanical Soft/Ground) **Food particle size 1/8 inch (fits through prongs of standard fork)** Food must be moist. Use a food processor to grind food particles into 1/8 inch prior to mixing. Moisten with broth as needed. Foods that do not process well should be omitted. Omit: Omit: green onion

Pureed: Smooth and cohesive. Use a food processor to puree to a smooth consistency. Foods are processed by grinding and then pureeing them. May add broth or sauce to puree. Do not add to much liquid. Puree should still hold its shape. Must not be firm or sticky. Puree foods while still hot. Appearance should be smooth like pudding. Foods that do not process well should be omitted. Omit: Omit: green onion Serve ½ c. puree chili and ½ cup puree peeled potato separately. No onions, Melt cheese on potato

Therapeutic Modified Diets:

Lowfat: No changes needed
Diabetic/No added Sugar/No Conc. Sweets/Calorie Controlled: No changes needed
Bland/Anti Reflux: omit chili powder, garlic powder, onion, sugar, ground cumin, paprika, kidney beans, tomatoes, green onions
Liberal House Renal: Omit salt, tomatoes and cheese
No Added Salt: No changes needed
2 Gram Sodium: omit salt, tomatoes and cheese. May use fresh tomatoes
Gluten Free: No changes needed. Prepare foods separately to prevent cross contamination.

Allergy Alerts: When an "X" is present, this indicates the allergen is present. Always read all food labels to ensure allergens are not present.

Wheat	Milk	Eggs	Fish Shellfish	Soy	Peanuts/Nuts	Other
	X					

Key: SF= Salt Free D= Diet or Sugarfree LF = Lowfat FF = Fat Free GF = Gluten Free

Copyright 2020 Jacqueline Larson M.S., R.D.N. and Associates.   All Rights Reserved

Recipe Name: Stuffing Hamburger Casserole
Recipe Category: Dinner Entrée
Portion Size: 1 1/2 cup
Ingredients: Yields: 8 servings

Ingredients	Notes:
2 1/2 pounds lean ground beef	
4 cups stuffing mixture or croutons	
1/2 teaspoon garlic powder	
1/2 teaspoon salt	
1 teaspoon poultry seasoning	
1/2 cup diced onions	
1/4 cup diced celery	
2 cans low sodium mixed vegetable, drained	
1 cup light sour cream	
2 cups low salt beef broth	
1 cup fat free evaporated milk	
2 cups reduce fat cheddar cheese	

Directions:

Steps:	Directions:	Critical Control Point /Quality Assurance
1	Brown ground beef in large skillet. Drain fat.	
2	Place hamburger in bottom of a baking pan.	
3	Spread croutons evenly over hamburger.	
4	Layer on the vegetables.	
5	Mix evaporated milk, broth, sour cream salt, poultry seasoning, onions, and celery.	
6	Pour over vegetable layer.	
7	Cover with cheese.	
8	Bake covered at 350 degrees for 40 to 45 minutes or until potatoes are done.	Cook until internal temperature reaches 165 F degrees for 15 seconds

Time Temperature Sensitive food. *Food safety Standards: hold food for service at an internal temperature above 140°F. Do not mix old product with new. Cool leftover product quickly (within 4 hours) to below 41°F. Follow proper cooling procedures. Store leftovers in a tightly sealed, labeled and dated container. Use leftover within 72 hours if stored in refrigerator or 30 days if stored in the freezer. Reheat leftover product quickly (within 2 hours) to 165 degrees F for 15 seconds. Reheat left over product only once; discard if not used. Cold holding at 41°F or colder or using time alone (less than four hours). Always wash hands and wash and sanitize counter tops utensils and containers between steps when working with raw meat.*

Texture Modified Diets:

Soft & Bite Size: (aka Bite size) **Food particle size ½ inch (~width of standard fork)** Food must be moist. Cut foods with a knife to a ½" particle size prior to mixing. Moisten with broth as needed. Foods that do not process well should be omitted.

Chopped: Food particle size ¼ inch (~ ½ width of standard fork) Food must be moist. Chop foods with a knife to 1/4" particle size prior to mixing. Moisten with broth as needed. Foods that do not process well should be omitted.

Minced and Moist:(aka Minced/Mechanical Soft/Ground) **Food particle size 1/8 inch (fits through prongs of standard fork)** Food must be moist. Use a food processor to grind food particles into 1/8 inch prior to mixing. Moisten with broth as needed. Foods that do not process well should be omitted.

Pureed: Smooth and cohesive. Use a food processor to puree to a smooth consistency. Foods are processed by grinding and then pureeing them. May add broth or sauce to puree. Do not add to much liquid. Puree should still hold its shape. Must not be firm or sticky. Puree foods while still hot. Appearance should be smooth like pudding. Foods that do not process well should be omitted. Serve ½ c. puree meat and ½ puree croutons separately.

Therapeutic Modified Diets:

Lowfat: No changes needed
Diabetic/No added Sugar/No Conc. Sweets/Calorie Controlled: No changes needed
Bland/Anti Reflux: Use plain croutons, Omit garlic powder, poultry seasoning, onions, and celery
Liberal House Renal: Serve 3 oz. SF hamburger patty and ½ cup SF pasta or rice and ½ cup SF green beans
No Added Salt: No changes needed.
2 Gram Sodium: Serve 3 oz. SF hamburger patty and ½ cup SF pasta or rice and ½ cup SF vegetables.
Gluten Free: Use gluten free stuffing mix or croutons. Use GF broth Prepare foods separately to prevent cross contamination.
**Allergy Alerts: When an "X" is present, this indicates the allergen is present.
Always read all food labels to ensure allergens are not present.**

Wheat	Milk	Eggs	Fish Shellfish	Soy	Peanuts/Nuts	Other
X	X	X				

Key: SF= Salt Free D= Diet or Sugarfree LF = Lowfat FF = Fat Free GF = Gluten Free

Recipe Name: Swedish Meatballs
Recipe Category: Dinner Entrée
Portion Size: 4 oz.
Ingredients: Yields: 8 servings

Ingredients	Notes:
1/2 cup chopped onion	Wash, peel and chop
1 tablespoons olive oil	
2 Eggs, beaten	
1 (14 oz.) can fat free evaporated milk	
1 1/2 cups soft crumbs	May use whole wheat bread crumbs
1/4 cup finely chopped parsley	
1 1/4 teaspoon salt	
1/4 teaspoon pepper	
1/4 teaspoon nutmeg	
1/4 teaspoon ground ginger	
2 1/2 pounds lean ground beef	
2 tablespoons flour	
1 teaspoon instant beef bouillon granules	
1 1/4 Cups water	

Directions:

Steps:	Directions:	Critical Control Point /Quality Assurance
1	Cook onion in oil.	
2	In mixing bowl combine egg and milk; stir in cooked onion, breadcrumbs, parsley, salt, pepper, nutmeg, and ginger. Add meat.	
3	Mix well by hand or on medium speed of electric mixer.	
4	Shape into 3/4 to 1 inch balls, referring to tip at right (mixture will be soft; for easier shaping, wet hands or chill mixture first).	
5	In large skillet brown meatballs, half at a time.	
6	Remove from skillet.	
7	Stir flour, and bouillon granules into pan juices; add water.	
	Cook and stir till thickened and bubbly. Add meatballs.	
8	Cover; simmer about 30 minutes, basting meatballs occasionally.	Cook until internal temperature reaches 165 F degrees for 15 seconds

Time Temperature Sensitive food. *Food safety Standards: hold food for service at an internal temperature above 140°F. Do not mix old product with new. Cool leftover product quickly (within 4 hours) to below 41°F. Follow proper cooling procedures. Store leftovers in a tightly sealed, labeled and dated container. Use leftover within 72 hours if stored in refrigerator or 30 days if stored in the freezer. Reheat leftover product quickly (within 2 hours) to 165 degrees F for 15 seconds. Reheat left over product only once; discard if not used. Cold holding at 41°F or colder or using time alone (less than four hours). Always wash hands and wash and sanitize counter tops utensils and containers between steps when working with raw meat.*

Texture Modified Diets:

Soft & Bite Size: (aka Bite size) **Food particle size ½ inch (~width of standard fork)** Food must be moist. Cut foods with a knife to a ½" particle size after cooking. Moisten with sauce as needed.

Chopped: Food particle size ¼ inch (~ ½ width of standard fork) Food must be moist. Chop foods with a knife to 1/4" particle size after cooking. Moisten with sauce as needed.

Minced and Moist:(aka Minced/Mechanical Soft/Ground) **Food particle size 1/8 inch (fits through prongs of standard fork)** Food must be moist. Use a food processor to grind food particles into 1/8 inch after cooking. Moisten with sauce as needed.

Pureed: Smooth and cohesive. Use a food processor to puree to a smooth consistency. Foods are processed by grinding and then pureeing them. May add broth or sauce to puree. Do not add to much liquid. Puree should still hold its shape. Must not be firm or sticky. Puree foods while still hot. Appearance should be smooth like pudding. Serve ½ c. meat serving topped with sauce.

Therapeutic Modified Diets:

Lowfat: No changes needed
Diabetic/No added Sugar/No Conc. Sweets/Calorie Controlled: No changes needed
Bland/Anti Reflux: omit onion, parsley, pepper, nutmeg
Liberal House Renal: Omit salt, bread crumbs and evaporated milk. Use SF beef granules or the omit sauce.
No Added Salt: No changes needed
2 Gram Sodium: omit salt and bread crumbs. Use SF beef granules or omit the sauce.
Gluten Free: Use gluten free soft bread crumbs or GF oat and GF flour. Use GF beef granules. Prepare foods separately to prevent cross contamination.

Allergy Alerts: When an "X" is present, this indicates the allergen is present. Always read all food labels to ensure allergens are not present.

Wheat	Milk	Eggs	Fish Shellfish	Soy	Peanuts/Nuts	Other
X	X	X				

Key: SF= Salt Free D= Diet or Sugarfree LF = Lowfat FF = Fat Free GF = Gluten Free

Recipe Name: Swiss Steak
Recipe Category: Dinner Entrée
Portion Size: 4 oz.
Ingredients: Yields: 8 servings

Ingredients	Notes:
2-2 1/2 pounds bottom round steak	Trim all visible fat
1/4 cup flour	
1 teaspoon garlic salt	
1 teaspoon pepper	
1 tablespoon vegetable oil	
1/2 cup diced carrots	Wash, peel and dice
1/4 cup diced celery	Wash, trim and dice
1/2 cup diced onion	Wash, peel and dice
1 cup water or low sodium beef stock	
1/2 cup low sodium tomato sauce	

Directions:

Steps:	Directions:	Critical Control Point /Quality Assurance
1	Pound meat on both sides with a mallet.	
2	Cut into serving size pieces.	
3	Combine garlic salt, pepper and flour.	
4	Dredge meat in flour mixture.	
5	Heat oil in a large pan.	
6	Sear meat on both sides until lightly brown.	
7	Add carrots, celery, onion, water or stock and tomato sauce.	
8	Place in a baking dish and bake in 300 degree oven for 1 1/2 to 2 hours.	Cook until internal temperature reaches 165 F degrees for 15 seconds

Time Temperature Sensitive food. *Food safety Standards: hold food for service at an internal temperature above 140° F. Do not mix old product with new. Cool leftover product quickly (within 4 hours) to below 41° F. Follow proper cooling procedures. Store leftovers in a tightly sealed, labeled and dated container. Use leftover within 72 hours if stored in refrigerator or 30 days if stored in the freezer. Reheat leftover product quickly (within 2 hours) to 165 degrees F for 15 seconds. Reheat left over product only once; discard if not used. Cold holding at 41°F or colder or using time alone (less than four hours). Always wash hands and wash and sanitize counter tops utensils and containers between steps when working with raw meat.*

<u>Texture Modified Diets:</u>

Soft & Bite Size: (aka Bite size) **Food particle size ½ inch (~width of standard fork)** Food must be moist. Cut foods with a knife to a ½" particle size prior to mixing. Moisten with broth as needed.

Chopped: Food particle size ¼ inch (~ ½ width of standard fork) Food must be moist. Chop foods with a knife to 1/4" particle size prior to mixing. Moisten with broth as needed.

Minced and Moist: (aka Minced/Mechanical Soft/Ground) **Food particle size 1/8 inch (fits through prongs of standard fork)** Food must be moist. Use a food processor to grind food particles into 1/8 inch prior to mixing. Moisten with broth as needed.

Pureed: Smooth and cohesive. Use a food processor to puree to a smooth consistency. Foods are processed by grinding and then pureeing them. May add broth or sauce to puree. Do not add to much liquid. Puree should still hold its shape. Must not be firm or sticky. Puree foods while still hot. Appearance should be smooth like pudding.

<u>Therapeutic Modified Diets</u>:
Lowfat: No changes needed
Diabetic/No added Sugar/No Conc. Sweets/Calorie Controlled: No changes needed
Bland/Anti Reflux: omit garlic salt, pepper, celery, onion and tomato sauce
Liberal House Renal: Omit garlic salt and tomato sauce. Use SF beef stock or water
No Added Salt: Replace garlic salt with granulated garlic.
2 Gram Sodium: omit garlic salt and tomato sauce. Use SF beef stock or water
Gluten Free: Use gluten free flour and GF beef stock. Prepare foods separately to prevent cross contamination.
Allergy Alerts: When an "X" is present, this indicates the allergen is present.
Always read all food labels to ensure allergens are not present.

Wheat	Milk	Eggs	Fish Shellfish	Soy	Peanuts/Nuts	Other
X						

Key: SF= Salt Free D= Diet or Sugarfree LF = Lowfat FF = Fat Free GF = Gluten Free

Recipe Name: Taco Beef Pizza
Recipe Category: Lunch Entrée
Portion Size: 1 Slice (1/8 pizza)
Ingredients: Yields: 8 servings

Ingredients	Notes:
1 pound lean ground beef	
1 taco seasoning package	
1 (1 pound) loaf frozen bread dough	Thawed
2 cups shredded lowfat cheddar cheese	
2 cups lettuce	Washed trimmed and chopped finely
½ cup diced tomatoes	Washed trimmed and diced
¼ cup low fat sour cream	

Directions:

Steps:	Directions:	Critical Control Point /Quality Assurance
1	In a skillet, cook beef over medium heat until no longer pink; drain.	Internal temperature of beef should reach 165 degree F
2	Add seasoning package and ¼ cup of water	
3	On a floured surface, roll dough into a 13-inch circle	
4	Press onto the bottom and up the sides of a greased 12-inch pizza pan.	
5	Spread beef over crust to within 1/2 inch of edge	
6	Top with cheese.	
7	Bake at 350 degrees F for 20-25 minutes or until crust is golden and cheese is melted	
8	Just before serving top with lettuce, tomato and sour cream	

Time Temperature Sensitive food. Food safety Standards: hold food for service at an internal temperature above 140°F. Do not mix old product with new. Cool leftover product quickly (within 4 hours) to below 41°F. Follow proper cooling procedures. Store leftovers in a tightly sealed, labeled and dated container. Use leftover within 72 hours if stored in refrigerator or 30 days if stored in the freezer. Reheat leftover product quickly (within 2 hours) to 165 degrees F for 15 seconds. Reheat left over product only once; discard if not used. Cold holding at 41°F or colder or using time alone (less than four hours). Always wash hands and wash and sanitize counter tops utensils and containers between steps when working with raw meat.

Texture Modified Diets:

Soft & Bite Size: (aka Bite size) **Food particle size ½ inch (~width of standard fork)** Food must be moist. Bake crust until soft. If crust is hard, it must be processed to 1/8 inch and moistened before adding the toppings. Cut foods with a knife to a ½" particle size prior to layering. Moisten with broth as needed.

Chopped: Food particle size ¼ inch (~ ½ width of standard fork) Food must be moist. Bake crust until soft. If crust is hard, it must be processed to 1/8 inch and moistened before adding the toppings Chop foods with a knife to 1/4" particle size prior to layering. Moisten with broth as needed.

Minced and Moist:(aka Minced/Mechanical Soft/Ground) **Food particle size 1/8 inch (fits through prongs of standard fork)** Food must be moist. Bake crust until soft. Use a food processor to grind food particles into 1/8 inch prior to layering. Moisten with broth as needed.

Pureed: Smooth and cohesive. Use a food processor to puree to a smooth consistency. Foods are processed by grinding and then pureeing them. May add broth or sauce to puree. Do not add to much liquid. Puree should still hold its shape. Must not be firm or sticky. Puree foods while still hot. Appearance should be smooth like pudding.

Therapeutic Modified Diets:

Lowfat: No changes
Diabetic/No added Sugar/No Conc. Sweets/Calorie Controlled: No changes needed
Bland/Anti Reflux: omit taco seasoning and tomatoes.
Liberal House Renal: Use alternate menu item
No Added Salt: No changes
2 Gram Sodium: Use alternate menu item
Gluten Free: Use gluten free seasoning and gluten free dough. Prepare foods separately to prevent cross contamination.

Allergy Alerts: When an "X" is present, this indicates the allergen is present. Always read all food labels to ensure allergens are not present.

Wheat	Milk	Eggs	Fish Shellfish	Soy	Peanuts/Nuts	Other
X	x					

Key: SF= Salt Free D= Diet or Sugarfree LF = Lowfat FF = Fat Free GF = Gluten Free

Recipe Name: Taco Pasta
Recipe Category: Dinner Entrée
Portion Size: 1 cup
Ingredients: Yields: 8 servings

Ingredients	Notes:
2 pounds lean ground beef	
1 teaspoon chili powder	
2 teaspoons cumin	
1-16 oz. pasta	Prepare according directions
1 small onion, chopped	Wash, peel and chop
1 cup fat free milk	
1 cup light sour cream	
2 cans (14 oz.) of low sodium tomato sauce	
1 cup shredded low fat cheddar cheese	

Directions:

Steps:	Directions:	Critical Control Point /Quality Assurance
1	Brown ground beef with onion. Drain excess fat.	
2	Prepare pasta according to directions on package. Drain.	
3	Combine ground beef, pasta, chili powder, cumin, milk, sour cream, and tomato sauce.	
4	Pour mixture into a baking dish.	
5	Sprinkle cheese on top.	
6	Bake in a 325 degree oven for about 30-35 minutes.	Cook until internal temperature reaches 165 F degrees for 15 seconds

Time Temperature Sensitive food. *Food safety Standards: hold food for service at an internal temperature above 140° F. Do not mix old product with new. Cool leftover product quickly (within 4 hours) to below 41° F. Follow proper cooling procedures. Store leftovers in a tightly sealed, labeled and dated container. Use leftover within 72 hours if stored in refrigerator or 30 days if stored in the freezer. Reheat leftover product quickly (within 2 hours) to 165 degrees F for 15 seconds. Reheat left over product only once; discard if not used. Cold holding at 41°F or colder or using time alone (less than four hours). Always wash hands and wash and sanitize counter tops utensils and containers between steps when working with raw meat.*

Texture Modified Diets: Tip: Use pasta that is the correct particle size.
Soft & Bite Size: (aka Bite size) **Food particle size ½ inch (~width of standard fork)** Food must be moist. Cut foods with a knife to a ½" particle size prior to mixing. Moisten with broth as needed.
Chopped: Food particle size ¼ inch (~ ½ width of standard fork) Food must be moist. Chop foods with a knife to 1/4" particle size prior to mixing. Moisten with broth as needed.
Minced and Moist: (aka Minced/Mechanical Soft/Ground) **Food particle size 1/8 inch (fits through prongs of standard fork)** Food must be moist. Use a food processor to grind food particles into 1/8 inch prior to mixing. Moisten with broth as needed.
Pureed: Smooth and cohesive. Use a food processor to puree to a smooth consistency. Foods are processed by grinding and then pureeing them. May add broth or sauce to puree. Do not add to much liquid. Puree should still hold its shape. Must not be firm or sticky. Puree foods while still hot. Appearance should be smooth like pudding. Foods that do not process well should be omitted. Serve 1 c. meat/ bean serving.

Therapeutic Modified Diets:
Lowfat: No changes needed
Diabetic/No added Sugar/No Conc. Sweets/Calorie Controlled: No changes needed
Bland/Anti Reflux: Serve plain hamburger patty and ½ c. plain pasta.
Liberal House Renal: Serve plain hamburger patty and ½ c. SF pasta. May season pasta with SF herbs and spices.
No Added Salt: No changes needed
2 Gram Sodium: Serve plain hamburger patty and ½ c. SF pasta. May season rice with SF herbs and spices
Gluten Free: Use GF pasta. Prepare foods separately to prevent cross contamination.
**Allergy Alerts: When an "X" is present, this indicates the allergen is present.
Always read all food labels to ensure allergens are not present.**

Wheat	Milk	Eggs	Fish Shellfish	Soy	Peanuts/Nuts	Other
X	X					

Key: SF= Salt Free D= Diet or Sugarfree LF = Lowfat FF = Fat Free GF = Gluten Free

Recipe Name: Taco Supreme
Recipe Category: Dinner Entrée
Portion Size: 1 Taco: ½ cup beef/potatoes mixture; 2 tablespoons cheese, tomato and lettuce
Ingredients: **Yields: 8 servings**

Ingredients	Notes:
3 large potatoes,	Washed, peeled and grated
1 large onion, grated	Washed, peeled and grated
2 pounds lean ground beef	
1 tablespoon chili powder	
Salt and Pepper to taste	
1/2 cup salad oil	
8 corn tortillas	
1 pound Low fat cheddar cheese	shredded
1 large tomato, chopped	Washed, trimmed and chopped
1 Head lettuce, shredded	Washed, trimmed and shredded

Directions:

Steps:	Directions:	Critical Control Point / Quality Assurance
1	Combine potatoes and onion in a large bowl.	
2	Add ground beef, chili powder, salt and pepper. Mix well.	
3	Heat 1/4 cup oil in a skillet, add meat mixture and cook over medium low heat, stirring frequently, until meat is browned and potatoes are tender. Drain off fat.	Cook until internal temperature reaches 165 F degrees for 15 seconds
4	Spread filling almost to edges of a tortilla.	
5	Fold tortilla in half forming a half circle.	
6	Heat remaining 1/4 cup oil in a skillet.	
7	With a spatula, place filled tortilla in hot oil; fry both sides until crisp.	
8	Repeat until all tortillas are fried.	
9	Open tacos slightly and stuff with cheese, tomatoes and lettuce.	

Time Temperature Sensitive food. *Food safety Standards: hold food for service at an internal temperature above 140° F. Do not mix old product with new. Cool leftover product quickly (within 4 hours) to below 41° F. Follow proper cooling procedures. Store leftovers in a tightly sealed, labeled and dated container. Use leftover within 72 hours if stored in refrigerator or 30 days if stored in the freezer. Reheat leftover product quickly (within 2 hours) to 165 degrees F for 15 seconds. Reheat left over product only once; discard if not used. Cold holding at 41°F or colder or using time alone (less than four hours). Always wash hands and wash and sanitize counter tops utensils and containers between steps when working with raw meat.*

Texture Modified Diets:

Soft & Bite Size: (aka Bite size) **Food particle size ½ inch (~width of standard fork)** Food must be moist. Cut foods with a knife to a ½" particle size prior to layering. Moisten with broth as needed.

Chopped: Food particle size ¼ inch (~ ½ width of standard fork) Food must be moist. Chop foods with a knife to 1/4" particle size prior to layering. Moisten with broth as needed.

Minced and Moist: (aka Minced/Mechanical Soft/Ground) **Food particle size 1/8 inch (fits through prongs of standard fork)** Food must be moist. Use a food processor to grind food particles into 1/8 inch prior to layering. Moisten with broth as needed.

Pureed: Smooth and cohesive. Use a food processor to puree to a smooth consistency. Foods are processed by grinding and then pureeing them. May add broth or sauce to puree. Do not add to much liquid. Puree should still hold its shape. Must not be firm or sticky. Puree foods while still hot. Appearance should be smooth like pudding. Serve ½ c. puree meat serving, ½ cup puree tortilla with cheese, lettuce and tomato, and ½ cup puree vegetable of choice.

Therapeutic Modified Diets:

Lowfat: No changes needed
Diabetic/No added Sugar/No Conc. Sweets/Calorie Controlled: No changes needed
Bland/Anti Reflux: omit onion, chili powder, pepper, tomato
Liberal House Renal: Omit salt, tomato and cheese. Use low sodium tortillas. (see recipe)
No Added Salt: No changes needed
2 Gram Sodium: omit salt and cheese. Use low sodium tortillas. (see recipe)
Gluten Free: No changes needed. Prepare foods separately to prevent cross contamination.

Allergy Alerts: When an "X" is present, this indicates the allergen is present. Always read all food labels to ensure allergens are not present.

Wheat	Milk	Eggs	Fish Shellfish	Soy	Peanuts/Nuts	Other
	X					

Key: SF= Salt Free D= Diet or Sugarfree LF = Lowfat FF = Fat Free GF = Gluten Free

Copyright 2020 Jacqueline Larson M.S., R.D.N. and Associates.   All Rights Reserved

Recipe Name: Teriyaki Beef
Recipe Category: Dinner Entrée
Portion Size: 3 oz. beef and ½ cup rice
Ingredients: **Yields: 8 servings**

Ingredients	Notes:
2 1/2 pounds beef top or bottom sirloin	Trim all visible fat, cut into thin strips
1 Bottle low sodium teriyaki baste and glaze sauce	Or see recipe in cookbook for sauce
1 teaspoon oil	
2 Garlic cloves, minced	
8 to 12 green onions	
4 cups hot cooked brown rice	

Directions:

Steps:	Directions:	Critical Control Point / Quality Assurance
1	Heat oil in a large skillet or wok.	
2	Add beef and garlic.	
3	Sauté until beef is no longer pink.	Cook until internal temperature reaches 145 F degrees for 15 seconds
4	Add green onions and sauté for 2 more minutes.	
5	Add teriyaki sauce and heat until bubbly.	
6	Serve over rice.	

Time Temperature Sensitive food. *Food safety Standards: hold food for service at an internal temperature above 140° F. Do not mix old product with new. Cool leftover product quickly (within 4 hours) to below 41° F. Follow proper cooling procedures. Store leftovers in a tightly sealed, labeled and dated container. Use leftover within 72 hours if stored in refrigerator or 30 days if stored in the freezer. Reheat leftover product quickly (within 2 hours) to 165 degrees F for 15 seconds. Reheat left over product only once; discard if not used. Cold holding at 41 °F or colder or using time alone (less than four hours). Always wash hands and wash and sanitize counter tops utensils and containers between steps when working with raw meat.*

Texture Modified Diets:
Soft & Bite Size: (aka Bite size) **Food particle size ½ inch (~width of standard fork)** Food must be moist. Cut foods with a knife to a ½" particle size prior to mixing. Moisten with broth as needed. Foods that do not process well should be omitted. Omit: green onions.
Chopped: Food particle size ¼ inch (~ ½ width of standard fork) Food must be moist. Chop foods with a knife to 1/4" particle size prior to mixing. Moisten with broth as needed. Foods that do not process well should be omitted. Omit: green onions.
Minced and Moist: (aka Minced/Mechanical Soft/Ground) **Food particle size 1/8 inch (fits through prongs of standard fork)** Food must be moist. Use a food processor to grind food particles into 1/8 inch prior to mixing. Moisten with broth as needed. Foods that do not process well should be omitted. Omit: green onions.
Pureed: Smooth and cohesive. Use a food processor to puree to a smooth consistency. Foods are processed by grinding and then pureeing them. May add broth or sauce to puree. Do not add to much liquid. Puree should still hold its shape. Must not be firm or sticky. Puree foods while still hot. Appearance should be smooth like pudding. Foods that do not process well should be omitted. Omit: green onions.
Therapeutic Modified Diets:
Lowfat: No changes needed
Diabetic/No added Sugar/No Conc. Sweets/Calorie Controlled: No changes needed
Bland/Anti Reflux: omit teriyaki sauce and onions
Liberal House Renal: Omit teriyaki sauce. May season with SF herb/spices.
No Added Salt: No changes needed
2 Gram Sodium: omit teriyaki sauce. May season with SF herb/spices.
Gluten Free: Use gluten free teriyaki sauce. Prepare foods separately to prevent cross contamination.
Allergy Alerts: When an "X" is present, this indicates the allergen is present.
Always read all food labels to ensure allergens are not present.

Wheat	Milk	Eggs	Fish Shellfish	Soy	Peanuts/Nuts	Other
X				X		

Key: SF= Salt Free D= Diet or Sugarfree LF = Lowfat FF = Fat Free GF = Gluten Free

Recipe Name: Vegetable Beef Soup
Recipe Category: Dinner Entrée
Portion Size: 2 cups
Ingredients: Yields: 8 servings

Ingredients	Notes:
2 1/2 Pounds lean stew meat	Trim all visible fat, cut into bite size pieces
1 Teaspoon vegetable oil	
4 Medium carrots (2 cups)	Wash, peel and slice
4 large potatoes (4 cups)	Wash, peel and chop
2 Medium onions (1 cup)	Wash, peel and dice
2 Celery stalks (1 cup)	Wash, trim and dice
2 Tablespoons parsley flakes	
2 (16 ounce) cans low sodium tomatoes	
2 ounces low sodium beef bouillon	
1 Teaspoon salt	
1/4 Teaspoon pepper	

Directions:

Steps:	Directions:	Critical Control Point / Quality Assurance
1	Peel and cut carrots and potatoes into large cubes.	
2	Coarsely chop onions, celery, and canned tomatoes.	
3	In a large soup pot heat oil.	
4	Add stew meat and brown.	
5	Drain excess fat.	
6	Add carrots, potatoes, onions, celery, parsley, tomatoes, beef bouillon salt and pepper.	
7	Add 8 cups water.	
8	Bring to boil.	
9	Reduce heat and simmer for 2 to 3 hours.	Cook until internal temperature reaches 165 F degrees for 15 seconds

Time Temperature Sensitive food. *Food safety Standards: hold food for service at an internal temperature above 140° F. Do not mix old product with new. Cool leftover product quickly (within 4 hours) to below 41° F. Follow proper cooling procedures. Store leftovers in a tightly sealed, labeled and dated container. Use leftover within 72 hours if stored in refrigerator or 30 days if stored in the freezer. Reheat leftover product quickly (within 2 hours) to 165 degrees F for 15 seconds. Reheat left over product only once; discard if not used. Cold holding at 41°F or colder or using time alone (less than four hours). Always wash hands and wash and sanitize counter tops utensils and containers between steps when working with raw meat.*

Texture Modified Diets:

Soft & Bite Size: (aka Bite size) **Food particle size ½ inch (~width of standard fork)** Food must be moist. Cut foods with a knife to a ½" particle size prior to mixing. Moisten with broth as needed.

Chopped: Food particle size ¼ inch (~ ½ width of standard fork) Food must be moist. Chop foods with a knife to 1/4" particle size prior to mixing. Moisten with broth as needed.

Minced and Moist:(aka Minced/Mechanical Soft/Ground) **Food particle size 1/8 inch (fits through prongs of standard fork)** Food must be moist. Use a food processor to grind food particles into 1/8 inch prior to mixing. Moisten with broth as needed.

Pureed: Smooth and cohesive. Use a food processor to puree to a smooth consistency. Foods are processed by grinding and then pureeing them. May add broth or sauce to puree. Do not add to much liquid. Puree should still hold its shape. Must not be firm or sticky. Puree foods while still hot. Appearance should be smooth like pudding. Serve ½ c. meat ½ cup potatoes, and ½ cup vegetables (onions, celery, carrots and tomatoes) servings pureed and served separately.

Therapeutic Modified Diets:

Lowfat: No changes needed
Diabetic/No added Sugar/No Conc. Sweets/Calorie Controlled: No changes needed
Bland/Anti Reflux: omit onion, celery, parsley flakes and pepper
Liberal House Renal: Omit salt and tomatoes. Use SF bouillon or water
No Added Salt: No changes
2 Gram Sodium: omit salt and Use SF broth or water. Omit tomatoes and add 2 cup fresh tomatoes
Gluten Free: Use gluten free bouillon Prepare foods separately to prevent cross contamination.
Allergy Alerts: When an "X" is present, this indicates the allergen is present.
Always read all food labels to ensure allergens are not present.

Wheat	Milk	Eggs	Fish Shellfish	Soy	Peanuts/Nuts	Other
X						

Key: SF= Salt Free D= Diet or Sugarfree LF = Lowfat FF = Fat Free GF = Gluten Free

Copyright 2020 Jacqueline Larson M.S., R.D.N. and Associates.   All Rights Reserved

BEEF LUNCH RECIPES

Recipe Name: Asian Pasta Salad with Beef and Broccoli
Recipe Category: Lunch Entrée
Portion Size: 1 ½ cup
Ingredients: Yields: 8 servings

Ingredients	Notes:
Soy-Ginger Dressing:	
3 medium garlic cloves	Wash, peel and mince
1/3 cup light soy sauce	
2 tablespoons rice wine vinegar	
1 tablespoon sugar	
1 tablespoon sesame oil	
1 teaspoon ground ginger	
3/4 teaspoon hot red pepper flakes (optional)	
2 tablespoons light mayonnaise	
1/4 cup vegetable oil	
Pasta Salad:	
1 pound pasta	May use whole grain
4 cups broccoli florets	Wash, trim and cut
1 pound rare deli roast beef	Sliced 1/8 inch thick and cut into bite-size strips
3 medium carrots	Wash, peel and shred
1 medium red bell pepper	Wash, trim and shred
4 green onions	Wash, trim and thinly slice
1/2 cup chopped unsalted roasted (or honey-roasted) peanuts	
1/4 cup chopped fresh cilantro	Wash, trim and chop fine

Directions:

Steps:	Directions:	Critical Control Point / Quality Assurance
1	Mix garlic, soy sauce, vinegar, sugar, sesame oil, ginger, and pepper flakes in a small bowl.	
2	Whisk in mayonnaise until smooth, then in a slow steady stream, whisk in oil to make an emulsified dressing	Keep chilled until ready to toss with salad
3	Bring water to boil in a large stock pot	
4	Add pasta and, using package times as a guide, boil, stirring frequently and adding broccoli the last 1 minute, cook until just tender	
5	Drain thoroughly (do not rinse) Set aside while preparing remaining salad ingredients	
6	In a large bowl add pasta, roast beef, carrots and red bell pepper.	
7	Add dressing and toss to coat	
8	Serve on individual plates and top with green onions, peanuts and cilantro	

Time Temperature Sensitive food. *Food safety Standards: Do not mix old product with new. Cool leftover product quickly (within 4 hours) to below 41°F. Follow proper cooling procedures. Store leftovers in a tightly sealed, labeled and dated container. Use leftover within 72 hours if stored in refrigerator or 30 days if stored in the freezer. Cold holding at 41°F or colder or using time alone (less than four hours).*

Texture Modified Diets: Tip; Use pasta in correct particle size.
Soft & Bite Size: (aka Bite size) **Food particle size ½ inch (~width of standard fork)** Food must be moist. Cut foods with a knife to a ½" particle size prior to mixing. Moisten with broth as needed. Foods that do not process well should be omitted. Omit: peanuts and green onions. Cook carrots, broccoli and peppers to soften

Chopped: Food particle size ¼ inch (~ ½ width of standard fork) Food must be moist. Chop foods with a knife to 1/4" particle size prior to mixing. Moisten with broth as needed. Foods that do not process well should be omitted. Omit: peanuts and green onions. Cook carrots, broccoli and peppers to soften

Minced and Moist:(aka Minced/Mechanical Soft/Ground) **Food particle size 1/8 inch (fits through prongs of standard fork)** Food must be moist. Use a food processor to grind food particles into 1/8 inch prior to mixing. Moisten with broth as needed. Foods that do not process well should be omitted. Omit: peanuts and green onions. Cook carrots, broccoli and peppers to soften

Pureed: Smooth and cohesive. Use a food processor to puree to a smooth consistency. Foods are processed by grinding and then pureeing them. May add broth or sauce to puree. Do not add to much liquid. Puree should still hold its shape. Must not be firm or sticky. Puree foods while still hot. Appearance should be smooth like pudding. Foods that do not process well should be omitted. Omit: peanuts and green onions. Cook carrots, broccoli and peppers to soften. Serve ½ c. meat, ½ c. puree noodles and ½ c. puree cooked broccoli separately.

<u>*Therapeutic Modified Diets:*</u>

Lowfat: Omit peanuts
Diabetic/No added Sugar/No Conc. Sweets/Calorie Controlled: No changes needed
Bland/Anti Reflux: omit garlic, red pepper, broccoli, red pepper flakes, green onions, cilantro and peanuts
Liberal House Renal: Omit soy ginger sauce. Toss with sesame oil and rice vinegar
No Added Salt: Omit soy ginger sauce. Toss with sesame oil and rice vinegar.
2 Gram Sodium: omit soy ginger sauce. Toss with sesame oil and rice vinegar
Gluten Free: Use gluten free pasta and soy sauce. Prepare foods separately to prevent cross contamination.
Allergy Alerts: When an "X" is present, this indicates the allergen is present.
Always read all food labels to ensure allergens are not present.

Wheat	Milk	Eggs	Fish Shellfish	Soy	Peanuts/Nuts	Other
X		X		X	X	

Key: SF= Salt Free D= Diet or Sugarfree LF = Lowfat FF = Fat Free GF = Gluten Free

Recipe Name: Beef Gyros
Recipe Category: Lunch Entrée
Portion Size: 1 wrap
Ingredients: **Yields: 8 servings**

Ingredients	Notes:
1 lb. beef top sirloin steak, cut into thin strips	Trim all visible fat and skin, cut into strips
½ cup cucumbers	Washed, trimmed and coarsely chopped
½ teaspoon dried dill weed	
2 tablespoons garlic (divided)	Washed, peeled, and minced
2 tablespoons cup distilled white vinegar	
2 tablespoons lemon juice (divided)	
1 teaspoon onion powder	
2 tablespoons olive oil (divided)	
1/4 teaspoon salt	
¼ teaspoon oregano, dried	
¼ teaspoon black ground pepper	
2 tablespoons red wine vinegar	
8 (6 inch) Pita bread rounds	
½ cup tomato diced	Washed, trimmed and diced
¼ cup red onion	Washed, trimmed and diced
1 cup lettuce	Washed, trimmed and shredded

Directions:

Steps:	Directions:	Critical Control Point /Quality Assurance
1	Place Greek yogurt, cucumber, dill weed, ½ garlic, ½ of lemon juice, white vinegar, 1/2 olive oil, pepper and salt in a blender. Blend until smooth. Chill.	
2	Wisk together, remaining garlic, lemon juice, red wine vinegar, remaining olive oil, and oregano in a large pan. Season with salt and pepper. Stir in beef strips and toss to evenly coat. Cover and marinate in refrigerator for 1 hour.	
3	Pre heat the oven's broiler and set the oven rack about 6 inches from the heat source.	
4	Remove beef from marinade and shake off excess. Discard the remaining marinade. Place beef on a large baking sheets. Broil 2- 4 minutes per side. Allow to rest for 5 minutes.	Cooked to minimum 155F degrees.
5	Heat oil in large skillet over medium heat. Heat pita bread in skillet until warm and soft. Serve warmed pita bread topped with beef strips, yogurt sauce, tomatoes, onions and lettuce.	Chilled internal temperature maintained at 41°F.

Time Temperature Sensitive food. *Food safety Standards: Do not mix old product with new. Cold holding at 41°F or colder or using time alone (less than four hours).*

Texture Modified Diets:
Soft & Bite Size: (aka Bite size) **Food particle size ½ inch (~width of standard fork)** Peel cucumber. Food must be moist. Cut foods with a knife to a ½" particle size prior to layering. Moisten with broth as needed.
Chopped: Food particle size ¼ inch (~ ½ width of standard fork) Peel cucumber. Food must be moist. Chop foods with a knife to 1/4" particle size prior to layering. Moisten with broth as needed.
Minced and Moist:(aka Minced/Mechanical Soft/Ground) **Food particle size 1/8 inch (fits through prongs of standard fork)** Peel cucumber. Food must be moist. Use a food processor to grind food particles into 1/8 inch prior to layering. Moisten with broth as needed.
Pureed: Smooth and cohesive. Peel cucumber. Use a food processor to puree to a smooth consistency. Foods are processed by grinding and then pureeing them. May add broth or sauce to puree. Do not add to much liquid.

Puree should still hold its shape. Must not be firm or sticky. Puree foods while still hot. Appearance should be smooth like pudding. Serve ½ c. puree meat, ½ cup puree vegetables with dressing and ½ cup puree pita separately.

Therapeutic Modified Diets:
Lowfat: No changes needed
Diabetic/No added Sugar/No Conc. Sweets/Calorie Controlled: No changes needed
Bland/Anti Reflux: Omit pepper, dill, garlic, vinegar, tomatoes, lemon juice, oregano and onion.
Liberal House Renal: Use SF tortilla (recipe in cookbook). Omit salt, and yogurt sauce.
No Added Salt: No changes
2 Gram Sodium: Use SF tortilla (recipe in cookbook). Omit salt
Gluten Free: Use GF corn tortilla Prepare foods separately to prevent cross contamination.
Allergy Alerts: When an "X" is present, this indicates the allergen is present.
Always read all food labels to ensure allergens are not present.

Wheat	Milk	Eggs	Fish Shellfish	Soy	Peanuts/Nuts	Other
X	X	X				

Key: SF= Salt Free D= Diet or Sugarfree LF = Lowfat FF = Fat Free GF = Gluten Free

Recipe Name: Beef Pizza
Recipe Category: Lunch Entrée
Portion Size: 1 slice (1/8 pizza)
Ingredients: **Yields: 8 servings**

Ingredients	Notes:
1 pound lean ground beef	
½ teaspoon garlic powder	
1 (1 pound) loaf frozen bread dough, thawed	
1 small jars low salt pizza sauce	
2 cups shredded low fat mozzarella cheese	
1/4 cup Parmesan Cheese	

Directions: Makes 1 pizza

Steps:	Directions:	Critical Control Point / Quality Assurance
1	In a skillet, cook beef over medium heat until no longer pink; drain.	Cook until internal temperature reaches 165 degrees F for 15 seconds.
2	Add garlic powder.	
3	On a floured surface, roll dough into a 13-in. circle.	
4	Press dough onto the bottom and up the sides of a greased 12-in. pizza pan.	
5	Spread sauce over crust to within 1/2 in. of edge.	
6	Top with beef mixture.	
7	Top with cheese.	
8	Bake at 350 degrees F for 20-25 minutes or until crust is golden and cheese is melted.	

Time Temperature Sensitive food. *Food safety Standards: hold food for service at an internal temperature above 140° F. Do not mix old product with new. Cool leftover product quickly (within 4 hours) to below 41° F. Follow proper cooling procedures. Store leftovers in a tightly sealed, labeled and dated container. Use leftover within 72 hours if stored in refrigerator or 30 days if stored in the freezer. Reheat leftover product quickly (within 2 hours) to 165 degrees F for 15 seconds. Reheat left over product only once; discard if not used. Cold holding at 41°F or colder or using time alone (less than four hours). Always wash hands and wash and sanitize counter tops utensils and containers between steps when working with raw meat.*

<u>Texture Modified Diets:</u>

Soft & Bite Size: (aka Bite size) **Food particle size ½ inch (~width of standard fork)** Food must be moist. Cut foods with a knife to a ½" particle size prior to layering. Moisten with broth as needed.

Chopped: Food particle size ¼ inch (~ ½ width of standard fork) Food must be moist. Chop foods with a knife to 1/4" particle size prior to layering. Moisten with broth as needed.

Minced and Moist:(aka Minced/Mechanical Soft/Ground) **Food particle size 1/8 inch (fits through prongs of standard fork)** Food must be moist. Use a food processor to grind food particles into 1/8 inch prior to layering. Moisten with broth as needed.

Pureed: Smooth and cohesive. Use a food processor to puree to a smooth consistency. Foods are processed by grinding and then pureeing them. May add broth or sauce to puree. Do not add to much liquid. Puree should still hold its shape. Must not be firm or sticky. Puree foods while still hot. Appearance should be smooth like pudding. Serve 1/3 cup puree beef and 1 c. puree crust and cheese with sauce separately.

<u>Therapeutic Modified Diets:</u>
Lowfat: No changes needed
Diabetic/No added Sugar/No Conc. Sweets/Calorie Controlled: No changes needed
Bland/Anti Reflux: omit tomato sauce
Liberal House Renal: Serve plain hamburger patty and Pasta seasoned with SF herbs/spices
No Added Salt: No changes needed
2 Gram Sodium: Serve plain hamburger patty and Pasta seasoned with SF herb/spices
Gluten Free: Substitute dough for gluten free dough. Prepare foods separately to prevent cross contamination.
Allergy Alerts: When an "X" is present, this indicates the allergen is presentAlways read all food labels to ensure allergens are not present.

Wheat	Milk	Eggs	Fish Shellfish	Soy	Peanuts/Nuts	Other
X	X					

Key: SF= Salt Free D= Diet or Sugarfree LF = Lowfat FF = Fat Free GF = Gluten Free

Recipe Name: Beef Salad
Recipe Category: Lunch Entrée
Portion Size: 1/3 cup on lettuce leaf
Ingredients: Yields: 8 servings

Ingredients	Notes:
4 cups lean sliced cooked Roast beef, diced	May use lean deli meat
1/2 cups celery	Wash, trim and mince
2 tablespoon chopped onions	Wash, peel and mince
2 tablespoons Dijon mustard	
2 teaspoons vinegar	
2/3 cup light mayonnaise	
2 teaspoons minced parsley	
8 Lettuce Greens leaves	Wash, trim and divide onto plates

Directions:

Steps:	Directions:	Critical Control Point / Quality Assurance
1	Combine the beef with celery, parsley, and onions.	Internal temperature of beef should reach 165 degree F or use deli meat
2	Mix the mustard and vinegar into the mayonnaise.	
3	Toss all together.	
4	Serve on a leaf of green.	

Time Temperature Sensitive food. Food safety Standards: Do not mix old product with new. Store leftovers in a tightly sealed, labeled and dated container. Use leftover within 72 hours if stored in refrigerator or 30 days if stored in the freezer. Cold holding at 41°F or colder or using time alone (less than four hours).

Texture Modified Diets:

Soft & Bite Size: (aka Bite size) **Food particle size ½ inch (~width of standard fork)** Food must be moist. Cut foods with a knife to a ½" particle size prior to mixing. Moisten with broth as needed.
Chopped: Food particle size ¼ inch (~ ½ width of standard fork) Food must be moist. Chop foods with a knife to 1/4" particle size prior to mixing. Moisten with broth as needed.
Minced and Moist: (aka Minced/Mechanical Soft/Ground) **Food particle size 1/8 inch (fits through prongs of standard fork)** Food must be moist. Use a food processor to grind food particles into 1/8 inch prior to mixing. Moisten with broth as needed.
Pureed: Smooth and cohesive. Use a food processor to puree to a smooth consistency. Foods are processed by grinding and then pureeing them. May add broth or sauce to puree. Do not add to much liquid. Puree should still hold its shape. Must not be firm or sticky. Puree foods while still hot. Appearance should be smooth like pudding. Puree with broth if needed. Serve 1/3 cup meat, may omit green leaf.

Therapeutic Modified Diets:

Lowfat: No changes needed
Diabetic/No added Sugar/No Conc. Sweets/Calorie Controlled: No changes needed
Bland/Anti Reflux: omit onions, celery, Dijon mustard, vinegar and parsley
Liberal House Renal: Use low sodium deli beef or other meat. (less than 140 mg. sodium per serving) Omit mayonnaise.
No Added Salt: No changes needed
2 Gram Sodium: Use low sodium deli beef or other meat. (less than 140 mg. sodium per serving) Omit mayonnaise
Gluten Free: No changes needed.
Allergy Alerts: When an "X" is present, this indicates the allergen is present.
Always read all food labels to ensure allergens are not present.

Wheat	Milk	Eggs	Fish Shellfish	Soy	Peanuts/Nuts	Other
		x				

Key: SF= Salt Free D= Diet or Sugarfree LF = Lowfat FF = Fat Free GF = Gluten Free

Recipe Name: Corn Beef Hash
Recipe Category: Lunch Entrée
Portion Size: 1 cup
Ingredients: Yields: 8 servings

Ingredients	Notes:
2 tablespoons oil	
2 onions, diced	Wash, peel and dice
4 large potatoes	Washed, peeled and chopped
2 (12 ounce) cans corned beef	
¼ teaspoon black pepper	
5 tablespoons cider vinegar	

Directions:

Steps:	Directions:	Critical Control Point /Quality Assurance
1	Heat the oil in a large skillet over medium high heat.	
2	Sauté the onions and potatoes until slightly browned, and stir in corned beef.	
3	Season the hash with pepper and vinegar.	
4	Partially cover skillet, reduce heat to medium low and cook stirring occasionally.	
5	Cook the hash for about 20 minutes or until potatoes are tender.	

Time Temperature Sensitive food. *Food safety Standards: hold food for service at an internal temperature above 140° F. Do not mix old product with new. Cool leftover product quickly (within 4 hours) to below 41° F. Follow proper cooling procedures. Store leftovers in a tightly sealed, labeled and dated container. Use leftover within 72 hours if stored in refrigerator or 30 days if stored in the freezer. Reheat leftover product quickly (within 2 hours) to 165 degrees F for 15 seconds. Reheat left over product only once; discard if not used. Cold holding at 41°F or colder or using time alone (less than four hours). Always wash hands and wash and sanitize counter tops utensils and containers between steps when working with raw meat.*

Texture Modified Diets:

Soft & Bite Size: (aka Bite size) **Food particle size ½ inch (~width of standard fork)** Food must be moist. Cut foods with a knife to a ½" particle size prior to mixing. Moisten with broth as needed.

Chopped: Food particle size ¼ inch (~ ½ width of standard fork) Food must be moist. Chop foods with a knife to 1/4" particle size prior to mixing. Moisten with broth as needed.

Minced and Moist: (aka Minced/Mechanical Soft/Ground) **Food particle size 1/8 inch (fits through prongs of standard fork)** Food must be moist. Use a food processor to grind food particles into 1/8 inch prior to mixing. Moisten with broth as needed.

Pureed: Smooth and cohesive. Use a food processor to puree to a smooth consistency. Foods are processed by grinding and then pureeing them. May add broth or sauce to puree. Do not add to much liquid. Puree should still hold its shape. Must not be firm or sticky. Puree foods while still hot. Appearance should be smooth like pudding.

Therapeutic Modified Diets:

Lowfat: Substitute lean ground beef for Corn Beef Hash.
Diabetic/No added Sugar/No Conc. Sweets/Calorie Controlled: no changes needed
Bland/Anti Reflux: omit onions, cider vinegar and pepper. Substitute lean ground beef for Corn Beef Hash.
Liberal House Renal: Substitute lean ground beef for Corn Beef Hash.
No Added Salt: Substitute lean ground beef for Corn Beef Hash.
2 Gram Sodium: Substitute lean ground beef for Corn Beef Hash.
Gluten Free: No changes needed
Allergy Alerts: When an "X" is present, this indicates the allergen is present.
Always read all food labels to ensure allergens are not present.

Wheat	Milk	Eggs	Fish Shellfish	Soy	Peanuts/Nuts	Other

Key: SF= Salt Free D= Diet or Sugarfree LF = Lowfat FF = Fat Free GF = Gluten Free

Copyright 2020 Jacqueline Larson M.S., R.D.N. and Associates.   All Rights Reserved

Recipe Name: French Dip Sandwich
Recipe Category: Lunch Entrée
Portion Size: 1 Sandwich
Ingredients: **Yields: 8 servings**

Ingredients	Notes:
8 Small French Rolls	May use whole grain
1 pound cooked and sliced lean deli roast beef	
8 oz. Shredded Low Fat Mozzarella Cheese	
14 oz. can reduced sodium beef broth	
1 tablespoon light soy sauce	
½ teaspoon garlic powder	

Directions:

Steps:	Directions:	Critical Control Point /Quality Assurance
1	In a sauce pan heat beef broth, soy sauce and garlic. Heat over medium high heat until boils. Reduce heat and simmer 5 minutes	
2	Add beef to broth and heat through.	Cook until internal temperature reaches 165 F degrees for 15 seconds
3	Place 2 oz. beef on each roll. Top with cheese. Serve immediately	

Time Temperature Sensitive food. *Do not mix old product with new. Store leftovers in a tightly sealed, labeled and dated container. Use leftover within 72 hours if stored in refrigerator or 30 days if stored in the freezer. Cold holding at 41°F or colder or using time alone (less than four hours)*

<u>*Texture Modified Diets:*</u>

Soft & Bite Size: (aka Bite size) **Food particle size ½ inch (~width of standard fork)** Food must be moist. Cut foods with a knife to a ½" particle size prior to mixing. Moisten with broth as needed.
Chopped: Food particle size ¼ inch (~ ½ width of standard fork) Food must be moist. Chop foods with a knife to 1/4" particle size prior to mixing. Moisten with broth as needed.
Minced and Moist:(aka Minced/Mechanical Soft/Ground) **Food particle size 1/8 inch (fits through prongs of standard fork)** Food must be moist. Use a food processor to grind food particles into 1/8 inch prior to mixing. Moisten with broth as needed.
Pureed: Smooth and cohesive. Use a food processor to puree to a smooth consistency. Foods are processed by grinding and then pureeing them. May add broth or sauce to puree. Do not add to much liquid. Puree should still hold its shape. Must not be firm or sticky. Puree foods while still hot. Appearance should be smooth like pudding. Serve 1/3 cup puree meat and 1 cup puree roll separately. Moisten with broth as needed.

<u>*Therapeutic Modified Diets:*</u>

Low fat: No changes needed
Diabetic/No added Sugar/No Conc. Sweets/Calorie Controlled: No changes needed
Bland/Anti Reflux: Omit Onions, tomato and spinach
Liberal House Renal: Use low sodium deli roast beef (less than 140 mg. sodium per serving). Use low sodium roll. Use SF broth. Omit soy sauce and cheese.
No Added Salt: Omit soy sauce
2 Gram Sodium: Use low sodium deli roast beef (less than 140 mg. sodium per serving). Use low sodium roll. Use SF broth. Omit soy sauce and cheese.
Gluten Free: Use gluten free roll and soy sauce. Prepare foods separately to prevent cross contamination.
Allergy Alerts: When an "X" is present, this indicates the allergen is present.
Always read all food labels to ensure allergens are not present.

Wheat	Milk	Eggs	Fish Shellfish	Soy	Peanuts/Nuts	Other
X	x	X		X		

Key: SF= Salt Free D= Diet or Sugarfree LF = Lowfat FF = Fat Free GF = Gluten Free

Recipe Name: French Onion Sandwiches
Recipe Category: Lunch Entrée
Portion Size: 1 sandwich (2 starch, 2 oz. beef cubed steaks, 1 oz. cheese)
Ingredients: Yields: 8 servings

Ingredients	Notes:
1 tablespoon olive oil	
4 (4-ounce) lean beef cubed steaks	
2 Medium onion	Washed, slice and separate into rings
2 cups low sodium beef broth	
2 tablespoon cornstarch	
3 teaspoons Worcestershire sauce	
1/4 teaspoon garlic powder	
4 French bread, rolls	Toasted and cut into half
4 1-ounce slices lowfat Swiss cheese	Halved

Directions:

Steps:	Directions:	Critical Control Point /Quality Assurance
1	Heat olive oil in pan	
2	Add steaks and cook over medium high heat for 2 to 3 minutes on each side or till done	Internal temperature should reach 165 degrees
3	Remove from skillet, reserving drippings	
4	Cook onion in drippings till tender	
5	Combine broth, cornstarch, Worcestershire sauce, garlic powder, and a dash of pepper	
6	Add to skillet. Cook and stir till bubbly	
7	Place steaks on bread with cheese and onion mixture	Use 2 oz. steak and 1 oz. cheese

Time Temperature Sensitive food. *Food safety Standards: hold food for service at an internal temperature above 140°F. Do not mix old product with new. Cool leftover product quickly (within 4 hours) to below 41°F. Follow proper cooling procedures. Store leftovers in a tightly sealed, labeled and dated container. Use leftover within 72 hours if stored in refrigerator or 30 days if stored in the freezer. Reheat leftover product quickly (within 2 hours) to 165 degrees F for 15 seconds. Reheat left over product only once; discard if not used. Cold holding at 41°F or colder or using time alone (less than four hours). Always wash hands and wash and sanitize counter tops utensils and containers between steps when working with raw meat.*

<u>**Texture Modified Diets:**</u>
Soft & Bite Size: (aka Bite size) **Food particle size ½ inch (~width of standard fork)** Food must be moist. Cut foods with a knife to a ½" particle size prior to mixing. No hard bread. Moisten with broth as needed.
Chopped: Food particle size ¼ inch (~ ½ width of standard fork) Food must be moist. Chop foods with a knife to 1/4" particle size prior to mixing. No hard bread. Moisten with broth as needed.
Minced and Moist:(aka Minced/Mechanical Soft/Ground) **Food particle size 1/8 inch (fits through prongs of standard fork)** Food must be moist. Use a food processor to grind food particles into 1/8 inch prior to mixing. No hard bread. Moisten with broth as needed.
Pureed: Smooth and cohesive. Use a food processor to puree to a smooth consistency. Foods are processed by grinding and then pureeing them. May add broth or sauce to puree. Do not add to much liquid. Puree should still hold its shape. Must not be firm or sticky. Puree foods while still hot. Appearance should be smooth like pudding. Serve ½ cup meat, 1 slice of bread/ Puree with broth if needed.

<u>**Therapeutic Modified Diets:**</u>
Lowfat: Omit cheese
Diabetic/No added Sugar/No Conc. Sweets/Calorie Controlled: No changes
Bland/Anti Reflux: omit onions, omit pepper, omit garlic, and omit Worcestershire
Liberal House Renal: omit beef broth, Worcestershire sauce, cornstarch and cheese
No Added Salt: omit beef broth, Worcestershire sauce, and cornstarch
2 Gram Sodium: omit beef broth, Worcestershire sauce, cornstarch and cheese
Gluten Free: Use gluten free bread and use GF beef broth. Prepare foods separately to prevent cross contamination
Allergy Alerts: When an "X" is present, this indicates the allergen is present. Always read all food labels to ensure allergens are not present.

Wheat	Milk	Eggs	Fish Shellfish	Soy	Peanuts/Nuts	Other
x	x		X			

Key: SF= Salt Free D= Diet or Sugarfree LF = Lowfat FF = Fat Free GF = Gluten Free

Recipe Name: Grilled Roast Beef and Cheese Sandwich
Recipe Category: Meatless
Portion Size: 1 sandwich
Ingredients: Yields: 8 servings

Ingredients	Notes:
1/4 cup margarine	Softened
8 Slices American cheese (1 oz.)	May use other low fat sliced cheese.
1 lb. sliced lean roast beef	
16 Slices bread	Wheat or white

Directions:

Steps:	Directions:	Critical Control Point /Quality Assurance
1	Put 1 slice of cheese and 2 oz. roast beef between 2 slices of bread.	
2	Spread margarine on the outside of each slice of bread.	
3	Heat a large skillet, and place sandwich in skillet.	
4	Cook until golden brown and then turn until both sides are golden brown.	
5	Repeat until each sandwich is made.	

Time Temperature Sensitive food. *Food safety Standards: Food safety Standards: hold food for service at an internal temperature above 140°F. Do not mix old product with new. Cool leftover product quickly (within 4 hours) to below 41°F. Follow proper cooling procedures. Store leftovers in a tightly sealed, labeled and dated container. Use leftover within 72 hours if stored in refrigerator or 30 days if stored in the freezer. Reheat leftover product quickly (within 2 hours) to 165 degrees F for 15 seconds. Reheat left over product only once; discard if not used. Cold holding at 41°F or colder or using time alone (less than four hours).*

Texture Modified Diets:
Soft & Bite Size: (aka Bite size) **Food particle size ½ inch (~width of standard fork) Do not grill bread.** Food must be moist. Cut foods with a knife to a ½" particle size prior to layering. Moisten with broth as needed.
Chopped: Food particle size ¼ inch (~ ½ width of standard fork) Do not grill bread. Food must be moist. Chop foods with a knife to 1/4" particle size prior to layering. Moisten with broth as needed.
Minced and Moist: (aka Minced/Mechanical Soft/Ground) **Food particle size 1/8 inch (fits through prongs of standard fork) Do not grill bread.** Food must be moist. Use a food processor to grind food particles into 1/8 inch prior to layering. Moisten with broth as needed.
Pureed: Smooth and cohesive. Do not grill bread. Use a food processor to puree to a smooth consistency. Foods are processed by grinding and then pureeing them. May add broth or sauce to puree. Do not add to much liquid. Puree should still hold its shape. Must not be firm or sticky. Puree foods while still hot. Appearance should be smooth like pudding. Puree bread and roast beef separately.

Therapeutic Modified Diets:
Lowfat: No changes needed
Diabetic/No added Sugar/No Conc. Sweets/Calorie Controlled: No changes needed
Bland/Anti Reflux: No changes needed
Liberal House Renal: Use SF bread and SF margarine. Use low sodium roast beef (less than 140 mg. per serving)
No Added Salt: Use low sodium roast beef.
2 Gram Sodium: Use SF bread and SF margarine. Use low sodium roast beef (less than 140 mg. per serving)
Gluten Free: Use gluten free bread. Prepare foods separately to prevent cross contamination.
Allergy Alerts: When an "X" is present, this indicates the allergen is present.
Always read all food labels to ensure allergens are not present.

Wheat	Milk	Eggs	Fish Shellfish	Soy	Peanuts/Nuts	Other
X	X			X		

Key: SF= Salt Free D= Diet or Sugarfree LF = Lowfat FF = Fat Free GF = Gluten Free

Recipe Name: Meatball Sandwich
Recipe Category: Lunch Entrée
Portion Size: 1 Sandwich
Ingredients: **Yields: 8 servings**

Ingredients	Notes:
8 Hoagie Rolls	May use whole grain
1 pound lean ground beef	
8 oz. shredded low fat Mozzarella	
2 cups prepared marinara sauce	
1 egg	
¼ cup onion	Wash, peel and diced
1/3 cup seasoned bread crumbs	

Directions:

Steps:	Directions:	Critical Control Point /Quality Assurance
1	Combine ground beef, onion, egg, and bread crumbs in a bowl. Shape into ½ inch balls.	
2	Cook in pan over medium high heat. Turning as you cook to brown. Drain excess fat from pan. Add marinara sauce and heat.	Cook until internal temperature reaches 165 F degrees for 15 seconds
3	To serve: add 3 oz. meatballs with sauce to each bun. Top with Mozzarella and serve warm. (may brown Mozzarella under broiler)	

Time Temperature Sensitive food. *Do not mix old product with new. Store leftovers in a tightly sealed, labeled and dated container. Use leftover within 72 hours if stored in refrigerator or 30 days if stored in the freezer. Cold holding at 41 °F or colder or using time alone (less than four hours*

Texture Modified Diets:
Soft & Bite Size: (aka Bite size) **Food particle size ½ inch (~width of standard fork)** Food must be moist. Cut foods with a knife to a ½" particle size prior to layering. Moisten with sauce as needed.
Chopped: Food particle size ¼ inch (~ ½ width of standard fork) Food must be moist. Chop foods with a knife to 1/4" particle size prior to layering. Moisten with sauce as needed.
Minced and Moist:(aka Minced/Mechanical Soft/Ground) **Food particle size 1/8 inch (fits through prongs of standard fork)** Food must be moist. Use a food processor to grind food particles into 1/8 inch prior to layering. Moisten with sauce as needed.
Pureed: Smooth and cohesive. Use a food processor to puree to a smooth consistency. Foods are processed by grinding and then pureeing them. May add broth or sauce to puree. Do not add to much liquid. Puree should still hold its shape. Must not be firm or sticky. Puree foods while still hot. Appearance should be smooth like pudding. Puree 1/3 cup puree meat and 1 cup puree bread separately.

Therapeutic Modified Diets:
Low fat: No changes needed
Diabetic/No added Sugar/No Conc. Sweets/Calorie Controlled: No changes needed
Bland/Anti Reflux: Omit marinara sauce, onions and use plain bread crumbs.
Liberal House Renal: Use low sodium rolls (less than 140 mg. sodium per serving). Omit cheese, marinara sauce and use low sodium bread crumbs.
No Added Salt: No changes needed
2 Gram Sodium: Use low sodium rolls (less than 140 mg. sodium per serving). Omit cheese and use low sodium bread crumbs. Use no added Salt tomato sauce seasoned with Italian herbs.
Gluten Free: Use gluten free rolls. Prepare foods separately to prevent cross contamination.
Allergy Alerts: When an "X" is present, this indicates the allergen is present.
Always read all food labels to ensure allergens are not present.

Wheat	Milk	Eggs	Fish Shellfish	Soy	Peanuts/Nuts	Other
X	X	x				

Key: SF= Salt Free D= Diet or Sugarfree LF = Lowfat FF = Fat Free GF = Gluten Free

Copyright 2020 Jacqueline Larson M.S., R.D.N. and Associates.   All Rights Reserved

Recipe Name: Pita Pocket Sandwiches
Recipe Category: Lunch Entrée
Portion Size: ½ pita
Ingredients: **Yields: 8 servings**

Ingredients	Notes:
1/2 cup light mayonnaise	
2 tablespoons prepared mustard	
16 oz. package thinly sliced lean corned beef, beef, ham, or turkey	
4 Pita bread rounds, cut in half	
3 tablespoons pickle relish	(Optional)
1 cup shredded Lowfat Swiss cheese	
8 Lettuce leaves	Washed, trimmed and chopped
Sliced tomatoes	Washed, trimmed and diced

Directions:

Steps:	Directions:	Critical Control Point / Quality Assurance
1	Mix mayonnaise, mustard, and relish	
2	Cut meat into thin strips.	
3	Add meat to mayonnaise mixture and stir until all meat is coated.	
4	Cut each piece of pita bread in half	
5	Open bread to make a pocket.	
6	Add 1/3 c. meat mixture, 2 T. Swiss cheese, tomatoes, and lettuce each to the pocket.	

Time Temperature Sensitive food. *Food safety Standards: Do not mix old product with new. Store leftovers in a tightly sealed, labeled and dated container. Use leftover within 72 hours if stored in refrigerator or 30 days if stored in the freezer. Cold holding at 41 °F or colder or using time alone (less than four hours).*

Texture Modified Diets:

Soft & Bite Size: (aka Bite size) **Food particle size ½ inch (~width of standard fork)** Food must be moist. Cut foods with a knife to a ½" particle size prior to layering. Moisten with broth as needed.

Chopped: Food particle size ¼ inch (~ ½ width of standard fork) Food must be moist. Chop foods with a knife to 1/4" particle size prior to layering. Moisten with broth as needed.

Minced and Moist:(aka Minced/Mechanical Soft/Ground) **Food particle size 1/8 inch (fits through prongs of standard fork)** Food must be moist. Use a food processor to grind food particles into 1/8 inch prior to layering. Moisten with broth as needed.

Pureed: Smooth and cohesive. Use a food processor to puree to a smooth consistency. Foods are processed by grinding and then pureeing them. May add broth or sauce to puree. Do not add to much liquid. Puree should still hold its shape. Must not be firm or sticky. Puree foods while still hot. Appearance should be smooth like pudding. Serve 1/3 puree cup meat separately from ½ cup puree pita with puree lettuce and puree tomato. Puree with broth if needed.

Therapeutic Modified Diets:

Lowfat: No changes needed
Diabetic/No added Sugar/No Conc. Sweets/Calorie Controlled: No changes needed
Bland/Anti Reflux: Omit mustard and pickle relish
Liberal House Renal: Omit mayonnaise, pickle relish and Swiss Cheese. Use low sodium meat (less than 140 mg per serving)
No Added Salt: Omit pickle relish
2 Gram Sodium: Omit mayonnaise, pickle relish and Swiss Cheese. Use low sodium meat (less than 140 mg per serving)
Gluten Free: Use gluten free bread or GF pita bread. Prepare foods separately to prevent cross contamination

Allergy Alerts: When an "X" is present, this indicates the allergen is present. Always read all food labels to ensure allergens are not present.

Wheat	Milk	Eggs	Fish Shellfish	Soy	Peanuts/Nuts	Other
x	x	x				

Key: SF= Salt Free D= Diet or Sugarfree LF = Lowfat FF = Fat Free GF = Gluten Free

Recipe Name: Reuben Sandwiches
Recipe Category: Lunch Entrée
Portion Size: 1 sandwich (2 slices bread, 2 oz. corned beef, 2 T. sauerkraut, 1 oz. Swiss Cheese, 1 T. dressing)
Ingredients: Yields: 8 servings

Ingredients	Notes:
16 Slices rye bread	
1 pound thinly sliced lean corned beef	
1 cup sauerkraut, drained	
8 Slices Lowfat Swiss cheese	
3/4 cup Reduced fat Russian or thousand island dressing	
Margarine	

Directions:

Steps:	Directions:	Critical Control Point / Quality Assurance
1	Preheat oven to 400 degree oven	
2	Lightly spread margarine on one side only of bread	
3	Layer corned beef, sauerkraut, and Swiss cheese. (Margarine needs to be on the outside of the bread)	
4	Spread thousand island dressing on cheese	
5	Wrap in foil and heat in oven until cheese is heated through	
6	You may also grill this sandwich under the broiler or brown in skillet	

Time Temperature Sensitive food. *Food safety Standards: Store leftovers in a tightly sealed, labeled and dated container. Use leftover within 72 hours if stored in refrigerator or 30 days if stored in the freezer. Cold holding at 41°F or colder or using time alone (less than four hours).*

<u>Texture Modified Diets</u>:

Soft & Bite Size: (aka Bite size) **Food particle size ½ inch (~width of standard fork) Do not grill bread.** Food must be moist. Cut foods with a knife to a ½" particle size prior to layering. Moisten with broth as needed.

Chopped: Food particle size ¼ inch (~ ½ width of standard fork) Do not grill bread. Food must be moist. Chop foods with a knife to 1/4" particle size prior to layering. Moisten with broth as needed.

Minced and Moist:(aka Minced/Mechanical Soft/Ground) **Food particle size 1/8 inch (fits through prongs of standard fork) Do not grill bread.** Food must be moist. Use a food processor to grind food particles into 1/8 inch prior to layering. Moisten with broth as needed.

Pureed: Smooth and cohesive. Do not grill bread. Use a food processor to puree to a smooth consistency. Foods are processed by grinding and then pureeing them. May add broth or sauce to puree. Do not add to much liquid. Puree should still hold its shape. Must not be firm or sticky. Puree foods while still hot. Appearance should be smooth like pudding.
Puree corn beef and Swiss Cheese with dressing for a 1/3 cup serving. Puree Rye bread separately with milk for ½ cup serving. Serve separately. Omit Sauerkraut.

<u>Therapeutic Modified Diets</u>:

Low fat: Omit margarine
Diabetic/No added Sugar/No Conc. Sweets/Calorie Controlled: No changes needed
Bland/Anti Reflux: Use lean roast beef or turkey for corned beef. Omit sauerkraut and dressing. May use light mayonnaise.
Liberal House Renal: Use low sodium roast beef or turkey for corned beef (less than 140 mg. sodium per serving). Omit sauerkraut and dressing. May add mustard.
No Added Salt: Use roast beef or turkey for corned beef. Omit sauerkraut.
2 Gram Sodium: Use low sodium roast beef or turkey for corned beef (less than 140 mg. sodium per serving). Omit sauerkraut and dressing. May add mustard.
Gluten Free: Use gluten free bread and dressing. Prepare foods separately to prevent cross contamination.

Allergy Alerts: When an "X" is present, this indicates the allergen is present. Always read all food labels to ensure allergens are not present.

Wheat	Milk	Eggs	Fish Shellfish	Soy	Peanuts/Nuts	Other
X	x	X	X			

Key: SF= Salt Free D= Diet or Sugarfree LF = Lowfat FF = Fat Free GF = Gluten Free

Recipe Name: Roast Beef Sandwich
Recipe Category: Lunch Entrée
Portion Size: 1 Sandwich
Ingredients: Yields: 8 servings

Ingredients	Notes:
16 slices bread	May use whole grain
1 pound cooked and sliced lean deli roast beef	
½ cup mayonnaise	
¼ cup mustard	
16 slices tomatoes	Wash, trim and sliced (optional)
1 Small red onion	Wash, peel and slice thin (optional)
2 cups fresh spinach leaves or lettuce	Washed, trimmed and chopped (optional

Directions:

Steps:	Directions:	Critical Control Point / Quality Assurance
1	Spread each slice bread with mayonnaise and mustard	
2	Top each sandwich with 2 oz. roast beef	
3	Arrange tomato, lettuce or spinach and onion on each sandwich. Cut in half diagonally. Chill in an airtight container until ready to serve.	

Time Temperature Sensitive food. *Do not mix old product with new. Store leftovers in a tightly sealed, labeled and dated container. Use leftover within 72 hours if stored in refrigerator or 30 days if stored in the freezer. Cold holding at 41°F or colder or using time alone (less than four hours*

Texture Modified Diets:

Soft & Bite Size: (aka Bite size) **Food particle size ½ inch (~width of standard fork)** Food must be moist. Cut foods with a knife to a ½" particle size prior to layering. Moisten with broth as needed.
Chopped: Food particle size ¼ inch (~ ½ width of standard fork) Food must be moist. Chop foods with a knife to 1/4" particle size prior to layering. Moisten with broth as needed.
Minced and Moist:(aka Minced/Mechanical Soft/Ground) **Food particle size 1/8 inch (fits through prongs of standard fork)** Food must be moist. Use a food processor to grind food particles into 1/8 inch prior to layering. Moisten with broth as needed.
Pureed: Smooth and cohesive. Use a food processor to puree to a smooth consistency. Foods are processed by grinding and then pureeing them. May add broth or sauce to puree. Do not add to much liquid. Puree should still hold its shape. Must not be firm or sticky. Puree foods while still hot. Appearance should be smooth like pudding. Puree 1/3 cup puree meat. 1 cup puree bread with sour mayonnaise and mustard mixture serve separately. Puree with milk if needed. Spinach, tomato and onion may be puree with bread.

Therapeutic Modified Diets:

Low fat: No changes needed
Diabetic/No added Sugar/No Conc. Sweets/Calorie Controlled: No changes needed
Bland/Anti Reflux: Omit Onions, tomato, mustard and spinach
Liberal House Renal: Use low sodium deli roast beef (less than 140 mg. sodium per serving). Omit mayonnaise May add mustard.
No Added Salt: No changes needed
2 Gram Sodium: Use low sodium deli roast beef (less than 140 mg. sodium per serving). Omit mayonnaise. May add mustard.
Gluten Free: Use gluten free bread. Prepare foods separately to prevent cross contamination.
Allergy Alerts: When an "X" is present, this indicates the allergen is present.
Always read all food labels to ensure allergens are not present.

Wheat	Milk	Eggs	Fish Shellfish	Soy	Peanuts/Nuts	Other
X		x				

Key: SF= Salt Free D= Diet or Sugarfree LF = Lowfat FF = Fat Free GF = Gluten Free

Recipe Name: Roast Beef Tortilla Wraps
Recipe Category: Lunch Entrée
Portion Size: 1 whole wrap (Approx. 2 oz. roast beef, 2 T. cream cheese/sour cream mixture, 1 T. tomatoes, 1 T. red onion and 2 T. spinach leaves)
Ingredients: Yields: 8 servings

Ingredients	Notes:
8 burrito sized flour tortillas	May use whole grain
1 pound cooked and sliced lean deli roast beef	
8 oz. light cream cheese, soften	
1/2 cup light sour cream	
1/2 cup chopped tomatoes	Wash, trim and chop
Small red onion	Wash, peel and slice thin
2 cups fresh spinach leaves	Washed, trimmed and chopped

Directions:

Steps:	Directions:	Critical Control Point /Quality Assurance
1	Heat each tortilla in a large skillet.	
2	Combine cream cheese and sour cream in a small bowl.	
3	Spread each tortilla with cream cheese mixture	
4	Arrange tomato, roast beef and onion on each tortilla	
5	Top with spinach leaves	
6	Roll up tight and cover each with plastic wrap. Refrigerate for 1 hour before serving	

Time Temperature Sensitive food. *Do not mix old product with new. Store leftovers in a tightly sealed, labeled and dated container. Use leftover within 72 hours if stored in refrigerator or 30 days if stored in the freezer. Cold holding at 41°F or colder or using time alone (less than four hours*

Texture Modified Diets:

Soft & Bite Size: (aka Bite size) **Food particle size ½ inch (~width of standard fork)** Food must be moist. Cut foods with a knife to a ½" particle size prior to layering. Moisten with broth as needed.
Chopped: Food particle size ¼ inch (~ ½ width of standard fork) Food must be moist. Chop foods with a knife to 1/4" particle size prior to layering. Moisten with broth as needed.
Minced and Moist:(aka Minced/Mechanical Soft/Ground) **Food particle size 1/8 inch (fits through prongs of standard fork)** Food must be moist. Use a food processor to grind food particles into 1/8 inch prior to layering. Moisten with broth as needed.
Pureed: Smooth and cohesive. Use a food processor to puree to a smooth consistency. Foods are processed by grinding and then pureeing them. May add broth or sauce to puree. Do not add to much liquid. Puree should still hold its shape. Must not be firm or sticky. Puree foods while still hot. Appearance should be smooth like pudding. Use 1/3 cup puree meat. 1 tortilla puree with sour cream and cream cheese mixture, and ½ c. per serving. Puree with milk if needed. Spinach, tomato and onion may be puree with tortilla.

Therapeutic Modified Diets:

Low fat: No changes needed
Diabetic/No added Sugar/No Conc. Sweets/Calorie Controlled: No changes needed
Bland/Anti Reflux: Omit Onions, tomato and spinach
Liberal House Renal: Use low sodium deli roast beef (less than 140 mg. sodium per serving). Omit tomato, sour cream, and cream cheese. May add mustard.
No Added Salt: No changes needed
2 Gram Sodium: Use low sodium deli roast beef (less than 140 mg. sodium per serving). Omit sour cream, and cream cheese. May add mustard.
Gluten Free: Use gluten free corn tortilla or omit. Prepare foods separately to prevent cross contamination.
Allergy Alerts: When an "X" is present, this indicates the allergen is present. Always read all food labels to ensure allergens are not present.

Wheat	Milk	Eggs	Fish Shellfish	Soy	Peanuts/Nuts	Other
X	x		X			

Key: SF= Salt Free D= Diet or Sugarfree LF = Lowfat FF = Fat Free GF = Gluten Free

Recipe Name: Sesame Steak Wraps
Recipe Category: Lunch Entrée
Portion Size: 1 whole wrap (Approx. 2 oz. steak, , 1 T. red onion and 2 T. spinach leaves)
Ingredients: Yields: 8 servings

Ingredients	Notes:
8 burrito sized flour tortillas	May use whole grain
1 pound round steak, thinly sliced	
½ cup honey	
2 tablespoons canola oil	
¼ cup lite soy sauce	
2 tablespoons cornstarch	
1 tablespoon sesame seeds	
2 teaspoons sesame oil	
1 teaspoon ground ginger	
½ teaspoon ground garlic powder	
Small red onion	Wash, peel and slice thin
2 cups fresh spinach leaves	Washed, trimmed and chopped

Directions:

Steps:	Directions:	Critical Control Point /Quality Assurance
1	In a small sauce pan combine honey, soy sauce, cornstarch, sesame seeds, sesame oil and garlic. Heat over medium high heat until thick and boiling.	
2	Heat oil in a pan over medium high heat. Sauté round steak until brown. Add onion and cook until tender. Add sauce. Heat until sauce is hot and thick.	Cook until internal temperature reaches 155 F degrees for 15 seconds
3	Spread each tortilla with spinach leaves and evenly distribute steak mixture on top. Serve warm immediately.	

Time Temperature Sensitive food. *Do not mix old product with new. Store leftovers in a tightly sealed, labeled and dated container. Use leftover within 72 hours if stored in refrigerator or 30 days if stored in the freezer. Cold holding at 41 °F or colder or using time alone (less than four hours*

Texture Modified Diets:
Soft & Bite Size: (aka Bite size) **Food particle size ½ inch (~width of standard fork)** Food must be moist. Cut foods with a knife to a ½" particle size prior to layering. Moisten with broth as needed.
Chopped: Food particle size ¼ inch (~ ½ width of standard fork) Food must be moist. Chop foods with a knife to 1/4" particle size prior to layering. Moisten with broth as needed.
Minced and Moist:(aka Minced/Mechanical Soft/Ground) **Food particle size 1/8-inch (fits through prongs of standard fork)** Food must be moist. Use a food processor to grind food particles into 1/8 inch prior to layering. Moisten with broth as needed.
Pureed: Smooth and cohesive. Use a food processor to puree to a smooth consistency. Foods are processed by grinding and then pureeing them. May add broth or sauce to puree. Do not add to much liquid. Puree should still hold its shape. Must not be firm or sticky. Puree foods while still hot. Appearance should be smooth like pudding. Omit sesame seeds.
Serve each item separately: meat/tortilla and spinach. Use 1/3 cup puree meat and sauce. 1 tortilla puree with milk top tortilla with 2 tablespoons puree spinach.

Therapeutic Modified Diets:
Low fat: No changes needed
Diabetic/No added Sugar/No Conc. Sweets/Calorie Controlled: No changes needed
Bland/Anti Reflux: Omit Onions, garlic, sesame seeds. and spinach
Liberal House Renal: Use low sodium tortillas (less than 140 mg. sodium per serving). Topped with SF thinly sliced SF steak. May add Dijon mustard.
No Added Salt: No changes needed
2 Gram Sodium: Use low sodium tortillas (less than 140 mg. sodium per serving). Topped with SF thinly sliced SF steak. May add Dijon mustard.

Gluten Free: Use gluten free corn tortilla or omit. Use GF soy sauce. Prepare foods separately to prevent cross contamination.
Allergy Alerts: When an "X" is present, this indicates the allergen is present.
Always read all food labels to ensure allergens are not present.

Wheat	Milk	Eggs	Fish Shellfish	Soy	Peanuts/Nuts	Other
X				X		

Key: SF= Salt Free D= Diet or Sugarfree LF = Lowfat FF = Fat Free GF = Gluten Free

Recipe Name: Taco Salad
Recipe Category: Lunch Entrée
Portion Size: 1 cup lettuce, 1/2 cup ground beef/bean mixture, 1-2 tablespoons onion, cheese, avocado, chips, dressing and tomato.
Ingredients: Yields: 8 servings

Ingredients	Notes:
1 pound lean ground beef	
1 can (15 oz.) kidney beans	Drain liquid
1 tablespoon Chili Powder	
½ teaspoon garlic powder	
½ teaspoon onion powder	
¼ teaspoon crushed red pepper flakes	(optional)
¼ teaspoon dried oregano	
½ teaspoon paprika	
1 teaspoon ground cumin	
1 teaspoon salt	
½ teaspoon black pepper	
1 Head lettuce	Wash, trim and shred lettuce
1 onion	Washed, peeled and diced
8 ounces Light Cheddar or Monterey Jack cheese, shredded	
1 Avocado, (optional)	Wash, peel, remove seed and cube
1 Bag (12 oz.) Baked tortilla chips, broken	
1 Bottle (8oz.) Light French, Ranch or Italian salad dressing	
Hot Sauce to taste	
1 Large Tomato	Washed, trimmed and diced

Directions:

Steps:	Directions:	Critical Control Point / Quality Assurance
1	Sauté ground beef. Drain fat	Internal temperature should reach 165 degrees
2	Add kidney beans and seasonings (chili powder, garlic powder, onion powder, red pepper flakes, dried oregano, paprika, cumin, salt and black pepper). Set aside. Heat through.	
3	Toss lettuce, onion cheese, cubed avocado, and tortilla chips.	
4	Add ground beef and beans to salad	
5	Toss with dressing and hot sauce	
6	Garnish with avocado, tortillas chips and tomato slices. Serve immediately	

Time Temperature Sensitive food. *Food safety Standards: hold food for service at an internal temperature above 140°F. Do not mix old product with new. Cool leftover product quickly (within 4 hours) to below 41°F. Follow proper cooling procedures. Store leftovers in a tightly sealed, labeled and dated container. Use leftover within 72 hours if stored in refrigerator. Do not freeze. Reheat leftover product quickly (within 2 hours) to 165 degrees F for 15 seconds. Reheat left over product only once; discard if not used. Cold holding at 41°F or colder or using time alone (less than four hours). Always wash hands and wash and sanitize counter tops utensils and containers between steps when working with raw meat.*

Texture Modified Diets:

Soft & Bite Size: (aka Bite size) **Food particle size ½ inch (~width of standard fork)** Food must be moist. Cut foods with a knife to a ½" particle size prior to mixing. Moisten with broth as needed. Foods **that do not process well should be omitted. Omit: tortilla chips.**

Chopped: Food particle size ¼ inch (~ ½ width of standard fork) Food must be moist. Chop foods with a knife to 1/4" particle size prior to mixing. Moisten with broth as needed. Foods that do not process well should be omitted. Omit: tortilla chips.

Copyright 2020 Jacqueline Larson M.S., R.D.N. and Associates. All Rights Reserved

Minced and Moist: (aka Minced/Mechanical Soft/Ground) **Food particle size 1/8 inch (fits through prongs of standard fork)** Food must be moist. Use a food processor to grind food particles into 1/8 inch prior to mixing. Moisten with broth as needed. Foods that do not process well should be omitted. Omit: tortilla chips.

Pureed: Smooth and cohesive. Use a food processor to puree to a smooth consistency. Foods are processed by grinding and then pureeing them. May add broth or sauce to puree. Do not add to much liquid. Puree should still hold its shape. Must not be firm or sticky. Puree foods while still hot. Appearance should be smooth like pudding. Foods that do not process well should be omitted. Omit: tortilla chips. Use ½ cup meat mixture per serving, ½ cup of lettuce mixture per serving. Top with puree dressing. Puree with broth if needed.

Therapeutic Modified Diets:

Low fat: Omit avocado

Diabetic/No added Sugar/No Conc. Sweets/Calorie Controlled: no changes need

Bland/Anti Reflux: omit chili powder, garlic powder, onion powder, red pepper flakes, dried oregano, paprika, cumin, salt, black pepper, kidney beans, hot sauce, dressing, tomato. Toss with small amount of light sour cream

Liberal House Renal: Omit salt, cheese, dressing and tomatoes.

No Added Salt: Omit chips

2 Gram Sodium: Omit salt, cheese and dressing

Gluten Free: No changes needed. Prepare foods separately to prevent cross contamination.

Allergy Alerts: When an "X" is present, this indicates the allergen is present.

Always read all food labels to ensure allergens are not present.

Wheat	Milk	Eggs	Fish Shellfish	Soy	Peanuts/Nuts	Other
X	x					

Key: SF= Salt Free D= Diet or Sugarfree LF = Lowfat FF = Fat Free GF = Gluten Free

HAM DINNER RECIPES

Recipe Name: Apricot Glazed Ham
Recipe Category: Dinner Entrée
Portion Size: 3 oz.
Ingredients: Yields: 8 servings

Ingredients	Notes:
2 lbs. fully cooked whole boneless ham	
1/3 cup packed brown sugar	
1 Tablespoon cornstarch	
½ teaspoon nutmeg	
1/8 teaspoon, ground cloves	
2/3 cup apricot nectar	
2 Tablespoons lemon juice	

Directions:

Steps:	Directions:	Critical Control Point / Quality Assurance
1	Pre heat oven to 325°F.	
2	Place ham on rack in shallow roasting pan.	
3	Bake uncovered for 40-45 minutes or until temperature reaches 140 degrees.	
4	For the glaze, in a small saucepan combine brown sugar, cornstarch, nutmeg, cloves, apricot nectar and lemon juice.	
5	Cook over medium heat until thickened and bubbly, stirring constantly.	
6	Remove ½ glaze and brush on ham.	
7	Bake for 15 minutes.	
8	Slice ham and serve with remaining glaze.	

Time Temperature Sensitive food. *Food safety Standards: hold food for service at an internal temperature above 140° F. Do not mix old product with new. Cool leftover product quickly (within 4 hours) to below 41° F. Follow proper cooling procedures. Store leftovers in a tightly sealed, labeled and dated container. Use leftover within 72 hours if stored in refrigerator or 30 days if stored in the freezer. Reheat leftover product quickly (within 2 hours) to 165 degrees F for 15 seconds. Reheat left over product only once; discard if not used. Cold holding at 41°F or colder or using time alone (less than four hours).*

Texture Modified Diets:
Soft & Bite Size: (aka Bite size) **Food particle size ½ inch (~width of standard fork)** Food must be moist. Cut foods with a knife to a ½" particle size prior to mixing. Moisten with broth as needed.
Chopped: Food particle size ¼ inch (~ ½ width of standard fork) Food must be moist. Chop foods with a knife to 1/4" particle size prior to mixing. Moisten with broth as needed. **Minced and Moist:** (aka Minced/Mechanical Soft/Ground) **Food particle size 1/8 inch (fits through prongs of standard fork)** Food must be moist. Use a food processor to grind food particles into 1/8 inch prior to mixing. Moisten with broth as needed.
Pureed: Smooth and cohesive. Use a food processor to puree to a smooth consistency. Foods are processed by grinding and then pureeing them. May add broth or sauce to puree. Do not add to much liquid. Puree should still hold its shape. Must not be firm or sticky. Puree foods while still hot. Appearance should be smooth like pudding. Serv ½ cup puree meat topped with glaze.

Therapeutic Modified Diets:
Lowfat: No changes needed
Diabetic/No added Sugar/No Conc. Sweets/Calorie Controlled: Omit glaze
Bland: omit nutmeg and cloves
Liberal House Renal: use alternate menu item
No Added Salt: use alternate menu item.
2 Gram Sodium: use alternate menu item
Gluten Free: No changes needed. Prepare foods separately to prevent cross contamination.
**Allergy Alerts: When an "X" is present, this indicates the allergen is present.
Always read all food labels to ensure allergens are not present.**

Wheat	Milk	Eggs	Fish Shellfish	Soy	Peanuts/Nuts	Other

Key: SF= Salt Free D= Diet or Sugarfree LF = Lowfat FF = Fat Free GF = Gluten Free

Recipe Name: Baked Ham
Recipe Category: Dinner Entrée
Portion Size: 3 oz.
Ingredients: Yields: 8 servings

Ingredients	Notes:
4 pounds ham, bone in or 2 lbs. boneless	Trim all visible fat
1 cup brown sugar	
¼ cup honey, maple syrup, or cider vinegar	
2 teaspoons dry mustard	
15 or more cloves	
1 can pineapple rings	(optional)

Directions:

Steps:	Directions:	Critical Control Point /Quality Assurance
1	Preheat the oven to 350° degree oven.	
2	Place the ham on a rack in a shallow roasting pan, fat side up.	
3	Bake the ham unglazed until the thermometer reads 130°F or until 1 hour before the ham is done.	
4	Prepare for glazing by scoring the outside fat in a diamond pattern, cutting ¼ inch deep with a sharp knife.	
5	Combine the brown sugar with the honey, syrup, or vinegar and the mustard.	
6	Mix well and spread over the outside of the ham.	
7	Stud with whole cloves set decoratively in the center of each diamond.	
8	Optional: Or if you like pineapple rings, set them in place with toothpicks, putting the cloves in the holes.	
9	Return to the oven for 1 hour to finish baking, brushing, if you wish, every 15 minutes with basting sauce.	Cook until internal temperature reaches 145°F for 4 minutes.
10	Let it rest 15 minutes before carving. Carve and serve hot.	

Time Temperature Sensitive food. *Food safety Standards: hold food for service at an internal temperature above 140° F. Do not mix old product with new. Cool leftover product quickly (within 4 hours) to below 41° F. Follow proper cooling procedures. Store leftovers in a tightly sealed, labeled and dated container. Use leftover within 72 hours if stored in refrigerator or 30 days if stored in the freezer. Reheat leftover product quickly (within 2 hours) to 165 degrees F for 15 seconds. Reheat left over product only once; discard if not used. Cold holding at 41°F or colder or using time alone (less than four hours).*

Texture Modified Diets:
Soft & Bite Size: (aka Bite size) **Food particle size ½ inch (~width of standard fork)** Food must be moist. Cut foods with a knife to a ½" particle size prior to mixing. Moisten with broth as needed. Foods that do not process well should be omitted. Omit: pineapple rings. May substitute canned peaches.
Chopped: Food particle size ¼ inch (~ ½ width of standard fork) Food must be moist. Chop foods with a knife to 1/4" particle size prior to mixing. Moisten with broth as needed. Foods that do not process well should be omitted. Omit: pineapple rings. May substitute canned peaches.
Minced and Moist: (aka Minced/Mechanical Soft/Ground) **Food particle size 1/8 inch (fits through prongs of standard fork)** Food must be moist. Use a food processor to grind food particles into 1/8 inch prior to mixing. Moisten with broth as needed. Foods that do not process well should be omitted. Omit: pineapple rings. May substitute canned peaches.
Pureed: Smooth and cohesive. Use a food processor to puree to a smooth consistency. Foods are processed by grinding and then pureeing them. May add broth or sauce to puree. Do not add to much liquid. Puree should still hold its shape. Must not be firm or sticky. Puree foods while still hot. Appearance should be smooth like pudding. Foods that do not process well should be omitted. Omit: pineapple rings. Serve ½ c. meat serving. May substitute canned peaches.

Therapeutic Modified Diets:
Lowfat: No changes needed
Diabetic/No added Sugar/No Conc. Sweets/Calorie Controlled: No brown sugar, honey or maple syrup
Bland/Anti Reflux: No pineapple rings and mustard

Copyright 2020 Jacqueline Larson M.S., R.D.N. and Associates.   All Rights Reserved

Liberal House Renal: Use alternate menu item
No Added Salt: Use alternate menu item
2 Gram Sodium: Use alternate menu item
Gluten Free: No changes needed.
**Allergy Alerts: When an "X" is present, this indicates the allergen is present.
Always read all food labels to ensure allergens are not present.**

Wheat	Milk	Eggs	Fish Shellfish	Soy	Peanuts/Nuts	Other

Key: SF= Salt Free D= Diet or Sugarfree LF = Lowfat FF = Fat Free GF = Gluten Free

Recipe Name: Baked Boneless Ham
Recipe Category: Dinner Entrée
Portion Size: 3 oz. boneless
Ingredients: Yields: 8 servings

Ingredients	Notes:
4-5 pounds fully cooked boneless ham	
Optional Glaze:	
½ cup honey	Combine glaze and glaze ham during last 15 minutes of reheating.
6 oz can thawed orange juice	

Directions:

Steps:	Directions:	Critical Control Point /Quality Assurance
1	Pre heat oven to 350°F.	
2	Place ham in large shallow roasting pan.	
3	Bake until meat thermometer inserted in thickest part registers 125° F; about 1 and ¼ hours. Serve hot.	

Time Temperature Sensitive food. *Food safety Standards: hold food for service at an internal temperature above 140°F. Do not mix old product with new. Cool leftover product quickly (within 4 hours) to below 41°F. Follow proper cooling procedures. Store leftovers in a tightly sealed, labeled and dated container. Use leftover within 72 hours if stored in refrigerator or 30 days if stored in the freezer. Reheat leftover product quickly (within 2 hours) to 165 degrees F for 15 seconds. Reheat left over product only once; discard if not used. Cold holding at 41°F or colder or using time alone (less than four hours).*

Texture Modified Diets:
Soft & Bite Size: (aka Bite size) **Food particle size ½ inch (~width of standard fork)** Food must be moist. Cut foods with a knife to a ½" particle size prior to mixing. Moisten with broth as needed.
Chopped: Food particle size ¼ inch (~ ½ width of standard fork) Food must be moist. Chop foods with a knife to 1/4" particle size prior to mixing. Moisten with broth as needed. **Minced and Moist:** (aka Minced/Mechanical Soft/Ground) **Food particle size 1/8 inch (fits through prongs of standard fork)** Food must be moist. Use a food processor to grind food particles into 1/8 inch prior to mixing. Moisten with broth as needed.
Pureed: Smooth and cohesive. Use a food processor to puree to a smooth consistency. Foods are processed by grinding and then pureeing them. May add broth or sauce to puree. Do not add to much liquid. Puree should still hold its shape. Must not be firm or sticky. Puree foods while still hot. Appearance should be smooth like pudding. Serv ½ cup puree meat topped with glaze. Serve ½ c. meat pureed. May top with glaze.

Therapeutic Modified Diets:
Lowfat: No changes needed
Diabetic/No added Sugar/No Conc. Sweets/Calorie Controlled: No glaze
Bland: no changes
Liberal House Renal: use alternate menu item
No Added Salt: use alternate menu item
2 Gram Sodium: use alternate menu item
Gluten Free: Use no changes needed. Prepare foods separately to prevent cross contamination.
Allergy Alerts: When an "X" is present, this indicates the allergen is present.
Always read all food labels to ensure allergens are not present.

Wheat	Milk	Eggs	Fish Shellfish	Soy	Peanuts/Nuts	Other

Key: SF= Salt Free D= Diet or Sugarfree LF = Lowfat FF = Fat Free GF = Gluten Free

Recipe Name: Cheese Ham and Pasta Bake
Recipe Category: Dinner Entrée
Portion Size: 1 1/2 cups (approx. ½ cup meat, pasta and vegetables)
Ingredients: Yields: 8 servings

Ingredients	Notes:
1 lb. pasta	May use whole grain pasta
2 cups fat free evaporated milk	
3½ tablespoons flour	
1 teaspoon thyme	Use fresh or dried
2 teaspoon marjoram	Use fresh or dried
1 tablespoon olive oil	
1 onion, finely chopped	
2 cups broccoli florets	Use fresh or frozen, Wash and trim
2 cups sliced mushrooms	Wash and trim
1 red bell pepper, chopped	Wash and trim
3 garlic cloves, crushed	
½ teaspoon pepper	
3 cups cooked lean ham, cubed	Trim all visible fat
1 cup low fat shredded cheddar or Monterey jack cheese	

Directions:

Steps:	Directions:	Critical Control Point / Quality Assurance
1	Prepare pasta according to package directions; drain well.	
2	Spray a baking dish with cooking spray.	
3	Place drained pasta in baking dish and set aside.	
4	Preheat oven to 350°F	
5	Combine milk, flour, thyme and marjoram in a small bowl and set aside.	
6	Heat a large, nonstick skillet over medium-high heat.	
7	Add oil and sauté onion, broccoli, mushroom, bell pepper, garlic, salt and pepper for 4 minutes, stirring frequently.	
8	Add ham and heat thoroughly, about 2 more minutes.	
9	Add reserved milk mixture and stir until thickened, about 4 minutes; do not boil.	
10	Sprinkle ham mixture over the pasta in the prepared baking.	
11	Sprinkle with cheese and bake uncovered for 15 minutes, or until cheese is melted.	Cook until internal temperature reaches 165°F for 15 seconds

Time Temperature Sensitive food. *Food safety Standards: hold food for service at an internal temperature above 140° F. Do not mix old product with new. Cool leftover product quickly (within 4 hours) to below 41° F. Follow proper cooling procedures. Store leftovers in a tightly sealed, labeled and dated container. Use leftover within 72 hours if stored in refrigerator or 30 days if stored in the freezer. Reheat leftover product quickly (within 2 hours) to 165 degrees F for 15 seconds. Reheat left over product only once; discard if not used. Cold holding at 41°F or colder or using time alone (less than four hours).*

Texture Modified Diets:

Soft & Bite Size: (aka Bite size) **Food particle size ½ inch (~width of standard fork)** Food must be moist. Cut foods with a knife to a ½" particle size prior to mixing. Moisten with broth as needed.
Chopped: Food particle size ¼ inch (~ ½ width of standard fork) Food must be moist. Chop foods with a knife to 1/4" particle size prior to mixing. Moisten with broth as needed. **Minced and Moist:**(aka Minced/Mechanical Soft/Ground) **Food particle size 1/8 inch (fits through prongs of standard fork)** Food must be moist. Use a food processor to grind food particles into 1/8 inch prior to mixing. Moisten with broth as needed.
Pureed: Smooth and cohesive. Use a food processor to puree to a smooth consistency. Foods are processed by grinding and then pureeing them. May add broth or sauce to puree. Do not add to much liquid. Puree should still hold its shape. Must not be firm or sticky. Puree foods while still hot. Appearance should be smooth like pudding. Foods that do not process well should be omitted. Omit: Serve ½ c. meat serving, ½ c. puree pasta and ½ c. puree broccoli separately. May puree pasta with cheese and seasonings for flavor.

Therapeutic Modified Diets:

Lowfat: No changes needed
Diabetic/No added Sugar/No Conc. Sweets/Calorie Controlled: Use fat free cheese
Bland/Anti Reflux: Omit bell pepper, broccoli, thyme, marjoram, garlic, onions and pepper
Liberal House Renal: Use alternate menu item
No Added Salt: Use alternate menu item
2 Gram Sodium: Use alternate menu item
Gluten Free: Use gluten free pasta and flour. Prepare foods separately to prevent cross contamination.
Allergy Alerts: When an "X" is present, this indicates the allergen is present.
Always read all food labels to ensure allergens are not present.

Wheat	Milk	Eggs	Fish Shellfish	Soy	Peanuts/Nuts	Other
X	X	X				

Key: SF= Salt Free D= Diet or Sugarfree LF = Lowfat FF = Fat Free GF = Gluten Free

Recipe Name: Cheesy Ham and Red Potato Bake
Recipe Category: Dinner Entrée
Portion Size: 1 cup
Ingredients: Yields: 8 servings

Ingredients	Notes:
2 lbs. cooked ham, diced	
4 cups red potatoes, diced	Wash and trim. May leave on peel.
2 tablespoons margarine or butter	
2 tablespoons all-purpose flour	
1 cup nonfat milk	
½ cup chopped green onion	
1 cup light sour cream	
½ cup bread crumbs	
1 cup lowfat cheddar cheese, shredded	

Directions:

Steps:	Directions:	Critical Control Point /Quality Assurance
1	Pre heat oven to 350 degrees	
2	Place potatoes in a large pot of water and bring to boil. Boil until slightly tender about 12 minutes. Drain and transfer to a large bowl.	
3	In a large saucepan, melt margarine or butter and add flour. Cook 1 minute.	
4	Stir in milk. Bring to boil and reduce heat to low. Stirring constantly.	
5	Add cheese and stir. Cook 1 minute.	
6	Add cheese sauce to potatoes. Add sour cream and onions. Stir.	
7	Arrange ham slices on bottom of baking dish. Top with bread crumbs.	
8	Bake for 40 minutes or until internal temperature reaches 160°F. Let stand for about 10 minutes.	

Time Temperature Sensitive food. *Food safety Standards: hold food for service at an internal temperature above 140° F. Do not mix old product with new. Cool leftover product quickly (within 4 hours) to below 41° F. Follow proper cooling procedures. Store leftovers in a tightly sealed, labeled and dated container. Use leftover within 72 hours if stored in refrigerator or 30 days if stored in the freezer. Reheat leftover product quickly (within 2 hours) to 165 degrees F for 15 seconds. Reheat left over product only once; discard if not used. Cold holding at 41°F or colder or using time alone (less than four hours).*

Texture Modified Diets:

Soft & Bite Size: (aka Bite size) **Food particle size ½ inch (~width of standard fork)** Food must be moist. Cut foods with a knife to a ½" particle size prior to mixing. Moisten with broth as needed. Foods that do not process well should be omitted. Omit: green onions. Peel potatoes. May add minced white onion.

Chopped: Food particle size ¼ inch (~ ½ width of standard fork) Food must be moist. Chop foods with a knife to 1/4" particle size prior to mixing. Moisten with broth as needed. Foods that do not process well should be omitted. Omit: green onions. May add minced white onion. Peel Potatoes.

Minced and Moist: (aka Minced/Mechanical Soft/Ground) **Food particle size 1/8 inch (fits through prongs of standard fork)** Food must be moist. Use a food processor to grind food particles into 1/8 inch prior to mixing. Moisten with broth as needed. Foods that do not process well should be omitted. Omit: green onions. May add minced white onion. Peel potatoes.

Pureed: Smooth and cohesive. Use a food processor to puree to a smooth consistency. Foods are processed by grinding and then pureeing them. May add broth or sauce to puree. Do not add to much liquid. Puree should still hold its shape. Must not be firm or sticky. Puree foods while still hot. Appearance should be smooth like pudding. Foods that do not process well should be omitted. Omit: green onions and peel potatoes. May add minced white onion. Serve ½ c. meat pureed with ½ c. pureed potato mixture on side

Therapeutic Modified Diets:

Lowfat: No changes needed
Diabetic/No added Sugar/No Conc. Sweets/Calorie Controlled: No changes needed
Bland: omit green onion. Use peeled potatoes
Liberal House Renal: use alternate menu item
No Added Salt: use alternate menu item or sub. Chicken or turkey for ham
2 Gram Sodium: use alternate menu item
Gluten Free: Use GF bread crumb or sub. With GF cornflakes. Use GF all-purpose flour. Prepare foods separately to prevent cross contamination.
Allergy Alerts: When an "X" is present, this indicates the allergen is present.
Always read all food labels to ensure allergens are not present.

Wheat	Milk	Eggs	Fish Shellfish	Soy	Peanuts/Nuts	Other
X	X			X		

Key: SF= Salt Free D= Diet or Sugarfree LF = Lowfat FF = Fat Free GF = Gluten Free

Recipe Name: Cheesy Ham and Broccoli Bake
Recipe Category: Dinner Entrée
Portion Size: 1 cup
Ingredients: Yields: 8 servings

Ingredients	Notes:
2 lbs. cooked ham, sliced	
1 (10 oz.) package chopped broccoli, thawed	
2 tablespoons margarine or butter	
2 tablespoons all-purpose flour	
1 cup nonfat milk	
4 cups cooked rice	Use brown or white rice
1 cup light sour cream	
½ cup bread crumbs	
1 cup lowfat cheddar cheese, shredded	

Directions:

Steps:	Directions:	Critical Control Point / Quality Assurance
1	Pre heat oven to 350°F.	
2	In a large saucepan, melt margarine or butter and add flour. Cook 1 minute.	
3	Stir in milk. Bring to boil and reduce heat to low. Stirring constantly.	
4	Add cheese and stir. Cook 1 minute.	
5	Remove from heat and stir in sour cream and broccoli	
6.	Arrange ham slices on bottom of baking dish. Top with broccoli mixture and then bread crumbs.	
7.	Bake for 40 minutes or until internal temperature reaches 160 °F. Let stand for about 10 minutes.	

Time Temperature Sensitive food. *Food safety Standards: hold food for service at an internal temperature above 140° F. Do not mix old product with new. Cool leftover product quickly (within 4 hours) to below 41° F. Follow proper cooling procedures. Store leftovers in a tightly sealed, labeled and dated container. Use leftover within 72 hours if stored in refrigerator or 30 days if stored in the freezer. Reheat leftover product quickly (within 2 hours) to 165 degrees F for 15 seconds. Reheat left over product only once; discard if not used. Cold holding at 41°F or colder or using time alone (less than four hours).*

Texture Modified Diets:

Soft & Bite Size: (aka Bite size) **Food particle size ½ inch (~width of standard fork)** Food must be moist. Cut foods with a knife to a ½" particle size prior to mixing. Moisten with broth as needed.
Chopped: Food particle size ¼ inch (~ ½ width of standard fork) Food must be moist. Chop foods with a knife to 1/4" particle size prior to mixing. Moisten with broth as needed.
Minced and Moist:(aka Minced/Mechanical Soft/Ground) **Food particle size 1/8 inch (fits through prongs of standard fork)** Food must be moist. Use a food processor to grind food particles into 1/8 inch prior to mixing. Moisten with broth as needed.
Pureed: Smooth and cohesive. Use a food processor to puree to a smooth consistency. Foods are processed by grinding and then pureeing them. May add broth or sauce to puree. Do not add to much liquid. Puree should still hold its shape. Must not be firm or sticky. Puree foods while still hot. Appearance should be smooth like pudding. Serve ½ c. meat pureed with ½ c. pureed rice mixture separately.

Therapeutic Modified Diets:

Lowfat: No changes needed
Diabetic/No added Sugar/No Conc. Sweets/Calorie Controlled: No changes needed
Bland: substitute green beans for broccoli
Liberal House Renal: use alternate menu item
No Added Salt: use alternate menu item or sub. Chicken or turkey for ham
2 Gram Sodium: use alternate menu item
Gluten Free: Use GF bread crumb or sub. With GF cornflakes. Use GF all-purpose flour. Prepare foods separately to prevent cross contamination.

Allergy Alerts: When an "X" is present, this indicates the allergen is present. Always read all food labels to ensure allergens are not present.

Wheat	Milk	Eggs	Fish Shellfish	Soy	Peanuts/Nuts	Other
X	X					

Key: SF= Salt Free D= Diet or Sugarfree LF = Lowfat FF = Fat Free GF = Gluten Free

Recipe Name: Florentine Ham Casserole
Recipe Category: Dinner Entrée
Portion Size: 1 cup total
Ingredients: Yields: 8 servings

Ingredients	Notes:
2 lbs. cooked ham, slices	
2 (10 oz.) package chopped spinach, thawed	May substitute fresh spinach for frozen, Washed trimmed and chopped.
12 oz. package mushrooms	Wash and slice
½ cup onion, chopped	Wash, peel and slice
1 teaspoon garlic powder	Or substitute 2 cloves minced
½ cup butter or margarine	
¼ cup all-purpose flour	
2 cups Nonfat milk	
4 eggs beaten	
½ teaspoon ground oregano	
1 teaspoon basil	
¼ teaspoon black pepper	
1 cup lowfat mozzarella cheese, shredded	

Directions:

Steps:	Directions:	Critical Control Point /Quality Assurance
1	Pre heat oven to 350°F.	
2	In a large saucepan cook mushroom, onion and garlic in margarine or butter, cook until tender but not brown.	
3	Stir in flour and milk.	
4	Cook and stir over medium low heat 4-5 minutes or until thickened and bubbly.	
5	Remove from heat and stir in oregano, pepper, basil, spinach and eggs.	
6	Arrange ham slices on bottom of baking dish. Top with spinach mixture and then cheese.	
7	Bake for 40 minutes or until internal temperature reaches 160°F. Let stand for about 10 minutes.	

Time Temperature Sensitive food. Food safety Standards: hold food for service at an internal temperature above 140° F. Do not mix old product with new. Cool leftover product quickly (within 4 hours) to below 41° F. Follow proper cooling procedures. Store leftovers in a tightly sealed, labeled and dated container. Use leftover within 72 hours if stored in refrigerator or 30 days if stored in the freezer. Reheat leftover product quickly (within 2 hours) to 165 degrees F for 15 seconds. Reheat left over product only once; discard if not used. Cold holding at 41°F or colder or using time alone (less than four hours).

Texture Modified Diets:

Soft & Bite Size: (aka Bite size) **Food particle size ½ inch (~width of standard fork)** Food must be moist. Cut foods with a knife to a ½" particle size prior to mixing. Moisten with broth as needed.

Chopped: Food particle size ¼ inch (~ ½ width of standard fork) Food must be moist. Chop foods with a knife to 1/4" particle size prior to mixing. Moisten with broth as needed.

Minced and Moist: (aka Minced/Mechanical Soft/Ground) **Food particle size 1/8 inch (fits through prongs of standard fork)** Food must be moist. Use a food processor to grind food particles into 1/8 inch prior to mixing. Moisten with broth as needed.

Pureed: Smooth and cohesive. Use a food processor to puree to a smooth consistency. Foods are processed by grinding and then pureeing them. May add broth or sauce to puree. Do not add to much liquid. Puree should still hold its shape. Must not be firm or sticky. Puree foods while still hot. Appearance should be smooth like pudding. Serve ½ c. meat pureed with ½ c. pureed mixture on side

Therapeutic Modified Diets:

Lowfat: No changes needed
Diabetic/No added Sugar/No Conc. Sweets/Calorie Controlled: No changes needed
Bland: omit pepper, garlic, oregano, and basil.
Liberal House Renal: use alternate menu item
No Added Salt: use alternate menu item or sub. Chicken or turkey for ham
2 Gram Sodium: use alternate menu item
Gluten Free: Use GF all purpose flour. Prepare foods separately to prevent cross contamination.

Allergy Alerts: When an "X" is present, this indicates the allergen is present. Always read all food labels to ensure allergens are not present.

Wheat	Milk	Eggs	Fish Shellfish	Soy	Peanuts/Nuts	Other
X	X	X		X		

Key: SF= Salt Free D= Diet or Sugarfree LF = Lowfat FF = Fat Free GF = Gluten Free

Recipe Name: Glazed Ham Loaf
Recipe Category: Dinner Entrée
Portion Size: 4 oz. boneless
Ingredients: Yields: 8 servings

Ingredients	Notes:
2 lbs. cooked ham, ground	
½ lb. lean ground pork	
½ cup Nonfat milk	
2 eggs	
½ cup bread crumbs	
½ cup catsup	
2 Tablespoons brown sugar	
1 Tablespoon chili powder	

Directions:

Steps:	Directions:	Critical Control Point /Quality Assurance
1	Pre heat oven to 350°F.	
2	In a large bowl, combine, ham, pork, milk, eggs, and bread crumbs.	
3	Spray loaf pan with nonstick cooking spray.	
4	Pat meat mixture into loaf and add to pan	
5	In a small bowl, combine catsup, brown sugar and chili powder	
6	Bake until internal temperature reaches 160°F. Let stand for about 10 minutes.	
7.	Slice and serve hot.	

Time Temperature Sensitive food. *Food safety Standards: hold food for service at an internal temperature above 140° F. Do not mix old product with new. Cool leftover product quickly (within 4 hours) to below 41° F. Follow proper cooling procedures. Store leftovers in a tightly sealed, labeled and dated container. Use leftover within 72 hours if stored in refrigerator or 30 days if stored in the freezer. Reheat leftover product quickly (within 2 hours) to 165 degrees F for 15 seconds. Reheat left over product only once; discard if not used. Cold holding at 41°F or colder or using time alone (less than four hours).*

Texture Modified Diets:

Soft & Bite Size: (aka Bite size) **Food particle size ½ inch (~width of standard fork)** Food must be moist. Cut foods with a knife to a ½" particle size after cooking. Moisten with milk as needed after cutting.

Chopped: Food particle size ¼ inch (~ ½ width of standard fork) Food must be moist. Chop foods with a knife to 1/4" particle size after cooking. Moisten with milk as needed after chopping.

Minced and Moist:(aka Minced/Mechanical Soft/Ground) **Food particle size 1/8 inch (fits through prongs of standard fork)** Food must be moist. Use a food processor to grind food particles into 1/8 inch after cooking. Moisten with milk as needed after processing.

Pureed: Smooth and cohesive. Use a food processor to puree to a smooth consistency. Foods are processed by grinding and then pureeing them. May add milk or sauce to puree. Do not add to much liquid. Puree should still hold its shape. Must not be firm or sticky. Puree foods while still hot. Appearance should be smooth like pudding. Serve ½ c. meat puree

Therapeutic Modified Diets:

Lowfat: No changes needed
Diabetic/No added Sugar/No Conc. Sweets/Calorie Controlled: No changes needed
Bland: omit chili powder
Liberal House Renal: use alternate menu item
No Added Salt: use alternate menu item
2 Gram Sodium: use alternate menu item
Gluten Free: Use GF bread crumbs or GF oats. Prepare foods separately to prevent cross contamination.
Allergy Alerts: When an "X" is present, this indicates the allergen is present.
Always read all food labels to ensure allergens are not present.

Wheat	Milk	Eggs	Fish Shellfish	Soy	Peanuts/Nuts	Other
X	X	X				

Key: SF= Salt Free D= Diet or Sugarfree LF = Lowfat FF = Fat Free GF = Gluten Free

Recipe Name: Grilled Ham Steak with Pineapple
Recipe Category: Dinner Entrée
Portion Size: 3 oz. ham
Ingredients: **Yields: 8 servings**

Ingredients	Notes:
1 large can pineapple rings in juice	Reserve ½ cup juice
¼ cup Dijon mustard	
¼ cup honey	
2 (1 Pound) cooked lean boneless ham steak, sliced	Trim all visible fat

Directions:

Steps:	Directions:	Critical Control Point /Quality Assurance
1	Drain juice from pineapple rings.	
2	In a small bowl mix pineapple juice with mustard and honey.	
3	Place ham steak on rack broiling pan and spread with ½ mustard mixture.	
4	Broil 3 to 4 minutes.	
5	Turn steak, top with pineapple slice, and spoon remaining mustard mixture over pineapple.	
6	Broil 3 to 4 minutes longer or until pineapple is lightly browned and steak is hot.	Cook until internal temperature reaches 165°F for 15 seconds

Time Temperature Sensitive food. Food safety Standards: hold food for service at an internal temperature above 140° F. Do not mix old product with new. Cool leftover product quickly (within 4 hours) to below 41° F. Follow proper cooling procedures. Store leftovers in a tightly sealed, labeled and dated container. Use leftover within 72 hours if stored in the refrigerator or 30 days if stored in the freezer. Reheat leftover product quickly (within 2 hours) to 165 degrees F for 15 seconds. Reheat left over product only once; discard if not used. Cold holding at 41°F or colder or using time alone (less than four hours).

<u>**Texture Modified Diets:**</u>

Soft & Bite Size: (aka Bite size) **Food particle size ½ inch (~width of standard fork)** Food must be moist. Cut foods with a knife to a ½" particle size prior to mixing. Moisten with broth as needed. Foods that do not process well should be omitted. Omit: pineapple rings. May substitute canned peaches.

Chopped: Food particle size ¼ inch (~ ½ width of standard fork) Food must be moist. Chop foods with a knife to 1/4" particle size prior to mixing. Moisten with broth as needed. Foods that do not process well should be omitted. Omit: pineapple rings. May substitute canned peaches.

Minced and Moist:(aka Minced/Mechanical Soft/Ground) **Food particle size 1/8 inch (fits through prongs of standard fork)** Food must be moist. Use a food processor to grind food particles into 1/8 inch prior to mixing. Moisten with broth as needed. Foods that do not process well should be omitted. Omit: pineapple rings. May substitute canned peaches.

Pureed: Smooth and cohesive. Use a food processor to puree to a smooth consistency. Foods are processed by grinding and then pureeing them. May add broth or sauce to puree. Do not add to much liquid. Puree should still hold its shape. Must not be firm or sticky. Puree foods while still hot. Appearance should be smooth like pudding. Foods that do not process well should be omitted. Omit: pineapple rings. Serve ½ c. meat serving. May substitute canned peaches.

<u>**Therapeutic Modified Diets:**</u>

Lowfat: No changes needed
Diabetic/No added Sugar/No Conc. Sweets/Calorie Controlled: omit honey
Bland/Anti Reflux: Substitute peaches for pineapple and omit mustard
Liberal House Renal: Use alternate menu item
No Added Salt: Use alternate menu item
2 Gram Sodium: Use alternate menu item
Gluten Free: No changes needed
Prepare foods separately to prevent cross contamination.

Allergy Alerts: When an "X" is present, this indicates the allergen is present. Always read all food labels to ensure allergens are not present.

Wheat	Milk	Eggs	Fish Shellfish	Soy	Peanuts/Nuts	Other

Key: SF= Salt Free D= Diet or Sugarfree LF = Lowfat FF = Fat Free GF = Gluten Free

Copyright 2020 Jacqueline Larson M.S., R.D.N. and Associates.   All Rights Reserved

Recipe Name: Ground Ham on Pineapple Slices or Peach Halves
Recipe Category: Dinner Entrée
Portion Size: 3 oz. ham
Ingredients: Yields: 8 servings

Ingredients	Notes:
4 cups lean ground ham, cooked	
3 teaspoons prepared mustard	
¼ cup light mayonnaise	
8 Slices drained, canned pineapple or 6 peach halves	Use water or juice packed

Directions:

Steps:	Directions:	Critical Control Point /Quality Assurance
1	Preheat oven to 400°F.	
2	Combine ham, mustard, and mayonnaise.	
3	Spray baking dish with nonstick vegetable spray.	
4	Place pineapple slices in baking dish.	
5	Top each pineapple with a mound of ham mixture.	
6	Bake in oven for 10 minutes. Serve hot.	Cook until internal temperature reaches 165°F for 15 seconds.

Time Temperature Sensitive food. *Food safety Standards: hold food for service at an internal temperature above 140° F. Do not mix old product with new. Cool leftover product quickly (within 4 hours) to below 41° F. Follow proper cooling procedures. Store leftovers in a tightly sealed, labeled and dated container. Use leftover within 72 hours if stored in refrigerator or 30 days if stored in the freezer. Reheat leftover product quickly (within 2 hours) to 165 degrees F for 15 seconds. Reheat left over product only once; discard if not used. Cold holding at 41°F or colder or using time alone (less than four hours).*

Texture Modified Diets:

Soft & Bite Size: (aka Bite size) **Food particle size ½ inch (~width of standard fork)** Food must be moist. Cut foods with a knife to a ½" particle size prior to mixing. Moisten with broth as needed. Foods that do not process well should be omitted. Omit: pineapple rings. May substitute canned peaches.

Chopped: Food particle size ¼ inch (~ ½ width of standard fork) Food must be moist. Chop foods with a knife to 1/4" particle size prior to mixing. Moisten with broth as needed. Foods that do not process well should be omitted. Omit: pineapple rings. May substitute canned peaches.

Minced and Moist: (aka Minced/Mechanical Soft/Ground) **Food particle size 1/8 inch (fits through prongs of standard fork)** Food must be moist. Use a food processor to grind food particles into 1/8 inch prior to mixing. Moisten with broth as needed. Foods that do not process well should be omitted. Omit: pineapple rings. May substitute canned peaches.

Pureed: Smooth and cohesive. Use a food processor to puree to a smooth consistency. Foods are processed by grinding and then pureeing them. May add broth or sauce to puree. Do not add to much liquid. Puree should still hold its shape. Must not be firm or sticky. Puree foods while still hot. Appearance should be smooth like pudding. Foods that do not process well should be omitted. Omit: pineapple rings. Serve ½ c. meat serving. May substitute canned peaches.

Therapeutic Modified Diets:

Lowfat: No changes
Diabetic/No added Sugar/No Conc. Sweets/Calorie Controlled: no changes
Bland/Anti Reflux: Use peach in place of pineapple; omit mustard
Liberal House Renal: Use alternate menu item
No Added Salt: Use alternate menu item
2 Gram Sodium: Use alternate menu item
Gluten Free: No changes needed. Prepare foods separately to prevent cross contamination.
Allergy Alerts: When an "X" is present, this indicates the allergen is present.
Always read all food labels to ensure allergens are not present.

Wheat	Milk	Eggs	Fish Shellfish	Soy	Peanuts/Nuts	Other
		X				

Key: SF= Salt Free D= Diet or Sugarfree LF = Lowfat FF = Fat Free GF = Gluten Free

Recipe Name: Ham and Bean Skillet
Recipe Category: Dinner Entrée
Portion Size: 1 cup
Ingredients: Yields: 8 servings

Ingredients	Notes:
2 pounds ham, cut into ½ inch cubes	
2 teaspoons vegetable oil	
4 medium carrots	Washed, peeled and diced.
1 large onion, diced	
2 (15 oz.) Great Northern beans	May use no added salt, rinsed and drained
1 cup reduced sodium chicken broth	
2 teaspoon thyme, crushed	
1 teaspoon dried oregano, crushed	
2 tablespoons dried parsley	

Directions:

Steps:	Directions:	Critical Control Point / Quality Assurance
1	In a large nonstick skillet over medium heat; sauté carrot and onion until onion is soft, about 5 minutes.	
2	Stir in ham, beans, broth, thyme, oregano and parsley.	
3	Bring to boil, cover and lower heat to a simmer; heat through about 10 minutes. Serve hot.	Internal temperature should reach 160°F.

Time Temperature Sensitive food. Food safety Standards: hold food for service at an internal temperature above 140° F. Do not mix old product with new. Cool leftover product quickly (within 4 hours) to below 41° F. Follow proper cooling procedures. Store leftovers in a tightly sealed, labeled and dated container. Use leftover within 72 hours if stored in refrigerator or 30 days if stored in the freezer. Reheat leftover product quickly (within 2 hours) to 165 degrees F for 15 seconds. Reheat left over product only once; discard if not used. Cold holding at 41°F or colder or using time alone (less than four hours).

Texture Modified Diets:
Soft & Bite Size: (aka Bite size) **Food particle size ½ inch (~width of standard fork)** Food must be moist. Cut foods with a knife to a ½" particle size prior to mixing. Moisten with broth as needed.
Chopped: Food particle size ¼ inch (~ ½ width of standard fork) Food must be moist. Chop foods with a knife to 1/4" particle size prior to mixing. Moisten with broth as needed.
Minced and Moist:(aka Minced/Mechanical Soft/Ground) **Food particle size 1/8 inch (fits through prongs of standard fork)** Food must be moist. Use a food processor to grind food particles into 1/8 inch prior to mixing. Moisten with broth as needed.
Pureed: Smooth and cohesive. Use a food processor to puree to a smooth consistency. Foods are processed by grinding and then pureeing them. May add broth or sauce to puree. Do not add to much liquid. Puree should still hold its shape. Must not be firm or sticky. Puree foods while still hot. Appearance should be smooth like pudding.

Therapeutic Modified Diets:
Lowfat: No changes needed
Diabetic/No added Sugar/No Conc. Sweets/Calorie Controlled: No changes needed
Bland: use alternate menu item
Liberal House Renal: use alternate menu item
No Added Salt: use alternate menu item
2 Gram Sodium: use alternate menu item
Gluten Free: Use GF broth. Prepare foods separately to prevent cross contamination.
Allergy Alerts: When an "X" is present, this indicates the allergen is present.
Always read all food labels to ensure allergens are not present.

Wheat	Milk	Eggs	Fish Shellfish	Soy	Peanuts/Nuts	Other
X						

Key: SF= Salt Free D= Diet or Sugarfree LF = Lowfat FF = Fat Free GF = Gluten Free

Recipe Name: Ham with Dijon Pineapple Sauce
Recipe Category: Dinner Entrée
Portion Size: 3 oz. ham
Ingredients: **Yields: 8 servings**

Ingredients	Notes:
1 (20 oz.) can crushed pineapple in 100% juice	Do not drain
2 ½ pounds lean cooked boneless ham	Trim all visible fat
1 cup firmly pack brown sugar	
½ cup maple syrup	
¼ cup Dijon mustard	
1 tablespoon cornstarch	

Directions:

Steps:	Directions:	Critical Control Point /Quality Assurance
1	Score ham. Line baking pan with foil.	
2	Place ham on rack in baking pan.	
3	Bake at 350°F for 2 hours or until internal temperature reaches 140°F. Combine sugar, syrup and mustard.	
4	Use ¾ cup glaze to baste ham every 10 minutes during last 35 to 40 minutes of baking.	Cook until internal temperature reaches 140°F for 12 minutes.
5	Dissolve cornstarch in remaining glaze; add undrained pineapple. Cook, stirring constantly, until thickened.	
6	Serve sauce with ham.	

Time Temperature Sensitive food. *Food safety Standards: hold food for service at an internal temperature above 140° F. Do not mix old product with new. Cool leftover product quickly (within 4 hours) to below 41° F. Follow proper cooling procedures. Store leftovers in a tightly sealed, labeled and dated container. Use leftover within 72 hours if stored in refrigerator or 30 days if stored in the freezer. Reheat leftover product quickly (within 2 hours) to 165 degrees F for 15 seconds. Reheat left over product only once; discard if not used. Cold holding at 41°F or colder or using time alone (less than four hours).*

Texture Modified Diets:

Soft & Bite Size: (aka Bite size) **Food particle size ½ inch (~width of standard fork)** Food must be moist. Cut foods with a knife to a ½" particle size prior to after cooking. Moisten with broth as needed. Foods that do not process well should be omitted. Omit: pineapple. May substitute canned peaches.

Chopped: Food particle size ¼ inch (~ ½ width of standard fork) Food must be moist. Chop foods with a knife to 1/4" particle size after cooking. Moisten with broth as needed. Foods that do not process well should be omitted. Omit: pineapple. May substitute canned peaches.

Minced and Moist:(aka Minced/Mechanical Soft/Ground) **Food particle size 1/8 inch (fits through prongs of standard fork)** Food must be moist. Use a food processor to grind food particles into 1/8 inch after cooking. Moisten with broth as needed. Foods that do not process well should be omitted. Omit: pineapple. May substitute canned peaches.

Pureed: Smooth and cohesive. Use a food processor to puree to a smooth consistency. Foods are processed by grinding and then pureeing them. May add broth or sauce to puree. Do not add to much liquid. Puree should still hold its shape. Must not be firm or sticky. Puree foods while still hot. Appearance should be smooth like pudding. Foods that do not process well should be omitted. Omit: pineapple . Serve ½ c. meat serving. May substitute canned peaches. Serve ½ c. meat serving.

Therapeutic Modified Diets:

Lowfat: No changes needed
Diabetic/No added Sugar/No Conc. Sweets/Calorie Controlled: omit brown sugar and maple sugar sauce.
Bland/Anti Reflux: omit pineapple and mustard
Liberal House Renal: Use alternate menu item
No Added Salt: Use alternate menu item
2 Gram Sodium: Use alternate menu item
Gluten Free: no changes needed
Prepare foods separately to prevent cross contamination.

Allergy Alerts: When an "X" is present, this indicates the allergen is present. Always read all food labels to ensure allergens are not present.

Wheat	Milk	Eggs	Fish Shellfish	Soy	Peanuts/Nuts	Other

Key: SF= Salt Free D= Diet or Sugarfree LF = Lowfat FF = Fat Free GF = Gluten Free

Copyright 2020 Jacqueline Larson M.S., R.D.N. and Associates.   All Rights Reserved

Recipe Name: Ham and Fettuccine
Recipe Category: Dinner Entrée
Portion Size: 1 cup
Ingredients: **Yields: 8 servings**

Ingredients	Notes:
1 (16 oz.) package fettuccine	May use whole grain pasta
2 pounds cooked ham, diced	Trim all visible fat
¼ cup oil	
¼ cup all-purpose flour	
2 cups fat free evaporated milk	
1 cup low salt chicken broth	
1 cup Parmesan cheese, grated	
1 cup low fat provolone cheese, shredded	
¼ teaspoon pepper	
2 cups frozen peas	

Directions:

Steps:	Directions:	Critical Control Point /Quality Assurance
1	Prepare pasta according to package directions. Set aside.	
2	Melt margarine in medium sauce pan. Stir in flour.	
3	Gradually add evaporated milk and chicken broth.	
4	Cook stirring constantly, until mixture comes to a boil and thickens.	
5	Stir in Parmesan cheese, provolone cheese, ham, peas, and pepper.	
6	Cook until cheese has melted and heated through.	Cook until internal temperature reaches 165°F for 15 seconds.
7	Toss the sauce with the pasta.	

Time Temperature Sensitive food. *Food safety Standards: hold food for service at an internal temperature above 140°F. Do not mix old product with new. Cool leftover product quickly (within 4 hours) to below 41°F. Follow proper cooling procedures. Store leftovers in a tightly sealed, labeled and dated container. Use leftover within 72 hours if stored in refrigerator or 30 days if stored in the freezer. Reheat leftover product quickly (within 2 hours) to 165 degrees F for 15 seconds. Reheat left over product only once; discard if not used. Cold holding at 41°F or colder or using time alone (less than four hours).*

Texture Modified Diets: TIP use pasta within correct particle size.
Soft & Bite Size: (aka Bite size) **Food particle size ½ inch (~width of standard fork)** Food must be moist. Cut foods with a knife to a ½" particle size prior to mixing. Moisten with broth as needed.
Chopped: Food particle size ¼ inch (~ ½ width of standard fork) Food must be moist. Chop foods with a knife to 1/4" particle size prior to mixing. Moisten with broth as needed.
Minced and Moist:(aka Minced/Mechanical Soft/Ground) **Food particle size 1/8 inch (fits through prongs of standard fork)** Food must be moist. Use a food processor to grind food particles into 1/8 inch prior to mixing. Moisten with broth as needed.
Pureed: Smooth and cohesive. Use a food processor to puree to a smooth consistency. Foods are processed by grinding and then pureeing them. May add broth or sauce to puree. Do not add to much liquid. Puree should still hold its shape. Must not be firm or sticky. Puree foods while still hot. Appearance should be smooth like pudding. . Serve ½ c. meat serving and pasta separately. May puree pasta puree with sauce for flavor.

Therapeutic Modified Diets:
Lowfat: no changes
Diabetic/No added Sugar/No Conc. Sweets/Calorie Controlled: no changes
Bland/Anti Reflux: omit pepper
Liberal House Renal: Use alternate menu item
No Added Salt: Omit ham, use chicken or turkey
2 Gram Sodium: omit ham, use chicken or turkey; use salt free broth
Gluten Free: Use gluten free broth, pasta, and flour. Prepare foods separately to prevent cross contamination.
Allergy Alerts: When an "X" is present, this indicates the allergen is present. Always read all food labels to ensure allergens are not present.

Wheat	Milk	Eggs	Fish Shellfish	Soy	Peanuts/Nuts	Other
X	X	X				

Key: SF= Salt Free D= Diet or Sugarfree LF = Lowfat FF = Fat Free GF = Gluten Free

Recipe Name: Ham and Macaroni Twists
Recipe Category: Dinner Entrée
Portion Size: 1 ½ cup (approx. 3 oz. meat, ½ c. pasta and ½ c vegetable)
Ingredients: Yields: 8 servings

Ingredients	Notes:
4 cups rotini or elbow macaroni	May use whole grain pasta
2 pounds lean cooked ham, cubed	Trim all visible fat
½ cup bread crumbs	
2 (10 oz.) packages frozen broccoli spears	Thawed and drained
3 cups nonfat milk	
¼ cup flour	
¼ cup oil	
1 large onion, diced	Wash, trim and dice
2 teaspoons thyme	
2 teaspoons parsley flakes	
2 cups low fat Cheddar cheese, shredded	
½ teaspoon garlic powder	
½ teaspoon pepper	

Directions:

Steps:	Directions:	Critical Control Point /Quality Assurance
1	Prepare pasta according to package directions; drain well.	
2	Preheat oven to 350°F.	
3	In a large baking dish, combine hot macaroni and ham.	
4	Divide broccoli spears into 8 small bunches.	
5	Arrange bunches of spears down center of dish, alternating direction of flowerets.	
6	In a small sauce pan, heat oil to medium high heat. Sauté onion until tender. Combine milk, flour, thyme, parsley, garlic and pepper. Heat to slow boil. Remove from heat. Pour over casserole.	
7	Sprinkle bread crumbs and cheese down the center of the dish.	
8	Bake, covered, at 350°F for 30 minutes or until heated through. Serve.	Cook until internal temperature reaches 165°F for 15 seconds.

Time Temperature Sensitive food. *Food safety Standards: hold food for service at an internal temperature above 140° F. Do not mix old product with new. Cool leftover product quickly (within 4 hours) to below 41° F. Follow proper cooling procedures. Store leftovers in a tightly sealed, labeled and dated container. Use leftover within 72 hours if stored in refrigerator or 30 days if stored in the freezer. Reheat leftover product quickly (within 2 hours) to 165 degrees F for 15 seconds. Reheat left over product only once; discard if not used. Cold holding at 41°F or colder or using time alone (less than four hours).*

Texture Modified Diets: TIP use pasta within correct particle size.
Soft & Bite Size: (aka Bite size) **Food particle size ½ inch (~width of standard fork)** Food must be moist. Cut foods with a knife to a ½" particle size prior to mixing. Moisten with broth as needed.
Chopped: Food particle size ¼ inch (~ ½ width of standard fork) Food must be moist. Chop foods with a knife to 1/4" particle size prior to mixing. Moisten with broth as needed.
Minced and Moist: (aka Minced/Mechanical Soft/Ground) **Food particle size 1/8 inch (fits through prongs of standard fork)** Food must be moist. Use a food processor to grind food particles into 1/8 inch prior to mixing. Moisten with broth as needed.
Pureed: Smooth and cohesive. Use a food processor to puree to a smooth consistency. Foods are processed by grinding and then pureeing them. May add broth or sauce to puree. Do not add to much liquid. Puree should still hold its shape. Must not be firm or sticky. Puree foods while still hot. Appearance should be smooth like pudding. . Serve ½ c. meat serving and pasta separately. May puree pasta puree with sauce for flavor.
Serve ½ c. meat serving, ½ c. pasta and ½ c. broccoli pureed separately. May add seasoning and cheese to pasta for flavor.
Therapeutic Modified Diets:

Lowfat: No changes needed.
Diabetic/No added Sugar/No Conc. Sweets/Calorie Controlled: No changes needed
Bland/Anti Reflux: Serve plan ham, carrots and pasta.
Liberal House Renal: Sub. Chicken or turkey for ham. Omit cheese
No Added Salt: Sub. Chicken or turkey for ham.
2 Gram Sodium: Sub. Chicken or turkey for ham. Omit cheese
Gluten Free: Use gluten free pasta and flour. Omit bread crumbs; May use crumbled plain potato chips. Prepare foods separately to prevent cross contamination.
Allergy Alerts: When an "X" is present, this indicates the allergen is present.
Always read all food labels to ensure allergens are not present.

Wheat	Milk	Eggs	Fish Shellfish	Soy	Peanuts/Nuts	Other
X	X	X				

Key: SF= Salt Free D= Diet or Sugarfree LF = Lowfat FF = Fat Free GF = Gluten Free

Recipe Name: Ham and Pasta Salad
Recipe Category: Dinner Entrée
Portion Size: 1 ½ cups (approx. 3 oz. meat, ½ c. pasta and ½ c. vegetables)
Ingredients: Yields: 8 servings

Ingredients	Notes:
1 (16 oz.) package dried pasta	May use whole grain pasta
2 pounds cooked lean ham, diced	Trim all visible fat
2 cups peas	
2 cups carrots, diced	Wash, peel and dice
8 green onions, sliced	Wash and trim
1 cup low fat plain yogurt	
½ cup low fat creamy cucumber dressing	or Ranch dressing
1 teaspoon dill	
4 medium tomatoes	Washed, trimmed, and sliced
1 red, green or yellow pepper, (optional)	Washed, trimmed and diced
Lettuce leaves	Wash and trim

Directions:

Steps:	Directions:	Critical Control Point /Quality Assurance
1	Cook pasta according to package directions.	
2	Drain pasta. Rinse with cold water and drain again.	
3	In small mixing bowl stir together yogurt, dressing and dill.	
4	Pour yogurt mixture over pasta and vegetable mixture. Toss until well coated.	
5	In a large mixing bowl combine pasta, peas and carrots, ham, yogurt, dressing, dill and green onions.	
6	Cover and chill for at least 1 hour.	
7	To serve, arrange the tomato slices, lettuce lined salad plates	
8	Stir the pasta mixture and divide mixture among plates	
9	Garnish with green peppers. Serve cold.	

Special Diets: Time Temperature Sensitive food. Food safety Standards: hold food for service at an internal temperature above 140° F. Do not mix old product with new. Cool leftover product quickly (within 4 hours) to below 41° F. Follow proper cooling procedures. Store leftovers in a tightly sealed, labeled and dated container. Use leftover within 72 hours if stored in refrigerator or 30 days if stored in the freezer. Cold holding at 41°F or colder or using time alone (less than four hours).

Texture Modified Diets:
Soft & Bite Size: (aka Bite size) **Food particle size ½ inch (~width of standard fork)** Food must be moist. Cut foods with a knife to a ½" particle size prior to mixing. Moisten with broth as needed. Foods that do not process well should be omitted. Omit: green onions. May substitute minced red onion. Cook carrots, bell pepper and peas to soften.
Chopped: Food particle size ¼ inch (~ ½ width of standard fork) Food must be moist. Chop foods with a knife to 1/4" particle size prior to mixing. Moisten with broth as needed. Foods that do not process well should be omitted. Omit: green onions. May substitute minced red onion. Cook carrots, bell pepper and peas to soften.
Minced and Moist: (aka Minced/Mechanical Soft/Ground) **Food particle size 1/8 inch (fits through prongs of standard fork)** Food must be moist. Use a food processor to grind food particles into 1/8 inch prior to mixing. Moisten with broth as needed. Foods that do not process well should be omitted. Omit: green onions. May substitute minced red onion. Cook carrots, bell pepper and peas to soften.
Pureed: Smooth and cohesive. Use a food processor to puree to a smooth consistency. Foods are processed by grinding and then pureeing them. May add broth or sauce to puree. Do not add to much liquid. Puree should still hold its shape. Must not be firm or sticky. Puree foods while still hot. Appearance should be smooth like pudding. Foods that do not process well should be omitted. Omit: green onions. May substitute minced red onion. Cook carrots, bell pepper and peas to soften.
Serve ½ c. puree ham, ½ c. puree pasta (with dill and mayonnaise) and ½ c. puree peas separately.

Therapeutic Modified Diets:

Lowfat: No changes needed
Diabetic/No added Sugar/No Conc. Sweets/Calorie Controlled: No changes.
Bland/Anti Reflux: omit dill, tomatoes and peppers
Liberal House Renal: replace ham with chicken or turkey; omit dressing
No Added Salt: replace ham with chicken or turkey
2 Gram Sodium: replace ham with chicken or turkey; omit dressing
Gluten Free: Use gluten free dressing and pasta. Prepare foods separately to prevent cross contamination.
Allergy Alerts: When an "X" is present, this indicates the allergen is present.
Always read all food labels to ensure allergens are not present.

Wheat	Milk	Eggs	Fish Shellfish	Soy	Peanuts/Nuts	Other
X	X	X				

Key: SF= Salt Free D= Diet or Sugarfree LF = Lowfat FF = Fat Free GF = Gluten Free

Recipe Name: Ham and Tortellini Alfredo
Recipe Category: Dinner Entrée
Portion Size: 1 ½ cups (approx. 3 oz. meat, ½ c. pasta and ½ c. peas and mushrooms)
Ingredients: **Yields: 8 servings**

Ingredients	Notes:
1 pound fresh tortellini pasta	
2 pounds lean cooked ham, diced	Trim all visible fat
3 cups frozen green peas	
2 cups fresh mushroom	Washed, trimmed and sliced
1 (32 oz.) low fat Alfredo style pasta sauce	

Directions:

Steps:	Directions:	Critical Control Point /Quality Assurance
1	Cook Tortellini according to the directions on the package. Drain.	
2	In a large skillet add ham, peas, and mushroom and heat thoroughly.	
3	Add sauce and tortellini to ham and stir all together.	
4	Heat to a slow boil. Simmer for 3 to 5 minutes. Serve hot.	Cook until internal temperature reaches 165°F for 15 seconds.

Time Temperature Sensitive food. *Food safety Standards: hold food for service at an internal temperature above 140° F. Do not mix old product with new. Cool leftover product quickly (within 4 hours) to below 41° F. Follow proper cooling procedures. Store leftovers in a tightly sealed, labeled and dated container. Use leftover within 72 hours if stored in refrigerator or 30 days if stored in the freezer. Reheat leftover product quickly (within 2 hours) to 165 degrees F for 15 seconds. Reheat left over product only once; discard if not used. Cold holding at 41°F or colder or using time alone (less than four hours).*

Texture Modified Diets: Tip: use pasta within correct particle size.
Soft & Bite Size: (aka Bite size) **Food particle size ½ inch (~width of standard fork)** Food must be moist. Cut foods with a knife to a ½" particle size prior to mixing. Moisten with broth as needed.
Chopped: Food particle size ¼ inch (~ ½ width of standard fork) Food must be moist. Chop foods with a knife to 1/4" particle size prior to mixing. Moisten with broth as needed.
Minced and Moist:(aka Minced/Mechanical Soft/Ground) **Food particle size 1/8 inch (fits through prongs of standard fork)** Food must be moist. Use a food processor to grind food particles into 1/8 inch prior to mixing. Moisten with broth as needed.
Pureed: Smooth and cohesive. Use a food processor to puree to a smooth consistency. Foods are processed by grinding and then pureeing them. May add broth or sauce to puree. Do not add to much liquid. Puree should still hold its shape. Must not be firm or sticky. Puree foods while still hot. Appearance should be smooth like pudding. Serve ½ c. meat serving, ½ c. pasta and ½ c. peas pureed separately

Therapeutic Modified Diets:
Lowfat: No changes needed
Diabetic/No added Sugar/No Conc. Sweets/Calorie Controlled: No changes needed
Bland/Anti Reflux: No changes needed
Liberal House Renal: Use alternate menu item
No Added Salt: Use alternate menu item
2 Gram Sodium: Use alternate menu item
Gluten Free: Use gluten free Alfredo sauce and pasta. Prepare foods separately to prevent cross contamination.
Allergy Alerts: When an "X" is present, this indicates the allergen is present.
Always read all food labels to ensure allergens are not present.

Wheat	Milk	Eggs	Fish Shellfish	Soy	Peanuts/Nuts	Other
X	X	X				

Key: SF= Salt Free D= Diet or Sugarfree LF = Lowfat FF = Fat Free GF = Gluten Free

Recipe Name: Ham Hocks and Beans
Recipe Category: Dinner Entrée
Portion Size: 1 cup (3 oz. meat, ½ cup beans)
Ingredients: Yields: 8 servings

Ingredients	Notes:
2 pounds lean ham, diced	Trim all visible fat
1 Ham hock bone	
2 large cans no added salt pinto beans	Rinsed and drained
½ cup onion	Washed, trimmed and chopped
4 cups water	
1 teaspoon pepper	
3 bay leaves	
1 teaspoon garlic powder	Or 2 cloves, minced

Directions:

Steps:	Directions:	Critical Control Point / Quality Assurance
1	In a large stock pot add ham bone, bay leaves, beans, onion and garlic.	
2	Bring to a boil.	
3	Reduce heat, cover, and cook over low heat for 1 hour.	
4	Remove bone and bay leaves. Add ham and beans.	
5	Heat through.	Cook until internal temperature reaches 165°F for 15 seconds.

Time Temperature Sensitive food. Food safety Standards: hold food for service at an internal temperature above 140°F. Do not mix old product with new. Cool leftover product quickly (within 4 hours) to below 41°F. Follow proper cooling procedures. Store leftovers in a tightly sealed, labeled and dated container. Use leftover within 72 hours if stored in refrigerator or 30 days if stored in the freezer. Reheat leftover product quickly (within 2 hours) to 165 degrees F for 15 seconds. Reheat left over product only once; discard if not used. Cold holding at 41°F or colder or using time alone (less than four hours).

<u>*Texture Modified Diets:*</u>
Soft & Bite Size: (aka Bite size) **Food particle size ½ inch (~width of standard fork)** Food must be moist. Cut foods with a knife to a ½" particle size prior to mixing. Moisten with broth as needed.
Chopped: Food particle size ¼ inch (~ ½ width of standard fork) Food must be moist. Chop foods with a knife to 1/4" particle size prior to mixing. Moisten with broth as needed.
Minced and Moist: (aka Minced/Mechanical Soft/Ground) **Food particle size 1/8 inch (fits through prongs of standard fork)** Food must be moist. Use a food processor to grind food particles into 1/8 inch prior to mixing. Moisten with broth as needed.
Pureed: Smooth and cohesive. Use a food processor to puree to a smooth consistency. Foods are processed by grinding and then pureeing them. May add broth or sauce to puree. Do not add to much liquid. Puree should still hold its shape. Must not be firm or sticky. Puree foods while still hot. Appearance should be smooth like pudding. Serve ½ c. meat serving and ½ c puree beans separately

<u>*Therapeutic Modified Diets:*</u>
Lowfat: No changes needed
Diabetic/No added Sugar/No Conc. Sweets/Calorie Controlled: No changes needed
Bland/Anti Reflux: Serve plain ham and rice
Liberal House Renal: Use alternate menu item
No Added Salt: Use alternate menu item
2 Gram Sodium: Use alternate menu item
Gluten Free: No changes needed. Prepare foods separately to prevent cross contamination.
Allergy Alerts: When an "X" is present, this indicates the allergen is present.
Always read all food labels to ensure allergens are not present.

Wheat	Milk	Eggs	Fish Shellfish	Soy	Peanuts/Nuts	Other

Key: SF= Salt Free D= Diet or Sugarfree LF = Lowfat FF = Fat Free GF = Gluten Free

Recipe Name: Ham Jambalaya
Recipe Category: Dinner Entrée
Portion Size: 3 oz.
Ingredients: Yields: 8 servings

Ingredients	Notes:
2 pounds lean cooked ham, diced	Trim all visible fat
1½ cups rice, uncooked	
1 large can stewed tomatoes	Do not drain
1 green pepper	Washed, trimmed and chopped
2 cups low salt beef broth	
¼ teaspoon paprika	
½ teaspoon thyme	
2 slices bacon, chopped	(optional)
3 green onions, chopped	Washed and Trimmed. Use both tops and bulbs
2 tablespoons dried parsley	

Directions:

Steps:	Directions:	Critical Control Point /Quality Assurance
1	Preheat oven to 375°F.	
2	Sauté bacon, onion, and pepper until light brown.	
3	Place uncooked rice in bottom of baking dish.	
4	Add ham, pepper, bacon, onions, tomatoes, broth, paprika, thyme, onions and parsley. Stir.	
5	Bake covered in 375°F oven until rice is done, about 1¼ hours.	Cook until internal temperature reaches 165°F for 15 seconds.
6	Stir before serving. Serve hot.	

Time Temperature Sensitive food. *Food safety Standards: hold food for service at an internal temperature above 140° F. Do not mix old product with new. Cool leftover product quickly (within 4 hours) to below 41° F. Follow proper cooling procedures. Store leftovers in a tightly sealed, labeled and dated container. Use leftover within 72 hours if stored in refrigerator or 30 days if stored in the freezer. Reheat leftover product quickly (within 2 hours) to 165 degrees F for 15 seconds. Reheat left over product only once; discard if not used. Cold holding at 41°F or colder or using time alone (less than four hours).*

Texture Modified Diets:

Soft & Bite Size: (aka Bite size) **Food particle size ½ inch (~width of standard fork)** Food must be moist. Cut foods with a knife to a ½" particle size prior to mixing. Moisten with broth as needed. Foods that do not process well should be omitted. Omit: bacon and green onion. May substitute white onion.

Chopped: Food particle size ¼ inch (~ ½ width of standard fork) Food must be moist. Chop foods with a knife to 1/4" particle size prior to mixing. Moisten with broth as needed. Foods that do not process well should be omitted. Omit: bacon and green onion. May substitute white onion.

Minced and Moist: (aka Minced/Mechanical Soft/Ground) **Food particle size 1/8 inch (fits through prongs of standard fork)** Food must be moist. Use a food processor to grind food particles into 1/8 inch prior to mixing. Moisten with broth as needed. Foods that do not process well should be omitted. Omit: bacon and green onion. May substitute white onion.

Pureed: Smooth and cohesive. Use a food processor to puree to a smooth consistency. Foods are processed by grinding and then pureeing them. May add broth or sauce to puree. Do not add to much liquid. Puree should still hold its shape. Must not be firm or sticky. Puree foods while still hot. Appearance should be smooth like pudding. Foods that do not process well should be omitted. Omit: bacon and green onion. May substitute white onion.
Serve ½ c. meat serving separately from ½ c. rice mixture.

Therapeutic Modified Diets:

Lowfat: Omit bacon
Diabetic/No added Sugar/No Conc. Sweets/Calorie Controlled: No changes
Bland/Anti Reflux: Serve plain ham and plain rice.
Liberal House Renal: Use alternate menu item
No Added Salt: Use alternate menu item
2 Gram Sodium: Use alternate menu item
Gluten Free: Use gluten free broth or bouillon. Prepare foods separately to prevent cross contamination.

Allergy Alerts: When an "X" is present, this indicates the allergen is present. Always read all food labels to ensure allergens are not present.

Wheat	Milk	Eggs	FishShellfish	Soy	Peanuts/Nuts	Other
X						

Key: SF= Salt Free D= Diet or Sugarfree LF = Lowfat FF = Fat Free GF = Gluten Free

Copyright 2020 Jacqueline Larson M.S., R.D.N. and Associates.   All Rights Reserved

Recipe Name: Ham Noodle Casserole
Recipe Category: Dinner Entrée
Portion Size: 1 ½ cups (approx. ½ c. meat ½ c. pasta and ½ c. vegetables
Ingredients: **Yields: 8 servings**

Ingredients	Notes:
1 lb pasta	May use whole grain
2 cups fat free evaporated milk	
3½ tablespoons flour	
1 teaspoon thyme	Use fresh or dried
2 teaspoon marjoram	Use fresh or dried
1 tablespoon olive oil	
1 onion, finely chopped	
2 cups broccoli florets	Use fresh or frozen, Wash and trim
2 cups sliced mushrooms	Use fresh or frozen, Wash and trim
1 red bell pepper, chopped	Use fresh or frozen, Wash and trim
3 garlic cloves, crushed	Or 1 teaspoon garlic powder
¾ tsp salt	
½ tsp pepper	
3 cups cooked lean ham, cubed	Trim all visible fat
1 cup low fat shredded cheddar or Monterey jack cheese	

Directions:

Steps:	Directions:	Critical Control Point / Quality Assurance
1	Prepare pasta according to package directions; drain well.	
2	Spray a baking dish with non stick cooking spray.	
3	Place drained pasta in baking and set aside.	
4	Preheat oven to 350°F	
5	Combine milk, flour, thyme and marjoram in a small bowl and set aside.	
6	Heat a large, nonstick skillet over medium-high heat.	
7	Add oil and sauté onion, broccoli, mushroom, bell pepper, garlic, salt and pepper for 4 minutes, stirring frequently.	
8	Add ham and heat thoroughly, about 2 more minutes.	
9	Add reserved milk mixture and stir until thickened, about 4 minutes; do not boil.	
10	Sprinkle ham mixture over the pasta in the prepared casserole.	
11	Sprinkle with cheese and bake uncovered for 15 minutes, or until cheese is melted.	Cook until internal temperature reaches 165°F for 15 seconds

Time Temperature Sensitive food. *Food safety Standards: hold food for service at an internal temperature above 140° F. Do not mix old product with new. Cool leftover product quickly (within 4 hours) to below 41° F. Follow proper cooling procedures. Store leftovers in a tightly sealed, labeled and dated container. Use leftover within 72 hours if stored in refrigerator or 30 days if stored in the freezer. Reheat leftover product quickly (within 2 hours) to 165 degrees F for 15 seconds. Reheat left over product only once; discard if not used. Cold holding at 41°F or colder or using time alone (less than four hours).*

Texture Modified Diets: TIP use pasta within correct particle size.

Soft & Bite Size: (aka Bite size) **Food particle size ½ inch (~width of standard fork)** Food must be moist. Cut foods with a knife to a ½" particle size prior to mixing. Moisten with broth as needed.

Chopped: Food particle size ¼ inch (~ ½ width of standard fork) Food must be moist. Chop foods with a knife to 1/4" particle size prior to mixing. Moisten with broth as needed.

Minced and Moist: (aka Minced/Mechanical Soft/Ground) **Food particle size 1/8 inch (fits through prongs of standard fork)** Food must be moist. Use a food processor to grind food particles into 1/8 inch prior to mixing. Moisten with broth as needed.

Pureed: Smooth and cohesive. Use a food processor to puree to a smooth consistency. Foods are processed by grinding and then pureeing them. May add broth or sauce to puree. Do not add to much liquid. Puree should still hold its shape. Must not be firm or sticky. Puree foods while still hot. Appearance should be smooth like pudding. . Serve ½ c. meat serving and pasta separately. May puree pasta puree with sauce for flavor.
Do not add ham in step 8. Puree meat and pasta separately.

Therapeutic Modified Diets:

Lowfat: No changes needed
Diabetic/No added Sugar/No Conc. Sweets/Calorie Controlled: no changes needed
Bland/Anti Reflux: Omit bell pepper peppers, garlic, onions, thyme and marjoram and pepper
Liberal House Renal: Use alternate menu item
No Added Salt: Use alternate menu item
2 Gram Sodium: Use alternate menu item
Gluten Free: Use gluten free pasta. Use gluten free flour. Prepare foods separately to prevent cross contamination.
Allergy Alerts: When an "X" is present, this indicates the allergen is present.
Always read all food labels to ensure allergens are not present.

Wheat	Milk	Eggs	Fish Shellfish	Soy	Peanuts/Nuts	Other
X	X	X				

Key: SF= Salt Free D= Diet or Sugarfree LF = Lowfat FF = Fat Free GF = Gluten Free

Recipe Name: Honey Dijon Ham
Recipe Category: Dinner Entrée
Portion Size: 3 oz. boneless
Ingredients: Yields: 8 servings

Ingredients	Notes:
1 smoked ham, rump or shank portions 2 ½ lbs.	
2/3 cup honey	
1/3 cup Dijon style mustard	
¼ teaspoon ground cloves	
¼ teaspoon ground nutmeg	

Directions:

Steps:	Directions:	Critical Control Point / Quality Assurance
1	Pre heat oven to 325°F.	
2	Place ham in large shallow roasting pan.	
3	Bake until meat thermometer inserted in thickest part registers 125°F; about 1 and ¼ hours	
4	Remove from oven, trim off rind, leaving very thin layer all around.	
5	Score ham by cutting diamond shapes ¼ inch deep into ham.	
6	In small bowl combine, honey, mustard, cloves and nutmeg. Spoon ½ mixture over ham.	
7.	Continue baking about 30 minutes or until meat thermometer registers 140°F. Serve with additional warm glaze.	

Time Temperature Sensitive food. Food safety Standards: hold food for service at an internal temperature above 140° F. Do not mix old product with new. Cool leftover product quickly (within 4 hours) to below 41° F. Follow proper cooling procedures. Store leftovers in a tightly sealed, labeled and dated container. Use leftover within 72 hours if stored in refrigerator or 30 days if stored in the freezer. Reheat leftover product quickly (within 2 hours) to 165 degrees F for 15 seconds. Reheat left over product only once; discard if not used. Cold holding at 41°F or colder or using time alone (less than four hours).

Texture Modified Diets:

Soft & Bite Size: (aka Bite size) **Food particle size ½ inch (~width of standard fork)** Food must be moist. Cut foods with a knife to a ½" particle size prior to mixing. Moisten with broth as needed.
Chopped: Food particle size ¼ inch (~ ½ width of standard fork) Food must be moist. Chop foods with a knife to 1/4" particle size prior to mixing. Moisten with broth as needed. **Minced and Moist:** (aka Minced/Mechanical Soft/Ground) **Food particle size 1/8 inch (fits through prongs of standard fork)** Food must be moist. Use a food processor to grind food particles into 1/8 inch prior to mixing. Moisten with broth as needed.
Pureed: Smooth and cohesive. Use a food processor to puree to a smooth consistency. Foods are processed by grinding and then pureeing them. May add broth or sauce to puree. Do not add to much liquid. Puree should still hold its shape. Must not be firm or sticky. Puree foods while still hot. Appearance should be smooth like pudding. Serv ½ cup puree meat topped with glaze. Serve ½ c. meat pureed. May top with glaze.

Therapeutic Modified Diets:

Lowfat: No changes needed
Diabetic/No added Sugar/No Conc. Sweets/Calorie Controlled: Omit honey
Bland: omit glaze.
Liberal House Renal: use alternate menu item
No Added Salt: use alternate menu item
2 Gram Sodium: use alternate menu item
Gluten Free: Use no changes needed. Prepare foods separately to prevent cross contamination.
Allergy Alerts: When an "X" is present, this indicates the allergen is present.
Always read all food labels to ensure allergens are not present.

Wheat	Milk	Eggs	Fish Shellfish	Soy	Peanuts/Nuts	Other

Key: SF= Salt Free D= Diet or Sugarfree LF = Lowfat FF = Fat Free GF = Gluten Free

HAM LUNCH RECIPES

Recipe Name: Chef Salad
Recipe Category: Lunch Entrée
Portion Size: 1 cup lettuce, 3 oz meat, 1 egg, ½ cup vegetables, 2 T. salad dressing
Ingredients: **Yields: 8 servings**

Ingredients	Notes:
8 Cups torn lettuce	Wash, trim and divide onto plates
8 Ounces sliced cooked ham	May use deli meat
8 Ounces sliced cooked turkey	May use deli meat
8 Ounces sliced lowfat cheese	
8 Hard Cooked eggs	Sliced
3 Medium tomatoes, cut into wedges	Wash, trim and cut into wedges
1 Medium bell pepper, cut into rings	Wash, remove seeds and cut into rings
1 Medium onion	Wash, peel and sliced thin
1/2 Cup seasoned croutons	Optional
Light or low fat Salad dressing of choice	(see recipes in cookbook)

Directions:

Steps:	Directions:	Critical Control Point / Quality Assurance
1	In a large bowl tear lettuce.	
2	Arrange ham, turkey, cheese, eggs, tomatoes, bell pepper, and onions on lettuce. Sprinkle with Croutons, if desired. Pour over dressing. Toss to coat. Serve.	

Time Temperature Sensitive food. *Food safety Standards: hold food for service at an internal temperature above 140° F. Do not mix old product with new. Cool leftover product quickly (within 4 hours) to below 41° F. Follow proper cooling procedures. Store leftovers in a tightly sealed, labeled and dated container. Use leftover within 72 hours if stored in refrigerator. Do not freeze.*

Texture Modified Diets:
Soft & Bite Size: (aka Bite size) **Food particle size ½ inch (~width of standard fork)** Food must be moist. Cut foods with a knife to a ½" particle size prior to mixing. Moisten with dressing as needed. Cook bell pepper, onion and tomatoes to soften or cut to 1/8 inch. Crush croutons
Chopped: Food particle size ¼ inch (~ ½ width of standard fork) Food must be moist. Chop foods with a knife to 1/4" particle size prior to mixing. Moisten with dressing as needed. Cook bell pepper, onion and tomatoes to soften or cut to 1/8 inch. Crush croutons
Minced and Moist: (aka Minced/Mechanical Soft/Ground) **Food particle size 1/8 inch (fits through prongs of standard fork)** Food must be moist. Use a food processor to grind food particles into 1/8 inch prior to mixing. Moisten with broth as needed. Lettuce must be cut into pieces no larger than ⅛" X ⅛" X ⅛ ". Cook bell pepper, onion and tomatoes to soften. Crush croutons
Pureed: Smooth and cohesive. Use a food processor to puree to a smooth consistency. Foods are processed by grinding and then pureeing them. May add broth or sauce to puree. Do not add to much liquid. Puree should still hold its shape. Must not be firm or sticky. Appearance should be smooth like pudding. Serve ½ cup puree meat and ½ cup puree vegetables separately. Top with puree dressing.

Therapeutic Modified Diets:
Lowfat: Use lowfat salad dressing. Omit croutons and eggs.
Diabetic/No added Sugar/No Conc. Sweets/Calorie Controlled: non changes needed
Bland/Anti Reflux: omit onions, bell peppers, and tomatoes.
Liberal House Renal: Use low sodium deli meat (less than 140 mg. sodium per serving) and SF salad dressing. Omit tomatoes and croutons.
No Added Salt: No changes needed.
2 Gram Sodium: Use low sodium meat. (less than 140 mg. sodium per serving) and SF salad dressing. Omit croutons
Gluten Free: Omit croutons. Use GF croutons . Prepare separately to prevent cross contamination.

Allergy Alerts: When an "X" is present, this indicates the allergen is present. Always read all food labels to ensure allergens are not present.

Wheat	Milk	Eggs	Fish Shellfish	Soy	Peanuts/Nuts	Other
x	x	x				

Key: SF= Salt Free D= Diet or Sugarfree LF = Lowfat FF = Fat Free GF = Gluten Free

Copyright 2020 Jacqueline Larson M.S., R.D.N. and Associates.   All Rights Reserved

Recipe Name: Ham and Cheese Sandwich
Recipe Category: Lunch Entrée
Portion Size: 1 Sandwich
Ingredients: Yields: 8 servings

Ingredients	Notes:
16 slices bread	May use whole grain
1 pound cooked and sliced lean deli ham	
8 slices cheese	
½ cup mayonnaise	
¼ cup mustard	
16 slices tomatoes	Wash, trim and sliced (optional)
1 small red onion	Wash, peel and slice thin (optional)
2 cups fresh spinach leaves or lettuce	Washed, trimmed and chopped (optional

Directions:

Steps:	Directions:	Critical Control Point /Quality Assurance
1	Spread each slice bread with mayonnaise and mustard	
2	Top each sandwich with 2 oz. ham and 1 slice cheese	
3	Arrange tomato, lettuce or spinach and onion on each sandwich. Cut in half diagonally. Chill in an airtight container until ready to serve.	

Time Temperature Sensitive food. *Do not mix old product with new. Store leftovers in a tightly sealed, labeled and dated container. Use leftover within 72 hours if stored in refrigerator or 30 days if stored in the freezer. Cold holding at 41°F or colder or using time alone (less than four hours*

Texture Modified Diets:

Soft & Bite Size: (aka Bite size) **Food particle size ½ inch (~width of standard fork)** Food must be moist. Cut foods with a knife to a ½" particle size prior to layering. Moisten with broth or water as needed.

Chopped: Food particle size ¼ inch (~ ½ width of standard fork) Food must be moist. Chop foods with a knife to 1/4" particle size prior to layering. Moisten with broth or water as needed.

Minced and Moist: (aka Minced/Mechanical Soft/Ground) **Food particle size 1/8 inch (fits through prongs of standard fork)** Food must be moist. Use a food processor to grind food particles into 1/8 inch prior to layering. Moisten with broth or water as needed.

Pureed: Smooth and cohesive. Use a food processor to puree to a smooth consistency. Foods are processed by grinding and then pureeing them. May add broth or milk to puree. Do not add to much liquid. Puree should still hold its shape. Must not be firm or sticky. Puree foods while still hot. Appearance should be smooth like pudding. Puree 1/3 cup puree meat. 1 cup puree bread with sour mayonnaise and mustard mixture serve separately. Puree with milk if needed. Spinach, tomato and onion may be puree with bread.

Therapeutic Modified Diets:

Low fat: No changes needed
Diabetic/No added Sugar/No Conc. Sweets/Calorie Controlled: No changes needed
Bland/Anti Reflux: Omit Onions, tomato, mustard and spinach
Liberal House Renal: Use low sodium deli roast beef or turkey (less than 140 mg. sodium per serving). Omit mayonnaise and cheese. May add mustard.
No Added Salt: Use roast beef or turkey in place of ham.
2 Gram Sodium: Use low sodium deli roast beef or turkey (less than 140 mg. sodium per serving). Omit mayonnaise and cheese. May add mustard.
Gluten Free: Use gluten free bread. Prepare foods separately to prevent cross contamination.
Allergy Alerts: When an "X" is present, this indicates the allergen is present.
Always read all food labels to ensure allergens are not present.

Wheat	Milk	Eggs	Fish Shellfish	Soy	Peanuts/Nuts	Other
X		x				

Key: SF= Salt Free D= Diet or Sugarfree LF = Lowfat FF = Fat Free GF = Gluten Free

Recipe Name: Ham and Linguine Primavera
Recipe Category: Lunch Entrée
Portion Size: 1 cup
Ingredients: Yields: 8 servings

Ingredients	Notes:
1 pound cooked ham, diced	
16 ounce linguine pasta	
4 cups broccoli florets	Washed
1 cup light mayonnaise	
½ cup grated parmesan cheese	
½ cup nonfat milk	
1 teaspoon garlic powder	
1 teaspoon dried basil leaves	
¼ teaspoon black pepper	

Directions:

Steps:	Directions:	Critical Control Point /Quality Assurance
1	Prepare pasta according to the directions on the package.	
2	Add broccoli during the last 4 minutes of pasta cooking time.	
3	Drain and return to pot.	
4	Add remaining ingredients and toss to coat.	
5	Serve hot.	

Time Temperature Sensitive food. Food safety Standards: hold food for service at an internal temperature above 140°F. Do not mix old product with new. Cool leftover product quickly (within 4 hours) to below 41°F. Follow proper cooling procedures. Store leftovers in a tightly sealed, labeled and dated container. Use leftover within 72 hours if stored in refrigerator or 30 days if stored in the freezer. Reheat leftover product quickly (within 2 hours) to 165 degrees F for 15 seconds. Reheat left over product only once; discard if not used. Cold holding at 41°F or colder or using time alone (less than four hours). Always wash hands and wash and sanitize counter tops utensils and containers between steps when working with raw meat.

Texture Modified Diets: TIP use pasta within correct particle size.
Soft & Bite Size: (aka Bite size) **Food particle size ½ inch (~width of standard fork)** Food must be moist. Cut foods with a knife to a ½" particle size prior to mixing. Moisten with broth as needed.
Chopped: Food particle size ¼ inch (~ ½ width of standard fork) Food must be moist. Chop foods with a knife to 1/4" particle size prior to mixing. Moisten with broth as needed.
Minced and Moist: (aka Minced/Mechanical Soft/Ground) **Food particle size 1/8 inch (fits through prongs of standard fork)** Food must be moist. Use a food processor to grind food particles into 1/8 inch prior to mixing. Moisten with broth as needed.
Pureed: Smooth and cohesive. Use a food processor to puree to a smooth consistency. Foods are processed by grinding and then pureeing them. May add broth or sauce to puree. Do not add to much liquid. Puree should still hold its shape. Must not be firm or sticky. Puree foods while still hot. Appearance should be smooth like pudding. Serve ½ c. meat serving and pasta separately. May puree pasta puree with sauce for flavor.

Therapeutic Modified Diets:
Lowfat: Omit Mayonnaise
Diabetic/No added Sugar/No Conc. Sweets/Calorie Controlled: No changes needed
Bland/Anti Reflux: omit broccoli. Substitute with spinach. Omit garlic powder, basil and black pepper.
Liberal House Renal: omit Parmesan cheese, mayonnaise, and milk. Sub. SF chicken for ham.
No Added Salt: No changes needed
2 Gram Sodium: omit Parmesan cheese, mayonnaise and milk. SF Chicken for ham.
Gluten Free: Use gluten free pasta Prepare foods separately to prevent cross contamination.
Allergy Alerts: When an "X" is present, this indicates the allergen is present.
Always read all food labels to ensure allergens are not present.

Wheat	Milk	Eggs	Fish Shellfish	Soy	Peanuts/Nuts	Other
X	x	X	X			

Key: SF= Salt Free D= Diet or Sugarfree LF = Lowfat FF = Fat Free GF = Gluten Free

Copyright 2020 Jacqueline Larson M.S., R.D.N. and Associates.   All Rights Reserved

Recipe Name: Ham Salad
Recipe Category: Lunch Entrée
Portion Size: 1/3 cup Ham Salad on lettuce leaf
Ingredients: Yields: 8 servings

Ingredients	Notes:
4 cups cooked ham, julienne strips or diced	
1 cups celery, diced or julienne strips	Wash, trim and diced or julienne strips
4 Small sweet pickles	Chopped
4 Hard cooked eggs	Quartered
2 tablespoons prepared mustard	
2 teaspoons pickle juice	
2/3 cup light mayonnaise	
8 Lettuce Greens leaves (garnish-optional)	Wash, trim and divide onto plates

Directions:

Steps:	Directions:	Critical Control Point /Quality Assurance
1	Combine the ham with celery, pickles, and eggs.	
2	Mix the mustard and pickle juice into the mayonnaise.	
3	Toss all together.	
4	Serve on a leaf of green. Serve chilled.	

Time Temperature Sensitive food. *Food safety Standards: Do not mix old product with new. Cool leftover product quickly (within 4 hours) to below 41°F. Follow proper cooling procedures. Store leftovers in a tightly sealed, labeled and dated container. Use leftover within 72 hours if stored in refrigerator. Do not freeze. Cold holding at 41°F or colder or using time alone (less than four hours). Always wash hands and wash and sanitize counter tops utensils and containers between steps when working with raw meat.*

Texture Modified Diets: TIP use pasta within correct particle size.
Soft & Bite Size: (aka Bite size) **Food particle size ½ inch (~width of standard fork)** Food must be moist. Cut foods with a knife to a ½" particle size prior to mixing. Moisten with broth as needed.
Chopped: Food particle size ¼ inch (~ ½ width of standard fork) Food must be moist. Chop foods with a knife to 1/4" particle size prior to mixing. Moisten with broth as needed.
Minced and Moist: (aka Minced/Mechanical Soft/Ground) **Food particle size 1/8 inch (fits through prongs of standard fork)** Food must be moist. Use a food processor to grind food particles into 1/8 inch prior to mixing. Moisten with broth as needed.
Pureed: Smooth and cohesive. Use a food processor to puree to a smooth consistency. Foods are processed by grinding and then pureeing them. May add broth or sauce to puree. Do not add to much liquid. Puree should still hold its shape. Must not be firm or sticky. Puree foods while still hot. Appearance should be smooth like pudding. . Serve ½ c. meat serving and pasta separately. May puree pasta puree with sauce for flavor.

Therapeutic Modified Diets:
Lowfat: Omit eggs
Diabetic/No added Sugar/No Conc. Sweets/Calorie Controlled: No changes needed
Bland/Anti Reflux: Omit pickles and mustard
Liberal House Renal: Use low sodium deli ham. (less than 140 mg. sodium per serving) or sub. with SF chicken. Omit mayonnaise, pickles, and pickle juice
No Added Salt: Use low sodium deli ham. (less than 140 mg. sodium per serving) or sub. With SF chicken
2 Gram Sodium: Use low sodium deli ham. (less than 140 mg. sodium per serving) or sub. With SF chicken Omit mayonnaise, pickles and pickle juice.
Gluten Free: No changes needed.
Allergy Alerts: When an "X" is present, this indicates the allergen is present.
Always read all food labels to ensure allergens are not present.

Wheat	Milk	Eggs	Fish Shellfish	Soy	Peanuts/Nuts	Other
		x				

Key: SF= Salt Free D= Diet or Sugarfree LF = Lowfat FF = Fat Free GF = Gluten Free

Recipe Name: Lima Beans & Ham Salad
Recipe Category: Lunch Entrée
Portion Size: 1 cup
Ingredients: **Yields: 8 servings**

Ingredients	Notes:
4 cups lima beans (frozen)	
1 lb. of diced cooked ham	
1/2 cup of celery	Wash, trim and finely dice
2 tablespoons of onions	Wash, peel and minced
¼ cup light sour cream	
1 tablespoon of white wine vinegar	
1/4 teaspoon of celery seed	Optional

Directions:

Steps:	Directions:	Critical Control Point /Quality Assurance
1	Cook the lima beans according to directions.	
2	Drain and rinse with cold water.	
3	Combine beans with ham, celery and onions in large bowl.	
4	Pour over dressing. Toss to coat. Chill until ready to serve.	

Time Temperature Sensitive food. *Food safety Standards: Do not mix old product with new. Cool leftover product quickly (within 4 hours) to below 41°F. Follow proper cooling procedures. Store leftovers in a tightly sealed, labeled and dated container. Use leftover within 72 hours if stored in refrigerator. Do not freeze Cold holding at 41°F or colder or using time alone (less than four hours). Always wash hands and wash and sanitize counter tops utensils and containers between steps when working with raw poultry.*

Texture Modified Diets: TIP use pasta within correct particle size.
Soft & Bite Size: (aka Bite size) **Food particle size ½ inch (~width of standard fork)** Food must be moist. Cut foods with a knife to a ½" particle size prior to mixing. Moisten with broth as needed.
Chopped: Food particle size ¼ inch (~ ½ width of standard fork) Food must be moist. Chop foods with a knife to 1/4" particle size prior to mixing. Moisten with broth as needed.
Minced and Moist:(aka Minced/Mechanical Soft/Ground) **Food particle size 1/8 inch (fits through prongs of standard fork)** Food must be moist. Use a food processor to grind food particles into 1/8 inch prior to mixing. Moisten with broth as needed.
Pureed: Smooth and cohesive. Use a food processor to puree to a smooth consistency. Foods are processed by grinding and then pureeing them. May add broth or sauce to puree. Do not add to much liquid. Puree should still hold its shape. Must not be firm or sticky. Puree foods while still hot. Appearance should be smooth like pudding. . Serve ½ c. meat serving and pasta separately. May puree pasta puree with sauce for flavor.
. Serve 1/3 cup puree ham and ½ cup puree lima beans separately.

Therapeutic Modified Diets:
Lowfat: No changes needed
Diabetic/No added Sugar/No Conc. Sweets/Calorie Controlled: No changes needed
Bland/Anti Reflux: omit onions, vinegar, celery seed and lima beans. Add peas in place of lima beans.
Liberal House Renal: Use low sodium ham(less than 140 mg. sodium per serving) or sub. SF chicken.
No Added Salt: Serve low sodium meat (less than 140 mg. sodium per serving)
2 Gram Sodium: Use low sodium ham (less than 140 mg. sodium per serving) or sub. SF chicken.
Gluten Free: No changes needed
Allergy Alerts: When an "X" is present, this indicates the allergen is present.
Always read all food labels to ensure allergens are not present.

Wheat	Milk	Eggs	Fish Shellfish	Soy	Peanuts/Nuts	Other
	x					

Key: SF= Salt Free D= Diet or Sugarfree LF = Lowfat FF = Fat Free GF = Gluten Free

Recipe Name: Submarine Sandwich
Recipe Category: Lunch Entrée
Portion Size: 1 sandwich (2 starch, 2 oz. meet, 1 oz. cheese)
Ingredients: Yields: 8 servings

Ingredients	Notes:
8 French style rolls	
1/4 Cup light mayonnaise	
3 Tablespoons prepared mustard	
8 Lettuce leaves	Washed, trimmed and separated
16 Ounces thinly sliced salami, pepperoni, summer sausage, fully cooked ham, or a combination of each	
8 Ounces sliced provolone, Swiss, or mozzarella cheese	
3 Medium tomatoes	Washed, trimmed and sliced

Directions:

Steps:	Directions:	Critical Control Point /Quality Assurance
1	Spilt rolls in half.	
2	Spread mayonnaise on the cut side of the bottoms; spread mustard on the cut side of the tops	Internal temperature should reach 165 degrees
3	On bottoms, layer lettuce, desired meat and cheese, and tomatoes.	Use 2 oz of meat, 1 oz of cheese

Time Temperature Sensitive food. *Food safety Standards: Do not mix old product with new. Cool leftover product quickly (within 4 hours) to below 41° F. Follow proper cooling procedures. Store leftovers in a tightly sealed, labeled and dated container. Use leftover within 72 hours if stored in refrigerator or 30 days if stored in the freezer. Cold holding at 41°F or colder or using time alone (less than four hours).*

Texture Modified Diets:

Soft & Bite Size: (aka Bite size) **Food particle size ½ inch (~width of standard fork)** Food must be moist. Cut foods with a knife to a ½" particle size prior to layering. Moisten with broth or water as needed. Use lean ham, roast beef or turkey

Chopped: Food particle size ¼ inch (~ ½ width of standard fork) Food must be moist. Chop foods with a knife to 1/4" particle size prior to layering. Moisten with broth or water as needed. Use lean ham, roast beef or turkey

Minced and Moist:(aka Minced/Mechanical Soft/Ground) **Food particle size 1/8 inch (fits through prongs of standard fork)** Food must be moist. Use a food processor to grind food particles into 1/8 inch prior to layering. Moisten with broth or water as needed. Use lean ham, roast beef or turkey

Pureed: Smooth and cohesive. Use a food processor to puree to a smooth consistency. Foods are processed by grinding and then pureeing them. May add broth or milk to puree. Do not add to much liquid. Puree should still hold its shape. Must not be firm or sticky. Puree foods while still hot. Appearance should be smooth like pudding. Use lean ham, roast beef or turkey

Puree 1/3 cup puree meat. 1 cup puree bread with sour mayonnaise and mustard mixture serve separately. Puree with milk if needed. Spinach, tomato and onion may be puree with bread.

Therapeutic Modified Diets:

Lowfat: Omit cheese. Use lean ham, roast beef or turkey
Diabetic/No added Sugar/No Conc. Sweets/Calorie Controlled: No changes
Bland/Anti Reflux: Omit mustard and tomatoes. Use lean ham, roast beef or turkey
Liberal House Renal: Serve SF bread or use 1 c. SF pasta and 2 oz. low sodium meat (less than 140 mg. sodium per serving). No cheese, mayonnase or tomatoes. May use mustard.
No Added Salt: Serve low sodium meat (less than 140 mg. sodium per serving)
2 Gram Sodium: Serve low sodium meat (less than 140 mg. sodium per serving). Serve SF bread or use 1 c. SF pasta. No cheese or mayonnaise. May use mustard.
Gluten Free: Use gluten free bread and lunch meat. Prepare foods separately to prevent cross contamination
Allergy Alerts: When an "X" is present, this indicates the allergen is present.
Always read all food labels to ensure allergens are not present.

Wheat	Milk	Eggs	Fish Shellfish	Soy	Peanuts/Nuts	Other
x	x	X				

Key: SF= Salt Free D= Diet or Sugarfree LF = Lowfat FF = Fat Free GF = Gluten Free

LAMB DINNER RECIPES

Recipe Name: Acorn Squash with Lamb
Recipe Category: Lamb
Portion Size: 1 cup lamb and rice, ½ c. squash
Ingredients: Yields: 8 servings

Ingredients	Notes:
3 cups water	
1 1/2 cups uncooked white rice	
2 pounds lamb, ground	May use ground turkey or beef
1 large onion	Washed, peeled and diced
2 gloves garlic	Washed, peeled and minced
1 teaspoon thyme	
1 teaspoon basil	
1 teaspoon dry ground mustard	
2 large acorn squash	Washed, cut in half and seeded removed
Salt and pepper to taste	

Directions:

Steps:	Directions:	Critical Control Point /Quality Assurance
1	In a medium saucepan bring water to boil	
2	Add rice and stir.	
3	Reduce heat, cover and simmer for 20 minutes.	
4	Preheat oven to 350 degrees F (175 degrees C).	
5	In a large skillet over medium heat, place the ground lamb, onion, garlic, thyme, basil and ground mustard. Cook until the lamb is evenly brown and the onion is soft. Stir the rice into the mixture.	Lamb temperature must reach 165 degrees.
6	Stuff the acorn squash halves with the ground lamb mixture. Season with salt and pepper.	
7	Place stuffed squash on a medium baking sheet	
8	Bake in the preheated oven 30 minutes, or until the squash is tender.	

Time Temperature Sensitive food. *Food safety Standards: hold food for service at an internal temperature above 140° F. Do not mix old product with new. Cool leftover product quickly (within 4 hours) to below 41° F. Follow proper cooling procedures. Store leftovers in a tightly sealed, labeled and dated container. Use leftover within 72 hours if stored in refrigerator or 30 days if stored in the freezer. Reheat leftover product quickly (within 2 hours) to 165 degrees F for 15 seconds. Reheat left over product only once; discard if not used. Cold holding at 41 °F or colder or using time alone (less than four hours). Always wash hands and wash and sanitize counter tops utensils and containers between steps when working with raw meat.*

Texture Modified Diets:
Soft & Bite Size: (aka Bite size) **Food particle size ½ inch (~width of standard fork)** Food must be moist. Cut foods with a knife to a ½" particle size after cooking. Peel squash. Moisten with milk as needed after cutting.
Chopped: Food particle size ¼ inch (~ ½ width of standard fork) Food must be moist. Chop foods with a knife to 1/4" particle size after cooking. Peel squash. Moisten with milk as needed after chopping.
Minced and Moist:(aka Minced/Mechanical Soft/Ground) **Food particle size 1/8 inch (fits through prongs of standard fork)** Food must be moist. Use a food processor to grind food particles into 1/8 inch after cooking. Peel squash. Moisten with milk as needed after processing.
Pureed: Smooth and cohesive. Use a food processor to puree to a smooth consistency. Foods are processed by grinding and then pureeing them. Peel squash. May add milk or sauce to puree. Do not add to much liquid. Puree should still hold its shape. Must not be firm or sticky. Puree foods while still hot. Appearance should be smooth like pudding. Serve ½ c. puree meat, ½ c. puree rice mixture and ½ c. puree squash separately.

Therapeutic Modified Diets:
Lowfat: No changes needed.
Diabetic/No added Sugar/No Conc. Sweets/Calorie Controlled: No changes needed
Bland/Anti Reflux: Omit onion, thyme, basil, garlic, mustard and pepper.
Liberal House Renal: Omit salt and squash. Serve 1/2 cup SF rice in place of squash.
No Added Salt: No changes needed
2 Gram Sodium: Omit salt
Gluten Free: No changes needed. Prepare foods separately to prevent cross contamination.

Allergy Alerts: When an "X" is present, this indicates the allergen is present. Always read all food labels to ensure allergens are not present.

Wheat	Milk	Eggs	Fish Shellfish	Soy	Peanuts/Nuts	Other

Key: SF= Salt Free D= Diet or Sugarfree LF = Lowfat FF = Fat Free GF = Gluten Free

Copyright 2020 Jacqueline Larson M.S., R.D.N. and Associates.   All Rights Reserved

Recipe Name: Lamb Chops with Mint Jelly
Recipe Category: Lamb
Portion Size: 3 oz. boneless, 5 oz. with bone
Ingredients: **Yields: 8 servings**

Ingredients	Notes:
8 (5 ounces each) lamb chops or 16 (2 1/2 oz.) lamb chops	
1 teaspoon garlic powder	
½ teaspoon salt	
1/2 teaspoon pepper	
1/2 cup Mint jelly	

Directions:

Steps:	Directions:	Critical Control Point /Quality Assurance
1	Preheat broiler.	Trim all visible fat
2	Season chops with garlic, salt and pepper.	
3	Place chops on unheated rack of a broiler pan.	
4	Broil for 4 to 5 inches from the heat for 10 to 15 minutes or until done, turning meat half way through broiling. Serve with mint jelly.	Cook until internal temperature reaches 145°F

Time Temperature Sensitive food. Food safety Standards: hold food for service at an internal temperature above 140°F. Do not mix old product with new. Cool leftover product quickly (within 4 hours) to below 41°F. Follow proper cooling procedures. Store leftovers in a tightly sealed, labeled and dated container. Use leftover within 72 hours if stored in refrigerator or 30 days if stored in the freezer. Reheat leftover product quickly (within 2 hours) to 165 degrees F for 15 seconds. Reheat left over product only once; discard if not used. Cold holding at 41°F or colder or using time alone (less than four hours). Always wash hands and wash and sanitize counter tops utensils and containers between steps when working with raw meat.

Texture Modified Diets:

Soft & Bite Size: (aka Bite size) **Food particle size ½ inch (~width of standard fork)** Food must be moist. Cut foods with a knife to a ½" particle size after cooking. Moisten with broth as needed after cutting.

Chopped: Food particle size ¼ inch (~ ½ width of standard fork) Food must be moist. Chop foods with a knife to 1/4" particle size after cooking. Moisten with broth as needed after chopping.

Minced and Moist:(aka Minced/Mechanical Soft/Ground) **Food particle size 1/8 inch (fits through prongs of standard fork)** Food must be moist. Use a food processor to grind food particles into 1/8 inch after cooking. Moisten with broth as needed after processing.

Pureed: Smooth and cohesive. Use a food processor to puree to a smooth consistency. Foods are processed by grinding and then pureeing them. May add milk or sauce to puree. Do not add to much liquid. Puree should still hold its shape. Must not be firm or sticky. Puree foods while still hot. Appearance should be smooth like pudding. Serve ½ c. serving topped with mint jelly.

Therapeutic Modified Diets:

Lowfat: Trim all visible fat.
Diabetic/No added Sugar/No Conc. Sweets/Calorie Controlled: Omit jelly
Bland/Anti Reflux: Omit garlic and pepper.
Liberal House Renal: Omit salt.
No Added Salt: No changes needed.
2 Gram Sodium: Omit salt
Gluten Free: No changes needed. Prepare foods separately to prevent cross contamination.
Allergy Alerts: When an "X" is present, this indicates the allergen is present.
Always read all food labels to ensure allergens are not present.

Wheat	Milk	Eggs	Fish Shellfish	Soy	Peanuts/Nuts	Other

Key: SF= Salt Free D= Diet or Sugarfree LF = Lowfat FF = Fat Free GF = Gluten Free

Recipe Name: Spicy Apricot Lamb Chops or Spicy Apricot Pork Chops.
Recipe Category: Lamb
Portion Size: 3 oz. boneless, 5 oz. with bone
Ingredients: Yields: 8 servings

Ingredients	Notes:
8 (5 ounces each) lamb chops or 16 (2 1/2 oz) lamb chops	Trim fat (or pork)
2 tablespoons packed brown sugar	
1 teaspoon garlic salt	
1/2 teaspoon chili powder	
1 teaspoon paprika	
1/2 teaspoon oregano	
1/4 teaspoon ground cinnamon	
1/4 teaspoon all spice	
1/4 teaspoon black pepper	
1/2 cup apricot preserves	

Directions:

Steps:	Directions:	Critical Control Point /Quality Assurance
1	Preheat broiler.	Trim all visible fat.
2	In a small bowl, combine brown sugar, garlic, salt, chili powder, paprika, oregano, cinnamon, all spice, and pepper.	
3	Rub spice mixture with seasoning.	
4	Place chops on unheated rack of a broiler pan.	
5	Broil for 4 to 5 inches from the heat for 10 to 15 minutes or until done, turning meat and brushing with preserves halfway through broiling.	Cook until internal temperature reaches *145°F*

Time Temperature Sensitive food. *Food safety Standards: hold food for service at an internal temperature above 140° F. Do not mix old product with new. Cool leftover product quickly (within 4 hours) to below 41° F. Follow proper cooling procedures. Store leftovers in a tightly sealed, labeled and dated container. Use leftover within 72 hours if stored in refrigerator or 30 days if stored in the freezer. Reheat leftover product quickly (within 2 hours) to 165 degrees F for 15 seconds. Reheat left over product only once; discard if not used. Cold holding at 41°F or colder or using time alone (less than four hours). Always wash hands and wash and sanitize counter tops utensils and containers between steps when working with raw meat.*

Texture Modified Diets:

Soft & Bite Size: (aka Bite size) **Food particle size ½ inch (~width of standard fork)** Food must be moist. Cut foods with a knife to a ½" particle size after cooking. Moisten with milk as needed after cutting.
Chopped: Food particle size ¼ inch (~ ½ width of standard fork) Food must be moist. Chop foods with a knife to 1/4" particle size after cooking. Moisten with milk as needed after chopping.
Minced and Moist: (aka Minced/Mechanical Soft/Ground) **Food particle size 1/8 inch (fits through prongs of standard fork)** Food must be moist. Use a food processor to grind food particles into 1/8 inch after cooking. Moisten with milk as needed after processing.
Pureed: Smooth and cohesive. Use a food processor to puree to a smooth consistency. Foods are processed by grinding and then pureeing them. May add milk or sauce to puree. Do not add to much liquid. Puree should still hold its shape. Must not be firm or sticky. Puree foods while still hot. Appearance should be smooth like pudding. Serve ½ c. serving topped with puree sauce.

Therapeutic Modified Diets:

Lowfat: No changes needed.
Diabetic/No added Sugar/No Conc. Sweets/Calorie Controlled: Omit apricot preserves
Bland/Anti Reflux: Omit garlic salt, chili powder, paprika, oregano, cinnamon, all spice and black pepper.
Liberal House Renal: Omit garlic salt.
No Added Salt: No changes needed.
2 Gram Sodium: Omit garlic salt.
Gluten Free: No changes needed.

Allergy Alerts: When an "X" is present, this indicates the allergen is present. Always read all food labels to ensure allergens are not present.

Wheat	Milk	Eggs	Fish Shellfish	Soy	Peanuts/Nuts	Other

Key: SF= Salt Free D= Diet or Sugarfree LF = Lowfat FF = Fat Free GF = Gluten Free

PORK DINNER RECIPES

Recipe Name: Asian Pork Tenderloin
Recipe Category: Dinner Entrée
Portion Size: 3 oz. boneless meat
Ingredients: **Yields: 8 servings**

Ingredients	Notes:
2 Pork Tenderloin (about 2-1/2 pounds), cut into 4 to 6-inch portions	Trim all visible fat.
1/2 cup reduced-sodium or regular soy sauce	
½ cup dark brown barbecue sauce	
¼ cup creamy peanut butter	
2 teaspoons garlic powder	
8 green onions, cut crosswise in half	Wash thoroughly before cutting

Directions:

Steps:	Directions:	Critical Control Point /Quality Assurance
1	Combine soy sauce, barbecue sauce, and peanut butter and garlic powder in small bowl; stir to combine thoroughly. Place pork tenderloin and soy sauce mixture in sealable container; turn to coat steaks. Close bag securely and marinate in refrigerator 1 hours or as long as overnight, turning occasionally	Store in refrigerator at less than 40 degrees F while marinating
2	Remove pork tenderloin from marinade; discard marinade. Place pork on rack of broiler pan so surface of pork is 2 to 3 inches from heat. Broil 10 to 13 minutes for medium rare (145°F) to medium (160°F) doneness, turning once. Carve steaks diagonally across grain into thin slices. During last 3 minutes of broiling top steaks with green onions.	Discard marinade. Minimum Temperature 145°F for 15 seconds

Time Temperature Sensitive food. *Food safety Standards: hold food for service at an internal temperature above 140° F. Do not mix old product with new. Cool leftover product quickly (within 4 hours) to below 41° F. Follow proper cooling procedures. Store leftovers in a tightly sealed, labeled and dated container. Use leftover within 72 hours if stored in refrigerator or 30 days if stored in the freezer. Reheat leftover product quickly (within 2 hours) to 165 degrees F for 15 seconds. Reheat left over product only once; discard if not used. Cold holding at 41°F or colder or using time alone (less than four hours).*

Texture Modified Diets:
Soft & Bite Size: (aka Bite size) **Food particle size ½ inch (~width of standard fork)** Food must be moist. Cut foods with a knife to a ½" particle size after cooking. Moisten with broth as needed. Foods that do not process well should be omitted. Omit: green onions.
Chopped: Food particle size ¼ inch (~ ½ width of standard fork) Food must be moist. Chop foods with a knife to 1/4" particle size after cooking. Moisten with broth as needed. Foods that do not process well should be omitted. Omit: green onions.
Minced and Moist:(aka Minced/Mechanical Soft/Ground) **Food particle size 1/8 inch (fits through prongs of standard fork)** Food must be moist. Use a food processor to grind food particles into 1/8 inch after cooking. Moisten with broth as needed. Foods that do not process well should be omitted. Omit: green onions
Pureed: Smooth and cohesive. Use a food processor to puree to a smooth consistency after cooking. Foods are processed by grinding and then pureeing them. May add broth or sauce to puree. Do not add to much liquid. Puree should still hold its shape. Must not be firm or sticky. Puree foods while still hot. Appearance should be smooth like pudding. Foods that do not process well should be omitted. Omit: green onions.

Therapeutic Modified Diets:
Lowfat: No changes needed
Diabetic/No added Sugar/No Conc. Sweets/Calorie Controlled: No changes needed
Bland: omit barbecue sauce, garlic powder and onion
Liberal House Renal: Omit soy sauce, barbeque sauce, peanut butter, season with no salt herbs
No Added Salt: Omit soy sauce
2 Gram Sodium: omit soy sauce, barbecue sauce, peanut butter, season with no salt herbs
Gluten Free: Use GF soy sauce and BBQ sauce. Prepare foods separately to prevent cross contamination.
Allergy Alerts: When an "X" is present, this indicates the allergen is present. Always read all food labels to ensure allergens are not present.

Wheat	Milk	Eggs	Fish Shellfish	Soy	Peanuts/Nuts	Other
X				X	X	

Key: SF= Salt Free D= Diet or Sugarfree LF = Lowfat   FF = Fat Free GF = Gluten Free

Copyright 2020 Jacqueline Larson M.S., R.D.N. and Associates.   All Rights Reserved

Recipe Name: Baked Pork Chops
Recipe Category: Dinner Entrée
Portion Size: 3 oz. boneless, 5 oz. with bone
Ingredients: **Yields: 8 servings**

Ingredients	Notes:
8 (3oz.) boneless lean pork chops, ½ inch thick or (5 oz.) bone in chop	Trim all visible fat
1 teaspoon salt	
½ teaspoon black pepper	
½ teaspoon garlic powder	
½ teaspoon rosemary	

Directions:

Steps:	Directions:	Critical Control Point / Quality Assurance
1	Season chops with salt, rosemary, garlic powder and pepper.	
2	Pre heat oven to 325 degrees	
3	Place chops in baking dish and bake for 1 hour or until temperature reaches 145 degrees.	Cook until internal temperature reaches 145 degrees with a 3 minute rest.

Time Temperature Sensitive food. *Food safety Standards: hold food for service at an internal temperature above 140° F. Do not mix old product with new. Cool leftover product quickly (within 4 hours) to below 41° F. Follow proper cooling procedures. Store leftovers in a tightly sealed, labeled and dated container. Use leftover within 72 hours if stored in refrigerator or 30 days if stored in the freezer. Reheat leftover product quickly (within 2 hours) to 165 degrees F for 15 seconds. Reheat left over product only once; discard if not used. Cold holding at 41 °F or colder or using time alone (less than four hours). Always wash hands and wash* and sanitize counter tops utensils and containers between steps when working with raw meat.

Special Diets:
Texture Modified Diets:
Soft & Bite Size: (aka Bite size) **Food particle size ½ inch (~width of standard fork)** Food must be moist. Cut foods with a knife to a ½" particle size after cooking. Moisten with broth as needed..
Chopped: Food particle size ¼ inch (~ ½ width of standard fork) Food must be moist. Chop foods with a knife to 1/4" particle size after cooking. Moisten with broth as needed.
Minced and Moist:(aka Minced/Mechanical Soft/Ground) **Food particle size 1/8 inch (fits through prongs of standard fork)** Food must be moist. Use a food processor to grind food particles into 1/8 inch after cooking. Moisten with broth as needed.
Pureed: Smooth and cohesive. Use a food processor to puree to a smooth consistency after cooking. Foods are processed by grinding and then pureeing them. May add broth or sauce to puree. Do not add to much liquid. Puree should still hold its shape. Must not be firm or sticky. Puree foods while still hot. Appearance should be smooth like pudding.
Therapeutic Modified Diets:
Lowfat: No changes needed
Diabetic/No added Sugar/No Conc. Sweets/Calorie Controlled: No changes needed
Bland: omit pepper, garlic, and rosemary
Liberal House Renal: Omit salt
No Added Salt: No changes needed
2 Gram Sodium: omit salt
Gluten Free: No changes needed. Prepare foods separately to prevent cross contamination.
Allergy Alerts: When an "X" is present, this indicates the allergen is present.
Always read all food labels to ensure allergens are not present.

Wheat	Milk	Eggs	Fish Shellfish	Soy	Peanuts/Nuts	Other

Key: SF= Salt Free D= Diet or Sugarfree LF = Lowfat FF = Fat Free GF = Gluten Free

Recipe Name: BBQ Pork Sandwich
Recipe Category: Dinner Entrée
Portion Size: 4 oz. boneless
Ingredients: Yields: 8 servings

Ingredients	Notes:
4 Pounds pork butt roast	Trim all visible fat.
1 teaspoon garlic powder	
½ teaspoon black pepper	
1 (18 oz) bottle barbeque sauce	Or see recipe in cookbook for barbeque sauce
8 hamburger buns or Kaiser rolls	

Directions:

Steps:	Directions:	Critical Control Point / Quality Assurance
1	Season roast with garlic and pepper.	
2	Cover with foil. Bake for 2 hours in 350°F oven.	
3	Remove roast from oven let rest 10 to 15 minutes.	
4	Shred pork with fork and knife.	
5	Stir in BBQ sauce and return to oven for 20 minutes. Spoon meat on buns	Cook until internal temperature reaches 165 degrees with a 3- minute rest.

Time Temperature Sensitive food. *Food safety Standards: hold food for service at an internal temperature above 140° F. Do not mix old product with new. Cool leftover product quickly (within 4 hours) to below 41° F. Follow proper cooling procedures. Store leftovers in a tightly sealed, labeled and dated container. Use leftover within 72 hours if stored in refrigerator or 30 days if stored in the freezer. Reheat leftover product quickly (within 2 hours) to 165 degrees F for 15 seconds. Reheat left over product only once; discard if not used. Cold holding at 41°F or colder or using time alone (less than four hours). Always wash hands and wash and sanitize counter tops utensils and containers between steps when working with raw meat.*

Texture Modified Diets:

Soft & Bite Size: (aka Bite size) **Food particle size ½ inch (~width of standard fork)** Food must be moist. Cut foods with a knife to a ½" particle size after cooking. Moisten with broth as needed.

Chopped: Food particle size ¼ inch (~ ½ width of standard fork) Food must be moist. Chop foods with a knife to 1/4" particle size after cooking. Moisten with broth as needed.

Minced and Moist: (aka Minced/Mechanical Soft/Ground) **Food particle size 1/8 inch (fits through prongs of standard fork)** Food must be moist. Use a food processor to grind food particles into 1/8 inch after cooking. Moisten with broth as needed.

Pureed: Smooth and cohesive. Use a food processor to puree to a smooth consistency after cooking. Foods are processed by grinding and then pureeing them. May add broth or sauce to puree. Do not add to much liquid. Puree should still hold its shape. Must not be firm or sticky. Puree foods while still hot. Appearance should be smooth like pudding.

Therapeutic Modified Diets:

Lowfat: No changes needed
Diabetic/No added Sugar/No Conc. Sweets/Calorie Controlled: No changes needed
Bland/Anti Reflux: omit garlic, pepper and sauce
Liberal House Renal: omit sauce. Use SF bread
No Added Salt: No changes needed
2 Gram Sodium: omit sauce. Use SF bread.
Gluten Free: Use gluten free buns and BBQ sauce. Prepare foods separately to prevent cross contamination.
Allergy Alerts: When an "X" is present, this indicates the allergen is present.
Always read all food labels to ensure allergens are not present.

Wheat	Milk	Eggs	Fish Shellfish	Soy	Peanuts/Nuts	Other
X	X	X				

Key: SF= Salt Free D= Diet or Sugarfree LF = Lowfat FF = Fat Free GF = Gluten Free

Recipe Name: Breaded Pork Chops
Recipe Category: Dinner Entrée
Portion Size: 4 oz. boneless, 6 oz. with bone (includes) breading
Ingredients: **Yields: 8 servings**

Ingredients	Notes:
8 (3oz.) boneless pork chops, ½ inch thick or (5 oz.) bone in chop	Trim all visible fat
1 teaspoon salt	
½ teaspoon black pepper	
½ teaspoon sage	
½ teaspoon thyme	
1 ½ cups Bread crumbs	
1 tablespoon Dijon mustard	
¾ cup light mayonnaise	
¼ cup Nonfat milk	

Directions:

Steps:	Directions:	Critical Control Point /Quality Assurance
1	Season chops with salt, sage, thyme and pepper.	
2	Place bread crumbs in small swallow dish	Discard excess
3	In a small swallow bowl combine, milk, mayonnaise and mustard. Coat each chop with mayonnaise and then bread crumbs.	Discard excess
4	Pre heat oven to 325° F. Place chops in baking dish and bake for 1 ½ hour or	Cook until internal temperature reaches 145° F for 15 seconds.

Time Temperature Sensitive food. Food safety Standards: hold food for service at an internal temperature above 140° F. Do not mix old product with new. Cool leftover product quickly (within 4 hours) to below 41° F. Follow proper cooling procedures. Store leftovers in a tightly sealed, labeled and dated container. Use leftover within 72 hours if stored in refrigerator or 30 days if stored in the freezer. Reheat leftover product quickly (within 2 hours) to 165 degrees F for 15 seconds. Reheat left over product only once; discard if not used. Cold holding at 41°F or colder or using time alone (less than four hours). Always wash hands and wash and sanitize counter tops utensils and containers between steps when working with raw meat.

Texture Modified Diets:

Soft & Bite Size: (aka Bite size) **Food particle size ½ inch (~width of standard fork)** Food must be moist. Cut foods with a knife to a ½" particle size after cooking. Moisten with broth as needed.

Chopped: Food particle size ¼ inch (~ ½ width of standard fork) Food must be moist. Chop foods with a knife to 1/4" particle size after cooking. Moisten with broth as needed.

Minced and Moist: (aka Minced/Mechanical Soft/Ground) **Food particle size 1/8 inch (fits through prongs of standard fork)** Food must be moist. Use a food processor to grind food particles into 1/8 inch after cooking. Moisten with broth as needed.

Pureed: Smooth and cohesive. Use a food processor to puree to a smooth consistency after cooking. Foods are processed by grinding and then pureeing them. May add broth or sauce to puree. Do not add to much liquid. Puree should still hold its shape. Must not be firm or sticky. Puree foods while still hot. Appearance should be smooth like pudding.
Serve ½ c. meat serving.

Therapeutic Modified Diets:

Lowfat: No changes needed
Diabetic/No added Sugar/No Conc. Sweets/Calorie Controlled: No changes needed
Bland/Anti Reflux: omit pepper, mustard, thyme and sage
Liberal House Renal: Omit salt and bread crumbs
No Added Salt: No changes needed
2 Gram Sodium: omit salt and bread crumbs
Gluten Free: Use gluten bread crumbs or crushed GF cornflakes. Prepare foods separately to prevent cross contamination.

Allergy Alerts: When an "X" is present, this indicates the allergen is present. Always read all food labels to ensure allergens are not present.

Wheat	Milk	Eggs	Fish Shellfish	Soy	Peanuts/Nuts	Other
X	X	X				

Key: SF= Salt Free D= Diet or Sugarfree LF = Lowfat FF = Fat Free GF = Gluten Free

Recipe Name: Lemon Garlic Pork Tenderloin
Recipe Category: Dinner Entrée
Portion Size: 3 oz. boneless
Ingredients: Yields: 8 servings

Ingredients	Notes:
3 ½ -4 lbs. boneless pork tenderloin	Trim all visible fat.
½ cup olive oil	Or vegetable oil
3 tablespoons lemon juice	
2 tablespoons grated lemon peel	
6 garlic cloves, mince	Wash, peel and mince
2 tablespoons dried oregano	
1 teaspoon salt	
1 teaspoon pepper	

Directions:

Steps:	Directions:	Critical Control Point / Quality Assurance
1	In a re sealable container, combine, oil, lemon juice, lemon peel, oregano, salt and pepper. Add Pork and Marinade for 1- 8 hours	
2	Heat oven to 450°F	
3	Remove pork from marinade. Spray with a baking stick nonstick cooking spray and add pork.	Discard marinate
4	Do not cover and do not add liquid.	
5	Add roast to oven and immediately reduce heat to 325°F. Roast 25 to 35 minutes to the pound.	A rolled roast or boned roast requires 5 to 10 minutes longer to the pound Slice thinly across the grain and serve. Heat to at least 145 degree with 4 minute rest

Time Temperature Sensitive food. *Food safety Standards: hold food for service at an internal temperature above 140° F. Do not mix old product with new. Cool leftover product quickly (within 4 hours) to below 41° F. Follow proper cooling procedures. Store leftovers in a tightly sealed, labeled and dated container. Use leftover within 72 hours if stored in the refrigerator or 30 days if stored in the freezer. Reheat leftover product quickly (within 2 hours) to 165 degrees F for 15 seconds. Reheat left over product only once; discard if not used. Cold holding at 41°F or colder or using time alone (less than four hours). Always wash hands and wash and sanitize counter tops utensils and containers between steps when working with raw meat.*

Texture Modified Diets:
Soft & Bite Size: (aka Bite size) **Food particle size ½ inch (~width of standard fork)** Food must be moist. Cut foods with a knife to a ½" particle size after cooking. Moisten with broth as needed.
Chopped: Food particle size ¼ inch (~ ½ width of standard fork) Food must be moist. Chop foods with a knife to 1/4" particle size after cooking. Moisten with broth as needed.
Minced and Moist: (aka Minced/Mechanical Soft/Ground) **Food particle size 1/8 inch (fits through prongs of standard fork)** Food must be moist. Use a food processor to grind food particles into 1/8 inch after cooking. Moisten with broth as needed. Foods that do not process well should be omitted. Omit: green onions
Pureed: Smooth and cohesive. Use a food processor to puree to a smooth consistency after cooking. Foods are processed by grinding and then pureeing them. May add broth or sauce to puree. Do not add to much liquid. Puree should still hold its shape. Must not be firm or sticky. Puree foods while still hot. Appearance should be smooth like pudding.

Therapeutic Modified Diets:
Lowfat: No changes needed
Diabetic/No added Sugar/No Conc. Sweets/Calorie Controlled: No changes needed
Bland/Anti Reflux: omit pepper and garlic
Liberal House Renal: omit salt, use SF broth
No Added Salt: No changes needed
2 Gram Sodium: omit salt, use SF broth
Gluten Free: Use gluten free broth. Prepare foods separately to prevent cross contamination.

Allergy Alerts: When an "X" is present, this indicates the allergen is present. Always read all food labels to ensure allergens are not present.

Wheat	Milk	Eggs	Fish Shellfish	Soy	Peanuts/Nuts	Other
X						

Key: SF= Salt Free D= Diet or Sugarfree LF = Lowfat FF = Fat Free GF = Gluten Free

Copyright 2020 Jacqueline Larson M.S., R.D.N. and Associates. All Rights Reserved

Recipe Name: Oriental Pork Tortillas or Oriental Chicken Tortillas
Recipe Category: Dinner Entrée
Portion Size: 1 1/2 cups over 1 tortilla
Ingredients: Yields: 8 servings

Ingredients	Notes:
2 ½ lbs. boneless pork chops	Trim all visible fat, cut into thin narrow strips. Or sub with boneless skin less chicken cut into thin strips.
1 cup plum jam	
2 Tablespoons cornstarch	
1 teaspoon ground ginger	
¼ cup lite soy sauce	
1 teaspoon dry mustard	
½ teaspoon garlic powder	
¼ cup red wine vinegar	
1 Tablespoon oil	
8 (10 inch) flour tortillas	
8 cups coleslaw blend	

Directions:

Steps:	Directions:	Critical Control Point / Quality Assurance
1	Partially freeze meat. Thinly slice across the grain into thin bite size strips.	
2	In a small bowl combine, jam, cornstarch, ginger, dry mustard, garlic powder, soy sauce and vinegar. Mix well. Set aside	
3	Heat large skillet over high heat. Add cooking oil.	
4	Add half the pork and cook for 2 to 3 minutes or till no pink remains. Remove from skillet and repeat with remaining pork.	Cook until internal temperature reaches 145° F for 15 seconds. If using chicken cook until internal temperature reaches 165°F for 15 seconds.
5	Return all meat to skillet. Push from the center of the skillet. Stir sauce and pour into center of skillet.	
6	Cook and stir till thickened and bubbly. Add coleslaw blend and cook until coleslaw is crisp tender	
7	Heat tortillas according to package directions. Spoon mixture evenly down center of each warm tortilla	

Time Temperature Sensitive food: Food safety Standards: hold food for service at an internal temperature above 140° F. Do not mix old product with new. Cool leftover product quickly (within 4 hours) to below 41° F. Follow proper cooling procedures. Store leftovers in a tightly sealed, labeled and dated container. Use leftover within 72 hours if stored in refrigerator or 30 days if stored in the freezer. Reheat leftover product quickly (within 2 hours) to 165 degrees F for 15 seconds. Reheat left over product only once; discard if not used. Cold holding at 41°F or colder or using time alone (less than four hours). Always wash hands and wash and sanitize counter tops utensils and containers between steps when working with raw meat.

Texture Modified Diets:

Soft & Bite Size: (aka Bite size) **Food particle size ½ inch (~width of standard fork)** Food must be moist. Cut foods with a knife to a ½" particle size after cooking. Moisten with broth as needed. Finely chop coleslaw blend.
Chopped: Food particle size ¼ inch (~ ½ width of standard fork) Food must be moist. Chop foods with a knife to 1/4" particle size after cooking. Moisten with broth as needed. Finely chop coleslaw blend.
Minced and Moist: (aka Minced/Mechanical Soft/Ground) **Food particle size 1/8 inch (fits through prongs of standard fork)** Food must be moist. Use a food processor to grind food particles into 1/8 inch after cooking. Moisten with broth as needed.
Pureed: Smooth and cohesive. Use a food processor to puree to a smooth consistency after cooking. Foods are processed by grinding and then pureeing them. May add broth or sauce to puree. Do not add to much liquid. Puree should still hold its shape. Must not be firm or sticky. Puree foods while still hot. Appearance should be smooth like pudding. Serve ½ cup puree pork, ½ puree tortilla and ¼ c. puree coleslaw separately.

Copyright 2020 Jacqueline Larson M.S., R.D.N. and Associates.   All Rights Reserved

Therapeutic Modified Diets:
Lowfat: No changes needed
Diabetic/No added Sugar/No Conc. Sweets/Calorie Controlled: No changes needed
Bland/Anti Reflux: use alternate menu item
Liberal House Renal: omit sauce. Use SF tortillas (see recipe in cookbook)
No Added Salt: omit soy sauce
2 Gram Sodium: omit sauce. Use SF tortillas (see recipe in cookbook)
Gluten Free: Use gluten free soy sauce. Use corn tortillas Prepare foods separately to prevent cross contamination.
Allergy Alerts: When an "X" is present, this indicates the allergen is present.
Always read all food labels to ensure allergens are not present.

Wheat	Milk	Eggs	Fish Shellfish	Soy	Peanuts/Nuts	Other
X				X		

Key: SF= Salt Free D= Diet or Sugarfree LF = Lowfat FF = Fat Free GF = Gluten Free

Recipe Name: Pork Carnitas
Recipe Category: Dinner Entrée
Portion Size: 3 oz. boneless, divided onto 2 tortillas (2 starches)
Ingredients: Yields: 8 servings

Ingredients	Notes:
2 ½ lbs. boneless pork shoulder, cut into bite size pieces	Trim all visible fat. Cut across the grain into thin bite size pieces
1 teaspoon salt	
½ teaspoon black pepper	
¼ cup all purpose flour	
¼ cup oil	
1 large sweet onion, cut into thin silvers	
1 (4 oz.) can diced green chilies, undrained	
1 teaspoon garlic powder	Or use 2 cloves, minced
1 cup chicken broth	
16 flour or corn tortillas	
1 cup shredded cheddar cheese	
1 cup fresh diced tomatoes	Or sub. Salsa
½ cup sour cream (optional)	
Fresh cilantro chopped (optional)	
1 large avocado, (optional)	

Directions:

Steps:	Directions:	Critical Control Point / Quality Assurance
1	Heat oven to 350 degrees	
2	In a large bowl, add pork, salt, pepper and flour. Toss to coat	
3	In a large pot add ½ of the oil and heat to medium high heat. Add ½ of the meat and cook until browned, stirring often. Remove pork and repeat with remaining pork.	
4	Drain excess fat.	
5	Return all pork to large pot and add onion, green chili, and chicken broth	
6	Cover and bake for 1 hour.	Cook until internal temperature reaches 165° F
7	Serve hot pork in warm tortillas, topped with cheese, tomatoes and optional items if desired.	

Time Temperature Sensitive food. Food safety Standards: hold food for service at an internal temperature above 140° F. Do not mix old product with new. Cool leftover product quickly (within 4 hours) to below 41° F. Follow proper cooling procedures. Store leftovers in a tightly sealed, labeled and dated container. Use leftover within 72 hours if stored in refrigerator or 30 days if stored in the freezer. Reheat leftover product quickly (within 2 hours) to 165 degrees F for 15 seconds. Reheat left over product only once; discard if not used. Cold holding at 41°F or colder or using time alone (less than four hours). Always wash hands and wash and sanitize counter tops utensils and containers between steps when working with raw meat.

Texture Modified Diets:

Soft & Bite Size: (aka Bite size) **Food particle size ½ inch (~width of standard fork)** Food must be moist. Cut foods with a knife to a ½" particle size prior to mixing. Moisten with broth as needed.

Chopped: Food particle size ¼ inch (~ ½ width of standard fork) Food must be moist. Chop foods with a knife to 1/4" particle size prior to mixing. Moisten with broth as needed.

Minced and Moist: (aka Minced/Mechanical Soft/Ground) **Food particle size 1/8 inch (fits through prongs of standard fork)** Food must be moist. Use a food processor to grind food particles into 1/8 inch prior to mixing. Moisten with broth as needed.

Pureed: Smooth and cohesive. Use a food processor to puree to a smooth consistency. Foods are processed by grinding and then pureeing them. May add broth or sauce to puree. Do not add to much liquid. Puree should still

Copyright 2020 Jacqueline Larson M.S., R.D.N. and Associates. All Rights Reserved

hold its shape. Must not be firm or sticky. Puree foods while still hot. Appearance should be smooth like pudding. Puree pork mixture and tortilla separately and serve separately

Therapeutic Modified Diets:
Lowfat: No changes needed
Diabetic/No added Sugar/No Conc. Sweets/Calorie Controlled: No changes needed
Bland/Anti Reflux: omit pepper, onion, chilies, garlic, tomato
Liberal House Renal: omit tomato/salsa, cheese, sour cream, green chilies and salt. Use SF broth or water. Use SF tortillas (see recipe in cookbook)
No Added Salt: No changes needed
2 Gram Sodium: omit salt, cheese, sour cream, green chilies and use salt free broth. Use SF tortillas (see recipe)
Gluten Free: Use gluten free broth and corn tortillas. No flour tortillas. Use gluten free all purpose flour. Prepare foods separately to prevent cross contamination.
Allergy Alerts: When an "X" is present, this indicates the allergen is present.
Always read all food labels to ensure allergens are not present.

Wheat	Milk	Eggs	Fish Shellfish	Soy	Peanuts/Nuts	Other
X	X					

Key: SF= Salt Free D= Diet or Sugarfree LF = Lowfat FF = Fat Free GF = Gluten Free

Recipe Name: Pork Chop Adobo
Recipe Category: Dinner Entrée
Portion Size: 3 oz. boneless, 5 oz. with bone
Ingredients: **Yields: 8 servings**

Ingredients	Notes:
8 boneless pork chops, ½ inch thick	Trim all visible fat
1 teaspoon salt	
½ teaspoon black pepper	
¼ cup oil	
1 cup orange juice	
¼ cup lime juice	
¼ cup red wine vinegar	
1 teaspoon garlic powder	
2 oz. can green chilies	
1 tablespoon oregano	
1 teaspoon ground cumin	
2 tablespoons cornstarch	

Directions:

Steps:	Directions:	Critical Control Point / Quality Assurance
1	Season chops with salt and pepper.	
2	Heat oil in large skillet over medium high heat. Brown chops, 7-8 minutes per side.	Cook until internal temperature reaches 145° F for 15 seconds.
3	In a small bowl combine, orange juice, lime juice, red wine vinegar, garlic, green chilies, oregano, cumin and cornstarch. Cook and stir until slightly thickened.	
4	Serve chops with sauce on top. Serve hot.	

Time Temperature Sensitive food. *Food safety Standards: hold food for service at an internal temperature above 140° F. Do not mix old product with new. Cool leftover product quickly (within 4 hours) to below 41° F. Follow proper cooling procedures. Store leftovers in a tightly sealed, labeled and dated container. Use leftover within 72 hours if stored in refrigerator or 30 days if stored in the freezer. Reheat leftover product quickly (within 2 hours) to 165 degrees F for 15 seconds. Reheat left over product only once; discard if not used. Cold holding at 41 °F or colder or using time alone (less than four hours). Always wash hands and wash and sanitize counter tops utensils and containers between steps when working with raw meat.*

Texture Modified Diets:
Soft & Bite Size: (aka Bite size) **Food particle size ½ inch (~width of standard fork)** Food must be moist. Cut foods with a knife to a ½" particle size after cooking. Moisten with sauce as needed after cutting.
Chopped: Food particle size ¼ inch (~ ½ width of standard fork) Food must be moist. Chop foods with a knife to 1/4" particle size after cooking. Moisten with sauce as needed after chopping.
Minced and Moist:(aka Minced/Mechanical Soft/Ground) **Food particle size 1/8 inch (fits through prongs of standard fork)** Food must be moist. Use a food processor to grind food particles into 1/8 inch after cooking. Moisten with sauce as needed after processing.
Pureed: Smooth and cohesive. Use a food processor to puree to a smooth consistency. Foods are processed by grinding and then pureeing them. May add milk or sauce to puree. Do not add to much liquid. Puree should still hold its shape. Must not be firm or sticky. Puree foods while still hot. Appearance should be smooth like pudding. Serve ½ c. meat serving. Top with puree sauce

Therapeutic Modified Diets:
Lowfat: No changes needed
Diabetic/No added Sugar/No Conc. Sweets/Calorie Controlled: No changes needed
Bland/Anti Reflux: use alternate menu item
Liberal House Renal: omit salt and green chilies
No Added Salt: No changes needed
2 Gram Sodium: omit salt and green chilies
Gluten Free: No changes needed. Prepare foods separately to prevent cross contamination.

Allergy Alerts: When an "X" is present, this indicates the allergen is present. Always read all food labels to ensure allergens are not present.

Wheat	Milk	Eggs	Fish Shellfish	Soy	Peanuts/Nuts	Other
X				X		

Key: SF= Salt Free D= Diet or Sugarfree LF = Lowfat FF = Fat Free GF = Gluten Free

Recipe Name: Pork Chops and Rice
Recipe Category: Dinner Entrée
Portion Size: 3 oz. boneless, plus 1/2 cup rice
Ingredients: Yields: 8 servings

Ingredients	Notes:
8 boneless pork chops, ½ inch thick	Trim all visible fat
1 teaspoon salt	
¼ teaspoon pepper	
2 cans tomato sauce	
3 teaspoons oregano	
1 medium green pepper	Wash, remove seeds and stem, and finely chop
4 cups cooked rice	Use white or brown rice
1 medium onion	Wash, peel and finely chopped
2 cups fresh mushrooms	Wash, trim and slice

Directions:

Steps:	Directions:	Critical Control Point /Quality Assurance
1	Season chops with salt and pepper.	
2	Heat oil in large skillet over medium high heat. Brown chops, 7-8 minutes per side.	Cook until internal temperature reaches 145° F for 15 seconds.
	Remove chops and keep warm. Saute' onions, pepper and mushrooms in same pan.	
3	Pre heat the oven to 350°F.	
4	Spray a baking dish with nonstick cooking spray.	
5	In a large bowl, add onions, pepper, and mushroom mixture. Stir in tomato sauce, rice and oregano.	
6	Transfer the chops mixture to baking dish.	
7	Arrange the rice, on top of the chops mixture. Bake until the rice mixture is hot and the temperature reaches 165°F. Bake 35 to 40 minutes.	

Time Temperature Sensitive food. *Food safety Standards: hold food for service at an internal temperature above 140° F. Do not mix old product with new. Cool leftover product quickly (within 4 hours) to below 41° F. Follow proper cooling procedures. Store leftovers in a tightly sealed, labeled and dated container. Use leftover within 72 hours if stored in refrigerator or 30 days if stored in the freezer. Reheat leftover product quickly (within 2 hours) to 165 degrees F for 15 seconds. Reheat left over product only once; discard if not used. Cold holding at 41°F or colder or using time alone (less than four hours). Always wash hands and wash and sanitize counter tops utensils and containers between steps when working with raw meat.*

<u>**Texture Modified Diets:** Serve Rice and pork chops separately. **Finely chop onions, peppers and mushroom mixture prior to baking.**</u>
Soft & Bite Size: (aka Bite size) **Food particle size ½ inch (~width of standard fork)** Food must be moist. Cut foods with a knife to a ½" particle size after cooking. Moisten with broth as needed after cutting.
Chopped: Food particle size ¼ inch (~ ½ width of standard fork) Food must be moist. Chop foods with a knife to 1/4" particle size after cooking. Moisten with broth as needed after chopping.
Minced and Moist:(aka Minced/Mechanical Soft/Ground) **Food particle size 1/8 inch (fits through prongs of standard fork)** Food must be moist. Use a food processor to grind food particles into 1/8 inch after cooking. Moisten with broth as needed after processing.
Pureed: Smooth and cohesive. Use a food processor to puree to a smooth consistency. Foods are processed by grinding and then pureeing them. May add milk or sauce to puree. Do not add to much liquid. Puree should still hold its shape. Must not be firm or sticky. Puree foods while still hot. Appearance should be smooth like pudding.
Serve ½ c. meat serving separate from puree rice mixture. Serve rice and meat separately.
<u>**Therapeutic Modified Diets:**</u>
Lowfat: No changes needed
Diabetic/No added Sugar/No Conc. Sweets/Calorie Controlled: No changes needed
Bland/Anti Reflux: Serve plain pork chop and ½ cup plain rice
Liberal House Renal: Serve plain SF pork chop and ½ cup SF plain rice
No Added Salt: No changes needed
2 Gram Sodium: Serve plain SF pork chop and ½ cup SF plain rice
Gluten Free: No changes needed
Allergy Alerts: When an "X" is present, this indicates the allergen is present. Always read all food labels to ensure allergens are not present.

Wheat	Milk	Eggs	Fish Shellfish	Soy	Peanuts/Nuts	Other

Key: SF= Salt Free D= Diet or Sugarfree LF = Lowfat FF = Fat Free GF = Gluten Free

Copyright 2020 Jacqueline Larson M.S., R.D.N. and Associates.   All Rights Reserved

Recipe Name: Pork Chop and Stuffing

Recipe Category: Dinner Entrée
Portion Size: 3 oz. boneless, plus 1/2 crouton mixture (stuffing)
Ingredients: Yields: 8 servings

Ingredients	Notes:
8 boneless pork chops, ½ inch thick	Trim all visible fat
1 teaspoon salt and ¼ teaspoon pepper	
2 teaspoons poultry seasoning	
2 cups light sour cream	
1 (8oz.) package fresh mushrooms	Wash and finely chop.
1 cup non-fat milk	
½ cup water	
4 cups seasoned croutons	
1/2 cup onion	Wash, peel and minced
1/2 cup celery	Wash, trim and minced

Directions:

Steps:	Directions:	Critical Control Point /Quality Assurance
1	Season chops with salt and pepper.	
2	Heat oil in large skillet over medium high heat. Brown chops, 7-8 minutes per side.	
3	Pre heat the oven to 350°F.	
4	Spray baking dish with nonstick cooking spray.	
5	In a large bowl, combine the poultry seasoning, sour cream, milk, water, onion, celery and stir in croutons	
6	Transfer the chops mixture to baking dish.	
7	Arrange the croutons, on top of the chops mixture. Bake until the crouton mixture is hot and the chops are cooked to 165°F. Bake 35 to 40 minutes. Serve hot.	Cook until internal temperature reaches 165° F for 15 seconds.

Time Temperature Sensitive food. Food safety Standards: hold food for service at an internal temperature above 140° F. Do not mix old product with new. Cool leftover product quickly (within 4 hours) to below 41° F. Follow proper cooling procedures. Store leftovers in a tightly sealed, labeled and dated container. Use leftover within 72 hours if stored in refrigerator or 30 days if stored in the freezer. Reheat leftover product quickly (within 2 hours) to 165 degrees F for 15 seconds. Reheat left over product only once; discard if not used. Cold holding at 41°F or colder or using time alone (less than four hours). Always wash hands and wash and sanitize counter tops utensils and containers between steps when working with raw meat.

Texture Modified Diets: Cook pork chops and cut, chop or mince prior to adding to casserole dish. Or may
Soft & Bite Size: (aka Bite size) **Food particle size ½ inch (~width of standard fork)** Food must be moist. Cut foods with a knife to a ½" particle size prior to mixing. Moisten with broth as needed.
Chopped: Food particle size ¼ inch (~ ½ width of standard fork) Food must be moist. Chop foods with a knife to 1/4" particle size prior to mixing. Moisten with broth as needed.
Minced and Moist: (aka Minced/Mechanical Soft/Ground) **Food particle size 1/8 inch (fits through prongs of standard fork)** Food must be moist. Use a food processor to grind food particles into 1/8 inch prior to mixing. Moisten with broth as needed.
Pureed: Smooth and cohesive. Use a food processor to puree to a smooth consistency. Foods are processed by grinding and then pureeing them. May add broth or sauce to puree. Do not add to much liquid. Puree should still hold its shape. Must not be firm or sticky. Puree foods while still hot. Appearance should be smooth like pudding. Do not combine and bake. Bake separately. Serve crouton mixture and meat separately.

Therapeutic Modified Diets:
Lowfat: No changes needed
Diabetic/No added Sugar/No Conc. Sweets/Calorie Controlled: No changes needed
Bland/Anti Reflux: Serve plain pork chop and ½ cup rice
Liberal House Renal: Serve plain pork chop and ½ cup rice
No Added Salt: No changes needed
2 Gram Sodium: Serve plain pork chop and ½ cup rice
Gluten Free: Serve plain pork chop and ½ cup rice. Or use gluten free croutons. Prepare foods separately to prevent cross contamination.

Allergy Alerts: When an "X" is present, this indicates the allergen is present. Always read all food labels to ensure allergens are not present.

Wheat	Milk	Eggs	Fish Shellfish	Soy	Peanuts/Nuts	Other
X	X					

Key: SF= Salt Free D= Diet or Sugarfree LF = Lowfat FF = Fat Free GF = Gluten Free

Recipe Name: Pork Chop with Dijon
Recipe Category: Dinner Entrée
Portion Size: 3 oz. boneless, 5 oz. with bone
Ingredients: Yields: 8 servings

Ingredients	Notes:
8 boneless pork chops, ½ inch thick	Trim all visible fat
¼ cup low fat Italian salad dressing	
¼ cup Dijon mustard	
¼ teaspoon pepper	
1 teaspoon onion powder	

Directions:

Steps:	Directions:	Critical Control Point /Quality Assurance
1	Pre oven to 350 F degrees.	
2	Spray baking dish with non-stick cooking spray.	
3	In a small bowl, blend Italian dressing, Dijon, pepper and onion powder.	
4	Place pork chops in baking dish and spread with ½ sauce. Bake for 30 minutes.	
5	Remove from oven. Turn over pork chops and spread on remaining sauce. Continue baking about 30 minutes or until internal temperature reaches 145 ° F with a 3 minute rest.	Cook until internal temperature reaches 145 ° F for 15 seconds. Discard unused mixture

Time Temperature Sensitive food. *Food safety Standards: hold food for service at an internal temperature above 140° F. Do not mix old product with new. Cool leftover product quickly (within 4 hours) to below 41° F. Follow proper cooling procedures. Store leftovers in a tightly sealed, labeled and dated container. Use leftover within 72 hours if stored in refrigerator or 30 days if stored in the freezer. Reheat leftover product quickly (within 2 hours) to 165 degrees F for 15 seconds. Reheat left over product only once; discard if not used. Cold holding at 41°F or colder or using time alone (less than four hours). Always wash hands and wash and sanitize counter tops utensils and containers between steps when working with raw meat.*

Texture Modified Diets:

Soft & Bite Size: (aka Bite size) **Food particle size ½ inch (~width of standard fork)** Food must be moist. Cut foods with a knife to a ½" particle size after cooking. Moisten with broth as needed after cutting.
Chopped: Food particle size ¼ inch (~ ½ width of standard fork) Food must be moist. Chop foods with a knife to 1/4" particle size after cooking. Moisten with broth as needed after chopping.
Minced and Moist:(aka Minced/Mechanical Soft/Ground) **Food particle size 1/8 inch (fits through prongs of standard fork)** Food must be moist. Use a food processor to grind food particles into 1/8 inch after cooking. Moisten with broth as needed after processing.
Pureed: Smooth and cohesive. Use a food processor to puree to a smooth consistency. Foods are processed by grinding and then pureeing them. May add milk or sauce to puree. Do not add to much liquid. Puree should still hold its shape. Must not be firm or sticky. Puree foods while still hot. Appearance should be smooth like pudding. Serve ½ c. meat serving.

Therapeutic Modified Diets:

Lowfat: No changes needed
Diabetic/No added Sugar/No Conc. Sweets/Calorie Controlled: No changes needed
Bland/Anti Reflux: omit Italian salad dressing, pepper, onion powder and mustard
Liberal House Renal: omit Italian dressing: substitute 2 T. oil and 2 T. vinegar.
No Added Salt: no changes
2 Gram Sodium: omit Italian dressing: substitute 2 T. oil and 2 T. vinegar
Gluten Free: Use gluten Italian dressing. Prepare foods separately to prevent cross contamination.
Allergy Alerts: When an "X" is present, this indicates the allergen is present.
Always read all food labels to ensure allergens are not present.

Wheat	Milk	Eggs	Fish Shellfish	Soy	Peanuts/Nuts	Other
X						

Key: SF= Salt Free D= Diet or Sugarfree LF = Lowfat FF = Fat Free GF = Gluten Free

Copyright 2020 Jacqueline Larson M.S., R.D.N. and Associates.   All Rights Reserved

Recipe Name: Pork Chop O Brien
Recipe Category: Dinner Entrée
Portion Size: 3 oz. boneless, plus 1/2 cup potatoes
Ingredients: **Yields: 8 servings**

Ingredients	Notes:
8 boneless pork chops, ½ inch thick	Trim all visible fat
1 teaspoon salt and ¼ teaspoon pepper	
1 teaspoon poultry seasoning	
1 cup celery	Wash, trim and dice.
½ cup nonfat milk	
½ cup light sour cream	
1 large bag (24 oz) Frozen O Brien or Hash brown potatoes	thawed
1 cup lowfat cheddar cheese	
1 can French Fried onion	(Optional)

Directions:

Steps:	Directions:	Critical Control Point /Quality Assurance
1	Season chops with salt and pepper.	
2	Heat oil in large skillet over medium high heat. Brown chops, 7-8 minutes per side.	
3	Pre heat the oven to 350 °F. Spray a baking dish with nonstick cooking spray.	Cook until internal temperature reaches 145 °F for 15 seconds.
4	In a large bowl, combine the poultry seasoning, celery, milk, sour cream, and stir in potatoes	
5	Transfer the chops mixture to casserole dish.	
6	Arrange the potatoes, on top of the chops mixture. Top with French Fried onions and cheddar cheese. Bake until the potatoes mixture is hot and the chops are cooked to 165°F. Bake 35 to 40 minutes. Serve hot.	Cook until internal temperature reaches 165 °F for 15 seconds.

Time Temperature Sensitive food. *Food safety Standards: hold food for service at an internal temperature above 140° F. Do not mix old product with new. Cool leftover product quickly (within 4 hours) to below 41° F. Follow proper cooling procedures. Store leftovers in a tightly sealed, labeled and dated container. Use leftover within 72 hours if stored in refrigerator or 30 days if stored in the freezer. Reheat leftover product quickly (within 2 hours) to 165 degrees F for 15 seconds. Reheat left over product only once; discard if not used. Cold holding at 41°F or colder or using time alone (less than four hours). Always wash hands and wash and sanitize counter tops utensils and containers between steps when working with raw meat.*

__Texture Modified Diets: Prepare and serve potatoes and pork chops separately.__
Soft & Bite Size: (aka Bite size) **Food particle size ½ inch (~width of standard fork)** Food must be moist. Cut foods with a knife to a ½" particle size after cooking. Moisten with milk as needed after cutting.
Chopped: Food particle size ¼ inch (~ ½ width of standard fork) Food must be moist. Chop foods with a knife to 1/4" particle size after cooking. Moisten with milk as needed after chopping.
Minced and Moist:(aka Minced/Mechanical Soft/Ground) **Food particle size 1/8 inch (fits through prongs of standard fork)** Food must be moist. Use a food processor to grind food particles into 1/8 inch after cooking. Moisten with milk as needed after processing.
Pureed: Smooth and cohesive. Use a food processor to puree to a smooth consistency. Foods are processed by grinding and then pureeing them. May add milk or sauce to puree. Do not add to much liquid. Puree should still hold its shape. Must not be firm or sticky. Puree foods while still hot. Appearance should be smooth like pudding. Serve potatoes and meat separately.
__Therapeutic Modified Diets:__
Lowfat: No changes needed
Diabetic/No added Sugar/No Conc. Sweets/Calorie Controlled: No changes needed
Bland/Anti Reflux: Serve plain pork chop and ½ cup plain hash brown potatoes
Liberal House Renal: Serve plain SF pork chop and ½ cup SF rice
No Added Salt: No changes needed
2 Gram Sodium: Serve plain SF pork chop and ½ cup hash brown potatoes
Gluten Free: Omit French fired onions. Prepare foods separately to prevent cross contamination.
Allergy Alerts: When an "X" is present, this indicates the allergen is present. Always read all food labels to ensure allergens are not present.

Wheat	Milk	Eggs	Fish Shellfish	Soy	Peanuts/Nuts	Other
X	X					

Key: SF= Salt Free D= Diet or Sugarfree LF = Lowfat FF = Fat Free GF = Gluten Free

Recipe Name: Pork Chops, Saute
Recipe Category: Dinner Entrée
Portion Size: 3 oz. boneless, 5 oz. with bone
Ingredients: Yields: 8 servings

Ingredients	Notes:
8 boneless pork chops, ½ inch thick	Trim all visible fat
1 teaspoon salt	
½ teaspoon black pepper	
3 Tablespoons olive oil	

Directions:

Steps:	Directions:	Critical Control Point /Quality Assurance
1	Season chops with salt and pepper.	
2	Heat 3 Tbsp. oil in large skillet over medium high heat. Brown chops, 7-8 minutes per side.	Cook until internal temperature reaches 145° F for 15 seconds.
3	Remove chops from pan. Serve hot.	

Time Temperature Sensitive food. *Food safety Standards: hold food for service at an internal temperature above 140° F. Do not mix old product with new. Cool leftover product quickly (within 4 hours) to below 41° F. Follow proper cooling procedures. Store leftovers in a tightly sealed, labeled and dated container. Use leftover within 72 hours if stored in refrigerator or 30 days if stored in the freezer. Reheat leftover product quickly (within 2 hours) to 165 degrees F for 15 seconds. Reheat left over product only once; discard if not used. Cold holding at 41°F or colder or using time alone (less than four hours). Always wash hands and wash and sanitize counter tops utensils and containers between steps when working with raw meat.*

Texture Modified Diets:

Soft & Bite Size: (aka Bite size) **Food particle size ½ inch (~width of standard fork)** Food must be moist. Cut foods with a knife to a ½" particle size after cooking. Moisten with broth as needed after cutting.

Chopped: Food particle size ¼ inch (~ ½ width of standard fork) Food must be moist. Chop foods with a knife to 1/4" particle size after cooking. Moisten with broth as needed after chopping.

Minced and Moist: (aka Minced/Mechanical Soft/Ground) **Food particle size 1/8 inch (fits through prongs of standard fork)** Food must be moist. Use a food processor to grind food particles into 1/8 inch after cooking. Moisten with broth as needed after processing.

Pureed: Smooth and cohesive. Use a food processor to puree to a smooth consistency. Foods are processed by grinding and then pureeing them. May add milk or sauce to puree. Do not add to much liquid. Puree should still hold its shape. Must not be firm or sticky. Puree foods while still hot. Appearance should be smooth like pudding. Serve ½ c. meat serving.

Therapeutic Modified Diets:

Lowfat: No changes needed
Diabetic/No added Sugar/No Conc. Sweets/Calorie Controlled: No changes needed
Bland/Anti Reflux: omit pepper
Liberal House Renal: Omit salt
No Added Salt: No changes needed
2 Gram Sodium: Omit salt
Gluten Free: No changes needed
Allergy Alerts: When an "X" is present, this indicates the allergen is present.
Always read all food labels to ensure allergens are not present.

Wheat	Milk	Eggs	FishShellfish	Soy	Peanuts/Nuts	Other

Key: SF= Salt Free D= Diet or Sugarfree LF = Lowfat FF = Fat Free GF = Gluten Free

Recipe Name: Pork Chop in Sour Cream
Recipe Category: Dinner Entrée
Portion Size: 3 oz. boneless, 5 oz. with bone
Ingredients: Yields: 8 servings

Ingredients	Notes:
8 boneless pork chops, ½ inch thick	Trim all visible fat
1 Tablespoon oil	
2 cups sliced onion	Washed, peeled and sliced
2 garlic gloves, minced	Washed, peeled and minced
1 teaspoon dill seed	
1 teaspoon caraway seeds	
2 teaspoons paprika	
1 teaspoon salt	
1 cup water	
2 cups light sour cream	

Directions:

Steps:	Directions:	Critical Control Point /Quality Assurance
1	In a large nonstick skillet, heat oil over medium high heat.	
2	Brown chops and season with salt and pepper.	
3	Cook chops on both sides, turning only for about 8-9 minutes total. Add onion, garlic, seasonings and water.	Cook to 145 °F for 15 seconds.
4	Bring to boil; reduce heat. Cover tightly and simmer until tender about 1 hour.	
5	Slowly stir in sour cream and heat for about 5 minutes. Serve hot.	

Time Temperature Sensitive food. Food safety Standards: hold food for service at an internal temperature above 140° F. Do not mix old product with new. Cool leftover product quickly (within 4 hours) to below 41° F. Follow proper cooling procedures. Store leftovers in a tightly sealed, labeled and dated container. Use leftover within 72 hours if stored in refrigerator or 30 days if stored in the freezer. Reheat leftover product quickly (within 2 hours) to 165 degrees F for 15 seconds. Reheat left over product only once; discard if not used. Cold holding at 41°F or colder or using time alone (less than four hours). Always wash hands and wash and sanitize counter tops utensils and containers between steps when working with raw meat.

Texture Modified Diets:

Soft & Bite Size: (aka Bite size) **Food particle size ½ inch (~width of standard fork)** Food must be moist. Cut foods with a knife to a ½" particle size after cooking. Moisten with sauce as needed after cutting.

Chopped: Food particle size ¼ inch (~ ½ width of standard fork) Food must be moist. Chop foods with a knife to 1/4" particle size after cooking. Moisten with sauce as needed after chopping.

Minced and Moist: (aka Minced/Mechanical Soft/Ground) **Food particle size 1/8 inch (fits through prongs of standard fork)** Food must be moist. Use a food processor to grind food particles into 1/8 inch after cooking. Moisten with sauce as needed after processing.

Pureed: Smooth and cohesive. Use a food processor to puree to a smooth consistency. Foods are processed by grinding and then pureeing them. May add milk or sauce to puree. Do not add to much liquid. Puree should still hold its shape. Must not be firm or sticky. Puree foods while still hot. Appearance should be smooth like pudding. Serve ½ c. meat serving. Serve puree sauce over meat.

Therapeutic Modified Diets:

Lowfat: No changes needed
Diabetic/No added Sugar/No Conc. Sweets/Calorie Controlled: No changes needed
Bland/Anti Reflux: omit dill seed, caraway, paprika, garlic, and onion
Liberal House Renal: omit salt
No Added Salt: No changes needed
2 Gram Sodium: omit salt
Gluten Free: No changes needed.

Allergy Alerts: When an "X" is present, this indicates the allergen is present.

Wheat	Milk	Eggs	Fish Shellfish	Soy	Peanuts/Nuts	Other
	X					

Key: SF= Salt Free D= Diet or Sugarfree LF = Lowfat FF = Fat Free GF = Gluten Free

Copyright 2020 Jacqueline Larson M.S., R.D.N. and Associates.   All Rights Reserved

Recipe Name: Pork Chop with Spiced Peaches
Recipe Category: Dinner Entrée
Portion Size: 3 oz. boneless, 5 oz. with bone
Ingredients: Yields: 8 servings

Ingredients	Notes:
8 boneless pork chops, ½ inch thick	Trim all visible fat
1 teaspoon paprika	
1 Tablespoon flour	
1 teaspoon salt	
½ teaspoon cinnamon	
½ teaspoon ground all spice	
1/8 teaspoon ground cloves	
¼ cup olive oil	
2 teaspoons Dijon mustard	
2 (16 oz.) cans sliced peaches, drained	Use peaches packed in fruit juice or rinse off excess syrup. Fresh peaches may be substituted.

Directions:

Steps:	Directions:	Critical Control Point /Quality Assurance
1	In a small bowl stir together paprika, flour, salt, cinnamon, all spice and cloves.	
2	Dredge pork chops in flour mixture and shake off excess.	Discard unused flour mixture.
3	In a large nonstick skillet, heat oil over medium high heat.	
4	Cook chops on both sides, turning only once. For about 8-9 total minutes.	Cook to 145°F for 15 seconds.
5	In a small bowl stir mustard and peach slices together.	
6	Add to skillet and cook until heated through.	
7	Serve with chops.	

Time Temperature Sensitive food. *Food safety Standards: hold food for service at an internal temperature above 140° F. Do not mix old product with new. Cool leftover product quickly (within 4 hours) to below 41° F. Follow proper cooling procedures. Store leftovers in a tightly sealed, labeled and dated container. Use leftover within 72 hours if stored in refrigerator or 30 days if stored in the freezer. Reheat leftover product quickly (within 2 hours) to 165 degrees F for 15 seconds. Reheat left over product only once; discard if not used. Cold holding at 41°F or colder or using time alone (less than four hours). Always wash hands and wash and sanitize counter tops utensils and containers between steps when working with raw meat.*

Texture Modified Diets:
Soft & Bite Size: (aka Bite size) **Food particle size ½ inch (~width of standard fork)** Food must be moist. Cut foods with a knife to a ½" particle size after cooking. Moisten with sauce as needed after cutting.
Chopped: Food particle size ¼ inch (~ ½ width of standard fork) Food must be moist. Chop foods with a knife to 1/4" particle size after cooking. Moisten with sauce as needed after chopping.
Minced and Moist:(aka Minced/Mechanical Soft/Ground) **Food particle size 1/8 inch (fits through prongs of standard fork)** Food must be moist. Use a food processor to grind food particles into 1/8 inch after cooking. Moisten with sauce as needed after processing.
Pureed: Smooth and cohesive. Use a food processor to puree to a smooth consistency. Foods are processed by grinding and then pureeing them. May add milk or sauce to puree. Do not add to much liquid. Puree should still hold its shape. Must not be firm or sticky. Puree foods while still hot. Appearance should be smooth like pudding. Serve ½ c. meat serving with fruit on top

Therapeutic Modified Diets:
Lowfat: No changes needed
Diabetic/No added Sugar/No Conc. Sweets/Calorie Controlled: No changes needed
Bland/Anti Reflux: omit paprika, cinnamon, all spice, cloves and mustard
Liberal House Renal: omit salt
No Added Salt: No changes needed
2 Gram Sodium: omit salt
Gluten Free: Use gluten free all purpose flour. Prepare foods separately to prevent cross contamination.

Allergy Alerts: When an "X" is present, this indicates the allergen is present. Always read all food labels to ensure allergens are not present.

Wheat	Milk	Eggs	Fish Shellfish	Soy	Peanuts/Nuts	Other
X						

Key: SF= Salt Free D= Diet or Sugarfree LF = Lowfat FF = Fat Free GF = Gluten Free

Copyright 2020 Jacqueline Larson M.S., R.D.N. and Associates.   All Rights Reserved

Recipe Name: Pork Chop with Tangy Sauce
Recipe Category: Dinner Entrée
Portion Size: 3 oz. boneless, 5 oz. with bone
Ingredients: **Yields: 8 servings**

Ingredients	Notes:
8 boneless pork chops, ½ inch thick	Trim all visible fat
2 Tablespoon lite soy sauce	
½ teaspoon black pepper	
3 Tablespoons oil	
3 Tablespoons Worcestershire sauce	
2 teaspoons lemon juice	
¼ cup ketchup	
¼ cup brown sugar	

Directions:

Steps:	Directions:	Critical Control Point /Quality Assurance
1	Pre oven to 350 °F	
2	Spray baking dish with nonstick cooking spray.	
3	In a small bowl, blend soy sauce, oil, Worcestershire sauce, lemon juice, brown sugar and ketchup.	
4	Place pork chops in baking dish and spread with ½ sauce. Bake for 30 minutes.	
5	Remove from oven. Turn over pork chops and spread on remaining sauce. Continue baking about 30 minutes or until internal temperature reaches 145 ° F with a 3 minute rest.	Cook until internal temperature reaches 145 ° F for 15 seconds. Discard unused mixture

Time Temperature Sensitive food. *Food safety Standards: hold food for service at an internal temperature above 140° F. Do not mix old product with new. Cool leftover product quickly (within 4 hours) to below 41° F. Follow proper cooling procedures. Store leftovers in a tightly sealed, labeled and dated container. Use leftover within 72 hours if stored in refrigerator or 30 days if stored in the freezer. Reheat leftover product quickly (within 2 hours) to 165 degrees F for 15 seconds. Reheat left over product only once; discard if not used. Cold holding at 41 °F or colder or using time alone (less than four hours). Always wash hands and wash and sanitize counter tops utensils and containers between steps when working with raw meat.*

Texture Modified Diets:

Soft & Bite Size: (aka Bite size) **Food particle size ½ inch (~width of standard fork)** Food must be moist. Cut foods with a knife to a ½" particle size after cooking. Moisten with sauce as needed after cutting.

Chopped: Food particle size ¼ inch (~ ½ width of standard fork) Food must be moist. Chop foods with a knife to 1/4" particle size after cooking. Moisten with sauce as needed after chopping.

Minced and Moist:(aka Minced/Mechanical Soft/Ground) **Food particle size 1/8 inch (fits through prongs of standard fork)** Food must be moist. Use a food processor to grind food particles into 1/8 inch after cooking. Moisten with sauce as needed after processing.

Pureed: Smooth and cohesive. Use a food processor to puree to a smooth consistency. Foods are processed by grinding and then pureeing them. May add milk or sauce to puree. Do not add to much liquid. Puree should still hold its shape. Must not be firm or sticky. Puree foods while still hot. Appearance should be smooth like pudding. Serve ½ c. meat serving

Therapeutic Modified Diets:

Lowfat: No changes needed
Diabetic/No added Sugar/No Conc. Sweets/Calorie Controlled: No changes needed
Bland/Anti Reflux: Omit black pepper, Worcestershire sauce, lemon juice and ketchup.
Liberal House Renal: omit soy sauce, catsup and Worcestershire sauce
No Added Salt: omit soy sauce and Worcestershire sauce
2 Gram Sodium: omit soy sauce, catsup and Worcestershire sauce
Gluten Free: Use gluten free soy sauce. Prepare foods separately to prevent cross contamination.

Allergy Alerts: When an "X" is present, this indicates the allergen is present. Always read all food labels to ensure allergens are not present.

Wheat	Milk	Eggs	Fish Shellfish	Soy	Peanuts/Nuts	Other
X			X	X		

Key: SF= Salt Free D= Diet or Sugarfree LF = Lowfat FF = Fat Free GF = Gluten Free

Recipe Name: Pork Chop with Apple Curry Sauce
Recipe Category: Dinner Entrée
Portion Size: 3 oz. boneless, 5 oz. with bone
Ingredients: Yields: 8 servings

Ingredients	Notes:
8 boneless pork chops, ½ inch thick	Trim all visible fat
1 teaspoon salt	
½ teaspoon black pepper	
¼ cup oil	
1 ½ cup apple cider or juice	
1 cup chicken broth, reduced salt	
1 Tablespoon cornstarch	
2 Tablespoons water	
1 teaspoon ground ginger	
1 teaspoon ground curry	

Directions:

Steps:	Directions:	Critical Control Point /Quality Assurance
1	In a large nonstick skillet, heat oil over medium high heat.	
2	Brown chops and season with salt and pepper.	Cook to 145° F for 15 seconds
3	Add apple cider, ginger and curry and broth. Cover and simmer for 8 minutes.	
4	In a small bowl combine cornstarch and water Add cornstarch mixture to chops and bring to boil. Cook until sauce thickens. Serve hot.	

Time Temperature Sensitive food. *Food safety Standards: hold food for service at an internal temperature above 140° F. Do not mix old product with new. Cool leftover product quickly (within 4 hours) to below 41° F. Follow proper cooling procedures. Store leftovers in a tightly sealed, labeled and dated container. Use leftover within 72 hours if stored in refrigerator or 30 days if stored in the freezer. Reheat leftover product quickly (within 2 hours) to 165 degrees F for 15 seconds. Reheat left over product only once; discard if not used. Cold holding at 41°F or colder or using time alone (less than four hours). Always wash hands and wash and sanitize counter tops utensils and containers between steps when working with raw meat.*

Texture Modified Diets:

Soft & Bite Size: (aka Bite size) **Food particle size ½ inch (~width of standard fork)** Food must be moist. Cut foods with a knife to a ½" particle size after cooking. Moisten with sauce as needed after cutting.

Chopped: Food particle size ¼ inch (~ ½ width of standard fork) Food must be moist. Chop foods with a knife to 1/4" particle size after cooking. Moisten with sauce as needed after chopping.

Minced and Moist:(aka Minced/Mechanical Soft/Ground) **Food particle size 1/8 inch (fits through prongs of standard fork)** Food must be moist. Use a food processor to grind food particles into 1/8 inch after cooking. Moisten with sauce as needed after processing.

Pureed: Smooth and cohesive. Use a food processor to puree to a smooth consistency. Foods are processed by grinding and then pureeing them. May add milk or sauce to puree. Do not add to much liquid. Puree should still hold its shape. Must not be firm or sticky. Puree foods while still hot. Appearance should be smooth like pudding. Serve ½ c. meat serving Serve ½ c. meat serving. Serve puree sauce over meat.

Therapeutic Modified Diets:

Lowfat: No changes needed
Diabetic/No added Sugar/No Conc. Sweets/Calorie Controlled: No changes needed
Bland/Anti Reflux: omit pepper and curry
Liberal House Renal: Omit salt. Use salt free broth or water
No Added Salt: No changes needed
2 Gram Sodium: Omit salt. Use salt free broth or water
Gluten Free: Use gluten free broth. Prepare foods separately to prevent cross contamination.

Allergy Alerts: When an "X" is present, this indicates the allergen is present. Always read all food labels to ensure allergens are not present.

Wheat	Milk	Eggs	Fish Shellfish	Soy	Peanuts/Nuts	Other
X						

Key: SF= Salt Free D= Diet or Sugarfree LF = Lowfat FF = Fat Free GF = Gluten Free

Copyright 2020 Jacqueline Larson M.S., R.D.N. and Associates.   All Rights Reserved

Recipe Name: Pork Chop with Apple Mustard Glaze
Recipe Category: Dinner Entrée
Portion Size: 3 oz. boneless, 5 oz. with bone
Ingredients: Yields: 8 servings

Ingredients	Notes:
8 boneless pork chops, ½ inch thick (3 oz. each)	Trim all visible fat.
½ teaspoon black pepper	
¼ cup oil	
1 teaspoon salt	
½ cup apple juice	
¼ cup apple jelly	
¼ cup Dijon mustard	

Directions:

Steps:	Directions:	Critical Control Point /Quality Assurance
1	Season pork chops with salt and pepper.	
2	In a large nonstick skillet, heat oil over medium high heat.	
3	Brown chops 2 minutes on one side	
4	In a small bowl combine apple juice, jelly and mustard	
5	Turn chops and add apple juice, jelly and mustard to skillet	
6	Reduce heat to low, cover and cook 5-6 minutes. To ensure doneness check with meat thermometer.	Cook to 145°F for 15 seconds
7	Serve hot.	

Time Temperature Sensitive food. *Food safety Standards: hold food for service at an internal temperature above 140° F. Do not mix old product with new. Cool leftover product quickly (within 4 hours) to below 41° F. Follow proper cooling procedures. Store leftovers in a tightly sealed, labeled and dated container. Use leftover within 72 hours if stored in refrigerator or 30 days if stored in the freezer. Reheat leftover product quickly (within 2 hours) to 165 degrees F for 15 seconds. Reheat left over product only once; discard if not used. Cold holding at 41 °F or colder or using time alone (less than four hours). Always wash hands and wash and sanitize counter tops utensils and containers between steps when working with raw meat.*

Texture Modified Diets:

Soft & Bite Size: (aka Bite size) **Food particle size ½ inch (~width of standard fork)** Food must be moist. Cut foods with a knife to a ½" particle size after cooking. Moisten with sauce as needed after cutting.

Chopped: Food particle size ¼ inch (~ ½ width of standard fork) Food must be moist. Chop foods with a knife to 1/4" particle size after cooking. Moisten with sauce as needed after chopping.

Minced and Moist: (aka Minced/Mechanical Soft/Ground) **Food particle size 1/8 inch (fits through prongs of standard fork)** Food must be moist. Use a food processor to grind food particles into 1/8 inch after cooking. Moisten with sauce as needed after processing.

Pureed: Smooth and cohesive. Use a food processor to puree to a smooth consistency. Foods are processed by grinding and then pureeing them. May add milk or sauce to puree. Do not add to much liquid. Puree should still hold its shape. Must not be firm or sticky. Puree foods while still hot. Appearance should be smooth like pudding. Serve ½ c. meat serving

Therapeutic Modified Diets:

Lowfat: No changes needed
Diabetic/No added Sugar/No Conc. Sweets/Calorie Controlled: No changes needed
Bland/Anti Reflux: omit pepper and mustard
Liberal House Renal: Omit salt
No Added Salt: No changes needed
2 Gram Sodium: Omit salt
Gluten Free: No changes needed.
Allergy Alerts: When an "X" is present, this indicates the allergen is present.
Always read all food labels to ensure allergens are not present.

Wheat	Milk	Eggs	Fish Shellfish	Soy	Peanuts/Nuts	Other

Key: SF= Salt Free D= Diet or Sugarfree LF = Lowfat FF = Fat Free GF = Gluten Free

Copyright 2020 Jacqueline Larson M.S., R.D.N. and Associates.   All Rights Reserved

Recipe Name: Pork Chop with Apricot Ginger Teriyaki Sauce
Recipe Category: Dinner Entrée
Portion Size: 3 oz. boneless, 5 oz. with bone
Ingredients: **Yields: 8 servings**

Ingredients	Notes:
8 boneless pork chops, ½ inch thick	Trim all visible fat
½ teaspoon black pepper	
¼ cup oil	
1 cup apricot fruit preserves	
½ cup lite soy sauce	
2 teaspoons ginger	
½ teaspoon garlic powder	Or used 2 cloves, minced
3 Tablespoons honey	
2 teaspoons, sesame seeds	
¼ cup chopped green onions (optional)	Wash, trim and slice.

Directions:

Steps:	Directions:	Critical Control Point /Quality Assurance
1	In a large nonstick skillet, heat oil over medium high heat. Brown chops and season with pepper.	
2	Cook chops on both sides, turning only for about 8-9 minutes total	Cook to 145°F for 15 seconds.
3	In a small bowl combine apricot preserves, soy sauce, ginger, garlic powder, honey and sesame seeds.	
4	Whisk thoroughly. Pour sauce over chops and heat until thick and bubbly. Serve chops and pour sauce over chops. Top with green onions.	

Time Temperature Sensitive food. Food safety Standards: hold food for service at an internal temperature above 140° F. Do not mix old product with new. Cool leftover product quickly (within 4 hours) to below 41° F. Follow proper cooling procedures. Store leftovers in a tightly sealed, labeled and dated container. Use leftover within 72 hours if stored in refrigerator or 30 days if stored in the freezer. Reheat leftover product quickly (within 2 hours) to 165 degrees F for 15 seconds. Reheat left over product only once; discard if not used. Cold holding at 41°F or colder or using time alone (less than four hours). Always wash hands and wash and sanitize counter tops utensils and containers between steps when working with raw meat.

<u>**Texture Modified Diets:**</u>
Soft & Bite Size: (aka Bite size) **Food particle size ½ inch (~width of standard fork)** Food must be moist. Cut foods with a knife to a ½" particle size prior to mixing. Moisten with broth as needed. Foods that do not process well should be omitted. Omit: green onions.
Chopped: Food particle size ¼ inch (~ ½ width of standard fork) Food must be moist. Chop foods with a knife to 1/4" particle size prior to mixing. Moisten with broth as needed. Foods that do not process well should be omitted. Omit: green onions.
Minced and Moist:(aka Minced/Mechanical Soft/Ground) **Food particle size 1/8 inch (fits through prongs of standard fork)** Food must be moist. Use a food processor to grind food particles into 1/8 inch prior to mixing. Moisten with broth as needed. Foods that do not process well should be omitted. Omit: green onions.
Pureed: Smooth and cohesive. Use a food processor to puree to a smooth consistency. Foods are processed by grinding and then pureeing them. May add broth or sauce to puree. Do not add to much liquid. Puree should still hold its shape. Must not be firm or sticky. Puree foods while still hot. Appearance should be smooth like pudding. Foods that do not process well should be omitted. Omit: sesame seeds and green onions. Serve ½ c. meat serving. Serve puree sauce over meat.
<u>**Therapeutic Modified Diets:**</u>
Lowfat: No changes needed
Diabetic/No added Sugar/No Conc. Sweets/Calorie Controlled: Use no added sugar preserves
Bland/Anti Reflux: omit pepper and sesame seeds
Liberal House Renal: Omit soy sauce.
No Added Salt: omit soy sauce
2 Gram Sodium: omit soy sauce
Gluten Free: Use gluten free soy sauce. Prepare foods separately to prevent cross contamination.
Allergy Alerts: When an "X" is present, this indicates the allergen is present.

Wheat	Milk	Eggs	Fish Shellfish	Soy	Peanuts/Nuts	Other
X				X		

Key: SF= Salt Free D= Diet or Sugarfree LF = Lowfat   FF = Fat Free GF = Gluten Free

Recipe Name: Pork Chop with Apple Raison Sauce
Recipe Category: Dinner Entrée
Portion Size: 3 oz. boneless, 5 oz. with bone
Ingredients: **Yields: 8 servings**

Ingredients	Notes:
8 boneless pork chops, ½ inch thick (3 oz. each)	Trim all visible fat.
1 teaspoon salt	
½ teaspoon black pepper	
¼ cup oil	
4 cups apple cider or juice	
½ cup coarse grain mustard	
6 large apples	Wash. Core and dice to ½ inch thickness
1 cup raisons	
½ cup sliced green onions	
¼ cup cornstarch	
½ cup water	

Directions:

Steps:	Directions:	Critical Control Point /Quality Assurance
1	In a large nonstick skillet, heat oil over medium high heat. Brown chops and season with salt and pepper.	
2	In a small bowl combine apple cider and mustard; pour over chops. Cover and simmer for 8 minutes	
3	Add apples and raisins. Reduce heat to low, cover and cook 5-10 minutes. To ensure doneness check with meat thermometer.	Cook to 145 ° F for 15 seconds.
4	Place pork chops and apples on serving platter; keep warm.	
5	In a small bowl combine cornstarch with water. Add to pork chops. Bring to boil; cook and stir until thickened	
6	Serve sauce over pork chops and apples. Stir.	
7	Top with green onion	

Time Temperature Sensitive food. *Food safety Standards: hold food for service at an internal temperature above 140° F. Do not mix old product with new. Cool leftover product quickly (within 4 hours) to below 41° F. Follow proper cooling procedures. Store leftovers in a tightly sealed, labeled and dated container. Use leftover within 72 hours if stored in refrigerator or 30 days if stored in the freezer. Reheat leftover product quickly (within 2 hours) to 165 degrees F for 15 seconds. Reheat left over product only once; discard if not used. Cold holding at 41°F or colder or using time alone (less than four hours). Always wash hands and wash and sanitize counter tops utensils and containers between steps when working with raw meat.*

Texture Modified Diets:
Soft & Bite Size: (aka Bite size) **Food particle size ½ inch (~width of standard fork)** Food must be moist. Cut foods with a knife to a ½" particle size after cooking. Moisten with sauce as needed after cutting. Omit raisons and green onions.
Chopped: Food particle size ¼ inch (~ ½ width of standard fork) Food must be moist. Chop foods with a knife to 1/4" particle size after cooking. Moisten with sauce as needed after chopping. Omit raisons and green onions.
Minced and Moist:(aka Minced/Mechanical Soft/Ground) **Food particle size 1/8 inch (fits through prongs of standard fork)** Food must be moist. Use a food processor to grind food particles into 1/8 inch after cooking. Moisten with sauce as needed after processing. Omit raisons and green onions.
Pureed: Smooth and cohesive. Use a food processor to puree to a smooth consistency. Foods are processed by grinding and then pureeing them. May add milk or sauce to puree. Do not add to much liquid. Puree should still hold its shape. Must not be firm or sticky. Puree foods while still hot. Appearance should be smooth like pudding. Serve ½ c. meat serving. Omit raisons and green onions.

Therapeutic Modified Diets:
Lowfat: No changes needed
Diabetic/No added Sugar/No Conc. Sweets/Calorie Controlled: No changes needed
Bland/Anti Reflux: omit pepper and mustard
Liberal House Renal: Omit salt and raisons
No Added Salt: No changes needed **2 Gram Sodium:** Omit salt
Gluten Free: No changes needed. Prepare foods separately to prevent cross contamination.
Allergy Alerts: When an "X" is present, this indicates the allergen is present. Always read all food labels to ensure allergens are not present.

Wheat	Milk	Eggs	Fish Shellfish	Soy	Peanuts/Nuts	Other

Key: SF= Salt Free D= Diet or Sugarfree LF = Lowfat FF = Fat Free GF = Gluten Free

Copyright 2020 Jacqueline Larson M.S., R.D.N. and Associates.   All Rights Reserved

Recipe Name: Pork Chop and Cheesy Rice Casserole
Recipe Category: Dinner Entrée
Portion Size: 3 oz. boneless, plus 1 cup rice and vegetable mixture
Ingredients: Yields: 8 servings

Ingredients	Notes:
8 boneless pork chops, ½ inch thick	Trim all visible fat
1 teaspoon salt	
½ teaspoon black pepper	
¼ cup oil	
4 cups cooked long grain rice	Use brown or white rice
4 cups frozen mixed vegetables, thawed	
2 cups shredded lowfat cheddar cheese	
2 cups lowfat cottage cheese	
½ cup Parmesan cheese, grated	
1 Tablespoon, parsley flakes	

Directions:

Steps:	Directions:	Critical Control Point / Quality Assurance
1	Season chops with salt and pepper.	
2	Heat oil in large skillet over medium high heat. Brown chops, 7-8 minutes per side.	Cook until internal temperature reaches 145 °F for 15 seconds.
3	Pre heat the oven to 375°F.	
4	Spray baking dish with nonstick cooking spray.	
5	In a large bowl, combine the rice, vegetable, cheddar cheese, and cottage cheese.	
6	Transfer the rice mixture to baking dish.	
7	Arrange the chops, on top of the rice mixture and bake until the rice mixture is hot and the chops are cooked to 145 degrees. Top with parsley.	
8	Serve the chops over the rice mixture. Serve hot.	

Time Temperature Sensitive food. *Food safety Standards: hold food for service at an internal temperature above 140°F. Do not mix old product with new. Cool leftover product quickly (within 4 hours) to below 41°F. Follow proper cooling procedures. Store leftovers in a tightly sealed, labeled and dated container. Use leftover within 72 hours if stored in refrigerator or 30 days if stored in the freezer. Reheat leftover product quickly (within 2 hours) to 165 degrees F for 15 seconds. Reheat left over product only once; discard if not used. Cold holding at 41°F or colder or using time alone (less than four hours). Always wash hands and wash and sanitize counter tops utensils and containers between steps when working with raw meat.*

<u>**Texture Modified Diets: Prepare size separately from pork chops.**</u>
Soft & Bite Size: (aka Bite size) **Food particle size ½ inch (~width of standard fork)** Food must be moist. Cut foods with a knife to a ½" particle size after cooking. Moisten with sauce or broth as needed after cutting.
Chopped: Food particle size ¼ inch (~ ½ width of standard fork) Food must be moist. Chop foods with a knife to 1/4" particle size after cooking. Moisten with sauce or broth as needed after chopping.
Minced and Moist: (aka Minced/Mechanical Soft/Ground) **Food particle size 1/8 inch (fits through prongs of standard fork)** Food must be moist. Use a food processor to grind food particles into 1/8 inch after cooking. Moisten with sauce or broth as needed after processing.
Pureed: Smooth and cohesive. Use a food processor to puree to a smooth consistency. Foods are processed by grinding and then pureeing them. May add milk or sauce to puree. Do not add to much liquid. Puree should still hold its shape. Must not be firm or sticky. Puree foods while still hot. Appearance should be smooth like pudding. Serve ½ c. meat serving

<u>**Therapeutic Modified Diets:**</u>
Lowfat: No changes needed
Carbohydrate Controlled:Diabetic/No added Sugar/No Conc. Sweets/Calorie Controlled: No changes needed
Bland/Anti Reflux: omit pepper, parsley and use peas and carrots for vegetables
Liberal House Renal: Serve 3 oz. SF Pork chop, SF rice and SF mixed vegetables
No Added Salt: No changes needed
2 Gram Sodium: Serve 3 oz. SF pork chop, SF rice and SF mixed vegetables
Gluten Free: No changes needed. Prepare foods separately to prevent cross contamination.
Allergy Alerts: When an "X" is present, this indicates the allergen is present. Always read all food labels to ensure allergens are not present.

Wheat	Milk	Eggs	Fish Shellfish	Soy	Peanuts/Nuts	Other
	X					

Key: SF= Salt Free D= Diet or Sugarfree LF = Lowfat FF = Fat Free GF = Gluten Free

Recipe Name: Pork Chop with Chili Rub and Topped with Pineapple Salsa
Recipe Category: Dinner Entrée
Portion Size: 3 oz. boneless, 5 oz. with bone
Ingredients: Yields: 8 servings

Ingredients	Notes:
8 boneless pork chops, ½ inch thick	Trim all visible fat
1 teaspoon salt	
½ teaspoon black pepper	
¼ cup oil	
1 teaspoon garlic powder	
1 teaspoon onion powder	
2 Tablespoons chili powder	
¼ cup brown sugar	
1 large can crushed pineapple, drained	
¼ cup minced red onion	
1 Tablespoon lime juice	Add zest of 1 fresh lime too. (optional)
¼ teaspoon salt	
Dash of cayenne pepper	

Directions:

Steps:	Directions:	Critical Control Point /Quality Assurance
1	In a small bowl stir together, salt, black pepper, garlic powder, onion powder, chili powder and brown sugar	
2	Dredge chops in mixture	Discard unused mixture
3	Heat oil in large skillet over medium high heat. Brown chops, 3-4 minutes per side.	Cook until internal temperature reaches 145°F for 15 seconds.
4	In a small bowl combine, pineapple, red onion, lime juice, salt and cayenne pepper	
5	Serve hot chops with 2 T. pineapple salsa on top.	

Time Temperature Sensitive food. Food safety Standards: hold food for service at an internal temperature above 140° F. Do not mix old product with new. Cool leftover product quickly (within 4 hours) to below 41° F. Follow proper cooling procedures. Store leftovers in a tightly sealed, labeled and dated container. Use leftover within 72 hours if stored in refrigerator or 30 days if stored in the freezer. Reheat leftover product quickly (within 2 hours) to 165 degrees F for 15 seconds. Reheat left over product only once; discard if not used. Cold holding at 41°F or colder or using time alone (less than four hours). Always wash hands and wash

<u>*Texture Modified Diets:*</u>
Soft & Bite Size: (aka Bite size) **Food particle size ½ inch (~width of standard fork)** Food must be moist. Cut foods with a knife to a ½" particle size after cooking. Moisten with sauce as needed after cutting. Omit pineapple salsa.
Chopped: Food particle size ¼ inch (~ ½ width of standard fork) Food must be moist. Chop foods with a knife to 1/4" particle size after cooking. Moisten with sauce as needed after chopping. Omit pineapple salsa.
Minced and Moist:(aka Minced/Mechanical Soft/Ground) **Food particle size 1/8 inch (fits through prongs of standard fork)** Food must be moist. Use a food processor to grind food particles into 1/8 inch after cooking. Moisten with sauce as needed after processing. Omit pineapple salsa.
Pureed: Smooth and cohesive. Use a food processor to puree to a smooth consistency. Foods are processed by grinding and then pureeing them. May add milk or sauce to puree. Do not add to much liquid. Puree should still hold its shape. Must not be firm or sticky. Puree foods while still hot. Appearance should be smooth like pudding. Serve ½ c. meat serving. Omit pineapple salsa.

<u>*Therapeutic Modified Diets:*</u>
Lowfat: No changes needed
Diabetic/No added Sugar/No Conc. Sweets/Calorie Controlled: No changes needed
Bland/Anti Reflux: use plain pork chop with brown sugar
Liberal House Renal: omit salt
No Added Salt: No changes needed
2 Gram Sodium: omit salt
Gluten Free: No changes needed.   Prepare foods separately to prevent cross contamination.

Allergy Alerts: When an "X" is present, this indicates the allergen is present. Always read all food labels to ensure allergens are not present.

Wheat	Milk	Eggs	Fish Shellfish	Soy	Peanuts/Nuts	Other

Key: SF= Salt Free D= Diet or Sugarfree LF = Lowfat FF = Fat Free GF = Gluten Free

Recipe Name: Pork Chop with Coriander
Recipe Category: Dinner Entrée
Portion Size: 3 oz. boneless, 5 oz. with bone
Ingredients: Yields: 8 servings

Ingredients	Notes:
8 boneless pork chops, ½ inch thick	Trim all visible fat
1 teaspoon salt	
½ teaspoon black pepper	
¼ cup oil	
1 Tablespoon coriander seeds, crushed	
3 Tablespoons brown sugar	
1/2 cup lite soy sauce	
1 cup low salt chicken broth	
1 1/2 Tablespoon cornstarch	

Directions:

Steps:	Directions:	Critical Control Point /Quality Assurance
1	Season chops with salt and pepper.	
2	Heat oil in large skillet over medium high heat. Brown chops, 7-8 minutes per side.	Cook until internal temperature reaches 145 °F for 15 seconds..
3	In a small bowl combine, coriander, brown sugar, soy sauce, chicken broth and cornstarch	
4	Cook and stir until slightly thickened in a small sauce pan. Pour over chops and baste.	
5	Serve chops with sauce on top.	

Time Temperature Sensitive food. *Food safety Standards: hold food for service at an internal temperature above 140° F. Do not mix old product with new. Cool leftover product quickly (within 4 hours) to below 41° F. Follow proper cooling procedures. Store leftovers in a tightly sealed, labeled and dated container. Use leftover within 72 hours if stored in refrigerator or 30 days if stored in the freezer. Reheat leftover product quickly (within 2 hours) to 165 degrees F for 15 seconds. Reheat left over product only once; discard if not used. Cold holding at 41°F or colder or using time alone (less than four hours). Always wash hands and wash and sanitize counter tops utensils and containers between steps when working with raw meat.*

Texture Modified Diets:
Soft & Bite Size: (aka Bite size) **Food particle size ½ inch (~width of standard fork)** Food must be moist. Cut foods with a knife to a ½" particle size after cooking. Moisten with sauce as needed after cutting. Omit Coconut.
Chopped: Food particle size ¼ inch (~ ½ width of standard fork) Food must be moist. Chop foods with a knife to 1/4" particle size after cooking. Moisten with sauce as needed after chopping. Omit Coconut
Minced and Moist:(aka Minced/Mechanical Soft/Ground) **Food particle size 1/8 inch (fits through prongs of standard fork)** Food must be moist. Use a food processor to grind food particles into 1/8 inch after cooking. Moisten with sauce as needed after processing.
Pureed: Smooth and cohesive. Use a food processor to puree to a smooth consistency. Foods are processed by grinding and then pureeing them. May add milk or sauce to puree. Do not add to much liquid. Puree should still hold its shape. Must not be firm or sticky. Puree foods while still hot. Appearance should be smooth like pudding. Serve ½ c. meat serving

Therapeutic Modified Diets:
Lowfat: No changes needed
Diabetic/No added Sugar/No Conc. Sweets/Calorie Controlled: No changes needed
Bland/Anti Reflux: omit coriander and pepper
Liberal House Renal: Omit salt, soy sauce and use SF broth or water
No Added Salt: No changes needed
2 Gram Sodium: Omit salt, soy sauce and use SF broth or water
Gluten Free: Use gluten free broth and soy sauce. Prepare foods separately to prevent cross contamination.
Allergy Alerts: When an "X" is present, this indicates the allergen is present. Always read all food labels to ensure allergens are not present.

Wheat	Milk	Eggs	Fish Shellfish	Soy	Peanuts/Nuts	Other
X				X		

Key: SF= Salt Free D= Diet or Sugarfree LF = Lowfat FF = Fat Free GF = Gluten Free

Recipe Name: Pork Chop with Cranberry Apple Sauce
Recipe Category: Dinner Entrée
Portion Size: 3 oz. boneless, 5 oz. with bone
Ingredients: **Yields: 8 servings**

Ingredients	Notes:
8 boneless pork chops, ½ inch thick	Trim all visible fat
1 teaspoon salt	
½ teaspoon black pepper	
¼ cup oil	
1 cup apple cider or juice	
1 cup cranberry sauce	May use canned.
¼ cup honey	
½ cup orange juice concentrate, thawed	
1 teaspoon ground ginger	

Directions:

Steps:	Directions:	Critical Control Point /Quality Assurance
1	In a large nonstick skillet, heat oil over medium high heat.	
2	Brown chops and season with salt and pepper.	
3	Add apple cider. Cover and simmer for 8 minutes.	Cook to 145° F for 15 seconds for Pork
4	In a small bowl combine cranberry sauce, honey, orange juice concentrate and ginger.	
5	Pour sauce over chops.	
6	Cook for 1-2 minutes until heated through.	

Time Temperature Sensitive food. Food safety Standards: hold food for service at an internal temperature above 140° F. Do not mix old product with new. Cool leftover product quickly (within 4 hours) to below 41° F. Follow proper cooling procedures. Store leftovers in a tightly sealed, labeled and dated container. Use leftover within 72 hours if stored in refrigerator or 30 days if stored in the freezer. Reheat leftover product quickly (within 2 hours) to 165 degrees F for 15 seconds. Reheat left over product only once; discard if not used. Cold holding at 41 °F or colder or using time alone (less than four hours). Always wash hands and wash and sanitize counter tops utensils and containers between steps when working with raw meat.

Texture Modified Diets:

Soft & Bite Size: (aka Bite size) **Food particle size ½ inch (~width of standard fork)** Food must be moist. Cut foods with a knife to a ½" particle size after cooking. Moisten with sauce as needed after cutting.

Chopped: Food particle size ¼ inch (~ ½ width of standard fork) Food must be moist. Chop foods with a knife to 1/4" particle size after cooking. Moisten with sauce as needed after chopping.

Minced and Moist:(aka Minced/Mechanical Soft/Ground) **Food particle size 1/8 inch (fits through prongs of standard fork)** Food must be moist. Use a food processor to grind food particles into 1/8 inch after cooking. Moisten with sauce as needed after processing.

Pureed: Smooth and cohesive. Use a food processor to puree to a smooth consistency. Foods are processed by grinding and then pureeing them. May add milk or sauce to puree. Do not add to much liquid. Puree should still hold its shape. Must not be firm or sticky. Puree foods while still hot. Appearance should be smooth like pudding. Serve ½ c. meat serving

Therapeutic Modified Diets:

Lowfat: No changes needed
Diabetic/No added Sugar/No Conc. Sweets/Calorie Controlled: No changes needed
Bland/Anti Reflux: omit pepper and ginger
Liberal House Renal: Omit salt
No Added Salt: No changes needed
2 Gram Sodium: omit salt
Gluten Free: No changes needed. Prepare foods separately to prevent cross contamination.

Allergy Alerts: When an "X" is present, this indicates the allergen is present.

Wheat	Milk	Eggs	Fish Shellfish	Soy	Peanuts/Nuts	Other

Key: SF= Salt Free D= Diet or Sugarfree LF = Lowfat FF = Fat Free GF = Gluten Free

Recipe Name: Pork Chop with Creamy Herb Sauce
Recipe Category: Dinner Entrée
Portion Size: 3 oz. boneless, 5 oz. with bone, 2 T. sauce
Ingredients: Yields: 8 servings

Ingredients	Notes:
8 boneless pork chops, ½ inch thick	Trim all visible fat
1 teaspoon salt	
½ teaspoon black pepper	
¼ cup oil	
½ cup finely, chopped carrots	
2 Tablespoons parsley flakes	Or ¼ cup finely chopped fresh parsley
2 T. flour	
1 teaspoon thyme	
1 teaspoon instant beef bouillon granules	
1 cup evaporated nonfat milk	
1 cup water	

Directions:

Steps:	Directions:	Critical Control Point /Quality Assurance
1	Season chops with salt and pepper.	
2	Heat oil in large skillet over medium high heat. Brown chops, 7-8 minutes per side.	Cook until internal temperature reaches 145 °F for 15 seconds
3	Remove chops from pan; reserve and keep chops warm	.
4	In the same large skillet, add oil and stir in flour. Add carrots, parsley, thyme, bouillon, milk and water.	
5	Cook and stir till thickened and bubbly.	
6	Return chops to pan and heat through.	
7	Serve chops with sauce on top. Serve hot.	

Time Temperature Sensitive food. *Food safety Standards: hold food for service at an internal temperature above 140°F. Do not mix old product with new. Cool leftover product quickly (within 4 hours) to below 41°F. Follow proper cooling procedures. Store leftovers in a tightly sealed, labeled and dated container. Use leftover within 72 hours if stored in refrigerator or 30 days if stored in the freezer. Reheat leftover product quickly (within 2 hours) to 165 degrees F for 15 seconds. Reheat left over product only once; discard if not used. Cold holding at 41°F or colder or using time alone (less than four hours). Always wash hands and wash and sanitize counter tops utensils and containers between steps when working with raw meat.*

Texture Modified Diets:
Soft & Bite Size: (aka Bite size) **Food particle size ½ inch (~width of standard fork)** Food must be moist. Cut foods with a knife to a ½" particle size after cooking. Moisten with sauce as needed after cutting.
Chopped: Food particle size ¼ inch (~ ½ width of standard fork) Food must be moist. Chop foods with a knife to 1/4" particle size after cooking. Moisten with sauce as needed after chopping.
Minced and Moist:(aka Minced/Mechanical Soft/Ground) **Food particle size 1/8 inch (fits through prongs of standard fork)** Food must be moist. Use a food processor to grind food particles into 1/8 inch after cooking. Moisten with sauce as needed after processing.
Pureed: Smooth and cohesive. Use a food processor to puree to a smooth consistency. Foods are processed by grinding and then pureeing them. May add milk or sauce to puree. Do not add to much liquid. Puree should still hold its shape. Must not be firm or sticky. Puree foods while still hot. Appearance should be smooth like pudding. Serve ½ c. meat serving

Therapeutic Modified Diets:
Lowfat: No changes needed
Diabetic/No added Sugar/No Conc. Sweets/Calorie Controlled: No changes needed
Bland/Anti Reflux: omit parsley, thyme and pepper
Liberal House Renal: omit salt and beef granules
No Added Salt: No changes needed
2 Gram Sodium: omit salt, and beef granules
Gluten Free: Use gluten free broth or beef granules. Use gluten free flour. Prepare foods separately to prevent cross contamination.

Allergy Alerts: When an "X" is present, this indicates the allergen is present.

Wheat	Milk	Eggs	Fish Shellfish	Soy	Peanuts/Nuts	Other
X	X					

Key: SF= Salt Free D= Diet or Sugarfree LF = Lowfat FF = Fat Free GF = Gluten Free

Recipe Name: Pork Chop with Curry Mango Sauce
Recipe Category: Dinner Entrée
Portion Size: 3 oz. boneless, 5 oz. with bone
Ingredients: **Yields: 8 servings**

Ingredients	Notes:
8 boneless pork chops, ½ inch thick	Trim all visible fat
1 teaspoon salt	
½ teaspoon black pepper	
¼ cup oil	
1 Tablespoon curry	
1 teaspoon onion powder	
6 green onions, sliced	
½ cup raisins	
1 cup low salt chicken broth	
1 Tablespoon cornstarch	
1 cup mango, diced	Use fresh or frozen
¼ cup flaked coconut	

Directions:

Steps:	Directions:	Critical Control Point /Quality Assurance
1	Season chops with curry powder, salt and pepper.	
2	Heat oil in large skillet over medium high heat. Brown chops, 7-8 minutes per side.	Cook until internal temperature reaches 145°F. for 15 seconds.
3	Remove chops from pan; reserve and keep chops warm	
4	In a small bowl combine, cornstarch well with chicken broth. Add raisins, mangos and chicken broth into skillet.	
5	Cook and stir until slightly thickened. Cook until sauce is thick.	
6	Return chops to pan and heat through. Add green onions and stir.	
7	Serve chops with hot sauce on top. Garnish with coconut.	

Time Temperature Sensitive food. *Food safety Standards: hold food for service at an internal temperature above 140° F. Do not mix old product with new. Cool leftover product quickly (within 4 hours) to below 41° F. Follow proper cooling procedures. Store leftovers in a tightly sealed, labeled and dated container. Use leftover within 72 hours if stored in refrigerator or 30 days if stored in the freezer. Reheat leftover product quickly (within 2 hours) to 165 degrees F for 15 seconds. Reheat left over product only once; discard if not used. Cold holding at 41°F or colder or using time alone (less than four hours). Always wash hands and wash and sanitize counter tops utensils and containers between steps when working with raw meat.*

Texture Modified Diets:
Soft & Bite Size: (aka Bite size) **Food particle size ½ inch (~width of standard fork)** Food must be moist. Cut foods with a knife to a ½" particle size after cooking. Moisten with sauce as needed after cutting. Omit coconut.
Chopped: Food particle size ¼ inch (~ ½ width of standard fork) Food must be moist. Chop foods with a knife to 1/4" particle size after cooking. Moisten with sauce as needed after chopping. Omit coconut.
Minced and Moist:(aka Minced/Mechanical Soft/Ground) **Food particle size 1/8 inch (fits through prongs of standard fork)** Food must be moist. Use a food processor to grind food particles into 1/8 inch after cooking. Moisten with sauce as needed after processing. Omit Coconut.
Pureed: Smooth and cohesive. Use a food processor to puree to a smooth consistency. Foods are processed by grinding and then pureeing them. May add milk or sauce to puree. Do not add to much liquid. Puree should still hold its shape. Must not be firm or sticky. Puree foods while still hot. Appearance should be smooth like pudding. Serve ½ c. meat serving topped with sauce. Omit coconut.

Therapeutic Modified Diets:
Lowfat: No changes needed
Diabetic/No added Sugar/No Conc. Sweets/Calorie Controlled: No changes needed
Bland: omit curry, green onions and pepper
Liberal House Renal: Omit salt and raisins. Use SF broth or water
No Added Salt: No changes needed
2 Gram Sodium: Omit salt and use salt free broth or water
Gluten Free: Use gluten free broth   Prepare foods separately to prevent cross contamination.
Allergy Alerts: When an "X" is present, this indicates the allergen is present.

Wheat	Milk	Eggs	Fish Shellfish	Soy	Peanuts/Nuts	Other
X						

Key: SF= Salt Free D= Diet or Sugarfree LF = Lowfat FF = Fat Free GF = Gluten Free

Copyright 2020 Jacqueline Larson M.S., R.D.N. and Associates.   All Rights Reserved

Recipe Name: Pork Chop with Fresh Plum Sauce
Recipe Category: Dinner Entrée
Portion Size: 3 oz. boneless, 5 oz. with bone
Ingredients: **Yields: 8 servings**

Ingredients	Notes:
8 boneless pork chops, ½ inch thick	Trim all visible fat
½ teaspoon salt	
1/4 teaspoon pepper	
1 teaspoon coriander seeds, crushed	
1 Tablespoon oil	
½ teaspoon ground ginger	
2 Tablespoon cider vinegar	
2 Tablespoon brown sugar	
2 lbs. fresh ripe plums	Wash, cut in halve and remove pit. Chop into ½ inch pieces. May use peaches if plums not available
1 sweet onion, diced	Wash, peel and dice

Directions:

Steps:	Directions:	Critical Control Point /Quality Assurance
1	In a medium saucepan, heat oil until hot. Add 1 tsp. oil. Cook coriander and mustard seeds in oil on high until mustard seeds begin to pop, about 1 minute	
2	Remove from heat.	
3	Stir in ginger, vinegar, brown sugar, and set aside.	
4	Place pork chops in baking dish and season with salt and pepper. Bake for 30 minutes.	
5	Remove from oven. Turn over pork chops and spread . Continue baking about 30 minutes or until internal temperature reaches 145 °F with a 3 minute rest.	Cook until internal temperature reaches 145 ° F for 15 seconds.
6	In small pan heat 1 tsp. oil. Add onion and cook until translucent.	
7	Add plums and sauté until slightly browned. Add spices to plums. Serve hot over pork chops.	

Time Temperature Sensitive food. *Food safety Standards: hold food for service at an internal temperature above 140° F. Do not mix old product with new. Cool leftover product quickly (within 4 hours) to below 41° F. Follow proper cooling procedures. Store leftovers in a tightly sealed, labeled and dated container. Use leftover within 72 hours if stored in refrigerator or 30 days if stored in the freezer. Reheat leftover product quickly (within 2 hours) to 165 degrees F for 15 seconds. Reheat left over product only once; discard if not used. Cold holding at 41°F or colder or using time alone (less than four hours). Always wash hands and wash and sanitize counter tops utensils and containers between steps when working with raw meat.*

Texture Modified Diets:
Soft & Bite Size: (aka Bite size) **Food particle size ½ inch (~width of standard fork)** Food must be moist. Cut foods with a knife to a ½" particle size after cooking. Moisten with sauce as needed after cutting. Puree plum sauce.
Chopped: Food particle size ¼ inch (~ ½ width of standard fork) Food must be moist. Chop foods with a knife to 1/4" particle size after cooking. Moisten with sauce as needed after chopping. Puree plum sauce.
Minced and Moist:(aka Minced/Mechanical Soft/Ground) **Food particle size 1/8 inch (fits through prongs of standard fork)** Food must be moist. Use a food processor to grind food particles into 1/8 inch after cooking. Moisten with sauce as needed after processing. Puree plum sauce.
Pureed: Smooth and cohesive. Use a food processor to puree to a smooth consistency. Foods are processed by grinding and then pureeing them. May add milk or sauce to puree. Do not add to much liquid. Puree should still hold its shape. Must not be firm or sticky. Puree foods while still hot. Appearance should be smooth like pudding. Serve ½ c. meat serving topped with sauce. Puree plum sauce.

Therapeutic Modified Diets:
Lowfat: No changes needed
Diabetic/No added Sugar/No Conc. Sweets/Calorie Controlled: No changes needed
Bland/Anti Reflux: omit sauce and pepper
Liberal House Renal: omit salt
No Added Salt: no changes

2 Gram Sodium: omit salt
Gluten Free: No changes needed
**Allergy Alerts: When an "X" is present, this indicates the allergen is present.
Always read all food labels to ensure allergens are not present.**

Wheat	Milk	Eggs	Fish Shellfish	Soy	Peanuts/Nuts	Other

Key: SF= Salt Free D= Diet or Sugarfree LF = Lowfat FF = Fat Free GF = Gluten Free

Recipe Name: Pork Chop with Honey Garlic Glaze
Recipe Category: Dinner Entrée
Portion Size: 3 oz. boneless, 5 oz. with bone
Ingredients: Yields: 8 servings

Ingredients	Notes:
8 boneless pork chops, ½ inch thick	Trim all visible fat
1 teaspoon salt	
½ teaspoon black pepper	
¼ cup oil	
½ cup lemon juice	
½ cup honey	
¼ cup lite soy sauce	
1 teaspoon garlic powder	
1 Tablespoon cornstarch	

Directions:

Steps:	Directions:	Critical Control Point /Quality Assurance
1	In a large nonstick skillet, heat oil over medium high heat. Brown chops and season with salt and pepper.	
2	Cook chops on both sides, turning only for about 8-9 minutes total.	Cook to 145 °F for 15 seconds.
3	In a small bowl, lemon juice, honey, soy sauce, garlic powder and cornstarch. Whisk thoroughly.	
4	Pour sauce over chops and heat.	
5	Serve chops and pour sauce over chops.	

Time Temperature Sensitive food. *Food safety Standards: hold food for service at an internal temperature above 140°F. Do not mix old product with new. Cool leftover product quickly (within 4 hours) to below 41°F. Follow proper cooling procedures. Store leftovers in a tightly sealed, labeled and dated container. Use leftover within 72 hours if stored in refrigerator or 30 days if stored in the freezer. Reheat leftover product quickly (within 2 hours) to 165 degrees F for 15 seconds. Reheat left over product only once; discard if not used. Cold holding at 41°F or colder or using time alone (less than four hours). Always wash hands and wash and sanitize counter tops utensils and containers between steps when working with raw meat.*

Texture Modified Diets:

Soft & Bite Size: (aka Bite size) **Food particle size ½ inch (~width of standard fork)** Food must be moist. Cut foods with a knife to a ½" particle size after cooking. Moisten with sauce as needed after cutting.
Chopped: Food particle size ¼ inch (~ ½ width of standard fork) Food must be moist. Chop foods with a knife to 1/4" particle size after cooking. Moisten with sauce as needed after chopping.
Minced and Moist: (aka Minced/Mechanical Soft/Ground) **Food particle size 1/8 inch (fits through prongs of standard fork)** Food must be moist. Use a food processor to grind food particles into 1/8 inch after cooking. Moisten with sauce as needed after processing.
Pureed: Smooth and cohesive. Use a food processor to puree to a smooth consistency. Foods are processed by grinding and then pureeing them. May add milk or sauce to puree. Do not add to much liquid. Puree should still hold its shape. Must not be firm or sticky. Puree foods while still hot. Appearance should be smooth like pudding. Serve ½ c. meat serving topped with sauce.

Therapeutic Modified Diets:

Lowfat: No changes needed
Diabetic/No added Sugar/No Conc. Sweets/Calorie Controlled: No changes needed
Bland/Anti Reflux: omit pepper and garlic
Liberal House Renal: Omit salt and soy sauce
No Added Salt: Omit soy sauce
2 Gram Sodium: Omit salt and soy sauce
Gluten Free: Use gluten free soy sauce. Prepare foods separately to prevent cross contamination.

Allergy Alerts: When an "X" is present, this indicates the allergen is present. Always read all food labels to ensure allergens are not present.

Wheat	Milk	Eggs	Fish Shellfish	Soy	Peanuts/Nuts	Other
X				X		

Key: SF= Salt Free D= Diet or Sugarfree LF = Lowfat FF = Fat Free GF = Gluten Free

Recipe Name: Pork Chop with Honey Orange Glaze
Recipe Category: Dinner Entrée
Portion Size: 3 oz. boneless, 5 oz. with bone
Ingredients: Yields: 8 servings

Ingredients	Notes:
8 boneless pork chops, ½ inch thick	Trim all visible fat
1 teaspoon orange zest	Wash and zest
1 cup orange juice	
½ cup pineapple juice	
¼ cup lite soy sauce	
2 Tablespoons honey	
¼ teaspoon pepper	
1/2 teaspoon garlic powder	
2 Tablespoons cornstarch	

Directions:

Steps:	Directions:	Critical Control Point /Quality Assurance
1	In a large nonstick skillet, heat oil over medium high heat. Brown chops and season with salt and pepper.	
2	Cook chops on both sides, turning once. Cook only for about 8-9 minutes total.	Cook to 145°F for 15 seconds.
3	In a small bowl, orange zest, orange juice, pineapple juice, pepper, honey, soy sauce, garlic powder and cornstarch. Whisk thoroughly.	
4	Pour sauce over chops and heat. Serve chops and pour sauce over chops.	Serve hot.

Time Temperature Sensitive food: Food safety Standards: hold food for service at an internal temperature above 140°F. Do not mix old product with new. Cool leftover product quickly (within 4 hours) to below 41°F. Follow proper cooling procedures. Store leftovers in a tightly sealed, labeled and dated container. Use leftover within 72 hours if stored in refrigerator or 30 days if stored in the freezer. Reheat leftover product quickly (within 2 hours) to 165 degrees F for 15 seconds. Reheat left over product only once; discard if not used. Cold holding at 41 °F or colder or using time alone (less than four hours). Always wash hands and wash and sanitize counter tops utensils and containers between steps when working with raw meat.

Texture Modified Diets:

Soft & Bite Size: (aka Bite size) **Food particle size ½ inch (~width of standard fork)** Food must be moist. Cut foods with a knife to a ½" particle size after cooking. Moisten with sauce as needed after cutting.
Chopped: Food particle size ¼ inch (~ ½ width of standard fork) Food must be moist. Chop foods with a knife to 1/4" particle size after cooking. Moisten with sauce as needed after chopping.
Minced and Moist:(aka Minced/Mechanical Soft/Ground) **Food particle size 1/8 inch (fits through prongs of standard fork)** Food must be moist. Use a food processor to grind food particles into 1/8 inch after cooking. Moisten with sauce as needed after processing.
Pureed: Smooth and cohesive. Use a food processor to puree to a smooth consistency. Foods are processed by grinding and then pureeing them. May add milk or sauce to puree. Do not add to much liquid. Puree should still hold its shape. Must not be firm or sticky. Puree foods while still hot. Appearance should be smooth like pudding. Serve ½ c. meat serving topped with sauce.

Therapeutic Modified Diets:

Lowfat: No changes needed
Diabetic/No added Sugar/No Conc. Sweets/Calorie Controlled: No changes needed
Bland/Anti Reflux: Serve plain pork chop
Liberal House Renal: Serve SF pork chope
No Added Salt: omit soy sauce
2 Gram Sodium: omit soy sauce
Gluten Free: Use gluten free soy sauce. Prepare foods separately to prevent cross contamination.
Allergy Alerts: When an "X" is present, this indicates the allergen is present.
Always read all food labels to ensure allergens are not present.

Wheat	Milk	Eggs	Fish Shellfish	Soy	Peanuts/Nuts	Other
X				X		

Key: SF= Salt Free D= Diet or Sugarfree LF = Lowfat FF = Fat Free GF = Gluten Free

Copyright 2020 Jacqueline Larson M.S., R.D.N. and Associates.   All Rights Reserved

Recipe Name: Pork Chop with Lemon Sauce
Recipe Category: Dinner Entrée
Portion Size: 3 oz. boneless, 5 oz. with bone
Ingredients: Yields: 8 servings

Ingredients	Notes:
8 boneless pork chops, ½ inch thick	Trim all visible fat
¼ cup lemon juice	
¼ cup catsup	
½ cup brown sugar	
1 teaspoon onion powder	
1 teaspoon garlic powder	

Directions:

Steps:	Directions:	Critical Control Point /Quality Assurance
1	Pre oven to 350°F	
2	Spray baking dish with nonstick cooking spray.	
3	In a small bowl, lemon juice, catsup and brown sugar, garlic powder and onion powder.	
4	Place pork chops in baking dish and spread with ½ sauce. Bake for 30 minutes.	
5	Remove from oven. Turn over pork chops and spread on remaining sauce. Continue baking about 30 minutes or until internal temperature reaches 145° F for 15 seconds.	Cook until internal temperature reaches 145 °F for 15 seconds. Discard unused mixture

Time Temperature Sensitive food. *Food safety Standards: hold food for service at an internal temperature above 140° F. Do not mix old product with new. Cool leftover product quickly (within 4 hours) to below 41° F. Follow proper cooling procedures. Store leftovers in a tightly sealed, labeled and dated container. Use leftover within 72 hours if stored in refrigerator or 30 days if stored in the freezer. Reheat leftover product quickly (within 2 hours) to 165 degrees F for 15 seconds. Reheat left over product only once; discard if not used. Cold holding at 41°F or colder or using time alone (less than four hours). Always wash hands and wash and sanitize counter tops utensils and containers between steps when working with raw meat.*

Texture Modified Diets:

Soft & Bite Size: (aka Bite size) **Food particle size ½ inch (~width of standard fork)** Food must be moist. Cut foods with a knife to a ½" particle size after cooking. Moisten with sauce as needed after cutting.
Chopped: Food particle size ¼ inch (~ ½ width of standard fork) Food must be moist. Chop foods with a knife to 1/4" particle size after cooking. Moisten with sauce as needed after chopping.
Minced and Moist: (aka Minced/Mechanical Soft/Ground) **Food particle size 1/8 inch (fits through prongs of standard fork)** Food must be moist. Use a food processor to grind food particles into 1/8 inch after cooking. Moisten with sauce as needed after processing.
Pureed: Smooth and cohesive. Use a food processor to puree to a smooth consistency. Foods are processed by grinding and then pureeing them. May add milk or sauce to puree. Do not add to much liquid. Puree should still hold its shape. Must not be firm or sticky. Puree foods while still hot. Appearance should be smooth like pudding. Serve ½ c. meat serving topped with sauce.

Therapeutic Modified Diets:

Lowfat: No changes needed
Diabetic/No added Sugar/No Conc. Sweets/Calorie Controlled: No changes needed
Bland/Anti Reflux: Serve plain pork chop.
Liberal House Renal: Omit lemon juice and catsup.
No Added Salt: no changes
2 Gram Sodium: omit catsup
Gluten Free: no changes needed.
Allergy Alerts: When an "X" is present, this indicates the allergen is present.
Always read all food labels to ensure allergens are not present.

Wheat	Milk	Eggs	FishShellfish	Soy	Peanuts/Nuts	Other

Key: SF= Salt Free D= Diet or Sugarfree LF = Lowfat FF = Fat Free GF = Gluten Free

Recipe Name: Pork Chop with Mexicali Sauce
Recipe Category: Dinner Entrée
Portion Size: 3 oz. boneless, 5 oz. with bone, 1 cup mixture (2 starches)
Ingredients: **Yields: 8 servings**

Ingredients	Notes:
8 boneless pork chops, ½ inch thick	Trim all visible fat
2 T. oil	
3 (14 oz.) cans stewed tomatoes, diced	
1 (16oz.) bag frozen whole kernel corn	
1 (16 oz.) can (no added Salt) kidney beans	Drained and rinsed
1 cup long grain rice	
2 (8 ounce) diced green chili peppers drained	Or 2 teaspoon chili powder
½ teaspoon salt	

Directions:

Steps:	Directions:	Critical Control Point /Quality Assurance
1	In a large skillet brown chops in oil about 5 minutes on each side. Remove from skillet. Drain fat. Keep warm.	Cook until internal temperature reaches 145 °F for 15 seconds.
2	In same skillet, combine tomatoes, corn, kidney beans, rice, chili peppers or chili powder, and salt.	
3	Bring to boil. Simmer for 30-40 minutes until rice is tender. Serve hot over chop.	

Time Temperature Sensitive food. *Food safety Standards: hold food for service at an internal temperature above 140° F. Do not mix old product with new. Cool leftover product quickly (within 4 hours) to below 41° F. Follow proper cooling procedures. Store leftovers in a tightly sealed, labeled and dated container. Use leftover within 72 hours if stored in refrigerator or 30 days if stored in the freezer. Reheat leftover product quickly (within 2 hours) to 165 degrees F for 15 seconds. Reheat left over product only once; discard if not used. Cold holding at 41°F or colder or using time alone (less than four hours). Always wash hands and wash and sanitize counter tops utensils and containers between steps when working with raw meat.*

Texture Modified Diets: Prepare and serve pork chop and rice mixture separately.
Soft & Bite Size: (aka Bite size) **Food particle size ½ inch (~width of standard fork)** Food must be moist. Cut pork chops with a knife to a ½" particle size after cooking. Moisten with sauce as needed after cutting. For rice mixture, food particles must be cut ½ inch or smaller before cooking.
Chopped: Food particle size ¼ inch (~ ½ width of standard fork) Food must be moist. Chop pork chops with a knife to 1/4" particle size after cooking. Moisten with sauce as needed after chopping. For rice mixture, food particles must be ¼ inch or small before cooking.
Minced and Moist:(aka Minced/Mechanical Soft/Ground) **Food particle size 1/8 inch (fits through prongs of standard fork)** Food must be moist. Use a food processor to grind pork chops particles into 1/8 inch after cooking. Moisten with sauce as needed after processing.
Pureed: Smooth and cohesive. Use a food processor to puree to a smooth consistency. Foods are processed by grinding and then pureeing them. May add milk or sauce to puree. Do not add to much liquid. Puree should still hold its shape. Must not be firm or sticky. Puree foods while still hot. Appearance should be smooth like pudding. Serve ½ c. meat serving and ½ c. puree rice mixture separately.
Therapeutic Modified Diets:
Lowfat: No changes needed
Diabetic/No added Sugar/No Conc. Sweets/Calorie Controlled: No changes needed
Bland/Anti Reflux: Serve plain pork chop and ½ cup rice
Liberal House Renal: Serve SF pork chop and ½ cup rice seasoned with SF herbs/spices
No Added Salt: no changes
2 Gram Sodium: Serve SF pork chop and ½ cup rice seasoned with SF herbs/spices
Gluten Free: No changes needed
Allergy Alerts: When an "X" is present, this indicates the allergen is present.
Always read all food labels to ensure allergens are not present.

Wheat	Milk	Eggs	Fish Shellfish	Soy	Peanuts/Nuts	Other

Key: SF= Salt Free D= Diet or Sugarfree LF = Lowfat FF = Fat Free GF = Gluten Free

Recipe Name: Pork Chop with Mexican Marinate
Recipe Category: Dinner Entrée
Portion Size: 3 oz. boneless, 5 oz. with bone
Ingredients: **Yields: 8 servings**

Ingredients	Notes:
8 boneless pork chops, ½ inch thick	Trim all visible fat
1 teaspoon salt	
½ teaspoon black pepper	
¼ cup oil	
8 ounces canned green chilies, chopped	
1 tablespoon dried oregano	
2 teaspoons garlic powder	Or use 4 cloves, minced
1 Tablespoon cumin	
Dash of cayenne pepper	
1 cup cider vinegar	
1 tablespoon cornstarch	

Directions:

Steps:	Directions:	Critical Control Point /Quality Assurance
1	In a blender combine, chilies, oregano, cumin, cayenne pepper and puree until smooth	
2	Marinate chops in ½ **of mixture** in refrigerator for 30 minutes-2 hours.	**Discard marinate.**
3	Brown chops and season with salt and pepper.	.
4	Cook chops on both sides, turning only for about 8-9 minutes total. Add cornstarch to remaining marinate. Top with remaining marinade and heat until sauce is thick.	Cook to 145 ° F for 15 seconds

Time Temperature Sensitive food: *Food safety Standards: hold food for service at an internal temperature above 140° F. Do not mix old product with new. Cool leftover product quickly (within 4 hours) to below 41° F. Follow proper cooling procedures. Store leftovers in a tightly sealed, labeled and dated container. Use leftover within 72 hours if stored in refrigerator or 30 days if stored in the freezer. Reheat leftover product quickly (within 2 hours) to 165 degrees F for 15 seconds. Reheat left over product only once; discard if not used. Cold holding at 41°F or colder or using time alone (less than four hours). Always wash hands and wash and sanitize counter tops utensils and containers between steps when working with raw meat.*

Texture Modified Diets:

Soft & Bite Size: (aka Bite size) **Food particle size ½ inch (~width of standard fork)** Food must be moist. Cut foods with a knife to a ½" particle size after cooking. Moisten with sauce as needed after cutting.
Chopped: Food particle size ¼ inch (~ ½ width of standard fork) Food must be moist. Chop foods with a knife to 1/4" particle size after cooking. Moisten with sauce as needed after chopping.
Minced and Moist:(aka Minced/Mechanical Soft/Ground) **Food particle size 1/8 inch (fits through prongs of standard fork)** Food must be moist. Use a food processor to grind food particles into 1/8 inch after cooking. Moisten with sauce as needed after processing.
Pureed: Smooth and cohesive. Use a food processor to puree to a smooth consistency. Foods are processed by grinding and then pureeing them. May add milk or sauce to puree. Do not add to much liquid. Puree should still hold its shape. Must not be firm or sticky. Puree foods while still hot. Appearance should be smooth like pudding. Serve ½ c. meat serving topped with sauce.

Therapeutic Modified Diets:

Lowfat: No changes needed
Diabetic/No added Sugar/No Conc. Sweets/Calorie Controlled: No changes needed
Bland/Anti Reflux: Serve plain pork chop
Liberal House Renal: Omit salt
No Added Salt: No changes needed
2 Gram Sodium: Omit salt
Gluten Free: No changes needed. Prepare foods separately to prevent cross contamination.

Allergy Alerts: When an "X" is present, this indicates the allergen is present. Always read all food labels to ensure allergens are not present.

Wheat	Milk	Eggs	Fish Shellfish	Soy	Peanuts/Nuts	Other

Key: SF= Salt Free D= Diet or Sugarfree LF = Lowfat FF = Fat Free GF = Gluten Free

Recipe Name: Pork Chop with Mushrooms
Recipe Category: Dinner Entrée
Portion Size: 3 oz. boneless, 5 oz. with bone
Ingredients: Yields: 8 servings

Ingredients	Notes:
8 boneless pork chops, ½ inch thick	Trim all visible fat
1 teaspoon salt	
½ teaspoon black pepper	
1 tablespoon plus 3 Tablespoons olive oil	
¼ cup flour	
12 oz. sliced mushrooms	Washed, trimmed and sliced
1 teaspoon thyme	
2 cups low salt chicken broth	

Directions:

Steps:	Directions:	Critical Control Point / Quality Assurance
1	Season chops with salt and pepper.	
2	Heat 1 T. oil in large skillet over medium high heat. Brown chops, 7-8 minutes per side.	Cook until internal temperature reaches 145° F for 15 seconds.
3	Remove chops from pan and add flour and 3T. oil. Stir and cook for 1 minute	
4	Whisk in chicken broth and bring to boil.	
5	Add chops, mushrooms and thyme and simmer 12-15 minutes. Puree mushroom sauce.	
6	Serve chops and pour sauce on top.	Serve hot.

Time Temperature Sensitive food. Food safety Standards: hold food for service at an internal temperature above 140°F. Do not mix old product with new. Cool leftover product quickly (within 4 hours) to below 41°F. Follow proper cooling procedures. Store leftovers in a tightly sealed, labeled and dated container. Use leftover within 72 hours if stored in refrigerator or 30 days if stored in the freezer. Reheat leftover product quickly (within 2 hours) to 165 degrees F for 15 seconds. Reheat left over product only once; discard if not used. Cold holding at 41°F or colder or using time alone (less than four hours). Always wash hands and wash and sanitize counter tops utensils and containers between steps when working with raw meat.

Texture Modified Diets:
Soft & Bite Size: (aka Bite size) **Food particle size ½ inch (~width of standard fork)** Food must be moist. Cut foods with a knife to a ½" particle size after cooking. Moisten with sauce as needed after cutting. Use puree sauce.
Chopped: Food particle size ¼ inch (~ ½ width of standard fork) Food must be moist. Chop foods with a knife to 1/4" particle size after cooking. Moisten with sauce as needed after chopping. Use puree sauce.
Minced and Moist:(aka Minced/Mechanical Soft/Ground) **Food particle size 1/8 inch (fits through prongs of standard fork)** Food must be moist. Use a food processor to grind food particles into 1/8 inch after cooking. Moisten with sauce as needed after processing.
Pureed: Smooth and cohesive. Use a food processor to puree to a smooth consistency. Foods are processed by grinding and then pureeing them. May add milk or sauce to puree. Do not add to much liquid. Puree should still hold its shape. Must not be firm or sticky. Puree foods while still hot. Appearance should be smooth like pudding. Serve ½ c. meat serving topped with sauce.

Therapeutic Modified Diets:
Lowfat: No changes needed
Diabetic/No added Sugar/No Conc. Sweets/Calorie Controlled: No changes needed
Bland/Anti Reflux: omit pepper and thyme
Liberal House Renal: Omit salt and use SF broth or water.
No Added Salt: No changes needed
2 Gram Sodium: Omit salt and use SF broth or water
Gluten Free: Use GF broth and GF all purpose flour. Prepare foods separately to prevent cross contamination.
Allergy Alerts: When an "X" is present, this indicates the allergen is present. Always read all food labels to ensure allergens are not present.

Wheat	Milk	Eggs	Fish Shellfish	Soy	Peanuts/Nuts	Other
X						

Key: SF= Salt Free D= Diet or Sugarfree LF = Lowfat FF = Fat Free GF = Gluten Free

Recipe Name: Pork Chop with Orange Mustard Sauce
Recipe Category: Dinner Entrée
Portion Size: 3 oz. boneless, 5 oz. with bone
Ingredients: Yields: 8 servings

Ingredients	Notes:
8 boneless pork chops, ½ inch thick	Trim all visible fat
1 teaspoon salt	
½ teaspoon black pepper	
¼ cup oil	
1 teaspoon ground ginger	
1 cup orange juice	Optional: add zest of 1 orange in addition to orange juice
¼ cup honey	
1 Tablespoon Dijon mustard	
2 teaspoons garlic powder	Or use 4 cloves, minced
½ cup lite soy sauce	
1 Tablespoon cornstarch	

Directions:

Steps:	Directions:	Critical Control Point /Quality Assurance
1	Season chops with salt and pepper	
2	Heat oil in large skillet over medium high heat. Brown chops, 3-4 minutes per side.	
3	In a small bowl stir together, ginger, orange juice, soy sauce, honey, mustard, garlic, and cornstarch. Pour sauce over chops and simmer cover for 8 minutes or until thick.	Cook to 145° F for 15 seconds.
4	Serve chops and pour sauce over chops.	

Time Temperature Sensitive food. *Food safety Standards: hold food for service at an internal temperature above 140° F. Do not mix old product with new. Cool leftover product quickly (within 4 hours) to below 41° F. Follow proper cooling procedures. Store leftovers in a tightly sealed, labeled and dated container. Use leftover within 72 hours if stored in refrigerator or 30 days if stored in the freezer. Reheat leftover product quickly (within 2 hours) to 165 degrees F for 15 seconds. Reheat left over product only once; discard if not used. Cold holding at 41°F or colder or using time alone (less than four hours). Always wash hands and wash and sanitize counter tops utensils and containers between steps when working with raw meat.*

Texture Modified Diets:
Soft & Bite Size: (aka Bite size) **Food particle size ½ inch (~width of standard fork)** Food must be moist. Cut foods with a knife to a ½" particle size after cooking. Moisten with sauce as needed after cutting.
Chopped: Food particle size ¼ inch (~ ½ width of standard fork) Food must be moist. Chop foods with a knife to 1/4" particle size after cooking. Moisten with sauce as needed after chopping.
Minced and Moist:(aka Minced/Mechanical Soft/Ground) **Food particle size 1/8 inch (fits through prongs of standard fork)** Food must be moist. Use a food processor to grind food particles into 1/8 inch after cooking. Moisten with sauce as needed after processing.
Pureed: Smooth and cohesive. Use a food processor to puree to a smooth consistency. Foods are processed by grinding and then pureeing them. May add milk or sauce to puree. Do not add to much liquid. Puree should still hold its shape. Must not be firm or sticky. Puree foods while still hot. Appearance should be smooth like pudding. Serve ½ c. meat serving topped with sauce.

Therapeutic Modified Diets:
Lowfat: No changes needed
Diabetic/No added Sugar/No Conc. Sweets/Calorie Controlled: No changes needed
Bland/Anti Reflux: omit pepper, mustard and garlic
Liberal House Renal: Omit salt, soy sauce and orange juice.
No Added Salt: Omit soy sauce.
2 Gram Sodium: Omit salt and soy sauce.
Gluten Free: Use gluten free soy sauce. Prepare foods separately to prevent cross contamination.

Allergy Alerts: When an "X" is present, this indicates the allergen is present. Always read all food labels to ensure allergens are not present.

Wheat	Milk	Eggs	Fish Shellfish	Soy	Peanuts/Nuts	Other
X				X		

Key: SF= Salt Free D= Diet or Sugarfree LF = Lowfat FF = Fat Free GF = Gluten Free

Recipe Name: Pork Chop with Quinoa Salad
Recipe Category: Dinner Entrée
Portion Size: 3 oz. boneless pork plus 1 cup lettuce and 1 cup quinoa mixture.
Ingredients: Yields: 8 servings

Ingredients	Notes:
8 boneless pork chops, ½ inch thick	Trim all visible fat.
1 teaspoon salt	
½ teaspoon black pepper	
¼ cup oil	
2 cups quinoa	May substitute cooked barley for quinoa (except for gluten free)
6 cups water	
¼ cup olive oil	
1 teaspoon paprika	
1 teaspoon garlic powder	Or 2 cloves minced
8 cups romaine lettuce	Wash, trim and chop
½ cup feta cheese (optional)	
2 limes, zested and juiced	
½ cup cider vinegar	
1 Tablespoon honey	
1 cup fresh tomatoes	Washed, trimmed and finely chopped
1 cucumber	Washed, trimmed and finely chopped

Directions:

Steps:	Directions:	Critical Control Point / Quality Assurance
1	Season chops with salt and pepper.	
2	Heat oil in large skillet over medium high heat. Brown chops, 7-8 minutes per side. Set aside and keep warm.	Cook until internal temperature reaches 145°F for 15 seconds
3	Combine the quinoa and water in a pot and bring to a boil. Once boiling, reduce to medium heat and let the quinoa cook until all the water is evaporated. (about 15 minutes)	
4	In a large bowl combine the quinoa, feta, red onion, lime juice and zest, cider vinegar, honey, tomatoes, cucumbers and toss to combine. Chill until ready to serve.	
5	Arrange 1 cup lettuce on each plate.	
6	Top lettuce with 1 cup quinoa mixture, and arrange thinly sliced warm pork on top of quinoa.	

Time Temperature Sensitive food. *Food safety Standards: hold food for service at an internal temperature above 140°F. Do not mix old product with new. Cool leftover product quickly (within 4 hours) to below 41°F. Follow proper cooling procedures. Store leftovers in a tightly sealed, labeled and dated container. Use leftover within 72 hours if stored in refrigerator or 30 days if stored in the freezer. Cold holding at 41°F or colder or using time alone (less than four hours). Always wash hands and wash and sanitize counter tops utensils and containers between steps when working with raw meat.*

Texture Modified Diets:

Soft & Bite Size: (aka Bite size) **Food particle size ½ inch (~width of standard fork)** Food must be moist. Cut foods with a knife to a ½" particle size prior to mixing. Moisten with dressing as needed. Foods that do not process well should be omitted. Omit: cucumber peel and seeds. Finely chop lettuce.

Chopped: Food particle size ¼ inch (~ ½ width of standard fork) Food must be moist. Chop foods with a knife to 1/4" particle size prior to mixing. Moisten with dressing as needed. Foods that do not process well should be omitted. Omit: cucumber peel and seeds. Finely chop lettuce.

Minced and Moist: (aka Minced/Mechanical Soft/Ground) **Food particle size 1/8 inch (fits through prongs of standard fork)** Food must be moist. Use a food processor to grind food particles into 1/8 inch prior to mixing. Moisten with dressing as needed. Foods that do not process well should be omitted. Omit: cucumber peel and seeds.

Pureed: Smooth and cohesive. Use a food processor to puree to a smooth consistency. Foods are processed by grinding and then pureeing them. May add broth or sauce to puree. Do not add to much liquid. Puree should still hold its shape. Must not be firm or sticky. Puree foods while still hot. Appearance should be smooth like pudding. Foods that do not process well should be omitted. Omit: cucumber peel and seeds. Serve ½ cup puree pork and ½ c. puree quinoa separately. Top with dressing.

<u>*Therapeutic Modified Diets:*</u>
Lowfat: No changes needed
Diabetic/No added Sugar/No Conc. Sweets/Calorie Controlled: No changes needed
Bland/Anti Reflux: omit pepper, paprika, garlic, tomato, cucumber and onion
Liberal House Renal: omit salt
No Added Salt: No changes needed
2 Gram Sodium: omit salt
Gluten Free: No changes needed. No barley. Prepare foods separately to prevent cross contamination.
Allergy Alerts: When an "X" is present, this indicates the allergen is present.
Always read all food labels to ensure allergens are not present.

Wheat	Milk	Eggs	Fish Shellfish	Soy	Peanuts/Nuts	Other
X if using barley						

Key: SF= Salt Free D= Diet or Sugarfree LF = Lowfat FF = Fat Free GF = Gluten Free

Recipe Name: Pork Chop with Ratatouille
Recipe Category: Dinner Entrée
Portion Size: 3 oz. boneless, ½ cup Ratatouille
Ingredients: Yields: 8 servings

Ingredients	Notes:
8 boneless pork chops, ½ inch thick	Trim all visible fat
1 teaspoon salt	
½ teaspoon black pepper	
¼ cup oil	
1 medium eggplant,	Washed, peeled and cubed
8 roma tomatoes	Washed, trimmed and chopped
1 large onion	Washed, peeled and chopped
1 bell pepper	Washed, trimmed and chopped
2 T. olive oil	
2 teaspoons basil	
1 teaspoon garlic powder	Or 2 cloves minced
1 teaspoon salt	
½ teaspoon black pepper.	

Directions:

Steps:	Directions:	Critical Control Point / Quality Assurance
1	Season chops with salt and pepper.	
2	Heat oil in large skillet over medium high heat. Brown chops, 7-8 minutes per side. Keep warm.	Cook until internal temperature reaches 145 ° F for 15 seconds.
3	In a large bowl combine, eggplant, tomatoes, onion, bell peppers, 2 T. olive oil, basil, garlic, 1 t. salt and ½ t. black pepper. Toss to coat.	
4	Pre oven to 350 °F.	
5	In large baking dish, add vegetable mixture and bake uncovered for 40 minutes, stirring occasionally. Remove from oven.	
6	Arrange chops on top of vegetable mixture and uncovered for 20 minutes until internal temperature reads 160°F.	
7	Serve chop with vegetable ratatouille.	Serve hot.

Time Temperature Sensitive food. *Food safety Standards: hold food for service at an internal temperature above 140° F. Do not mix old product with new. Cool leftover product quickly (within 4 hours) to below 41° F. Follow proper cooling procedures. Store leftovers in a tightly sealed, labeled and dated container. Use leftover within 72 hours if stored in refrigerator or 30 days if stored in the freezer. Reheat leftover product quickly (within 2 hours) to 165 degrees F for 15 seconds. Reheat left over product only once; discard if not used. Cold holding at 41 °F or colder or using time alone (less than four hours). Always wash hands and wash and sanitize counter tops utensils and containers between steps when working with raw meat.*

<u>**Texture Modified Diets: Serve pork chop and ratatouille separately.**</u>
Soft & Bite Size: (aka Bite size) **Food particle size ½ inch (~width of standard fork)** Food must be moist. Cut foods with a knife to a ½" particle size prior to mixing. Moisten with broth as needed.
Chopped: Food particle size ¼ inch (~ ½ width of standard fork) Food must be moist. Chop foods with a knife to 1/4" particle size prior to mixing. Moisten with broth as needed.
Minced and Moist: (aka Minced/Mechanical Soft/Ground) **Food particle size 1/8 inch (fits through prongs of standard fork)** Food must be moist. Use a food processor to grind food particles into 1/8 inch prior to mixing. Moisten with broth as needed.
Pureed: Smooth and cohesive. Use a food processor to puree to a smooth consistency. Foods are processed by grinding and then pureeing them. May add broth or sauce to puree. Do not add to much liquid. Puree should still hold its shape. Must not be firm or sticky. Puree foods while still hot. Appearance should be smooth like pudding. Serve ½ c. meat serving. Serve with ½ c. ratatouille puree on side.

Copyright 2020 Jacqueline Larson M.S., R.D.N. and Associates.   All Rights Reserved

Therapeutic Modified Diets:
Lowfat: No changes needed
Diabetic/No added Sugar/No Conc. Sweets/Calorie Controlled: No changes needed
Bland/Anti Reflux: Serve plain pork chop and ½ cup green beans or peas
Liberal House Renal: omit tomatoes and salt
No Added Salt: No changes needed
2 Gram Sodium: omit salt
Gluten Free: No changes needed. Prepare foods separately to prevent cross contamination.
Allergy Alerts: When an "X" is present, this indicates the allergen is present.
Always read all food labels to ensure allergens are not present.

Wheat	Milk	Eggs	Fish Shellfish	Soy	Peanuts/Nuts	Other

Key: SF= Salt Free D= Diet or Sugarfree LF = Lowfat FF = Fat Free GF = Gluten Free

Recipe Name: Pork Chow Mein
Recipe Category: Dinner Entrée
Portion Size: 1 cup; Pork/ vegetables over ½ c. noodles
Ingredients: Yields: 8 servings

Ingredients	Notes:
2 ½ lbs. boneless pork shoulder, pork blade, or arm steak, cut into ½ inch size pieces	Trim all visible fat. Cut across the grain into ½ inch size pieces
2 tablespoons oil	
4 cups low sodium beef broth	
¼ cup lite soy sauce	
4 Medium stalks, celery	Wash, trim and thinly slice
1 Medium onion	Wash, trim and chop
6 tablespoons cornstarch	
1 lb. frozen Chinese vegetables	
6 oz. jar sliced mushrooms	Or 1 package, sliced fresh mushrooms
4 cups Chow Mein Noodles or spaghetti	Prepare according to directions on package

Directions:

Steps:	Directions:	Critical Control Point /Quality Assurance
1	In large skillet, heat oil over medium high heat. Add pork and sauté until brown.	
2	Stir in broth, soy sauce, celery, mushrooms and onion. Heat to boiling. Reduce heat	
3	Cover and simmer 30 minutes.	
4	Mix cornstarch with 1 cup cold water.	
5	Slowly stir into mixture. Return heat to medium high and heat to boiling stirring constantly. Boil and Stir 1 minute.	
6	Add Vegetables and heat to boiling.	Minimum Pork Cook until internal temperature reaches 145° for 15 seconds.
7	Toss with noodles. Serve hot.	

Time Temperature Sensitive food. *Food safety Standards: hold food for service at an internal temperature above 140° F. Do not mix old product with new. Cool leftover product quickly (within 4 hours) to below 41° F. Follow proper cooling procedures. Store leftovers in a tightly sealed, labeled and dated container. Use leftover within 72 hours if stored in refrigerator or 30 days if stored in the freezer. Reheat leftover product quickly (within 2 hours) to 165 degrees F for 15 seconds. Reheat left over product only once; discard if not used. Cold holding at 41°F or colder or using time alone (less than four hours). Always wash hands and wash and sanitize counter tops utensils and containers between steps when working with raw meat.*

Texture Modified Diets: **TIP: Use pasta that is the correct particle size.**
Soft & Bite Size: (aka Bite size) **Food particle size ½ inch (~width of standard fork)** Food must be moist. Cut foods with a knife to a ½" particle size prior to mixing. Moisten with broth as needed.
Chopped: Food particle size ¼ inch (~ ½ width of standard fork) Food must be moist. Chop foods with a knife to 1/4" particle size prior to mixing. Moisten with broth as needed.
Minced and Moist: (aka Minced/Mechanical Soft/Ground) **Food particle size 1/8 inch (fits through prongs of standard fork)** Food must be moist. Use a food processor to grind food particles into 1/8 inch prior to mixing. Moisten with broth as needed.
Pureed: Smooth and cohesive. Use a food processor to puree to a smooth consistency. Foods are processed by grinding and then pureeing them. May add broth or sauce to puree. Do not add to much liquid. Puree should still hold its shape. Must not be firm or sticky. Puree foods while still hot. Appearance should be smooth like pudding.
Puree each item individually and serve separately (meat, vegetables and noodles). May add broth to moisten meat.

Therapeutic Modified Diets:
Lowfat: No changes needed
Diabetic/No added Sugar/No Conc. Sweets/Calorie Controlled: No changes needed
Bland/Anti Reflux: omit celery and onion, use green beans and carrots for vegetables
Liberal House Renal: omit soy sauce and use low sodium broth or water
No Added Salt: No changes needed
2 Gram Sodium: omit soy sauce and use low sodium broth or water
Gluten Free: Use gluten free broth, soy sauce, and noodles. Prepare foods separately to prevent cross contamination.

Allergy Alerts: When an "X" is present, this indicates the allergen is present. Always read all food labels to ensure allergens are not present.

Wheat	Milk	Eggs	Fish Shellfish	Soy	Peanuts/Nuts	Other
X		X		X		

Key: SF= Salt Free D= Diet or Sugarfree LF = Lowfat FF = Fat Free GF = Gluten Free

Recipe Name: Pork Fajitas
Recipe Category: Dinner Entrée
Portion Size: 2 fajitas with 1 (1 whole grain tortilla) plus 1 1/2 oz. Meat for a total of 2 tortillas and 3 oz. meat.
Ingredients: Yields: 8 servings

Ingredients	Notes:
2 1/2 Pounds pork tenderloin, cut into thin strips	Trim all visible fat.
16 (6 inch) flour tortillas	May use whole grain
2 teaspoons vegetable oil	
3 Green bell peppers	Wash, trim and slice into strips
1 tablespoon cornstarch	
2 teaspoons chili powder	
1 teaspoon salt	
1 teaspoon sugar	
½ teaspoon onion powder	
½ teaspoon garlic powder	
¼ teaspoon cayenne pepper	
½ teaspoon ground cumin	
2/3 cup water	
1 cup tomato, diced	Wash, trim and dice
1 cup shredded low fat cheddar cheese	
½ cup light sour cream	
avocado	(optional)

Directions:

Steps:	Directions:	Critical Control Point / Quality Assurance
1	Sauté onions and peppers in 1 teaspoon oil in a large pan until tender crisp on medium high heat. Remove from pan.	
2	In the same pan on medium high heat, sauté pork in 1 teaspoon oil until lightly browned.	Minimum Temperature 145°F for 15 seconds
3	In a small bowl combine cornstarch, chili powder, salt, paprika, sugar, onion powder, garlic powder, cayenne pepper, cumin and water.	
4	Combine seasoning mix with cooked pork.	
5	Simmer 10 to 15 minutes.	
6	Heat tortilla according to package directions.	
7	To serve, spoon meat mixture evenly down center of each warm tortilla. Top with green peppers and onions.	
8	Sprinkle with cheese and roll up. Serve with s cheddar cheese, sour cream, and tomato	

Time Temperature Sensitive food. *Food safety Standards: hold food for service at an internal temperature above 140° F. Do not mix old product with new. Cool leftover product quickly (within 4 hours) to below 41° F. Follow proper cooling procedures. Store leftovers in a tightly sealed, labeled and dated container. Use leftover within 72 hours if stored in refrigerator or 30 days if stored in the freezer. Reheat leftover product quickly (within 2 hours) to 165 degrees F for 15 seconds. Reheat left over product only once; discard if not used. Cold holding at 41°F or colder or using time alone (less than four hours). Always wash hands and wash and sanitize counter tops utensils and containers between steps when working with raw meat.*

Texture Modified Diets:
Soft & Bite Size: (aka Bite size) **Food particle size ½ inch (~width of standard fork)** Food must be moist. Cut foods with a knife to a ½" particle size prior to mixing/layering. Moisten with broth as needed.
Chopped: Food particle size ¼ inch (~ ½ width of standard fork) Food must be moist. Chop foods with a knife to 1/4" particle size prior to mixing/layering Moisten with broth as needed.
Minced and Moist: (aka Minced/Mechanical Soft/Ground) **Food particle size 1/8 inch (fits through prongs of standard fork)** Food must be moist. Use a food processor to grind food particles into 1/8 inch prior to mixing/layering. Moisten with broth as needed.

Pureed: Smooth and cohesive. Use a food processor to puree to a smooth consistency. Foods are processed by grinding and then pureeing them. May add broth or sauce to puree. Do not add to much liquid. Puree should still hold its shape. Must not be firm or sticky. Puree foods while still hot. Appearance should be smooth like pudding. Serve 1/2 c. puree meat mixture separately.1 cup puree tortilla separately. May puree tomato and add to sour cream and tomato top of tortilla to moisten. May melt cheese on meat mixture.

Therapeutic Modified Diets:

Lowfat: No changes needed

Diabetic/No added Sugar/No Conc. Sweets/Calorie Controlled: No changes needed

Bland: omit all seasonings except salt

Liberal House Renal: Omit tomato, salt, cheddar cheese, sour cream and bell pepper, Use low sodium tortillas. (see recipe)

No Added Salt: no changes

2 Gram Sodium: Omit salt, cheddar cheese, sour cream. Use low sodium tortillas. (See recipe)

Gluten Free: Use GF corn tortillas. Prepare foods separately to prevent cross contamination.

Allergy Alerts: When an "X" is present, this indicates the allergen is present.

Always read all food labels to ensure allergens are not present.

Wheat	Milk	Eggs	Fish Shellfish	Soy	Peanuts/Nuts	Other
X	X					

Key: SF= Salt Free D= Diet or Sugarfree LF = Lowfat FF = Fat Free GF = Gluten Free

Recipe Name: Pork Lettuce Wraps

Recipe Category: Dinner Entrée
Portion Size: 2 wraps (approx. 1 lettuce leave, ¼ c. meat mixture, ¼ c. carrots, green onion and red bell pepper per wrap)
Ingredients: Yields: 8 servings

Ingredients	Notes:
2 lbs. pork tenderloin	Trim all fat. Dice into very small pieces.
2 tablespoons lite soy sauce	
2 teaspoons garlic powder	
1 teaspoon ground ginger	
1 teaspoon cornstarch	
16 lettuce leaves	Washed and trimmed
1 cup carrots	Washed, peeled and shredded
I cup green onions	Washed, trimmed and thinly sliced
1 cup red bell pepper	Washed, trimmed and thinly sliced
2/3 light soy sauce	
1/3 cup water	
¼ cup lemon juice	
2 teaspoon garlic powder	
1 teaspoon ginger	
3 teaspoon honey	
2 tablespoons cornstarch	
1 large head lettuce	Washed, trimmed and leaves removed.

Directions:

Steps:	Directions:	Critical Control Point / Quality Assurance
1	In a large size pan, heat oil over medium high heat. Add pork and cook until lightly browned.	
2	Add 2 tablespoons soy sauce, 2 teaspoons garlic powder, 1-teaspoon cornstarch and 1 teaspoon ginger, over medium high heat.	
3	Bring to boil. Reduce heat and simmer for 5 minutes.	Cook until internal temperature reaches 145°F. for 15 seconds.
4	In a small sauce pan add 2/3 cup soy sauce, ½ cup water, ¼ lemon juice, garlic powder, ground ginger, honey and cornstarch. Stir to combine.	
5	Heat on medium high to a boil. Reduce heat and simmer for 10 minutes or until desired thickness.	
6	Top lettuce leave with pork, carrots, bell peppers and green onions. Roll up and spoon sauce over.	

Time Temperature Sensitive food. *Food safety Standards: hold food for service at an internal temperature above 140°F. Do not mix old product with new. Cool leftover product quickly (within 4 hours) to below 41°F. Follow proper cooling procedures. Store leftovers in a tightly sealed, labeled and dated container. Use leftover within 72 hours if stored in refrigerator or 30 days if stored in the freezer. Reheat leftover product quickly (within 2 hours) to 165 degrees F for 15 seconds. Reheat left over product only once; discard if not used. Cold holding at 41°F or colder or using time alone (less than four hours).*

Texture Modified Diets:

Soft & Bite Size: (aka Bite size) **Food particle size ½ inch (~width of standard fork)** Food must be moist. Cut foods with a knife to a ½" particle size prior to mixing. Moisten with broth as needed. Foods that do not process well should be omitted. Omit: green onions.

Chopped: Food particle size ¼ inch (~ ½ width of standard fork) Food must be moist. Chop foods with a knife to 1/4" particle size prior to mixing. Moisten with broth as needed. Foods that do not process well should be omitted. Omit: green onions.

Minced and Moist: (aka Minced/Mechanical Soft/Ground) **Food particle size 1/8 inch (fits through prongs of standard fork)** Food must be moist. Use a food processor to grind food particles into 1/8 inch prior to mixing. Moisten with broth as needed. Foods that do not process well should be omitted. Omit: green onions.

Pureed: Smooth and cohesive. Use a food processor to puree to a smooth consistency. Foods are processed by grinding and then pureeing them. May add broth or sauce to puree. Do not add to much liquid. Puree should still hold its shape. Must not be firm or sticky. Puree foods while still hot. Appearance should be smooth like pudding. Foods that do not process well should be omitted. Omit: green onions.
Serve ½ c. puree meat mixture, and ½ c. puree cooked carrots and bell pepper.

Therapeutic Modified Diets:
Lowfat: No changes needed.
Diabetic/No added Sugar/No Conc. Sweets/Calorie Controlled: No changes needed.
Bland/Anti Reflux: Omit onions, red bell pepper, green onion, lemon juice and garlic.
Liberal House Renal: Use alternate menu item
No Added Salt: Use alternate menu item
2 Gram Sodium: Use alternate menu item.
Gluten Free: Use GF soy sauce and imitation ground beef.
**Allergy Alerts: When an "X" is present, this indicates the allergen is present.
Always read all food labels to ensure allergens are not present.**

Wheat	Milk	Eggs	Fish Shellfish	Soy	Peanuts/Nuts	Other
X		X		X		

Key: SF= Salt Free D= Diet or Sugarfree LF = Lowfat FF = Fat Free GF = Gluten Free

Recipe Name: Pork Tenderloin Lo Mein

Recipe Category: Dinner Entrée
Portion Size: 3 oz. boneless meat, ½ cup pasta, ½ cup vegetables (approx. 1 ½ cups)
Ingredients: Yields: 8 servings

Ingredients	Notes:
2 ½ pounds pork tenderloin	Cut into small thin strips
1 lb. spaghetti	May use whole grain
1/2 cup reduced-sodium soy sauce	
1 tablespoon sesame oil	
¼ cup hot water	
1 tablespoon chicken bouillon	
¼ cup brown sugar	
2 teaspoons garlic powder or garlic cloves minced	
2 tablespoon oil	
2 cups carrots	Wash thoroughly, peeled, and sliced thin
2 cups broccoli	Wash thoroughly, cut into bite size pieces
1 large onion	Wash thoroughly before cutting, sliced
2 tablespoons sesame seeds, toasted	

Directions:

Steps:	Directions:	Critical Control Point / Quality Assurance
1	In a small bowl, dissolve bouillon in hot water. Add soy sauce, brown sugar, sesame oil and garlic in the small bowl. Stir.	
2	Prepare pasta according to directions on package. Drain reserving 1 cup water	
3	In a medium high heated skillet, add oil. Add pork and cook until lightly browned	
4	Add sauce mixture, cook all together for about 2 minutes and remove from pan.	Minimum Temperature 145°F for 15 seconds for shrimp
5	In the same pan, sauté onions until golden brown. Remove from heat.	
6	In a separate skillet, stir fry carrot until just tender. Add broccoli and cook until just tender.	
7	In a large pot combine reserved water, pasta, vegetables and pork. Toss to coat.	
8	Top with sesame seeds. Serve hot.	

Time Temperature Sensitive food. *Food safety Standards: hold food for service at an internal temperature above 140°F. Do not mix old product with new. Cool leftover product quickly (within 4 hours) to below 41°F. Follow proper cooling procedures. Store leftovers in a tightly sealed, labeled and dated container. Use leftover within 72 hours if stored in refrigerator or 30 days if stored in the freezer. Reheat leftover product quickly (within 2 hours) to 165 degrees F for 15 seconds. Reheat left over product only once; discard if not used. Cold holding at 41°F or colder or using time alone (less than four hours). Always wash hands and wash and sanitize counter tops utensils and containers between steps when working with raw meat.*

Texture Modified Diets: TIP: Use pasta with correct particle size.
Soft & Bite Size: (aka Bite size) **Food particle size ½ inch (~width of standard fork)** Food must be moist. Cut foods with a knife to a ½" particle size prior to mixing. Moisten with broth as needed.
Chopped: Food particle size ¼ inch (~ ½ **width of standard fork)** Food must be moist. Chop foods with a knife to 1/4" particle size prior to mixing. Moisten with broth as needed.
Minced and Moist:(aka Minced/Mechanical Soft/Ground) **Food particle size 1/8 inch (fits through prongs of standard fork)** Food must be moist. Use a food processor to grind food particles into 1/8 inch prior to mixing. Moisten with broth as needed.
Pureed: Smooth and cohesive. Use a food processor to puree to a smooth consistency. Foods are processed by grinding and then pureeing them. May add broth or sauce to puree. Do not add to much liquid. Puree should still hold its shape. Must not be firm or sticky. Puree foods while still hot. Appearance should be smooth like pudding. Serve ½ c. puree meat serving, ½ cup puree pasta and ½ cup puree vegetables separately. Omit sesame seeds.

Copyright 2020 Jacqueline Larson M.S., R.D.N. and Associates.   All Rights Reserved

Therapeutic Modified Diets:
Lowfat: No changes needed
Diabetic/No added Sugar/No Conc. Sweets/Calorie Controlled: No changes needed
Bland: omit sesame seeds, garlic powder, broccoli and onion
Liberal House Renal: Omit sauce, season with no salt herbs
No Added Salt: Omit sauce
2 Gram Sodium: omit sauce, season with no salt herbs
Gluten Free: Use GF soy sauce. Use gluten free pasta. Prepare foods separately to prevent cross contamination.
Allergy Alerts: When an "X" is present, this indicates the allergen is present.
Always read all food labels to ensure allergens are not present.

Wheat	Milk	Eggs	Fish Shellfish	Soy	Peanuts/Nuts	Other
X		X	x	X		

Key: SF= Salt Free D= Diet or Sugarfree LF = Lowfat FF = Fat Free GF = Gluten Free

Recipe Name: Pork Mediterranean
Recipe Category: Dinner Entrée
Portion Size: ½ c. pork mixture, ½ c. noodles
Ingredients: **Yields: 8 servings**

Ingredients	Notes:
2 ½ lbs. boneless pork	Trim all visible fat. Cut across the grain into ½ inch size pieces
1 tablespoon oil	
2 large onions	Wash, slice and separate into rings
½ teaspoon garlic powder	Or use 1 glove, minced
2 (16 oz.) can tomatoes, cut up	
2 teaspoons instant chicken bouillon granules	
2 teaspoons dried thyme, crushed	
6 oz. can mushrooms, drained	Or 1 (6 oz.) package, fresh sliced mushrooms
½ cup pitted, sliced olive	(optional)
2 tablespoons, dried parsley flakes	Or ¼ cup chopped fresh parsley
2 tablespoons flour	
½ cup water	
4 cups. Hot cooked noodles	May use high fiber noodles. Prepare according to directions on package.

Directions:

Steps:	Directions:	Critical Control Point / Quality Assurance
1	In a large skillet brown half of the pork in hot oil over medium high heat. Remove from heat.	
2	Brown remaining pork with onion rings and garlic. Return all pork to skillet	
3	Stir in un-drained tomatoes, bouillon granules, thyme, mushrooms, olives and parsley. Cover. Bring to boil; reduce heat. Simmer 45 minutes or until meat is tender.	Minimum Cooking until internal temperature reaches 145 degrees for 15 seconds.
4	In small bowl, combine water and flour. Stir into mixture. Cook and stir until thick and bubbly. Serve hot over noodles.	

Time Temperature Sensitive food. *Food safety Standards: hold food for service at an internal temperature above 140°F. Do not mix old product with new. Cool leftover product quickly (within 4 hours) to below 41°F. Follow proper cooling procedures. Store leftovers in a tightly sealed, labeled and dated container. Use leftover within 72 hours if stored in refrigerator or 30 days if stored in the freezer. Reheat leftover product quickly (within 2 hours) to 165 degrees F for 15 seconds. Reheat left over product only once; discard if not used. Cold holding at 41°F or colder or using time alone (less than four hours). Always wash hands and wash and sanitize counter tops utensils and containers between steps when working with raw meat.*

Texture Modified Diets: TIP: use pasta that is the correct particle size.
Soft & Bite Size: (aka Bite size) **Food particle size ½ inch (~width of standard fork)** Food must be moist. Cut foods with a knife to a ½" particle size prior to mixing. Moisten with broth as needed.
Chopped: Food particle size ¼ inch (~ ½ width of standard fork) Food must be moist. Chop foods with a knife to 1/4" particle size prior to mixing. Moisten with broth as needed.
Minced and Moist: (aka Minced/Mechanical Soft/Ground) **Food particle size 1/8 inch (fits through prongs of standard fork)** Food must be moist. Use a food processor to grind food particles into 1/8 inch prior to mixing. Moisten with broth as needed.
Pureed: Smooth and cohesive. Use a food processor to puree to a smooth consistency. Foods are processed by grinding and then pureeing them. May add broth or sauce to puree. Do not add to much liquid. Puree should still hold its shape. Must not be firm or sticky. Puree foods while still hot. Appearance should be smooth like pudding. Puree meat mixture and noodles individually and serve separately. May add broth to moisten meat.

Therapeutic Modified Diets:
Lowfat: No changes needed
Diabetic/No added Sugar/No Conc. Sweets/Calorie Controlled: No changes needed
Bland/Anti Reflux: omit garlic, tomatoes, thyme, and parsley
Liberal House Renal: omit chicken granules, tomatoes and olives
No Added Salt: No changes needed
2 Gram Sodium: omit chicken granules and olives. Use fresh tomatoes for canned
Gluten Free: Use gluten free granules or broth. Use gluten free flour. Serve over gluten free noodles or rice. Prepare foods separately to prevent cross contamination.

Allergy Alerts: When an "X" is present, this indicates the allergen is present. Always read all food labels to ensure allergens are not present.

Wheat	Milk	Eggs	Fish Shellfish	Soy	Peanuts/Nuts	Other
X						

Key: SF= Salt Free D= Diet or Sugarfree LF = Lowfat FF = Fat Free GF = Gluten Free

Recipe Name: Pork Roast with Sauerkraut
Recipe Category: Dinner Entrée
Portion Size: 3 oz. boneless, ½ c. sauerkraut
Ingredients: **Yields: 8 servings**

Ingredients	Notes:
3 ½-4 lbs. boneless pork roast	Trim all visible fat. Cut across the grain into thin bite size pieces
½ teaspoon garlic powder	
½ teaspoon black pepper	
4 cups sauerkraut	
½ teaspoon caraway seeds	
½ cup peeled and diced apple	
1 small onion, diced	

Directions:

Steps:	Directions:	Critical Control Point /Quality Assurance
1	Heat oven to 350 degrees	
2	Place roast in a roasting pan and season with garlic powder and pepper.	
3	Add sauerkraut, caraway seeds, apple and onion. Cover. Bake for 2 ½ hours to 3 hours	Cook until internal temperature reaches 145 ° F with a 3-minute rest. Or longer.

Time Temperature Sensitive food. *Food safety Standards: hold food for service at an internal temperature above 140° F. Do not mix old product with new. Cool leftover product quickly (within 4 hours) to below 41° F. Follow proper cooling procedures. Store leftovers in a tightly sealed, labeled and dated container. Use leftover within 72 hours if stored in refrigerator or 30 days if stored in the freezer. Reheat leftover product quickly (within 2 hours) to 165 degrees F for 15 seconds. Reheat left over product only once; discard if not used. Cold holding at 41°F or colder or using time alone (less than four hours). Always wash hands and wash and sanitize counter tops utensils and containers between steps when working with raw meat.*

Texture Modified Diets: Prepare and serve pork roast and sauerkraut separately.
Soft & Bite Size: (aka Bite size) **Food particle size ½ inch (~width of standard fork)** Food must be moist. Cut foods with a knife to a ½" particle size prior to mixing. Moisten with broth as needed. Omit seeds.
Chopped: Food particle size ¼ inch (~ ½ width of standard fork) Food must be moist. Chop foods with a knife to 1/4" particle size prior to mixing. Moisten with broth as needed. Omit seeds.
Minced and Moist:(aka Minced/Mechanical Soft/Ground) **Food particle size 1/8 inch (fits through prongs of standard fork)** Food must be moist. Use a food processor to grind food particles into 1/8 inch prior to mixing. Moisten with broth as needed. Omit seeds.
Pureed: Smooth and cohesive. Use a food processor to puree to a smooth consistency. Foods are processed by grinding and then pureeing them. May add broth or sauce to puree. Do not add to much liquid. Puree should still hold its shape. Must not be firm or sticky. Puree foods while still hot. Appearance should be smooth like pudding. Omit caraway seeds. Puree each item individually and serve separately. (meat and sauerkraut) May add broth to moisten meat.

Therapeutic Modified Diets:
Lowfat: No changes needed
Diabetic/No added Sugar/No Conc. Sweets/Calorie Controlled: No changes needed
Bland/Anti Reflux: omit pepper, garlic powder, sauerkraut
Liberal House Renal: omit sauerkraut
No Added Salt: omit sauerkraut
2 Gram Sodium: omit sauerkraut
Gluten Free: No changes needed.

Allergy Alerts: When an "X" is present, this indicates the allergen is present. Always read all food labels to ensure allergens are not present.

Wheat	Milk	Eggs	Fish Shellfish	Soy	Peanuts/Nuts	Other

Key: SF= Salt Free D= Diet or Sugarfree LF = Lowfat FF = Fat Free GF = Gluten Free

Copyright 2020 Jacqueline Larson M.S., R.D.N. and Associates.   All Rights Reserved

Recipe Name: Pork Stir Fry with Vegetables
Recipe Category: Dinner Entrée
Portion Size: 1 cup
Ingredients: Yields: 8 servings

Ingredients	Notes:
2 pounds lean boneless pork loin	Trim all visible fat.
2 Tablespoons lite soy sauce	
1 Tablespoon rice vinegar	
1 Tablespoon oil	
1 teaspoon garlic powder	Or 2 cloves minced
1 teaspoon ground ginger	
20 oz. package stir fry vegetables	
1 Tablespoon low salt chicken broth or water	
1 Tablespoon sesame seeds	

Directions:

Steps:	Directions:	Critical Control Point /Quality Assurance
1	Slice pork across grain into 1/8 inch strips.	
2	Marinate in soy sauce, vinegar, oil, garlic and ginger for 10 minutes.	
3	Heat oil in nonstick pan until hot	
4	Add pork and stir fry for 3-5 minutes until pork is no longer pink	Cook to 145°F for 15 seconds
5	Add frozen vegetables and chicken broth or water. Stir Mixture. Cover. Cook until vegetables are tender crisp.	
6	Sprinkle with sesame seeds.	

Time Temperature Sensitive food. *Food safety Standards: hold food for service at an internal temperature above 140° F. Do not mix old product with new. Cool leftover product quickly (within 4 hours) to below 41° F. Follow proper cooling procedures. Store leftovers in a tightly sealed, labeled and dated container. Use leftover within 72 hours if stored in refrigerator or 30 days if stored in the freezer. Reheat leftover product quickly (within 2 hours) to 165 degrees F for 15 seconds. Reheat left over product only once; discard if not used. Cold holding at 41°F or colder or using time alone (less than four hours). Always wash hands and wash and sanitize counter tops utensils and containers between steps when working with raw meat.*

Texture Modified Diets:

Soft & Bite Size: (aka Bite size) **Food particle size ½ inch (~width of standard fork)** Food must be moist. Cut foods with a knife to a ½" particle size prior to mixing. Moisten with broth as needed.
Chopped: Food particle size ¼ inch (~ ½ width of standard fork) Food must be moist. Chop foods with a knife to 1/4" particle size prior to mixing. Moisten with broth as needed.
Minced and Moist:(aka Minced/Mechanical Soft/Ground) **Food particle size 1/8 inch (fits through prongs of standard fork)** Food must be moist. Use a food processor to grind food particles into 1/8 inch prior to mixing. Moisten with broth as needed.
Pureed: Smooth and cohesive. Use a food processor to puree to a smooth consistency. Foods are processed by grinding and then pureeing them. May add broth or sauce to puree. Do not add to much liquid. Puree should still hold its shape. Must not be firm or sticky. Puree foods while still hot. Appearance should be smooth like pudding. Omit sesame seeds. Remove meat before adding vegetables. Serve ½ c. meat separate from ½ c. vegetables.

Therapeutic Modified Diets:

Lowfat: No changes needed
Diabetic/No added Sugar/No Conc. Sweets/Calorie Controlled: No changes needed
Bland/Anti Reflux: omit garlic, sesame seeds, use peas, carrots and green beans for vegetables
Liberal House Renal: Omit soy sauce and use SF broth or water
No Added Salt: No changes needed
2 Gram Sodium: Omit soy sauce and use SF broth or water
Gluten Free: Use gluten free soy sauce and broth. . Prepare foods separately to prevent cross contamination.
Allergy Alerts: When an "X" is present, this indicates the allergen is present. Always read all food labels to ensure allergens are not present.

Wheat	Milk	Eggs	Fish Shellfish	Soy	Peanuts/Nuts	Other
X				X		

Key: SF= Salt Free D= Diet or Sugarfree LF = Lowfat   FF = Fat Free GF = Gluten Free

Copyright 2020 Jacqueline Larson M.S., R.D.N. and Associates.   All Rights Reserved

Recipe Name: Pork Tenderloin and Brown Rice Salad
Recipe Category: Dinner Entrée
Portion Size: 1 ½ cups (3 oz. meat, ½ cup starch, ½ cup vegetables)
Ingredients: Yields: 8 servings

Ingredients	Notes:
2 1/2 lbs. Pork Tenderloin, cut 3/4 inch thick	Trim all visible fat.
2 teaspoons olive oil	
2 cups asparagus pieces (2-inch pieces)	Wash all produce, prior to cutting
2 cups medium yellow squash,	Wash and cut lengthwise in half, then crosswise into 1/4-inch thick slices
4 cups hot cooked brown rice	See recipe for brown rice
1 cup diced, seeded tomatoes	Wash, seeded and diced
1 cup canned garbanzo beans	Rinsed and drained
1/4 cup fresh basil, thinly sliced	Or 2 Tablespoons dried
1/2 teaspoon salt	
Marinade Ingredients ½ cup olive oil ¾ cup soy sauce ½ cup lemon juice ½ cup Worcestershire sauce 2 tablespoons Dijon mustard 1 clove garlic, minced ¼ teaspoon pepper to taste	

Directions:

Steps:	Directions:	Critical Control Point / Quality Assurance
1	Combine marinade ingredients in small bowl. Place tenderloin and 1/4 cup marinade in food-safe plastic bag; turn pork to coat. Close bag securely and marinate in refrigerator 1 hour or as long as overnight. Reserve remaining marinade in refrigerator for dressing.	Store marinate and pork in refrigerator at 40F degrees or less.
2	Remove tenderloin from marinade; discard marinade. Place pork on rack in broiler pan so surface of beef is 2 to 3 inches from heat. Broil 12 to 13 minutes for medium rare (145°F) doneness, turning once. Remove; keep warm.	Discard Marinade. Check Temperature. Minimum Temperature 145°F for 15 seconds pork
3	Heat oil in large nonstick skillet over medium-high heat until hot. Add asparagus and squash; cook and stir 7 to 8 minutes or until tender. Toss with rice, tomatoes, beans, basil, salt and reserved marinade in large bowl. Chill.	
4	Carve pork tenderloin into thin slices. Serve warm over chilled rice salad.	

Time Temperature Sensitive food. *Food safety Standards: hold food for service at an internal temperature above 140° F. Do not mix old product with new. Cool leftover product quickly (within 4 hours) to below 41° F. Follow proper cooling procedures. Store leftovers in a tightly sealed, labeled and dated container. Use leftover within 72 hours if stored in refrigerator or 30 days if stored in the freezer. Reheat leftover product quickly (within 2 hours) to 165 degrees F for 15 seconds. Reheat left over product only once; discard if not used. Cold holding at 41°F or colder or using time alone (less than four hours). Always wash hands and wash and sanitize counter tops utensils and containers between steps when working with raw meat.*

Texture Modified Diets:
Soft & Bite Size: (aka Bite size) **Food particle size ½ inch (~width of standard fork)** Food must be moist. Cut foods with a knife to a ½" particle size prior to mixing. Moisten with marinade as needed.
Chopped: Food particle size ¼ inch (~ ½ width of standard fork) Food must be moist. Chop foods with a knife to 1/4" particle size prior to mixing. Moisten with marinade as needed.

Minced and Moist: (aka Minced/Mechanical Soft/Ground) **Food particle size 1/8 inch (fits through prongs of standard fork)** Food must be moist. Use a food processor to grind food particles into 1/8 inch prior to mixing. Moisten with marinade as needed.

Pureed: Smooth and cohesive. Use a food processor to puree to a smooth consistency. Foods are processed by grinding and then pureeing them. May add broth or sauce to puree. Do not add to much liquid. Puree should still hold its shape. Must not be firm or sticky. Puree foods while still hot. Appearance should be smooth like pudding. Serve ½ c. meat serving, ½ cup vegetables, and ½ cup rice separately.

Therapeutic Modified Diets:

Lowfat: No changes needed
Diabetic/No added Sugar/No Conc. Sweets/Calorie Controlled: No changes needed
Bland: omit garbanzo beans, basil, tomatoes, lemon juice, Dijon mustard, and pepper
Liberal House Renal: Omit salt, tomatoes, soy sauce, and Worcestershire sauce
No Added Salt: No changes
2 Gram Sodium: omit salt, soy sauce and Worcestershire sauce
Gluten Free: Use gluten free soy sauce. Prepare separately to prevent cross contamination.
Allergy Alerts: When an "X" is present, this indicates the allergen is present.
Always read all food labels to ensure allergens are not present.

Wheat	Milk	Eggs	FishShellfish	Soy	Peanuts/Nuts	Other
X			X			

Key: SF= Salt Free D= Diet or Sugarfree LF = Lowfat FF = Fat Free GF = Gluten Free

Recipe Name: Pork Tenderloin Medallions
Recipe Category: Dinner Entrée
Portion Size: 3 oz. boneless
Ingredients: Yields: 8 servings

Ingredients	Notes:
2 lbs. boneless pork tenderloin	Trim all visible fat, Thinly slice into thin slices across the grain.
1/4 cup olive oil	Or vegetable oil
1 teaspoon garlic salt	
1 teaspoon pepper	

Directions:

Steps:	Directions:	Critical Control Point / Quality Assurance
1	Season Meat with garlic salt and pepper	
2	Heat oil to medium high heat.	
3	Add pork slices	
4	Cook for 2 minutes until slightly brown	DO NOT OVER COOK
5	Turn slices and cook until brown	Heat to at least 145 degree with 4 minute rest
6	Slice thinly across the grain and serve.	

Time Temperature Sensitive food. *Food safety Standards: hold food for service at an internal temperature above 140° F. Do not mix old product with new. Cool leftover product quickly (within 4 hours) to below 41° F. Follow proper cooling procedures. Store leftovers in a tightly sealed, labeled and dated container. Use leftover within 72 hours if stored in refrigerator or 30 days if stored in the freezer. Reheat leftover product quickly (within 2 hours) to 165 degrees F for 15 seconds. Reheat left over product only once; discard if not used. Cold holding at 41°F or colder or using time alone (less than four hours). Always wash hands and wash and sanitize counter tops utensils and containers between steps when working with raw meat.*

Texture Modified Diets:

Soft & Bite Size: (aka Bite size) **Food particle size ½ inch (~width of standard fork)** Food must be moist. Cut foods with a knife to a ½" particle size after cooking. Moisten with broth as needed after cutting.

Chopped: Food particle size ¼ inch (~ ½ width of standard fork) Food must be moist. Chop foods with a knife to 1/4" particle size after cooking. Moisten with broth as needed after chopping.

Minced and Moist: (aka Minced/Mechanical Soft/Ground) **Food particle size 1/8 inch (fits through prongs of standard fork)** Food must be moist. Use a food processor to grind food particles into 1/8 inch after cooking. Moisten with milk as needed after processing.

Pureed: Smooth and cohesive. Use a food processor to puree to a smooth consistency. Foods are processed by grinding and then pureeing them. May add milk or sauce to puree. Do not add to much liquid. Puree should still hold its shape. Must not be firm or sticky. Puree foods while still hot. Appearance should be smooth like pudding.

Therapeutic Modified Diets:

Lowfat: No changes needed
Diabetic/No added Sugar/No Conc. Sweets/Calorie Controlled: No changes needed
Bland/Anti Reflux: omit pepper and garlic salt
Liberal House Renal: omit garlic salt and use garlic powder
No Added Salt: No changes needed
2 Gram Sodium: omit garlic salt and use garlic powder
Gluten Free: No changes. Prepare foods separately to prevent cross contamination.
Allergy Alerts: When an "X" is present, this indicates the allergen is present.
Always read all food labels to ensure allergens are not present.

Wheat	Milk	Eggs	Fish Shellfish	Soy	Peanuts/Nuts	Other

Key: SF= Salt Free D= Diet or Sugarfree LF = Lowfat FF = Fat Free GF = Gluten Free

Recipe Name: Pork Tenderloin Piccata'
Recipe Category: Dinner Entrée
Portion Size: 3 oz meat plus 2 T topping
Ingredients: Yields: 8 servings

Ingredients	Notes:
2 1/2 lbs. boneless, lean, pork tenderloin, thinly sliced into ¼ inch thickness	Trim any fat.
1/2 cup flour	
1 teaspoon salt	
1/4 teaspoon pepper	
1/4 cup vegetable oil	
1/4 cup water	
1/4 cup lemon juice	
1 lemon	Washed and thinly sliced.
1/4 cup capers	
1/4 cup chopped fresh parsley	

Directions:

Steps:	Directions:	Critical Control Point /Quality Assurance
1	Combine flour, salt, pepper in a shallow dish. Dredge pork in flour mixture; shake off excess.	
2	In a large frying pan, heat vegetable oil over medium heat.	
3	Add pork. Cook about 3 minutes a side until tender and opaque. Remove and keep warm.	Cook pork until internal temperature reaches 155 degrees F.
4	Add water to pan juices. Cook 1 minute scraping up brown bits from bottom of pan. Add lemon juice and heat to boiling.	
5	Return pork to pan and cook until sauce thickens slightly, about 3 minutes.	
6	Serve chicken on a large platter garnished with lemon slices, capers, and parsley.	

Time Temperature Sensitive food. *Food safety Standards: hold food for service at an internal temperature above 140°F. Do not mix old product with new. Cool leftover product quickly (within 4 hours) to below 41°F. Follow proper cooling procedures. Store leftovers in a tightly sealed, labeled and dated container. Use leftover within 72 hours if stored in refrigerator or 30 days if stored in the freezer. Reheat leftover product quickly (within 2 hours) to 165 degrees F for 15 seconds. Reheat left over product only once; discard if not used. Cold holding at 41°F or colder or using time alone (less than four hours). Always wash hands and wash and sanitize counter tops utensils and containers between steps when working with raw poultry.*

Texture Modified Diets:
Soft & Bite Size: (aka Bite size) **Food particle size ½ inch (~width of standard fork)** Food must be moist. Cut foods with a knife to a ½" particle size after cooking. Moisten with broth as needed. Foods that do not process well should be omitted. Omit: capers.
Chopped: Food particle size ¼ inch (~ ½ width of standard fork) Food must be moist. Chop foods with a knife to 1/4" particle size after cooking. Moisten with broth as needed. Foods that do not process well should be omitted. Omit: capers.
Minced and Moist: (aka Minced/Mechanical Soft/Ground) **Food particle size 1/8 inch (fits through prongs of standard fork)** Food must be moist. Use a food processor to grind food particles into 1/8 inch prior to after cooking. Moisten with broth as needed. Foods that do not process well should be omitted. Omit: capers.
Pureed: Smooth and cohesive. Use a food processor to puree to a smooth consistency. Foods are processed by grinding and then pureeing them. May add broth or sauce to puree. Do not add to much liquid. Puree should still hold its shape. Must not be firm or sticky. Puree foods while still hot. Appearance should be smooth like pudding. Foods that do not process well should be omitted. Omit: capers.

Therapeutic Modified Diets:
Lowfat: No changes needed.
Diabetic/No added Sugar/No Conc. Sweets/Calorie Controlled: No changes needed.
Bland/Anti Reflux: Serve 3 oz. plain cooked pork
Liberal House Renal: Omit salt and capers.
No Added Salt: Omit capers.
2 Gram Sodium: Omit salt and capers.
Gluten Free: Use gluten free flour. Prepare foods separately to prevent cross contamination.

Allergy Alerts: When an "X" is present, this indicates the allergen is present. Always read all food labels to ensure allergens are not present.

Wheat	Milk	Eggs	Fish Shellfish	Soy	Peanuts/Nuts	Other
X						

Key: SF= Salt Free D= Diet or Sugarfree LF = Lowfat FF = Fat Free GF = Gluten Free

Recipe Name: Pork Tenderloin with Cranberry Glaze
Recipe Category: Dinner Entrée
Portion Size: 3 oz. boneless
Ingredients: Yields: 8 servings

Ingredients	Notes:
2 lbs. boneless pork tenderloin	Trim all visible fat.
2 tablespoons olive oil	
½ teaspoon salt	
1 teaspoon pepper	
1 can (12 oz.) jellied cranberry sauce	
½ cup orange juice	
¼ cup brown sugar	

Directions:

Steps:	Directions:	Critical Control Point /Quality Assurance
1	Pre Heat. Oven to 350 degrees F. Season pork with salt and pepper. Rub on olive oil	
2	Bake uncovered for 40 minutes.	
3	In a small saucepan combine, cranberry sauce, orange juice, and brown sugar. Cook over medium heat until cranberry sauce is melted. Drizzle ¼ sauce over roast.	
4	Bake 20 minutes longer. Baste with sauce every 10 minutes. Let stand for 10 minutes.	Heat to at least 145 degree with 4 minute rest DO NOT OVER COOK
5	Slice thinly across the grain and serve. Serve with remaining glaze drizzled over slices.	

Time Temperature Sensitive food. *Food safety Standards: hold food for service at an internal temperature above 140° F. Do not mix old product with new. Cool leftover product quickly (within 4 hours) to below 41° F. Follow proper cooling procedures. Store leftovers in a tightly sealed, labeled and dated container. Use leftover within 72 hours if stored in refrigerator or 30 days if stored in the freezer. Reheat leftover product quickly (within 2 hours) to 165 degrees F for 15 seconds. Reheat left over product only once; discard if not used. Cold holding at 41 °F or colder or using time alone (less than four hours). Always wash hands and wash and sanitize counter tops utensils and containers between steps when working with raw meat.*

Texture Modified Diets:

Soft & Bite Size: (aka Bite size) **Food particle size ½ inch (~width of standard fork)** Food must be moist. Cut foods with a knife to a ½" particle size after cooking. Moisten with sauce as needed after cutting.
Chopped: Food particle size ¼ inch (~ ½ width of standard fork) Food must be moist. Chop foods with a knife to 1/4" particle size after cooking. Moisten with sauce as needed after chopping.
Minced and Moist: (aka Minced/Mechanical Soft/Ground) **Food particle size 1/8 inch (fits through prongs of standard fork)** Food must be moist. Use a food processor to grind food particles into 1/8 inch after cooking. Moisten with sauce as needed after processing.
Pureed: Smooth and cohesive. Use a food processor to puree to a smooth consistency. Foods are processed by grinding and then pureeing them. May add milk or sauce to puree. Do not add to much liquid. Puree should still hold its shape. Must not be firm or sticky. Puree foods while still hot. Appearance should be smooth like pudding. Serve ½ c. meat serving

Therapeutic Modified Diets:

Lowfat: No changes needed
Diabetic/No added Sugar/No Conc. Sweets/Calorie Controlled: No changes needed
Bland/Anti Reflux: omit pepper and orange juice
Liberal House Renal: omit salt
No Added Salt: No changes needed
2 Gram Sodium: omit salt
Gluten Free: Use GF cranberry sauce. . Prepare foods separately to prevent cross contamination.

Allergy Alerts: When an "X" is present, this indicates the allergen is present. Always read all food labels to ensure allergens are not present.

Wheat	Milk	Eggs	Fish Shellfish	Soy	Peanuts/Nuts	Other
X						

Key: SF= Salt Free D= Diet or Sugarfree LF = Lowfat FF = Fat Free GF = Gluten Free

Copyright 2020 Jacqueline Larson M.S., R.D.N. and Associates.   All Rights Reserved

Recipe Name: Pork Tetrazzini
Recipe Category: Dinner Entree
Portion Size: 1 cup
Ingredients: Yields: 8 servings

Ingredients	Notes:
1/2 pound fresh mushrooms	
2 lbs. cooked pork tenderloin (see recipe for pork tenderloin medallions)	Cut into 1/2 inch pieces
3 tablespoons dry white wine	(Optional)
3 tablespoons margarine	
2 tablespoon flour	
2 cups reduced sodium chicken broth	
1 (14 oz.) can nonfat evaporated milk	
1 pound spaghetti	May use whole grain
1/2 c. Parmesan cheese	Grated

Directions:

Steps:	Directions:	Critical Control Point /Quality Assurance
1	Prepare pork tenderloin according to direction in pork tenderloin recipe. Prepare spaghetti according to directions on the package.	
2	Melt margarine in a saucepan. Add mushrooms and sauté	
3	Add flour. Cook and stir until well coated.	
4	Add chicken broth. Heat over low heat.	
5	Slowly add evaporated milk. Add half the sauce to the pork and half to spaghetti and mushrooms.	
6	Place the spaghetti in a vegetable non stick sprayed casserole dish. Make a hole in the center. Place the pork in the hole with the spaghetti.	
7	Sprinkle with parmesan cheese. Bake in a 375 degree oven for about 40 minutes or until lightly browned and heated through.	Instant read thermometer should read 165.

Time Temperature Sensitive food. *Food safety Standards: hold food for service at an internal temperature above 140° F. Do not mix old product with new. Cool leftover product quickly (within 4 hours) to below 41° F. Follow proper cooling procedures. Store leftovers in a tightly sealed, labeled and dated container. Use leftover within 72 hours if stored in refrigerator or 30 days if stored in the freezer. Reheat leftover product quickly (within 2 hours) to 165 degrees F for 15 seconds. Reheat left over product only once; discard if not used. Cold holding at 41°F or colder or using time alone (less than four hours). Always wash hands and wash and sanitize counter tops utensils and containers between steps when working with raw meat.*

Texture Modified Diets: TIP: Use pasta that is the correct particle size.
Soft & Bite Size: (aka Bite size) **Food particle size ½ inch (~width of standard fork)** Food must be moist. Cut foods with a knife to a ½" particle size prior to mixing. Moisten with broth as needed.
Chopped: Food particle size ¼ inch (~ ½ width of standard fork) Food must be moist. Chop foods with a knife to 1/4" particle size prior to mixing. Moisten with broth as needed.
Minced and Moist: (aka Minced/Mechanical Soft/Ground) **Food particle size 1/8 inch (fits through prongs of standard fork)** Food must be moist. Use a food processor to grind food particles into 1/8 inch prior to mixing. Moisten with broth as needed.
Pureed: Smooth and cohesive. Use a food processor to puree to a smooth consistency. Foods are processed by grinding and then pureeing them. May add broth or sauce to puree. Do not add to much liquid. Puree should still hold its shape. Must not be firm or sticky. Puree foods while still hot. Appearance should be smooth like pudding.
Puree each item individually and serve separately (meat, vegetables and noodles). May add broth to moisten meat. Serve ½ c. puree pork and ½ c. puree pasta separately.

Therapeutic Modified Diets:
Lowfat: No changes needed
Diabetic/No added Sugar/No Conc. Sweets/Calorie Controlled: No changes needed
Bland/Anti Reflux: Omit the dry white wine.
Liberal House Renal: Omit the evaporated milk and Parmesan cheese. Use SF chicken broth or water
No Added Salt: No changes needed.
2 Gram Sodium: Omit Parmesan cheese. Use SF chicken broth or water
Gluten Free: Use gluten free noodles, gluten free all purpose flour and gluten free chicken broth. Prepare foods separately to prevent cross contamination.

Allergy Alerts: When an "X" is present, this indicates the allergen is present. Always read all food labels to ensure allergens are not present.

Wheat	Milk	Eggs	Fish Shellfish	Soy	Peanuts/Nuts	Other
X	X	X		X		

Key: SF= Salt Free D= Diet or Sugarfree LF = Lowfat FF = Fat Free GF = Gluten Free

Copyright 2020 Jacqueline Larson M.S., R.D.N. and Associates. All Rights Reserved

Recipe Name: Spicy Apricot Pork Chops.
Recipe Category: Pork Dinner
Portion Size: 3 oz. boneless, 5 oz. with bone
Ingredients: Yields: 8 servings

Ingredients	Notes:
8 (5 ounces each) lamb chops or 16 (2 1/2 oz) lamb chops	Trim fat (or pork)
2 tablespoons packed brown sugar	
1 teaspoon garlic salt	
1/2 teaspoon chili powder	
1 teaspoon paprika	
1/2 teaspoon oregano	
1/4 teaspoon ground cinnamon	
1/4 teaspoon all spice	
1/4 teaspoon black pepper	
1/2 cup apricot preserves	

Directions:

Steps:	Directions:	Critical Control Point /Quality Assurance
1	Preheat broiler.	Trim all visible fat.
2	In a small bowl combine brown sugar, garlic, salt, chili powder, paprika, oregano, cinnamon, all spice, and pepper. Rub spice mixture on chops.	
3	Place chops on unheated rack of a broiler pan.	
4	Broil for 4 to 5 inches from the heat for 10 to 15 minutes or until done, turning meat and brushing with preserves halfway through broiling.	Cook until internal temperature reaches *145° F*

Time Temperature Sensitive food. Food safety Standards: hold food for service at an internal temperature above 140° F. Do not mix old product with new. Cool leftover product quickly (within 4 hours) to below 41° F. Follow proper cooling procedures. Store leftovers in a tightly sealed, labeled and dated container. Use leftover within 72 hours if stored in refrigerator or 30 days if stored in the freezer. Reheat leftover product quickly (within 2 hours) to 165 degrees F for 15 seconds. Reheat left over product only once; discard if not used. Cold holding at 41°F or colder or using time alone (less than four hours). Always wash hands and wash and sanitize counter tops utensils and containers between steps when working with raw meat.

Texture Modified Diets:

Soft & Bite Size: (aka Bite size) **Food particle size ½ inch (~width of standard fork)** Food must be moist. Cut foods with a knife to a ½" particle size after cooking. Moisten with milk as needed after cutting.

Chopped: Food particle size ¼ inch (~ ½ width of standard fork) Food must be moist. Chop foods with a knife to 1/4" particle size after cooking. Moisten with milk as needed after chopping.

Minced and Moist: (aka Minced/Mechanical Soft/Ground) **Food particle size 1/8 inch (fits through prongs of standard fork)** Food must be moist. Use a food processor to grind food particles into 1/8 inch after cooking. Moisten with milk as needed after processing.

Pureed: Smooth and cohesive. Use a food processor to puree to a smooth consistency. Foods are processed by grinding and then pureeing them. May add milk or sauce to puree. Do not add to much liquid. Puree should still hold its shape. Must not be firm or sticky. Puree foods while still hot. Appearance should be smooth like pudding. Serve ½ c. serving topped with puree sauce.

Therapeutic Modified Diets:

Lowfat: No changes needed.
Diabetic/No added Sugar/No Conc. Sweets/Calorie Controlled: Omit apricot preserves
Bland/Anti Reflux: Omit garlic salt, chili powder, paprika, oregano, cinnamon, all spice and black pepper.
Liberal House Renal: Omit garlic salt.
No Added Salt: No changes needed.
2 Gram Sodium: Omit garlic salt.
Gluten Free: No changes needed.

Allergy Alerts: When an "X" is present, this indicates the allergen is present. Always read all food labels to ensure allergens are not present.

Wheat	Milk	Eggs	Fish Shellfish	Soy	Peanuts/Nuts	Other

Key: SF= Salt Free D= Diet or Sugarfree LF = Lowfat FF = Fat Free GF = Gluten Free

Recipe Name: Sweet and Sour Pork
Recipe Category: Dinner Entrée
Portion Size: 3 oz. pork, 1 c. serving size with sauce and vegetables
Ingredients: Yields: 8 servings

Ingredients	Notes:
2 ½ lb. Boneless lean pork cut into ½ inch size pieces	Trim all visible fat,
1 16 ounce can pineapple chunks (juice packed)	
2/3 cup sugar	
½ cup vinegar	
¼ cup cornstarch	
2 teaspoons instant chicken bouillon granules	
¼ cup lite soy sauce	
2 eggs, beaten	
½ cup cornstarch	
½ cup flour	
½ cup water	
¼ teaspoon black pepper	
2 Tablespoon oil	
4 medium carrots	Wash, Peel, and thinly sliced at an angle
4 cloves garlic, minced	
2 Large bell peppers, green or red	Wash, remove stem and seeds, and cut into ½ inch pieces
4 Cups, hot cooked rice	May use brown or white enriched rice

Directions:

Steps:	Directions:	Critical Control Point /Quality Assurance
1	For sauce, drain pineapple, reserving juice. Cut pineapple into ½ inch pieces.	
2	Add water to reserved juice to equal 1 ½ cups	
3	Stir in sugar, vinegar, the 2 Tablespoons cornstarch, soy sauce and bouillon and set aside	
4	For batter: In a small bowl, combine egg the ¼ cup cornstarch, flour, water and pepper.	
5	Whisk thoroughly, until smooth.	
6	Dip pork pieces into batter. In small amount of oil, sauté about 1/3 of the pork. Cook pieces for 4-5 minutes on medium high heat. Batter Should be golden brown. Repeat until all pork is cooked. Drain any excess oil on paper towels.	Cook 165° F degrees for chicken
7	In a large skillet or wok, Add 1 Tablespoon oil, and heat over medium high heat.	
8	Stir fry carrots and garlic for 1 minute.	
9	Add sweet peppers and stir fry for 1 to 2 minutes, or till tender crisp	
10	Push from center of pan. Stir in sauce into center of pan or wok. Cook until thick and bubbly	
11	Stir in all pineapple and pork. Stir together all ingredients to coat with sauce. Heat through.	Cook until temperature reaches 165°F. Serve.

Time Temperature Sensitive food. Food safety Standards: hold food for service at an internal temperature above 140° F. Do not mix old product with new. Cool leftover product quickly (within 4 hours) to below 41° F. Follow proper cooling procedures. Store leftovers in a tightly sealed, labeled and dated container. Use leftover within 72 hours if stored in refrigerator or 30 days if stored in the freezer. Reheat leftover product quickly (within 2 hours) to 165 degrees F for 15 seconds. Reheat left over product only once; discard if not used. Cold holding at 41°F or colder or using time alone (less than four hours). Always wash hands and wash and sanitize counter tops utensils and containers between steps when working with raw meat.

Copyright 2020 Jacqueline Larson M.S., R.D.N. and Associates.   All Rights Reserved

Texture Modified Diets: TIP: Use pasta that is the correct particle size.

Soft & Bite Size: (aka Bite size) **Food particle size ½ inch (~width of standard fork)** Food must be moist. Cut foods with a knife to a ½" particle size prior to mixing. Moisten with sauce as needed. Omit pineapples.

Chopped: Food particle size ¼ inch (~ ½ width of standard fork) Food must be moist. Chop foods with a knife to 1/4" particle size prior to mixing. Moisten with sauce as needed. Omit pineapples.

Minced and Moist: (aka Minced/Mechanical Soft/Ground) **Food particle size 1/8 inch (fits through prongs of standard fork)** Food must be moist. Use a food processor to grind food particles into 1/8 inch prior to mixing. Moisten with sauce as needed. Omit pineapples.

Pureed: Smooth and cohesive. Use a food processor to puree to a smooth consistency. Foods are processed by grinding and then pureeing them. May add broth or sauce to puree. Do not add to much liquid. Puree should still hold its shape. Must not be firm or sticky. Puree foods while still hot. Appearance should be smooth like pudding. Omit pineapples.

Puree each item individually and serve separately (meat, vegetables andrice). May add broth to moisten meat.

Therapeutic Modified Diets:

Lowfat: No changes needed

Diabetic/No added Sugar/No Conc. Sweets/Calorie Controlled: No changes needed

Bland/Anti Reflux: omit pepper and garlic

Liberal House Renal: omit chicken granules and soy sauce

No Added Salt: omit chicken granules and soy sauce

2 Gram Sodium: omit chicken granules and soy sauce

Gluten Free: Use gluten free soy sauce. Use gluten free flour. Omit chicken granules and use gluten free chicken broth in place of water. Prepare foods separately to prevent cross contamination.

Allergy Alerts: When an "X" is present, this indicates the allergen is present. Always read all food labels to ensure allergens are not present.

Wheat	Milk	Eggs	Fish Shellfish	Soy	Peanuts/Nuts	Other
X		X		X		

Key: SF= Salt Free D= Diet or Sugarfree LF = Lowfat FF = Fat Free GF = Gluten Free

PORK LUNCH RECIPES

Recipe Name: Asian Pork and Noodles Soup
Recipe Category: Lunch entree
Portion Size: 2 cups
Ingredients: **Yields: 8 servings**

Ingredients	Notes:
3/4 lbs. dry Chinese noodles or spaghetti	May use whole grain
2 Tablespoons olive oil	
2 cups cabbage	Wash, remove core and shredded
1 small l onion, diced	Wash, peel and dice
½ cup carrots	Wash, peel and shredded
2 Tablespoon lite soy sauce	
¼ teaspoon black pepper	
1 lb. lean pork tenderloin	Cut into thin strips
2 gallons reduced sodium chicken broth	
2 tablespoons garlic clove, minced	
1 tablespoon ground ginger	
2 tablespoons fresh green onions	Wash, trim and slice thin. (including green tops)

Directions:

Steps:	Directions:	Critical Control Point /Quality Assurance
1	In a large stock pot heat oil to medium high heat. Add pork tenderloin and cook until lightly browned. Stir in cabbage, carrots, garlic and onion. Cook until tender	
2	Stir in chicken broth, soy sauce, pepper and ginger. Bring to boil. Add noodles and cook until tender. About 8-10 minutes Serve hot. Top with green onions.	Temperature check must reach 165 °F degrees

Time Temperature Sensitive food. Food safety Standards: hold food for service at an internal temperature above 140° F. Do not mix old product with new. Cool leftover product quickly (within 4 hours) to below 41° F. Follow proper cooling procedures. Store leftovers in a tightly sealed, labeled and dated container. Use leftover within 72 hours if stored in refrigerator or 30 days if stored in the freezer. Reheat leftover product quickly (within 2 hours) to 165 degrees F for 15 seconds. Reheat left over product only once; discard if not used. Cold holding at 41 °F or colder or using time alone (less than four hours).

<u>**Texture Modified Diets: TIP: Use pasta that is the correct particle size.**</u>
Soft & Bite Size: (aka Bite size) **Food particle size ½ inch (~width of standard fork)** Food must be moist. Cut foods with a knife to a ½" particle size prior to mixing. Moisten with broth as needed. Omit green onions.
Chopped: Food particle size ¼ inch (~ ½ width of standard fork) Food must be moist. Chop foods with a knife to 1/4" particle size prior to mixing. Moisten with broth as needed. Omit green onions.
Minced and Moist:(aka Minced/Mechanical Soft/Ground) **Food particle size 1/8 inch (fits through prongs of standard fork)** Food must be moist. Use a food processor to grind food particles into 1/8 inch prior to mixing. Moisten with broth as needed. Omit green onions.
Pureed: Smooth and cohesive. Use a food processor to puree to a smooth consistency. Foods are processed by grinding and then pureeing them. May add broth or sauce to puree. Do not add to much liquid. Puree should still hold its shape. Must not be firm or sticky. Puree foods while still hot. Appearance should be smooth like pudding. Omit green onions.
Puree each item individually and serve separately (meat, vegetables and noodles). May add broth to moisten meat. Serve ½ c. puree pork and ½ c. puree pasta separately.
Serve ½ cup puree pork, ½ cup puree noodles and ½ cup puree carrots separately.
<u>**Therapeutic Modified Diets:**</u>
Lowfat: no changes
Diabetic/No added Sugar/No Conc. Sweets/Calorie Controlled: No changes needed
Bland/Anti Reflux: Omit pepper, garlic, and onions. Sub. Green beans for cabbage.
Liberal House Renal: Omit soy sauce. Use SF chicken broth or water.
No Added Salt: Omit soy sauce
2 Gram Sodium: Omit soy sauce. Use SF chicken broth or water
Gluten Free: Use gluten free noodles, GF soy sauce and GF chicken broth. Prepare foods separately to prevent cross contamination.
Allergy Alerts: When an "X" is present, this indicates the allergen is present. Always read all food labels to ensure allergens are not present.

Wheat	Milk	Eggs	Fish Shellfish	Soy	Peanuts/Nuts	Other
X		X		X		

Key: SF= Salt Free D= Diet or Sugarfree LF = Lowfat FF = Fat Free GF = Gluten Free

Recipe Name: Bacon, Lettuce, Cheese and Tomato Sandwich
Recipe Category: Pork Lunch
Portion Size: 1 sandwich
Ingredients: Yields: 8 servings

Ingredients	Notes:
16 Slices bacon	
8 Lettuce leaves	Washed, trimmed and any tough stems removed.
3 Large tomatoes	Washed, trimmed and sliced.
1/2 Cup light mayonnaise	
16 Slices bread	
8 Slices of lowfat cheese	American or cheddar

Directions:

Steps:	Directions:	Critical Control Point / Quality Assurance
1	Sauté bacon until crisp.	
2	Drain fat.	
3	Toast bread slices.	
4	Slice tomatoes.	
5	Top each sandwich with mayonnaise, lettuce leaves, tomato slices, cheese, and bacon. Serve immediately.	

Time Temperature Sensitive food. Food safety Standards: Do not mix old product with new. Store leftovers in a tightly sealed, labeled and dated container. Use leftover within 72 hours if stored in refrigerator. Do not freeze. Cold holding at 41°F or colder or using time alone (less than four hours).

Special Diets:

Texture Modified Diets:

Soft & Bite Size: (aka Bite size) **Food particle size ½ inch (~width of standard fork)** Food must be moist. Cut foods with a knife to a ½" particle size prior to layering. Moisten with broth or milk as needed. Foods that do not process well should be omitted. Omit: bacon. May use lean ham.

Chopped: Food particle size ¼ inch (~ ½ width of standard fork) Food must be moist. Chop foods with a knife to 1/4" particle size prior to layering. Moisten with broth as needed. Foods that do not process well should be omitted. Omit: bacon. May use lean ham.

Minced and Moist: (aka Minced/Mechanical Soft/Ground) **Food particle size 1/8 inch (fits through prongs of standard fork)** Food must be moist. Use a food processor to grind food particles into 1/8 inch prior to layering. Moisten with broth as needed. Foods that do not process well should be omitted. Omit: bacon. May use lean ham.

Pureed: Smooth and cohesive. Use a food processor to puree to a smooth consistency. Foods are processed by grinding and then pureeing them. May add broth or sauce to puree. Do not add to much liquid. Puree should still hold its shape. Must not be firm or sticky. Puree foods while still hot. Appearance should be smooth like pudding. Foods that do not process well should be omitted. Omit: bacon. May use lean ham. Serve 1/3 cup puree ham, 1 cup puree bread with mayonnaise and tomato separately.

Therapeutic Modified Diets:

Lowfat: Replace bacon with lean ham slices and use light mayonnaise
Diabetic/No added Sugar/No Conc. Sweets/Calorie Controlled: No changes need. **Bland/Anti Reflux:** Serve a cheese sandwich with light mayonnaise.
Liberal House Renal: Serve alternate menu item.
No Added Salt: Replace bacon with low sodium lean deli meat.
2 Gram Sodium: Use alternate menu item.
Gluten Free: Use gluten free bread. Prepare foods separately to prevent cross contamination.
Allergy Alerts: When an "X" is present, this indicates the allergen is present.
Always read all food labels to ensure allergens are not present.

Wheat	Milk	Eggs	Fish Shellfish	Soy	Peanuts/Nuts	Other
X	X					

Key: SF= Salt Free D= Diet or Sugarfree LF = Lowfat FF = Fat Free GF = Gluten Free

Recipe Name: Bacon Lettuce and Tomato Wraps
Recipe Category: Lunch Entree
Portion Size: 1 wrap
Ingredients: Yields: 8 servings

Ingredients	Notes:
6 inch flour tortillas	
1 pound shredded lowfat cheddar cheese	
½ pound bacon	Cooked crisp and crumbled
8 oz. light cream cheese,	Soften
1/2 cup light mayonnaise	
1 cup chopped tomatoes	
2 cups shredded lettuce	

Directions:

Steps:	Directions:	Critical Control Point /Quality Assurance
1	Heat each tortilla in a large skillet. Remove tortilla from skillet.	
2	Combine cream cheese and mayonnaise in a small bowl. Spread each tortilla with cream cheese mixture.	
3	Arrange tomato, cheese and bacon on each tortilla. Top with lettuce.	
4	Roll up tight and cover each with plastic wrap Refrigerate for 1 hour before serving. Chill.	

Time Temperature Sensitive food. *Food safety Standards: Do not mix old product with new. Store leftovers in a tightly sealed, labeled and dated container. Use leftover within 72 hours if stored in refrigerator. Do not freeze. Cold holding at 41°F or colder or using time alone (less than four hours).*

<u>**Texture Modified Diets:**</u>

Soft & Bite Size: (aka Bite size) **Food particle size ½ inch (~width of standard fork)** Food must be moist. Cut foods with a knife to a ½" particle size prior to layering. Moisten with broth or milk as needed. Foods that do not process well should be omitted. Omit: bacon. May use lean ham.

Chopped: Food particle size ¼ inch (~ ½ width of standard fork) Food must be moist. Chop foods with a knife to 1/4" particle size prior to layering. Moisten with broth as needed. Foods that do not process well should be omitted. Omit: bacon. May use lean ham.

Minced and Moist: (aka Minced/Mechanical Soft/Ground) **Food particle size 1/8 inch (fits through prongs of standard fork)** Food must be moist. Use a food processor to grind food particles into 1/8 inch prior to layering. Moisten with broth as needed. Foods that do not process well should be omitted. Omit: bacon. May use lean ham.

Pureed: Smooth and cohesive. Use a food processor to puree to a smooth consistency. Foods are processed by grinding and then pureeing them. May add broth or sauce to puree. Do not add to much liquid. Puree should still hold its shape. Must not be firm or sticky. Puree foods while still hot. Appearance should be smooth like pudding. Foods that do not process well should be omitted. Omit: bacon. May use lean ham. Serve 1/3 cup puree ham, 1 cup puree bread with mayonnaise and tomato separately. Puree ¼ cup ham and 1/4 cup cheese to serve as ½ cup meat. Puree tortillas with all other ingredients and serve ½ cup separately

<u>**Therapeutic Modified Diets:**</u>

Lowfat: Omit bacon and substitute lean ham.
Diabetic/No added Sugar/No Conc. Sweets/Calorie Controlled: no changes needed. **Bland/Anti Reflux:** Omit bacon and substitute lean ham. Omit tomatoes
Liberal House Renal: Use alternative recipe.
No Added Salt: Replace bacon with lean chicken slices.
2 Gram Sodium: Use alternate menu item.
Gluten Free: Use gluten free corn tortillas. Prepare foods separately to prevent cross contamination.

Allergy Alerts: When an "X" is present, this indicates the allergen is present. Always read all food labels to ensure allergens are not present.

Wheat	Milk	Eggs	Fish Shellfish	Soy	Peanuts/Nuts	Other
X	X					

Key: SF= Salt Free D= Diet or Sugarfree LF = Lowfat FF = Fat Free GF = Gluten Free

Recipe Name: Grilled Ham and Cheese Sandwich
Recipe Category: Pork Lunch
Portion Size: 1 sandwich
Ingredients: Yields: 8 servings

Ingredients	Notes:
1/4 Cup margarine	Softened
8 Slices American cheese (1 oz.)	May use other low fat sliced cheese
1 lb. sliced lean ham	
16 Slices bread	Wheat or white

Directions:

Steps:	Directions:	Critical Control Point /QualityAssurance
1	Put 1 slice of cheese and 2 oz. ham between 2 slices of bread.	
2	Spread margarine on the outside of each slice of bread.	
3	Heat a large skillet, and place sandwich in skillet.	
4	Cook until golden brown and then turn until both sides are golden brown.	
5	Repeat until 8 sandwiches are made.	

Time Temperature Sensitive food. *Food safety Standards: Food safety Standards: hold food for service at an internal temperature above 140° F. Do not mix old product with new. Cool leftover product quickly (within 4 hours) to below 41° F. Follow proper cooling procedures. Store leftovers in a tightly sealed, labeled and dated container. Use leftover within 72 hours if stored in refrigerator or 30 days if stored in the freezer. Reheat leftover product quickly (within 2 hours) to 165 degrees F for 15 seconds. Reheat left over product only once; discard if not used. Cold holding at 41°F or colder or using time alone (less than four hours).*

Texture Modified Diets:

Soft & Bite Size: (aka Bite size) **Food particle size ½ inch (~width of standard fork)** Food must be moist. Cut foods with a knife to a ½" particle size after cooking. Moisten with milk as needed after cutting.

Chopped: Food particle size ¼ inch (~ ½ width of standard fork) Food must be moist. Chop foods with a knife to 1/4" particle size after cooking. Moisten with milk as needed after chopping.

Minced and Moist: (aka Minced/Mechanical Soft/Ground) **Food particle size 1/8 inch (fits through prongs of standard fork)** Food must be moist. Use a food processor to grind food particles into 1/8 inch after cooking. Moisten with milk as needed after processing.

Pureed: Smooth and cohesive. Use a food processor to puree to a smooth consistency. Foods are processed by grinding and then pureeing them. May add milk or sauce to puree. Do not add to much liquid. Puree should still hold its shape. Must not be firm or sticky. Puree foods while still hot. Appearance should be smooth like pudding. Serve 1 c. serving.

Therapeutic Modified Diets:

Lowfat: No changes needed
Diabetic/No added Sugar/No Conc. Sweets/Calorie Controlled: No changes needed
Bland/Anti Reflux: No changes needed
Liberal House Renal: Use SF bread and SF margarine. Use low sodium ham meat (less than 140 mg. per serving)
No Added Salt: Use low sodium ham.
2 Gram Sodium: Use SF bread and SF margarine. Use low sodium ham meat (less than 140 mg. per serving)
Gluten Free: Use gluten free bread. Prepare foods separately to prevent cross contamination.
Allergy Alerts: When an "X" is present, this indicates the allergen is present.
Always read all food labels to ensure allergens are not present.

Wheat	Milk	Eggs	Fish Shellfish	Soy	Peanuts/Nuts	Other
X	X			X		

Key: SF= Salt Free D= Diet or Sugarfree LF = Lowfat FF = Fat Free GF = Gluten Free

Recipe Name: Pork and Corn Salad or Chicken and Corn Salad
Recipe Category: Lunch Entrée
Portion Size: 1/2 cup vegetables with 2 oz. meat on top
Ingredients: Yields: 8 servings

Ingredients	Notes:
1 pound cooked pork loin roast, sliced thin across the grain or 1 lb. cooked sliced chicken	(see recipe in cookbook for pork loin roast)(may use pork tenderloin)
4 cups frozen corn, thawed	
1 cup fresh tomatoes, chopped	Washed, trimmed and chopped
¼ cup oil	
½ cup red wine vinegar	
1 teaspoon dried cilantro	
1/2 cup green onion, chopped	Washed, trimmed and chopped
½ teaspoon garlic	
1 Tablespoon Dijon mustard	
½ teaspoon pepper	
½ teaspoon salt	
1 Avocado, diced (optional)	
Lettuce leaves (optional)	

Directions:

Steps:	Directions:	Critical Control Point /Quality Assurance
1	In a small bowl, whisk together oil, red wine vinegar, garlic, cilantro, mustard, pepper and salt. Chill	
2	In large bowl corn tomato and green onions, toss gently. Chill.	
3	Pour dressing over and toss gently.	
4	Serve on lettuce leave. Top with pork (or chicken)	
5	Top with avocado. Serve chilled.	

Time Temperature Sensitive food. *Food safety Standards: Do not mix old product with new. Cool leftover product quickly (within 4 hours) to below 41°F. Follow proper cooling procedures. Store leftovers in a tightly sealed, labeled and dated container. Use leftover within 72 hours if stored in refrigerator. Do not freeze. Cold holding at 41°F or colder or using time alone (less than four hours).*

Texture Modified Diets:

Soft & Bite Size: (aka Bite size) **Food particle size ½ inch (~width of standard fork)** Food must be moist. Cut foods with a knife to a ½" particle size prior to mixing. Moisten with broth as needed. Foods that do not process well should be omitted. Omit: green onions and corn. May sub. black beans for corn.

Chopped: Food particle size ¼ inch (~ ½ width of standard fork) Food must be moist. Chop foods with a knife to 1/4" particle size prior to mixing. Moisten with broth as needed. Foods that do not process well should be omitted. Omit: green onions and corn. May sub. black beans for corn.

Minced and Moist: (aka Minced/Mechanical Soft/Ground) **Food particle size 1/8 inch (fits through prongs of standard fork)** Food must be moist. Use a food processor to grind food particles into 1/8 inch prior to mixing. Moisten with broth as needed. Foods that do not process well should be omitted. Omit: green onions and corn. May sub. black beans for corn.

Pureed: Smooth and cohesive. Use a food processor to puree to a smooth consistency. Foods are processed by grinding and then pureeing them. May add broth or sauce to puree. Do not add to much liquid. Puree should still hold its shape. Must not be firm or sticky. Puree foods while still hot. Appearance should be smooth like pudding. Foods that do not process well should be omitted. Omit: green onions and corn. May sub. black beans for corn.

Serve ½ c. meat serving. And ½ c. puree bean mixture separately.

Therapeutic Modified Diets:

Lowfat: No changes needed
Diabetic/No added Sugar/No Conc. Sweets/Calorie Controlled: No changes needed
Bland: use alternate menu item
Liberal House Renal: Omit tomatoes and salt.
No Added Salt: No changes needed
2 Gram Sodium: omit salt
Gluten Free: No changes needed. Prepare foods separately to prevent cross contamination.

Allergy Alerts: When an "X" is present, this indicates the allergen is present.

Wheat	Milk	Eggs	Fish Shellfish	Soy	Peanuts/Nuts	Other

Key: SF= Salt Free D= Diet or Sugarfree LF = Lowfat FF = Fat Free GF = Gluten Free

Copyright 2020 Jacqueline Larson M.S., R.D.N. and Associates. All Rights Reserved

Recipe Name: Pork Tenderloin and Couscous Salad with Raisins and Walnuts
Recipe Category: Lunch Entrée
Portion Size: 1 cup (approx. 2 oz. chicken and ½ c. pasta)
Ingredients: Yields: 8 servings

Ingredients	Notes:
1 pound cooked pork tenderloin, cut into thin slices across the grain.	
2 cups uncooked couscous	
1 cup lowfat buttermilk	
2 teaspoons cumin	
1 teaspoon salt	
½ teaspoon black pepper	
½ cup chopped unsalted walnuts	Or almonds
2 tablespoons dried mint or cilantro	Or ¼ cup of fresh. Wash and minced
½ cup raisons	
4 green onions	Wash, trim and slice (including greens)
2 teaspoon olive oil	
1 clove garlic, minced	Wash, peel and mince

Directions:

Steps:	Directions:	Critical Control Point /Quality Assurance
1	Bring broiler to high. Brush pork with oil. Arrange chicken or pork on single layer in a large oven proof pan. Season with salt and pepper Broil on top rack for 5 minutes and turn. Broil an additional 3 minutes or until done.	Cook until internal temperature reaches 145°F for 15 seconds for pork.
2	Bring 3 cups of water to boil in a large pot. Stir in couscous and remove from heat. Let stand covered for 5 minutes. Fluff couscous with a fork.	
3	In a small bowl, combine cumin and buttermilk. Add couscous, garlic, chopped walnuts, mint, or cilantro, and raison. Toss to coast	
4	Serve couscous topped with pork. Top with green onions	
5	Serve immediately or chilled.	

Time Temperature Sensitive food. *Food safety Standards: Do not mix old product with new. Cool leftover product quickly (within 4 hours) to below 41°F. Follow proper cooling procedures. Store leftovers in a tightly sealed, labeled and dated container. Use leftover within 72 hours if stored in refrigerator or 30 days if stored in the freezer. seconds. Cold holding at 41°F or colder or using time alone (less than four hours).*

Texture Modified Diets:

Soft & Bite Size: (aka Bite size) **Food particle size ½ inch (~width of standard fork)** Food must be moist. Cut foods with a knife to a ½" particle size prior to mixing. Moisten with broth as needed. Foods that do not process well should be omitted. Omit: nuts, green onions, and raisons

Chopped: Food particle size ¼ inch (~ ½ width of standard fork) Food must be moist. Chop foods with a knife to 1/4" particle size prior to mixing. Moisten with broth as needed. Foods that do not process well should be omitted. Omit: nuts, green onions, and raisons

Minced and Moist:(aka Minced/Mechanical Soft/Ground) **Food particle size 1/8 inch (fits through prongs of standard fork)** Food must be moist. Use a food processor to grind food particles into 1/8 inch prior to mixing. Moisten with broth as needed. Foods that do not process well should be omitted. Omit: nuts, green onions, and raisons

Pureed: Smooth and cohesive. Use a food processor to puree to a smooth consistency. Foods are processed by grinding and then pureeing them. May add broth or sauce to puree. Do not add to much liquid. Puree should still hold its shape. Must not be firm or sticky. Puree foods while still hot. Appearance should be smooth like pudding. Foods that do not process well should be omitted. Omit: nuts, green onions, and raisons. Serve ½ c. puree meat serving and ½ c. puree couscous mixture separately.

Therapeutic Modified Diets:
Lowfat: No changes needed
Diabetic/No added Sugar/No Conc. Sweets/Calorie Controlled: No changes needed
Bland: omit nuts, raison, cumin, pepper, garlic, mint, cilantro, and green onions
Liberal House Renal: omit salt
No Added Salt: No changes needed
2 Gram Sodium: omit salt
Gluten Free: Use GF pasta in place of couscous. Prepare foods separately to prevent cross contamination.
Allergy Alerts: When an "X" is present, this indicates the allergen is present.

Wheat	Milk	Eggs	Fish Shellfish	Soy	Peanuts/Nuts	Other
X	X	X			X	

Key: SF= Salt Free D= Diet or Sugarfree LF = Lowfat FF = Fat Free GF = Gluten Free

SAUSAGE DINNER RECIPES

Recipe Name: Brats Sandwich
Recipe Category: Dinner Entrée
Portion Size: 1 Brats with bun
Ingredients: Yields: 8 servings

Ingredients	Notes:
8 Brats (3 oz.)	
8 Hot dog buns	
Catsup, mustard, relish, onions, sauerkraut	optional

Directions:

Steps:	Directions:	Critical Control Point / Quality Assurance
1	Cover brats with a small amount of water in saucepan. Bring to a boil.	
2	Let water evaporate. Cook to brown on sides	
3	Reduce heat and simmer 3 to 4 minutes	Cook until temperature reaches 165 degrees.
4	Place well drained Brats in a hot dog bun	
5	Top with catsup, mustard, relish, sauerkraut, and onions as desired.	

Time Temperature Sensitive food. *Food safety Standards: hold food for service at an internal temperature above 140° F. Do not mix old product with new. Cool leftover product quickly (within 4 hours) to below 41° F. Follow proper cooling procedures. Store leftovers in a tightly sealed, labeled and dated container. Use leftover within 72 hours if stored in refrigerator or 30 days if stored in the freezer. Reheat leftover product quickly (within 2 hours) to 165 degrees F for 15 seconds. Reheat left over product only once; discard if not used. Cold holding at 41°F or colder or using time alone (less than four hours).*

Texture Modified Diets: NO Brats: skin is too tough.
Soft & Bite Size: (aka Bite size) **Food particle size ½ inch (~width of standard fork)** Food must be moist. Cut foods with a knife to a ½" particle size prior to mixing. Moisten with broth as needed. Foods that do not process well should be omitted. Omit: Brats and sub. ground turkey or bulk. Italian sausage. Top with condiments.
Chopped: Food particle size ¼ inch (~ ½ width of standard fork) Food must be moist. Chop foods with a knife to 1/4" particle size prior to mixing. Moisten with broth as needed. Foods that do not process well should be omitted. Omit: Brats and sub. ground turkey or bulk. Italian sausage. Top with condiments.
Minced and Moist: (aka Minced/Mechanical Soft/Ground) **Food particle size 1/8 inch (fits through prongs of standard fork)** Food must be moist. Use a food processor to grind food particles into 1/8 inch prior to mixing. Moisten with broth as needed. Foods that do not process well should be omitted. Omit: Brats and sub. ground turkey or bulk. Italian sausage. Top with condiments.
Pureed: Smooth and cohesive. Use a food processor to puree to a smooth consistency. Foods are processed by grinding and then pureeing them. May add broth or sauce to puree. Do not add to much liquid. Puree should still hold its shape. Must not be firm or sticky. Puree foods while still hot. Appearance should be smooth like pudding. Foods that do not process well should be omitted. Omit: hot dogs and sub. ground turkey or bulk Italian sausage. Top with condiments. Serve ½ puree ground turkey or puree bulk Italian sausage and 1/2 cup puree bread with toppings.

Therapeutic Modified Diets:
Low fat: Omit cheese. Use lowfat brats dogs.
Diabetic/No added Sugar/No Conc. Sweets/Calorie Controlled: No changes needed
Bland/Anti Reflux: Use alternate menu item
Liberal House Renal: Use alternate menu item
No Added Salt: Use alternate menu item
2 Gram Sodium: Use alternate menu item
Gluten Free: Use gluten free bun or bread. Use gluten free hot dogs. Prepare foods separately to prevent cross contamination.
Allergy Alerts: When an "X" is present, this indicates the allergen is present.
Always read all food labels to ensure allergens are not present.

Wheat	Milk	Eggs	Fish Shellfish	Soy	Peanuts/Nuts	Other
X	X					

Key: SF= Salt Free D= Diet or Sugarfree LF = Lowfat FF = Fat Free GF = Gluten Free

Recipe Name: Cheese Sausage Quiche
Recipe Category: Sausage
Portion Size: 1 slice (1/8 of pie or ¾ cup)
Ingredients: Yields: 8 servings

Ingredients	Notes:
1 pastry shell (8 inch)	unbaked
2 pounds lean pork or turkey sausage	
1 green pepper	Washed, trimmed and chopped
2 cups low fat cheddar cheese	shredded
3 eggs	
2 Tablespoon all-purpose flour	
1 Tablespoon parsley flakes	
1/2 teaspoon salt	
1/4 teaspoon garlic salt	
1/4 teaspoon black pepper	
2 cups fat free evaporated milk	

Directions:

Steps:	Directions:	Critical Control Point /Quality Assurance
1	Preheat oven to 425 degrees.	
2	Prepare pastry shell. Bake 7 minutes; remove from oven. Reduce heat to 350 degrees.	
3	In a medium skillet, brown sausage. Reserve 2 tablespoons fat; drain off remaining fat.	
4	Saute onion and green pepper in reserved fat until crisp tender, about 2 minutes. Stir in drained sausage.	
5	Spoon into partially baked shell; sprinkle with cheese.	
6	In a medium sized bowl, beat eggs until well blended.	
7	Add remaining ingredients; mix well. Pour over cheese.	
8	Bake at 350 degrees for 30-35 minutes. Cool for 5 to 10 minutes; cut into wedges to serve.	Bake until knife inserted comes out clean. Cook until internal temperature reaches 165 F.

Time Temperature Sensitive food. Food safety Standards: hold food for service at an Do not mix old product with new. Cool leftover product quickly (within 4 hours) to below 41°F. Follow proper cooling procedures. Store leftovers in a tightly sealed, labeled and dated container. Use leftover within 72 hours if stored in refrigerator or 30 days if stored in the freezer. Reheat leftover product quickly (within 2 hours) to 165 degrees F for 15 seconds. Reheat left over product only once; discard if not used. Cold holding at 41°F or colder or using time alone (less than four hours). Always wash hands and wash and sanitize counter tops utensils and containers between steps when working with raw meat.

Texture Modified Diets:
Soft & Bite Size: (aka Bite size) **Food particle size ½ inch (~width of standard fork)** Food must be moist. Cut foods with a knife to a ½" particle size prior to mixing. Moisten with milk as needed.
Chopped: Food particle size ¼ inch (~ ½ width of standard fork) Food must be moist. Chop foods with a knife to 1/4" particle size prior to mixing. Moisten with milk as needed.
Minced and Moist: (aka Minced/Mechanical Soft/Ground) **Food particle size 1/8 inch (fits through prongs of standard fork)** Food must be moist. Use a food processor to grind food particles into 1/8 inch prior to mixing. Moisten with milk as needed.
Pureed: Smooth and cohesive. Use a food processor to puree to a smooth consistency. Foods are processed by grinding and then pureeing them. May add broth or sauce to puree. Do not add to much liquid. Puree should still hold its shape. Must not be firm or sticky. Puree foods while still hot. Appearance should be smooth like pudding. Serve 3/4 c. serving.

Therapeutic Modified Diets:
Lowfat: Omit pie crust.
Diabetic/No added Sugar/No Conc. Sweets/Calorie Controlled: No changes needed
Bland/Anti Reflux: Omit pie crust, parsley, green pepper, garlic, and black pepper.
Liberal House Renal: Use alternate menu item.
No Added Salt: No changes needed
2 Gram Sodium: Use alternate menu item
Gluten Free: Use gluten free all-purpose flour and GF pie crust or omit. Prepare foods separately to prevent cross contamination.

Allergy Alerts: When an "X" is present, this indicates the allergen is present. Always read all food labels to ensure allergens are not present.

Wheat	Milk	Eggs	Fish Shellfish	Soy	Peanuts/Nuts	Other
X	X	X				

Key: SF= Salt Free D= Diet or Sugarfree LF = Lowfat FF = Fat Free GF = Gluten Free

Recipe Name: Hawaiian Pineapple with Sweet and Sour Turkey Sausage
Recipe Category: Sausage Dinner
Portion Size: 1 cup (1/2 cup rice and ½ cup meat mixture)
Ingredients: Yields: 8 servings
Directions:

Steps:	Directions:	Critical Control Point /Quality Assurance
1	Cook and stir the bell peppers in oil over medium-high heat for 5 minutes	
2	Add the sausage and cook until lightly browned and peppers are tender.	
3	Add chili garlic sauce and pineapple; cook and stir for 5 minutes. Serve over cooked rice.	Cook until internal temperature reaches 165 F.

Time Temperature Sensitive food. *Food safety Standards: hold food for service at an internal temperature above 140° F. Do not mix old product with new. Cool leftover product quickly (within 4 hours) to below 41° F. Follow proper cooling procedures. Store leftovers in a tightly sealed, labeled and dated container. Use leftover within 72 hours if stored in refrigerator or 30 days if stored in the freezer. Reheat leftover product quickly (within 2 hours) to 165 degrees F for 15 seconds. Reheat left over product only once; discard if not used. Cold holding at 41 °F or colder or using time alone (less than four hours). Always wash hands and wash and sanitize counter tops utensils and containers between steps when working with raw meat.*

Texture Modified Diets:

Soft & Bite Size: (aka Bite size) **Food particle size ½ inch (~width of standard fork)** Food must be moist. Cut foods with a knife to a ½" particle size prior to mixing. Moisten with broth as needed. Substitute chicken for turkey sausage and green beans for pineapple.

Chopped: Food particle size ¼ inch (~ ½ width of standard fork) Food must be moist. Chop foods with a knife to 1/4" particle size prior to mixing. Moisten with broth as needed. Substitute chicken for turkey sausage and green beans for pineapple.

Minced and Moist: (aka Minced/Mechanical Soft/Ground) **Food particle size 1/8 inch (fits through prongs of standard fork)** Food must be moist. Use a food processor to grind food particles into 1/8 inch prior to mixing. Moisten with broth as needed. Substitute chicken for turkey sausage and green beans for pineapple.

Pureed: Smooth and cohesive. Use a food processor to puree to a smooth consistency. Foods are processed by grinding and then pureeing them. May add broth or sauce to puree. Do not add to much liquid. Puree should still hold its shape. Must not be firm or sticky. Puree foods while still hot. Appearance should be smooth like pudding. Substitute chicken for turkey sausage and green beans for pineapple. Serve ½ c. puree chicken topped with puree sauce and ½ cup puree rice separately.

Therapeutic Modified Diets:

Lowfat: No changes needed.
Diabetic/No added Sugar/No Conc. Sweets/Calorie Controlled: Omit sweet Chili Sauce
Bland/Anti Reflux: Use alternate menu item.
Liberal House Renal: Use alternate menu item.
No Added Salt: Use alternate menu items.
2 Gram Sodium: Use alternate menu item.
Gluten Free: Use GF turkey sausage and GF sweet chili garlic sauce. Prepare separately to prevent cross contamination.
Allergy Alerts: When an "X" is present, this indicates the allergen is present.
Always read all food labels to ensure allergens are not present.

Wheat	Milk	Eggs	Fish Shellfish	Soy	Peanuts/Nuts	Other
X						

Key: SF= Salt Free D= Diet or Sugarfree LF = Lowfat FF = Fat Free GF = Gluten Free

Copyright 2020 Jacqueline Larson M.S., R.D.N. and Associates.   All Rights Reserved

Recipe Name: Italian Sausage Soup Minestrone
Recipe Category: Sausage
Portion Size: 2 cups
Ingredients: Yields: 8 servings

Ingredients	Notes:
2 pounds lean sweet Italian sausage	Use links or bulk
1 medium onion	Washed, peeled and chopped
1 teaspoon garlic powder	
5 cups beef broth	
1 cup water	
1 can (14 oz.) tomatoes sauce	
1 cup carrots	Washed, peeled and sliced thin
1 can (14 oz.) dark kidney beans	
1 can (14 oz.) garbanzo beans	
1 teaspoon basil	
1 teaspoon oregano	
1 ½ cup zucchini	Washed, trimmed and sliced.
1 cup cauliflower	Washed, trimmed and cut up
8 ounces pasta	May use whole grain
2 Tablespoon parsley flakes	
1 bag fresh baby spinach	Washed and trimmed
¼ cup Parmesan cheese	

Directions:

Steps:	Directions:	Critical Control Point / Quality Assurance
1	In a large stock pot, add sausage and brown.	Cook until internal temperature reaches 165 F.
2	Remove sausage and drain, reserving 1 T. of the drippings. Slice links.	
3	Saute onion and garlic in the drippings.	
4	Stir in flour.	
5	Stir in beef broth, water, tomato sauce, garbanzo beans, kidney beans, cauliflower, carrots, basil, oregano, tomato sauce and sausage.	
6	Bring to a boil.	
7	Reduce heat; simmer uncovered for 30 minutes.	
8	Stir in zucchini and parsley.	
9	Simmer covered for 30 minutes.	
10	Add pasta and simmer for 10 minutes.	
11	Add spinach and cook for 2 minutes with the lid off. Serve in bowls.	
12	Top with Parmesan cheese.	

Time Temperature Sensitive food. *Food safety Standards: hold food for service at an internal temperature above 140° F. Do not mix old product with new. Cool leftover product quickly (within 4 hours) to below 41° F. Follow proper cooling procedures. Store leftovers in a tightly sealed, labeled and dated container. Use leftover within 72 hours if stored in refrigerator or 30 days if stored in the freezer. Reheat leftover product quickly (within 2 hours) to 165 degrees F for 15 seconds. Reheat left over product only once; discard if not used. Cold holding at 41°F or colder or using time alone (less than four hours). Always wash hands and wash and sanitize counter tops utensils and containers between steps when working with raw meat.*

Texture Modified Diets: TIP: use pasta within the correct particle size and ground bulk Italian sausage.
Soft & Bite Size: (aka Bite size) **Food particle size ½ inch (~width of standard fork)** Food must be moist. Cut foods with a knife to a ½" particle size prior to mixing. Moisten with broth as needed.
Chopped: Food particle size ¼ inch (~ ½ width of standard fork) Food must be moist. Chop foods with a knife to 1/4" particle size prior to mixing. Moisten with broth as needed.
Minced and Moist:(aka Minced/Mechanical Soft/Ground) **Food particle size 1/8 inch (fits through prongs of standard fork)** Food must be moist. Use a food processor to grind food particles into 1/8 inch prior to mixing. Moisten with broth as needed.

Copyright 2020 Jacqueline Larson M.S., R.D.N. and Associates.   All Rights Reserved

Pureed: Smooth and cohesive. Use a food processor to puree to a smooth consistency. Foods are processed by grinding and then pureeing them. May add broth or sauce to puree. Do not add to much liquid. Puree should still hold its shape. Must not be firm or sticky. Puree foods while still hot. Appearance should be smooth like pudding. Serve ½ c. puree Italian sausage, ½ c. puree pasta and ½ cup puree vegetables separately.

<u>Therapeutic Modified Diets:</u>
Lowfat: No changes needed
Diabetic/No added Sugar/No Conc. Sweets/Calorie Controlled: No changes needed
Bland/Anti Reflux: Use alternate menu item.
Liberal House Renal: Use alternate menu item.
No Added Salt: No changes needed
2 Gram Sodium: Use alternate menu item.
Gluten Free: Use GF turkey sausage, GF pasta, GF flour and GF broth . Prepare foods separately to prevent cross contamination.
Allergy Alerts: When an "X" is present, this indicates the allergen is present.
Always read all food labels to ensure allergens are not present.

Wheat	Milk	Eggs	Fish Shellfish	Soy	Peanuts/Nuts	Other
X	X	X				

Key: SF= Salt Free D= Diet or Sugarfree LF = Lowfat FF = Fat Free GF = Gluten Free

Recipe Name: Italian Sausage Sandwich
Recipe Category: Sausage
Portion Size: ½ cup meat mixture on 1 roll
Ingredients: Yields: 8 servings

Ingredients	Notes:
8 French style rolls	
2 pounds bulk lean Italian sausage (turkey)	(Use bulk for texture modified diets)
1 16-ounce can pizza sauce	
1 8-ounce can mushrooms stems and pieces	Drained. (optional)
2 medium green peppers	Washed, trimmed and diced
12 ounces sliced low fat mozzarella cheese	

Directions:

Steps:	Directions:	Critical Control Point / Quality Assurance
1	In a skillet, cook sausage till no ink remains. Drain fat.	Cook until internal temperature reaches 165 F.
2	Stir in pizza sauce, green pepper, and mushrooms; heat through.	
3	Slice rolls in half. Spoon in meat mixture.	
4	Top with and cheese.	
5	Place sandwiches in a shallow baking pan or on a baking sheet.	
6	Cover tightly with foil and heat in a 375 degree oven for 15 minutes or till cheese melts and sandwiches are hot.	

Time Temperature Sensitive food. Food safety Standards: hold food for service at an internal temperature above 140° F. Do not mix old product with new. Cool leftover product quickly (within 4 hours) to below 41° F. Follow proper cooling procedures. Store leftovers in a tightly sealed, labeled and dated container. Use leftover within 72 hours if stored in refrigerator or 30 days if stored in the freezer. Reheat leftover product quickly (within 2 hours) to 165 degrees F for 15 seconds. Reheat left over product only once; discard if not used. Cold holding at 41°F or colder or using time alone (less than four hours). Always wash hands and wash and sanitize counter tops utensils and containers between steps when working with raw meat.

Texture Modified Diets: TIP: bulk Italian sausage without skin.
Soft & Bite Size: (aka Bite size) **Food particle size ½ inch (~width of standard fork)** Food must be moist. Cut foods with a knife to a ½" particle size prior to mixing and layering. Moisten with broth as needed.
Chopped: Food particle size ¼ inch (~ ½ width of standard fork) Food must be moist. Chop foods with a knife to 1/4" particle size prior to mixing and layering. Moisten with broth as needed.
Minced and Moist: (aka Minced/Mechanical Soft/Ground) **Food particle size 1/8 inch (fits through prongs of standard fork)** Food must be moist. Use a food processor to grind food particles into 1/8 inch prior to mixing and layering. Moisten with broth as needed.
Pureed: Smooth and cohesive. Use a food processor to puree to a smooth consistency. Foods are processed by grinding and then pureeing them. May add broth or sauce to puree. Do not add to much liquid. Puree should still hold its shape. Must not be firm or sticky. Puree foods while still hot. Appearance should be smooth like pudding. Puree with sauce if needed. Serve ½ c. serving meat mixture and ½ c. puree bun separately.

Therapeutic Modified Diets:
Lowfat: No changes needed.
Diabetic/No added Sugar/No Conc. Sweets/Calorie Controlled: No changes needed.
Bland/Anti Reflux: Serve plain turkey sandwich.
Liberal House Renal: Use alternate menu item.
No Added Salt: No changes needed
2 Gram Sodium: Use alternate menu item.
Gluten Free: Use gluten-free bread, GF turkey sausage and GF pizza sauce. Prepare separately to prevent cross contamination.
Allergy Alerts: When an "X" is present, this indicates the allergen is present.
Always read all food labels to ensure allergens are not present.

Wheat	Milk	Eggs	Fish Shellfish	Soy	Peanuts/Nuts	Other
X	X	X				

Key: SF= Salt Free D= Diet or Sugarfree LF = Lowfat FF = Fat Free GF = Gluten Free

Recipe Name: Italian Sausage Soup with Tortellini
Recipe Category: Sausage
Portion Size: 2 cups
Ingredients: Yields: 8 servings

Ingredients	Notes:
2 pounds lean sweet Italian sausage (turkey)	Use bulk or links.
1 medium onion	Washed, peeled and chopped fine
1 teaspoon garlic powder	
2 tablespoon all purpose flour	
5 cups beef broth	
1 cup water	
1 large can (16 oz.) chopped tomatoes	
1 cup sliced thin carrots	Washed, peeled and sliced
1 teaspoon basil	
1/2 teaspoon oregano	
1 (8 oz.) can tomato sauce	
1 1/2 cup sliced zucchini	Washed, trimmed and sliced.
8 ounces tortellini pasta	
2 tablespoons parsley flakes	
1 bag fresh baby spinach	Washed and trimmed
1/4 cup Parmesan cheese	

Directions:

Steps:	Directions:	Critical Control Point / Quality Assurance
1	In a large stock pot add sausage and brown.	
2	Remove sausage and drain, reserving 1 tablespoon of the drippings.	
3	Slice sausage.	
4	Saute onion and garlic in the drippings. Add flour.	
5	Stir in beef broth, water, tomatoes, carrots, basil, oregano, tomato sauce, and sausage.	
6	Bring to a boil.	
7	Reduce heat; simmer uncovered for 30 minutes.	
8	Stir in zucchini and parsley.	
9	Simmer covered for 30 minutes.	
10	Add tortellini and simmer for 10 minutes.	
11	Add spinach and cook for 3 minutes with lid off.	
12	Top with Parmesan cheese.	

Time Temperature Sensitive food. *Food safety Standards: hold food for service at an internal temperature above 140° F. Do not mix old product with new. Cool leftover product quickly (within 4 hours) to below 41° F. Follow proper cooling procedures. Store leftovers in a tightly sealed, labeled and dated container. Use leftover within 72 hours if stored in refrigerator or 30 days if stored in the freezer. Reheat leftover product quickly (within 2 hours) to 165 degrees F for 15 seconds. Reheat left over product only once; discard if not used. Cold holding at 41°F or colder or using time alone (less than four hours). Always wash hands and wash and sanitize counter tops utensils and containers between steps when working with raw meat.*

<u>**Texture Modified Diets: TIP: use pasta within the correct particle size and ground bulk Italian sausage.**</u>
Soft & Bite Size: (aka Bite size) **Food particle size ½ inch (~width of standard fork)** Food must be moist. Cut foods with a knife to a ½" particle size prior to mixing. Moisten with broth as needed.
Chopped: Food particle size ¼ inch (~ ½ width of standard fork) Food must be moist. Chop foods with a knife to 1/4" particle size prior to mixing. Moisten with broth as needed.
Minced and Moist: (aka Minced/Mechanical Soft/Ground) **Food particle size 1/8 inch (fits through prongs of standard fork)** Food must be moist. Use a food processor to grind food particles into 1/8 inch prior to mixing. Moisten with broth as needed.
Pureed: Smooth and cohesive. Use a food processor to puree to a smooth consistency. Foods are processed by grinding and then pureeing them. May add broth or sauce to puree. Do not add to much liquid. Puree should still hold its shape. Must not be firm or sticky. Puree foods while still hot. Appearance should be smooth like pudding.

Copyright 2020 Jacqueline Larson M.S., R.D.N. and Associates.   All Rights Reserved

Serve ½ c. puree Italian sausage, ½ c. puree pasta and ½ cup puree vegetables separately.

Therapeutic Modified Diets:
Lowfat: No changes needed.
Diabetic/No added Sugar/No Conc. Sweets/Calorie Controlled: No changes needed.
Bland/Anti Reflux: Use alternate menu item.
Liberal House Renal: Use alternate menu item
No Added Salt: No changes needed.
2 Gram Sodium: Use alternate menu item.
Gluten Free: Use gluten-free pasta, GF broth, and GF Italian sausage. Prepare separately to prevent cross contamination
Allergy Alerts: When an "X" is present, this indicates the allergen is present.
Always read all food labels to ensure allergens are not present.

Wheat	Milk	Eggs	Fish Shellfish	Soy	Peanuts/Nuts	Other
X	X	X				

Key: SF= Salt Free D= Diet or Sugarfree LF = Lowfat FF = Fat Free GF = Gluten Free

Recipe Name: Italian Sausage with Sweet Peppers and Pasta
Recipe Category: Sausage
Portion Size: 1 cup
Ingredients: **Yields: 8 servings**

Ingredients	Notes:
2 pounds mild Italian Sausage (turkey)	Use bulk for texture modified diets. No links
1 pound bow tie pasta	May use whole grain
3 medium red sweet pepper	Cut into 3/4 inch pieces
1 cup vegetable or beef broth	
1/2 teaspoon black pepper	
2 tablespoons parsley	
Grated Parmesan cheese	

Directions:

Steps:	Directions:	Critical Control Point /Quality Assurance
1	Prepare pasta according to directions on the package.	
2	Cut sausage into 1 inch pieces.	
3	In a large skillet cook sausage and sweet peppers over medium-high heat until sausage is brown.	Cook until internal temperature reaches 165 F.
4	Drain well.	
5	Stir in the broth and black pepper into skillet.	
6	Bring to boiling; reduce heat.	
7	Simmer uncovered for 5 minutes.	
8	Sprinkle with Parmesan cheese.	

Time Temperature Sensitive food: *Food safety Standards: hold food for service at an internal temperature above 140° F. Do not mix old product with new. Cool leftover product quickly (within 4 hours) to below 41° F. Follow proper cooling procedures. Store leftovers in a tightly sealed, labeled and dated container. Use leftover within 72 hours if stored in refrigerator or 30 days if stored in the freezer. Reheat leftover product quickly (within 2 hours) to 165 degrees F for 15 seconds. Reheat left over product only once; discard if not used. Cold holding at 41°F or colder or using time alone (less than four hours). Always wash hands and wash and sanitize counter tops utensils and containers between steps when working with raw meat.*

__Texture Modified Diets: TIP: use pasta within the correct particle size and ground bulk Italian sausage.__
Soft & Bite Size: (aka Bite size) **Food particle size ½ inch (~width of standard fork)** Food must be moist. Cut foods with a knife to a ½" particle size prior to mixing. Moisten with sauce as needed.
Chopped: Food particle size ¼ inch (~ ½ width of standard fork) Food must be moist. Chop foods with a knife to 1/4" particle size prior to mixing. Moisten with sauce as needed.
Minced and Moist:(aka Minced/Mechanical Soft/Ground) **Food particle size 1/8 inch (fits through prongs of standard fork)** Food must be moist. Use a food processor to grind food particles into 1/8 inch prior to mixing. Moisten with sauce as needed.
Pureed: Smooth and cohesive. Use a food processor to puree to a smooth consistency. Foods are processed by grinding and then pureeing them. May add broth or sauce to puree. Do not add to much liquid. Puree should still hold its shape. Must not be firm or sticky. Puree foods while still hot. Appearance should be smooth like pudding.
Serve ½ c. puree sausage and ½ c. puree pasta separately.
__Therapeutic Modified Diets:__
Lowfat: No changes needed.
Diabetic/No added Sugar/No Conc. Sweets/Calorie Controlled: No changes needed.
Bland/Anti Reflux: Use chicken in place of sausage. Omit pepper, parsley and black pepper.
Liberal House Renal: Use SF chicken in place of sausage. Use SF broth or water.
No Added Salt: No changes needed.
2 Gram Sodium: Use SF chicken in place of sausage. Use SF. Broth or water.
Gluten Free: Use gluten-free pasta, GF broth and GF turkey sausage. Prepare foods separately to prevent cross contamination.
Allergy Alerts: When an "X" is present, this indicates the allergen is present. Always read all food labels to ensure allergens are not present.

Wheat	Milk	Eggs	Fish Shellfish	Soy	Peanuts/Nuts	Other
X	X	X				

Key: SF= Salt Free D= Diet or Sugarfree LF = Lowfat FF = Fat Free GF = Gluten Free

Copyright 2020 Jacqueline Larson M.S., R.D.N. and Associates.   All Rights Reserved

Recipe Name: Jambalaya
Recipe Category: Sausage Dinner
Portion Size: 1 cup (1/2 c. rice and ½ c. meat mixture)
Ingredients: Yields: 8 servings

Ingredients	Notes:
1 lb boneless skinless chicken breast or thighs	
1 lb. lean kielbasa	Sliced
2 tablespoons cooking oil	
2 green bell peppers	Washed, trimmed and diced.
1 cup celery	Washed, trimmed and diced.
1 teaspoon garlic powder	
1/2 teaspoon cayenne pepper	
1 teaspoon onion powder	
Salt and pepper to taste	
4 cups cooked white rice	
6 cups low sodium chicken stock	
2 cups tomato sauce	
3 bay leaves	
2 teaspoons Worcestershire sauce	

Directions:

Steps:	Directions:	Critical Control Point / Quality Assurance
1	Heat oil in a large pot over medium high heat.	
2	Sauté chicken and kielbasa until lightly browned, about 5 minutes.	Cook until internal temperature reaches 165 F.
3	Stir in onion, bell pepper, celery and garlic.	
4	Season with cayenne, onion powder, salt and pepper.	
5	Cook 5 minutes o r until onion is translucent.	
6	Stir in chicken stock, tomato sauce, and bay leaves.	
7	Bring to a boil, then reduce heat, cover and simmer 5 minutes.	
8	Stir in Worcestershire sauce. Remove bay leaf.	
9	Serve over rice	

Time Temperature Sensitive food. *Food safety Standards: hold food for service at an internal temperature above 140° F. Do not mix old product with new. Cool leftover product quickly (within 4 hours) to below 41° F. Follow proper cooling procedures. Store leftovers in a tightly sealed, labeled and dated container. Use leftover within 72 hours if stored in refrigerator or 30 days if stored in the freezer. Reheat leftover product quickly (within 2 hours) to 165 degrees F for 15 seconds. Reheat left over product only once; discard if not used. Cold holding at 41°F or colder or using time alone (less than four hours). Always wash hands and wash and sanitize counter tops utensils and containers between steps when working with raw meat.*

Texture Modified Diets:

Soft & Bite Size: (aka Bite size) **Food particle size ½ inch (~width of standard fork)** Food must be moist. Cut foods with a knife to a ½" particle size prior to mixing. Moisten with broth as needed. Foods that do not process well should be omitted. Omit: Kielbasa and double chicken.

Chopped: Food particle size ¼ inch (~ ½ width of standard fork) Food must be moist. Chop foods with a knife to 1/4" particle size prior to mixing. Moisten with broth as needed. Foods that do not process well should be omitted. Omit: Kielbasa and double chicken

Minced and Moist: (aka Minced/Mechanical Soft/Ground) **Food particle size 1/8 inch (fits through prongs of standard fork)** Food must be moist. Use a food processor to grind food particles into 1/8 inch prior to mixing. Moisten with broth as needed. Foods that do not process well should be omitted. Omit: Kielbasa and double chicken

Pureed: Smooth and cohesive. Use a food processor to puree to a smooth consistency. Foods are processed by grinding and then pureeing them. May add broth or sauce to puree. Do not add to much liquid. Puree should still hold its shape. Must not be firm or sticky. Puree foods while still hot. Appearance should be smooth like pudding. Foods that do not process well should be omitted. Omit: Kielbasa and double chicken.
Serve ½ c. puree chicken mixture and ½ c. puree rice separately.

Therapeutic Modified Diets:
Lowfat: No changes needed.
Diabetic/No added Sugar/No Conc. Sweets/Calorie Controlled: No changes needed.
Bland/Anti Reflux: Serve ½ c. plain rice and ½ c. plain chicken.
Liberal House Renal: Serve ½ c. SF rice and ½ C. SF chicken
No Added Salt: No changes needed.
2 Gram Sodium: Serve ½ c. SF rice and ½ c. SF chicken.
Gluten Free: Use gluten-free stock and kielbasa. Prepare foods separately to prevent cross contamination.
Allergy Alerts: When an "X" is present, this indicates the allergen is present.
Always read all food labels to ensure allergens are not present.

Wheat	Milk	Eggs	Fish Shellfish	Soy	Peanuts/Nuts	Other
X			X			

Key: SF= Salt Free D= Diet or Sugarfree LF = Lowfat FF = Fat Free GF = Gluten Free

Recipe Name: Kielbasa and Potato Bake
Recipe Category: Sausage
Portion Size: 1 cup
Ingredients: Yields: 8 servings

Ingredients	Notes:
2 pounds rings lean turkey sausage (Kielbasa)	Diced
2 (14 oz.) cans fat free evaporated milk	
2 cloves garlic	Washed, peeled and minced
2 cups low fat shredded cheddar cheese	
1/2 teaspoon black pepper	
1 teaspoon poultry seasoning	
4 large russet potatoes	Washed, peeled and diced

Directions:

Steps:	Directions:	Critical Control Point / Quality Assurance
1	Preheat oven to 375 degrees.	
2	In a large mixing bowl, mix together cheese, milk, garlic and pepper.	
3	Stir in potatoes and kielbasa.	
4	Spoon the mixture into a large baking dish.	
5	Bake uncovered for 1 hour, or until potatoes are tender.	Cook until internal temperature reaches 165 F.

Time Temperature Sensitive food. *Food safety Standards: hold food for service at an internal temperature above 140° F. Do not mix old product with new. Cool leftover product quickly (within 4 hours) to below 41° F. Follow proper cooling procedures. Store leftovers in a tightly sealed, labeled and dated container. Use leftover within 72 hours if stored in refrigerator or 30 days if stored in the freezer. Reheat leftover product quickly (within 2 hours) to 165 degrees F for 15 seconds. Reheat left over product only once; discard if not used. Cold holding at 41°F or colder or using time alone (less than four hours). Always wash hands and wash and sanitize counter tops utensils and containers between steps when working with raw meat.*

Texture Modified Diets:

Soft & Bite Size: (aka Bite size) **Food particle size ½ inch (~width of standard fork)** Food must be moist. Cut foods with a knife to a ½" particle size prior to mixing. Moisten with broth as needed. Foods that do not process well should be omitted. Omit: Kielbasa and use chicken

Chopped: Food particle size ¼ inch (~ ½ width of standard fork) Food must be moist. Chop foods with a knife to 1/4" particle size prior to mixing. Moisten with broth as needed. Foods that do not process well should be omitted. Omit: Kielbasa and use chicken

Minced and Moist: (aka Minced/Mechanical Soft/Ground) **Food particle size 1/8 inch (fits through prongs of standard fork)** Food must be moist. Use a food processor to grind food particles into 1/8 inch prior to mixing. Moisten with broth as needed. Foods that do not process well should be omitted. Omit: Kielbasa and use chicken

Pureed: Smooth and cohesive. Use a food processor to puree to a smooth consistency. Foods are processed by grinding and then pureeing them. May add broth or sauce to puree. Do not add to much liquid. Puree should still hold its shape. Must not be firm or sticky. Puree foods while still hot. Appearance should be smooth like pudding. Foods that do not process well should be omitted. Omit: Kielbasa and use chicken.

Therapeutic Modified Diets:

Lowfat: No changes needed.
Diabetic/No added Sugar/No Conc. Sweets/Calorie Controlled: No changes needed.
Bland/Anti Reflux: Use alternate menu item.
Liberal House Renal: Use alternate menu item.
No Added Salt: No changes needed.
2 Gram Sodium: Use alternate menu item.
Gluten Free: Use GF kielbasa. Prepare separately to prevent cross contamination.

Allergy Alerts: When an "X" is present, this indicates the allergen is present. Always read all food labels to ensure allergens are not present.

Wheat	Milk	Eggs	Fish Shellfish	Soy	Peanuts/Nuts	Other
X	X					

Key: SF= Salt Free D= Diet or Sugarfree LF = Lowfat FF = Fat Free GF = Gluten Free

Recipe Name: Kielbasa, Sauerkraut and Red Potato Stew
Recipe Category: Sausage
Portion Size: 1 cup
Ingredients: Yields: 8 servings

Ingredients	Notes:
2 pounds lean kielbasa	Sliced
2 cups sauerkraut	Drained and diced
2 Granny Smith apples	Washed, peeled, cored and diced
1 medium onion	Washed, peeled, and chopped fine
2 pounds red potatoes	Washed, trimmed and quartered
1 1/2 cups low sodium chicken broth	
1/2 teaspoon caraway seeds	
1/2 cup low fat Swiss Cheese	

Directions:

Steps:	Directions:	Critical Control Point /Quality Assurance
1	In a large stock pot, cook kielbasa until lightly browned.	
2	Add the sauerkraut.	
3	Cover with apples, onions, potatoes, and chicken broth.	
4	Sprinkle on caraway seeds.	
5	Cover and bring to boil. Cook for 40 minutes or until potatoes are tender.	Cook until internal temperature reaches 165 F.
6	Serve in a bowl. Top with Swiss cheese.	

Time Temperature Sensitive food. *Food safety Standards: hold food for service at an internal temperature above 140° F. Do not mix old product with new. Cool leftover product quickly (within 4 hours) to below 41° F. Follow proper cooling procedures. Store leftovers in a tightly sealed, labeled and dated container. Use leftover within 72 hours if stored in refrigerator or 30 days if stored in the freezer. Reheat leftover product quickly (within 2 hours) to 165 degrees F for 15 seconds. Reheat left over product only once; discard if not used. Cold holding at 41°F or colder or using time alone (less than four hours). Always wash hands and wash and sanitize counter tops utensils and containers between steps when working with raw meat.*

<u>Texture Modified Diets:</u>

Soft & Bite Size: (aka Bite size) **Food particle size ½ inch (~width of standard fork)** Food must be moist. Cut foods with a knife to a ½" particle size prior to mixing. Moisten with broth as needed. Foods that do not process well should be omitted. Omit: Kielbasa and use chicken. Peel potatoes. Omit caraway seeds.

Chopped: Food particle size ¼ inch (~ ½ width of standard fork) Food must be moist. Chop foods with a knife to 1/4" particle size prior to mixing. Moisten with broth as needed. Foods that do not process well should be omitted. Omit: Kielbasa and use chicken. Peel potatoes. Omit caraway seeds

Minced and Moist:(aka Minced/Mechanical Soft/Ground) **Food particle size 1/8 inch (fits through prongs of standard fork)** Food must be moist. Use a food processor to grind food particles into 1/8 inch prior to mixing. Moisten with broth as needed. Foods that do not process well should be omitted. Omit: Kielbasa and use chicken. Peel Potatoes. Omit caraway seeds.

Pureed: Smooth and cohesive. Use a food processor to puree to a smooth consistency. Foods are processed by grinding and then pureeing them. May add broth or sauce to puree. Do not add to much liquid. Puree should still hold its shape. Must not be firm or sticky. Puree foods while still hot. Appearance should be smooth like pudding. Foods that do not process well should be omitted. Omit: Kielbasa and use chicken. Peel potatoes. Omit caraway seeds. Serve ½ c. puree chicken and ½ c. puree potatoes separately.

<u>Therapeutic Modified Diets:</u>

Lowfat: No changes needed.
Diabetic/No added Sugar/No Conc. Sweets/Calorie Controlled: No changes needed.
Bland/Anti Reflux: Use alternate menu item.
Liberal House Renal: Use alternate menu item.
No Added Salt: Use alternate menu item.
2 Gram Sodium: Use alternate menu item.
Gluten Free: Use gluten-free chicken broth and GF kielbasa. Prepare foods separately to prevent cross contamination.

Allergy Alerts: When an "X" is present, this indicates the allergen is present.
Always read all food labels to ensure allergens are not present.

Wheat	Milk	Eggs	Fish Shellfish	Soy	Peanuts/Nuts	Other
X	X					

Key: SF= Salt Free D= Diet or Sugarfree LF = Lowfat FF = Fat Free GF = Gluten Free

Recipe Name: Pasta and Italian Sausage in a Creamy Basil Tomato Sauce
Recipe Category: Dinner Entrée
Portion Size: ½ cup sauce and ½ c. pasta
Ingredients: **Yields: 8 servings**

Ingredients	Notes:
2 1/2 Pounds lean Sweet Italian Sausage links	Use bulk for texture modified diets. No tough skin.
1 Teaspoon garlic powder	
3/4 Teaspoon salt	
1/8 Teaspoon pepper	
4 Cups low sodium tomato sauce	
2 Teaspoons basil	
2 (8 oz.) light cream cheese	
1 Teaspoon oregano	
1 Pound pasta	May use whole wheat pasta
¼ cup Grated Parmesan cheese	

Directions:

Steps:	Directions:	Critical Control Point / Quality Assurance
1	Prepare pasta according to directions on the package.	
2	Sauté ground Italian sausage links in a medium size sauce pan until brown on all sides. Remove and slice into thin slices. Drain grease.	
3	Add garlic powder, salt, pepper, basil, oregano, and tomato sauce. Simmer over low heat for 20 minutes. Add cream cheese and stir until melted.	Cook until internal temperature reaches 165 F degrees for 15 seconds
4	Serve pasta on a hot platter.	
5	First a layer of pasta, then a layer of sauce.	
6	Sprinkle with parmesan cheese.	

Time Temperature Sensitive food. *Food safety Standards: hold food for service at an internal temperature above 140° F. Do not mix old product with new. Cool leftover product quickly (within 4 hours) to below 41° F. Follow proper cooling procedures. Store leftovers in a tightly sealed, labeled and dated container. Use leftover within 72 hours if stored in refrigerator or 30 days if stored in the freezer. Reheat leftover product quickly (within 2 hours) to 165 degrees F for 15 seconds. Reheat left over product only once; discard if not used. Cold holding at 41°F or colder or using time alone (less than four hours). Always wash hands and wash and sanitize counter tops utensils and containers between steps when working with raw meat.*

Texture Modified Diets: Tip: Use pasta in correct particle size. Use bulk Italian sausage.

Soft & Bite Size: (aka Bite size) **Food particle size ½ inch (~width of standard fork)** Food must be moist. Cut foods with a knife to a ½" particle size prior to layering. Moisten with broth as needed.

Chopped: Food particle size ¼ inch (~ ½ width of standard fork) Food must be moist. Chop foods with a knife to 1/4" particle size prior to layering. Moisten with broth as needed.

Minced and Moist:(aka Minced/Mechanical Soft/Ground) **Food particle size 1/8 inch (fits through prongs of standard fork)** Food must be moist. Use a food processor to grind food particles into 1/8 inch prior to layering. Moisten with broth as needed.

Pureed: Smooth and cohesive. Use a food processor to puree to a smooth consistency. Foods are processed by grinding and then pureeing them. May add broth or sauce to puree. Do not add to much liquid. Puree should still hold its shape. Must not be firm or sticky. Puree foods while still hot. Appearance should be smooth like pudding. Serve ½ c. meat serving and ½ cup puree pasta separately.

Therapeutic Modified Diets:
Lowfat: No changes needed
Diabetic/No added Sugar/No Conc. Sweets/Calorie Controlled: No changes needed
Bland/Anti Reflux: omit garlic powder, pepper, tomato sauce, basil, oregano
Liberal House Renal: Omit salt, cream cheese. tomato sauce and Parmesan cheese
No Added Salt: No changes needed
2 Gram Sodium: omit salt, cream cheese and Parmesan cheese.
Gluten Free: Use gluten free pasta. Prepare foods separately to prevent cross contamination.
Allergy Alerts: When an "X" is present, this indicates the allergen is present. Always read all food labels to ensure allergens are not present.

Wheat	Milk	Eggs	Fish Shellfish	Soy	Peanuts/Nuts	Other
X	X	X				

Key: SF= Salt Free D= Diet or Sugarfree LF = Lowfat FF = Fat Free GF = Gluten Free

Recipe Name: Pepperoni Stromboli
Recipe Category: Sausage Dinner
Portion Size: 1 slice (approx. 1 cup)
Ingredients: Yields: 8 servings

Ingredients	Notes:
2 (1 pounds) loaves frozen bread dough	Thawed and allowed to rise.
2 cups spaghetti sauce	
1/2 teaspoon dried oregano	
8 ounces sliced low-fat pepperoni sausage	
4 cups shredded mozzarella cheese	
1/2 cup grated Parmesan cheese	

Directions:

Steps:	Directions:	Critical Control Point /QualityAssurance
1	Preheat oven to 350 degrees F (175 degrees C).	
2	Punch dough down. On a lightly floured surface, roll each loaf into 20X8 inch rectangle. Place one rectangle on a greased baking sheet. Spread spaghetti sauce in an 18X4 inch strip down the center. Sprinkle with oregano, pepperoni and mozzarella cheese. Fold long sides of dough up toward filling; set aside. Cut the remaining rectangle into three strips. Loosely braid strips; pinch ends to seal. Place bread on top of the cheese; pinch braid to dough to seal. Sprinkle with Parmesan cheese.	
3	Bake in preheated oven for 30 minutes, or until golden brown.	

Time Temperature Sensitive food. Food safety Standards: hold food for service at an internal temperature above 140° F. Do not mix old product with new. Cool leftover product quickly (within 4 hours) to below 41° F. Follow proper cooling procedures. Store leftovers in a tightly sealed, labeled and dated container. Use leftover within 72 hours if stored in refrigerator or 30 days if stored in the freezer. Reheat leftover product quickly (within 2 hours) to 165 degrees F for 15 seconds. Reheat left over product only once; discard if not used. Cold holding at 41°F or colder or using time alone (less than four hours

Texture Modified Diets:

Soft & Bite Size: (aka Bite size) **Food particle size ½ inch (~width of standard fork)** Food must be moist and SOFT. Cut foods with a knife to a ½" particle size after cooking. Moisten with milk as needed after cutting. If the crust is overcook it will turn hard. If this happens, process turnover in a food processor and process to minced and moist consistency and serve in a souffle dish topped with extra sauce.

Chopped: Food particle size ¼ inch (~ ½ width of standard fork) Food must be moist and SOFT. Chop foods with a knife to 1/4" particle size after cooking. Moisten with milk as needed after chopping. If the crust is overcook it will turn hard. If this happens, process turnover in a food processor and process to minced and moist consistency and serve in a souffle dish topped with extra sauce.

Minced and Moist:(aka Minced/Mechanical Soft/Ground) **Food particle size 1/8 inch (fits through prongs of standard fork)** Food must be moist and soft. Use a food processor to grind food particles into 1/8 inch after cooking. Moisten with milk as needed after processing topped with extra sauce.

Pureed: Smooth and cohesive. Use a food processor to puree to a smooth consistency. Foods are processed by grinding and then pureeing them. May add milk or sauce to puree. Do not add to much liquid. Puree should still hold its shape. Must not be firm or sticky. Puree foods while still hot. Appearance should be smooth like pudding. Puree all ingredients together. 1 cup serving.
Serve 1 c. puree serving.

Therapeutic Modified Diets:

Lowfat: No changes needed.
Diabetic/No added Sugar/No Conc. Sweets/Calorie Controlled: No changes needed.
Bland/Anti Reflux: Served cheese sandwich.
Liberal House Renal: Use alternate menu item.
No Added Salt: No changes needed.
2 Gram Sodium: Use alternate menu item.
Gluten Free: Use gluten-free bread dough or substitute GF pizza. Prepare foods separately to prevent cross contamination.

Allergy Alerts: When an "X" is present, this indicates the allergen is present. Always read all food labels to ensure allergens are not present.

Wheat	Milk	Eggs	Fish Shellfish	Soy	Peanuts/Nuts	Other
X	X	X				

Key: SF= Salt Free D= Diet or Sugarfree LF = Lowfat FF = Fat Free GF = Gluten Free

Copyright 2020 Jacqueline Larson M.S., R.D.N. and Associates.   All Rights Reserved

Recipe Name: Rigatoni with Creamy Basil Tomato Sauce and Italian Sausage
Recipe Category: Dinner Entrée
Portion Size: ½ cup Meat Sauce and ½ cup Pasta Total 1 cup
Ingredients: Yields: 8 servings

Ingredients	Notes:
32 oz. Spaghetti sauce	
2 lbs. Low fat Italian Style Mild Sausage Links	
1 lb. rigatoni pasta	
2 (8 oz.) packages light cream cheese	
2 tablespoons dried basil	
½ c. Parmesan cheese	

Directions:

Steps:	Directions:	Critical Control Point /Quality Assurance
1	Brown Italian sausage in large skillet. Drain. Remove and slice into ½ inch slices.	Minimum Temperature 165°F for 15 seconds
2	Add spaghetti sauce to sausage in large skillet. Cook for 10 minutes until hot. Stir in cream cheese and basil.	
3	Cook pasta according to directions on package. Drain.	
4	Combine pasta with meat mixture.	
5	Garnish with Parmesan cheese and serve hot.	

Time Temperature Sensitive food. Food safety Standards: hold food for service at an internal temperature above 140°F. Do not mix old product with new. Cool leftover product quickly (within 4 hours) to below 41°F. Follow proper cooling procedures. Store leftovers in a tightly sealed, labeled and dated container. Use leftover within 72 hours if stored in refrigerator or 30 days if stored in the freezer. Reheat leftover product quickly (within 2 hours) to 165 degrees F for 15 seconds. Reheat left over product only once; discard if not used. Cold holding at 41°F or colder or using time alone (less than four hours). Always wash hands and wash and sanitize counter tops utensils and containers between steps when working with raw meat.

Texture Modified Diets: TIP ; use pasta that is correct particle size. May use bulk Italian sausage instead of links.
Soft & Bite Size: (aka Bite size) **Food particle size ½ inch (~width of standard fork)** Food must be moist. Cut foods with a knife to a ½" particle size prior to mixing. Moisten with broth as needed.
Chopped: Food particle size ¼ inch (~ ½ width of standard fork) Food must be moist. Chop foods with a knife to 1/4" particle size prior to mixing. Moisten with broth as needed.
Minced and Moist: (aka Minced/Mechanical Soft/Ground) **Food particle size 1/8 inch (fits through prongs of standard fork)** Food must be moist. Use a food processor to grind food particles into 1/8 inch prior to mixing. Moisten with broth as needed.
Pureed: Smooth and cohesive. Use a food processor to puree to a smooth consistency. Foods are processed by grinding and then pureeing them. May add broth or sauce to puree. Do not add to much liquid. Puree should still hold its shape. Must not be firm or sticky. Puree foods while still hot. Appearance should be smooth like pudding. Puree Pasta while hot for best results. Serve ½ c. meat sauce serving and ½ cup pasta separately

Therapeutic Modified Diets:
Lowfat: No changes needed
Diabetic/No added Sugar/No Conc. Sweets/Calorie Controlled: No changes needed
Bland: omit spaghetti sauce, serve hamburger patty plain and plain pasta
Liberal House Renal: Omit spaghetti sauce Mozzarella cheese, cream cheese, and Parmesan cheese. Serve hamburger patty plain and SF plain pasta. May toss pasta with salt free herbs/spices.
No Added Salt: No changes
2 Gram Sodium: Omit spaghetti sauce, cream cheese and Parmesan. . Serve hamburger patty plain and plain SF pasta. May toss pasta with salt free herbs/spices, and fresh tomatoes
Gluten Free: Use GF spaghetti sauce and GF pasta. Prepare foods separately to prevent cross contamination.
Allergy Alerts: When an "X" is present, this indicates the allergen is present. Always read all food labels to ensure allergens are not present.

Wheat	Milk	Eggs	Fish Shellfish	Soy	Peanuts/Nuts	Other
X	X	X				

Key: SF= Salt Free D= Diet or Sugarfree LF = Lowfat FF = Fat Free GF = Gluten Free

Copyright 2020 Jacqueline Larson M.S., R.D.N. and Associates.   All Rights Reserved

Recipe Name: Turkey Sausage and Pasta with Alfredo Sauce
Recipe Category: Sausage
Portion Size: 1 cup
Ingredients: Yields: 8 servings

Ingredients	Notes:
1 package (16 oz.) low fat turkey sausage	Cut into 1/2 inch slices. Use bulk sausage without skin for texture modified diets.
1 pound package penne pasta	May use whole grain.
1 (14 oz.) fat free evaporated milk	
2 cloves garlic	Washed, peeled and minced
1 cup nonfat milk	
1 (8 oz.) light cream cheese	Cut into small cubes
1/2 cup Parmesan cheese	
1 cup frozen peas	

Directions:

Steps:	Directions:	Critical Control Point/Quality Assurance
1	Prepare pasta according to package directions; drain and set aside.	
2	Sauté sausage in a large skillet over medium-high heat for 5 minutes, turning occasionally until lightly browned.	Cook until internal temperature reaches 165 F.
3	Add milk, evaporated milk, garlic, cream cheese and stir.	
4	Bring to a boil over medium-high heat. Reduce heat.	
5	Add peas, simmer gently for 3-4 minutes or until mixture begins to thicken.	
6	Remove from heat, stir in Parmesan cheese.	
7	Add pasta to sauce and toss.	

Time Temperature Sensitive food. *Food safety Standards: hold food for service at an internal temperature above 140° F. Do not mix old product with new. Cool leftover product quickly (within 4 hours) to below 41° F. Follow proper cooling procedures. Store leftovers in a tightly sealed, labeled and dated container. Use leftover within 72 hours if stored in refrigerator or 30 days if stored in the freezer. Reheat leftover product quickly (within 2 hours) to 165 degrees F for 15 seconds. Reheat left over product only once; discard if not used. Cold holding at 41°F or colder or using time alone (less than four hours). Always wash hands and wash and sanitize counter tops utensils and containers between steps when working with raw meat.*

Texture Modified Diets: TIP: use pasta within the correct particle size and ground bulk Italian sausage.
Soft & Bite Size: (aka Bite size) **Food particle size ½ inch (~width of standard fork)** Food must be moist. Cut foods with a knife to a ½" particle size prior to mixing. Moisten with broth as needed.
Chopped: Food particle size ¼ inch (~ ½ width of standard fork) Food must be moist. Chop foods with a knife to 1/4" particle size prior to mixing. Moisten with broth as needed.
Minced and Moist:(aka Minced/Mechanical Soft/Ground) **Food particle size 1/8 inch (fits through prongs of standard fork)** Food must be moist. Use a food processor to grind food particles into 1/8 inch prior to mixing. Moisten with broth as needed.
Pureed: Smooth and cohesive. Use a food processor to puree to a smooth consistency. Foods are processed by grinding and then pureeing them. May add broth or sauce to puree. Do not add to much liquid. Puree should still hold its shape. Must not be firm or sticky. Puree foods while still hot. Appearance should be smooth like pudding.
Serve ½ c. puree Italian sausage, ½ c. puree pasta and ½ cup puree vegetables separately.
Therapeutic Modified Diets:
Lowfat: No changes needed
Diabetic/No added Sugar/No Conc. Sweets/Calorie Controlled: No changes needed.
Bland/Anti Reflux: Omit garlic.
Liberal House Renal: Serve ½ c. SF pasta and 3 oz. SF chicken or SF turkey.
No Added Salt: No changes needed.
2 Gram Sodium: Serve ½ c. SF pasta and 3 oz. SF chicken or SF turkey
Gluten Free: Use gluten-free penne pasta. Prepare foods separately to prevent cross contamination.
Allergy Alerts: When an "X" is present, this indicates the allergen is present. Always read all food labels to ensure allergens are not present.

Wheat	Milk	Eggs	Fish Shellfish	Soy	Peanuts/Nuts	Other
X	X	X				

Key: SF= Salt Free D= Diet or Sugarfree LF = Lowfat FF = Fat Free GF = Gluten Free

Recipe Name: Turkey Sausage and Pasta with Sun Dried Tomatoes
Recipe Category: Sausage
Portion Size: 1 cup
Ingredients: Yields: 8 servings

Ingredients	Notes:
2 (1pound) low fat turkey sausage (kielbasa)	Cut into 1/2 inch slices
1 pound package pasta	May use whole grain
1/2 cup sun dried tomatoes or 1 c. fresh tomatoes	Washed, trimmed and chopped
4 cups baby spinach	Washed, trimmed and chopped
1/2 cup Parmesan cheese	

Directions:

Steps:	Directions:	Critical Control Point /Quality Assurance
1	Prepare pasta according to package directions; drain and set aside.	
2	Sauté Turkey sausage in oil in a large skillet over medium-high heat for 15 minutes, turning occasionally until lightly browned and temperature reaches 165 degrees F.	
3	Add sun dried tomatoes and spinach.	
4	Stir gently until spinach wilts.	
5	Remove from heat, stir in Parmesan cheese.	
6	Add pasta to sauce and toss.	

Time Temperature Sensitive food. *Food safety Standards: hold food for service at an internal temperature above 140° F. Do not mix old product with new. Cool leftover product quickly (within 4 hours) to below 41° F. Follow proper cooling procedures. Store leftovers in a tightly sealed, labeled and dated container. Use leftover within 72 hours if stored in refrigerator or 30 days if stored in the freezer. Reheat leftover product quickly (within 2 hours) to 165 degrees F for 15 seconds. Reheat left over product only once; discard if not used. Cold holding at 41°F or colder or using time alone (less than four hours). Always wash hands and wash and sanitize counter tops utensils and containers between steps when working with raw meat.*

Texture Modified Diets: **TIP: use pasta within the correct particle size and ground bulk Italian sausage.**
Soft & Bite Size: (aka Bite size) **Food particle size ½ inch (~width of standard fork)** Food must be moist. Cut foods with a knife to a ½" particle size prior to mixing. Moisten with broth as needed. Foods that do not process well should be omitted. Omit: sundried tomatoes. Use fresh tomatoes. Avoid tough stems and membranes with spinach.
Chopped: Food particle size ¼ inch (~ ½ width of standard fork) Food must be moist. Chop foods with a knife to 1/4" particle size prior to mixing. Moisten with broth as needed. Foods that do not process well should be omitted. Omit: sundried tomatoes. Use fresh tomatoes. Avoid tough stems and membranes with spinach.
Minced and Moist: (aka Minced/Mechanical Soft/Ground) **Food particle size 1/8 inch (fits through prongs of standard fork)** Food must be moist. Use a food processor to grind food particles into 1/8 inch prior to mixing. Moisten with broth as needed. Foods that do not process well should be omitted. Omit: sundried tomatoes. Use fresh tomatoes. Avoid tough stems and membranes with spinach.
Pureed: Smooth and cohesive. Use a food processor to puree to a smooth consistency. Foods are processed by grinding and then pureeing them. May add broth or sauce to puree. Do not add to much liquid. Puree should still hold its shape. Must not be firm or sticky. Puree foods while still hot. Appearance should be smooth like pudding. Foods that do not process well should be omitted. Omit: sundried tomatoes. Use fresh tomatoes. Avoid tough stems and membranes with spinach. Serve ½ c. puree turkey sausage, ½ cup puree pasta and ½ c. puree spinach and tomato mixture separately.

Therapeutic Modified Diets:
Lowfat: No changes needed.
Diabetic/No added Sugar/No Conc. Sweets/Calorie Controlled: No changes needed.
Bland/Anti Reflux: Omit tomatoes.
Liberal House Renal: Serve 3 oz. SF turkey, ½ c. SF pasta and ½ c. SF carrots.
No Added Salt: No changes needed.
2 Gram Sodium: Serve 3 oz. SF turkey, ½ c. SF pasta and ½ c. cooked spinach and tomato.
Gluten Free: Use gluten-free pasta and GF sausage. Prepare foods separately to prevent cross contamination.

Allergy Alerts: When an "X" is present, this indicates the allergen is present. Always read all food labels to ensure allergens are not present.

Wheat	Milk	Eggs	Fish Shellfish	Soy	Peanuts/Nuts	Other
X	X	X				

Key: SF= Salt Free D= Diet or Sugarfree LF = Lowfat FF = Fat Free GF = Gluten Free

Copyright 2020 Jacqueline Larson M.S., R.D.N. and Associates.   All Rights Reserved

Recipe Name: Turkey Sausage Skillet Dinner
Recipe Category: Sausage
Portion Size: 1 ½ cups
Ingredients: Yields: 8 servings

Ingredients	Notes:
3 tablespoons vegetable oil	
1 package (24 ounces) frozen potatoes O'Brien	
1 teaspoon dried oregano leaves	
1/2 teaspoon black pepper	
4 cups chopped broccoli	Washed, trimmed and chopped
2 (2pounds) rings lean turkey sausage (Kielbasa)	
1/2 cup low fat shredded Cheddar Cheese	

Directions:

Steps:	Directions:	Critical Control Point /Quality Assurance
1	Heat oil in a large skill until hot.	
2	Add potatoes, oregano and pepper.	
3	Cover and cook 8 to 10 minutes, stirring until potatoes are light brown.	
4	Add broccoli and sausage.	
5	Cover and cook about 15 minutes until hot.	Cook until internal temperature reaches 165 F.
6	Top with cheese.	
7	Cover and heat until cheese is melted.	

Time Temperature Sensitive food. *Food safety Standards: hold food for service at an internal temperature above 140° F. Do not mix old product with new. Cool leftover product quickly (within 4 hours) to below 41° F. Follow proper cooling procedures. Store leftovers in a tightly sealed, labeled and dated container. Use leftover within 72 hours if stored in refrigerator or 30 days if stored in the freezer. Reheat leftover product quickly (within 2 hours) to 165 degrees F for 15 seconds. Reheat left over product only once; discard if not used. Cold holding at 41°F or colder or using time alone (less than four hours). Always wash hands and wash and sanitize counter tops utensils and containers between steps when working with raw meat.*

Texture Modified Diets:

Soft & Bite Size: (aka Bite size) **Food particle size ½ inch (~width of standard fork)** Food must be moist. Cut foods with a knife to a ½" particle size prior to mixing. Moisten with broth as needed. Foods that do not process well should be omitted. Omit: Kielbasa and substitute ground turkey.

Chopped: Food particle size ¼ inch (~ ½ width of standard fork) Food must be moist. Chop foods with a knife to 1/4" particle size prior to mixing. Moisten with broth as needed. Foods that do not process well should be omitted. Omit: Kielbasa and substitute ground turkey.

Minced and Moist:(aka Minced/Mechanical Soft/Ground) **Food particle size 1/8 inch (fits through prongs of standard fork)** Food must be moist. Use a food processor to grind food particles into 1/8 inch prior to mixing. Moisten with broth as needed. Foods that do not process well should be omitted. Omit: Kielbasa and substitute ground turkey.

Pureed: Smooth and cohesive. Use a food processor to puree to a smooth consistency. Foods are processed by grinding and then pureeing them. May add broth or sauce to puree. Do not add to much liquid. Puree should still hold its shape. Must not be firm or sticky. Puree foods while still hot. Appearance should be smooth like pudding. Foods that do not process well should be omitted. Omit: Kielbasa and substitute ground turkey. Serve ½ c. puree turkey, ½ c. puree potatoes and ½ c. puree broccoli separately.

Therapeutic Modified Diets:

Low fat: No changes needed.
Diabetic/No added Sugar/No Conc. Sweets/Calorie Controlled: No changes needed.
Bland/Anti Reflux: Use alternate menu item.
Liberal House Renal: Use alternate menu item.
No Added Salt: No changes needed.
2 Gram Sodium: Use alternate menu item.
Gluten Free: Use GF kielbasa. Prepare separately to prevent cross contamination.

Allergy Alerts: When an "X" is present, this indicates the allergen is present. Always read all food labels to ensure allergens are not present.

Wheat	Milk	Eggs	Fish Shellfish	Soy	Peanuts/Nuts	Other
X	X					

Key: SF= Salt Free D= Diet or Sugarfree LF = Lowfat FF = Fat Free GF = Gluten Free

Copyright 2020 Jacqueline Larson M.S., R.D.N. and Associates.   All Rights Reserved

Recipe Name: Zucchini Stuffed with Italian Sausage
Recipe Category: Sausage
Portion Size: 1 medium (1/2 cup meat)
Ingredients: **Yields: 8 servings**

Ingredients	Notes:
4 medium zucchini	
1 pound lean ground beef	
1 pound lean bulk Italian Sausage (sweet or spicy)	
1 small onion	Washed, peeled and chopped
1 teaspoon fennel	
2 teaspoons dried basil	
1/2 teaspoon ground oregano	
3 gloves fresh garlic	Minced
2 eggs	
1 cup dried bread crumbs	
1 (15 oz) tomato sauce	
1 (6 oz) can tomato paste	
2 teaspoon sugar	
1 cup Mozzarella cheese	
1/4 cup Parmesan	

Directions:

Steps:	Directions:	Critical Control Point / Quality Assurance
1	Preheat oven to 375 degrees.	
2	Spray a large baking dish with non stick cooking spray.	
3	Cut zucchini in half lengthwise.	
4	With a spoon, scoop out the seeds.	
5	Chop seeds and save.	
6	In a large bowl, mix together ground beef, sausage, chopped onion, bread crumbs, eggs and the zucchini seeds.	
7	Scoop meat mixture equally into all the zucchini halves into the prepared baking dish.	
8	In a bowl, stir together fennel, basil, oregano, garlic, tomato sauce, tomato paste, and sugar.	
9	Spoon tomato mixture over filled zucchini.	
10	Bake in oven for 1 hour.	Cook until internal temperature reaches 165 F.
11	Remove from oven.	
12	Top with cheese.	
13	Return to oven and bake for 10 minutes.	

Time Temperature Sensitive food. Food safety Standards: hold food for service at an internal temperature above 140° F. Do not mix old product with new. Cool leftover product quickly (within 4 hours) to below 41° F. Follow proper cooling procedures. Store leftovers in a tightly sealed, labeled and dated container. Use leftover within 72 hours if stored in refrigerator or 30 days if stored in the freezer. Reheat leftover product quickly (within 2 hours) to 165 degrees F for 15 seconds. Reheat left over product only once; discard if not used. Cold holding at 41°F or colder or using time alone (less than four hours). Always wash hands and wash and sanitize counter tops utensils and containers between steps when working with raw meat.

Texture Modified Diets:

Soft & Bite Size: (aka Bite size) **Food particle size ½ inch (~width of standard fork)** Food must be moist. Cut foods with a knife to a ½" particle size prior to mixing. Moisten with broth as needed.

Chopped: Food particle size ¼ inch (~ ½ width of standard fork) Food must be moist. Chop foods with a knife to 1/4" particle size prior to mixing. Moisten with broth as needed.

Minced and Moist:(aka Minced/Mechanical Soft/Ground) **Food particle size 1/8 inch (fits through prongs of standard fork)** Food must be moist. Use a food processor to grind food particles into 1/8 inch prior to mixing. Moisten with broth as needed.

Pureed: Smooth and cohesive. Use a food processor to puree to a smooth consistency. Foods are processed by grinding and then pureeing them. May add broth or sauce to puree. Do not add to much liquid. Puree should still hold its shape. Must not be firm or sticky. Puree foods while still hot. Appearance should be smooth like pudding. Serve ½ c. puree meat and ½ cup puree zucchini separately.

Therapeutic Modified Diets:
Low fat: No changes needed.
Diabetic/No added Sugar/No Conc. Sweets/Calorie Controlled: No changes needed
Bland/Anti Reflux: Serve ½ c. plain zucchini and 3 oz. beef patty.
Liberal House Renal: Serve ½ c. SF zucchini and 3 oz. SF beef patty.
No Added Salt: No changes needed.
2 Gram Sodium: Serve ½ c. SF zucchini and 3 oz. SF beef patty.
Gluten Free: Use gluten-free bread crumbs or oats. Use GF sausage. Prepare foods separately to prevent cross contamination.
Allergy Alerts: When an "X" is present, this indicates the allergen is present.
Always read all food labels to ensure allergens are not present.

Wheat	Milk	Eggs	Fish Shellfish	Soy	Peanuts/Nuts	Other
X	X	X				

Key: SF= Salt Free D= Diet or Sugarfree LF = Lowfat FF = Fat Free GF = Gluten Free

SAUSAGE LUNCH

Recipe Name: Hot Dogs
Recipe Category: Lunch Entrée
Portion Size: 1 Hot Dog with bun
Ingredients: Yields: 8 servings

Ingredients	Notes:
8 Hot dogs	
8 Hot dog buns	
Catsup, mustard, relish, onions	optional

Directions:

Steps:	Directions:	Critical Control Point /Quality Assurance
1	Cover hot dogs with water in saucepan	
2	Bring to a boil	
3	Reduce heat and simmer 3 to 4 minutes	Cook until temperature reaches 165 degrees.
4	Place well drained hot dog in a hot dog bun	
5	Top with catsup, mustard, relish and onions as desired.	

Time Temperature Sensitive food. *Food safety Standards: hold food for service at an internal temperature above 140° F. Do not mix old product with new. Cool leftover product quickly (within 4 hours) to below 41° F. Follow proper cooling procedures. Store leftovers in a tightly sealed, labeled and dated container. Use leftover within 72 hours if stored in refrigerator or 30 days if stored in the freezer. Reheat leftover product quickly (within 2 hours) to 165 degrees F for 15 seconds. Reheat left over product only once; discard if not used. Cold holding at 41 °F or colder or using time alone (less than four hours).*

Texture Modified Diets: NO Hot dogs: skin is too tough.

Soft & Bite Size: (aka Bite size) **Food particle size ½ inch (~width of standard fork)** Food must be moist. Cut foods with a knife to a ½" particle size prior to mixing. Moisten with broth as needed. Foods that do not process well should be omitted. Omit: hot dogs and sub. ground turkey or bulk. Italian sausage. Top with condiments.

Chopped: Food particle size ¼ inch (~ ½ width of standard fork) Food must be moist. Chop foods with a knife to 1/4" particle size prior to mixing. Moisten with broth as needed. Foods that do not process well should be omitted. Omit: hot dogs and sub. ground turkey or bulk. Italian sausage. Top with condiments.

Minced and Moist: (aka Minced/Mechanical Soft/Ground) **Food particle size 1/8 inch (fits through prongs of standard fork)** Food must be moist. Use a food processor to grind food particles into 1/8 inch prior to mixing. Moisten with broth as needed. Foods that do not process well should be omitted. Omit: hot dogs and sub. ground turkey or bulk. Italian sausage. Top with condiments.

Pureed: Smooth and cohesive. Use a food processor to puree to a smooth consistency. Foods are processed by grinding and then pureeing them. May add broth or sauce to puree. Do not add to much liquid. Puree should still hold its shape. Must not be firm or sticky. Puree foods while still hot. Appearance should be smooth like pudding. Foods that do not process well should be omitted. Omit: hot dogs and sub. ground turkey or bulk Italian sausage. Top with condiments. Serve ½ puree ground turkey or puree bulk Italian sausage and 1/2 cup puree bread with toppings.

Therapeutic Modified Diets:

Low fat: Omit cheese . Use lowfat hot dogs.
Diabetic/No added Sugar/No Conc. Sweets/Calorie Controlled: No changes needed
Bland/Anti Reflux: Use alternate menu item
Liberal House Renal: Use alternate menu item
No Added Salt: Use alternate menu item
2 Gram Sodium: Use alternate menu item
Gluten Free: Use gluten free bun or bread. Use gluten free hot dogs. Prepare foods separately to prevent cross contamination.

Allergy Alerts: When an "X" is present, this indicates the allergen is present. Always read all food labels to ensure allergens are not present.

Wheat	Milk	Eggs	Fish Shellfish	Soy	Peanuts/Nuts	Other
X	X					

Key: SF= Salt Free D= Diet or Sugarfree LF = Lowfat FF = Fat Free GF = Gluten Free

Copyright 2020 Jacqueline Larson M.S., R.D.N. and Associates.   All Rights Reserved

Recipe Name: Hot Dogs with Chili
Recipe Category: Lunch Entrée
Portion Size: 1 Hot Dog with bun
Ingredients: Yields: 8 servings

Ingredients	Notes:
8 Hot dogs	
8 Hot dog buns	
1 Can (20 ounce) prepared chili without bean	
½ Cup shredded Cheddar cheese	
¼ Cup thinly sliced green onion , white onion OR red onion	Optional

Directions:

Steps:	Directions:	Critical Control Point /Quality Assurance
1	Cover hot dogs with water in saucepan	
2	Bring to a boil	
3	Reduce heat and simmer 3 to 4 minutes	Cook until temperature reaches 165 degrees.
4	In a separate sauce pan, heat chili until warm	Cook until temperature reaches 165 degrees.
5	Place well drained hot dog in a hot dog bun	
6	Top with chili, cheese, and onions.	

Time Temperature Sensitive food. Food safety Standards: hold food for service at an internal temperature above 140°F. Do not mix old product with new. Cool leftover product quickly (within 4 hours) to below 41°F. Follow proper cooling procedures. Store leftovers in a tightly sealed, labeled and dated container. Use leftover within 72 hours if stored in refrigerator or 30 days if stored in the freezer. Reheat leftover product quickly (within 2 hours) to 165 degrees F for 15 seconds. Reheat left over product only once; discard if not used. Cold holding at 41°F or colder or using time alone (less than four hours).

Texture Modified Diets: NO Hot dogs: skin is too tough. Serve chili with meat sauce on top of bun.
Soft & Bite Size: (aka Bite size) **Food particle size ½ inch (~width of standard fork)** Food must be moist. Cut foods with a knife to a ½" particle size prior to mixing. Moisten with broth as needed. Foods that do not process well should be omitted. Omit: hot dogs and give chili with ground beef on top bun. Omit green onions.
Chopped: Food particle size ¼ inch (~ ½ width of standard fork) Food must be moist. Chop foods with a knife to 1/4" particle size prior to mixing. Moisten with broth as needed. Foods that do not process well should be omitted. Omit: hot dogs. Serve chili with ground beef on top with bun. Omit green onions.
Minced and Moist:(aka Minced/Mechanical Soft/Ground) **Food particle size 1/8 inch (fits through prongs of standard fork)** Food must be moist. Use a food processor to grind food particles into 1/8 inch prior to mixing. Moisten with broth as needed. Foods that do not process well should be omitted. Omit: hot dogs. Serve chili with ground on top with bun. Omit with green onions.
Pureed: Smooth and cohesive. Use a food processor to puree to a smooth consistency. Foods are processed by grinding and then pureeing them. May add broth or sauce to puree. Do not add to much liquid. Puree should still hold its shape. Must not be firm or sticky. Puree foods while still hot. Appearance should be smooth like pudding. Foods that do not process well should be omitted. Omit: hot dogs and sub. ground turkey or bulk Italian sausage. Top with melted cheese. Omit green onions. Serve ½ puree ground beef chili and 1/2 cup puree bread with toppings.
Therapeutic Modified Diets:
Low fat: Omit cheese . Use lowfat hot dogs.
Diabetic/No added Sugar/No Conc. Sweets/Calorie Controlled: No changes needed
Bland/Anti Reflux: Use alternate menu item
Liberal House Renal: Use alternate menu item
No Added Salt: Use alternate menu item
2 Gram Sodium: Use alternate menu item
Gluten Free: Use gluten free bun or bread. Use gluten free chili and hot dogs. Prepare foods separately to prevent cross contamination.

Allergy Alerts: When an "X" is present, this indicates the allergen is present. Always read all food labels to ensure allergens are not present.

Wheat	Milk	Eggs	Fish Shellfish	Soy	Peanuts/Nuts	Other
X	X					

Key: SF= Salt Free D= Diet or Sugarfree LF = Lowfat FF = Fat Free GF = Gluten Free

Copyright 2020 Jacqueline Larson M.S., R.D.N. and Associates.   All Rights Reserved

Recipe Name: Kale and Sausage Soup
Recipe Category: Lunch entree
Portion Size: 1 ½ cup
Ingredients: Yields: 8 servings

Ingredients	Notes:
4 red potatoes	Wash, trimmed and diced (may leave on skin)
2 tablespoons olive oil	
4 cups kale	Wash, peel and torn into bite size pieces. Remove tough membranes
1 large onion, diced	Wash, peel and dice
1 teaspoon salt	
½ teaspoon black pepper	
1 (14 oz.) can nonfat evaporated milk	
8 cups reduced sodium chicken broth	
1 garlic clove, minced	
¼ cup flour	
1 ½ lbs. lean ground turkey Italian sausage	(bulk no links for texture modified diets)
¼ cup parmesan cheese	

Directions:

Steps:	Directions:	Critical Control Point Quality Assurance
1	In a large stock pot heat oil to medium high heat. Add ground turkey sausage and cook until lightly browned.	
2	Add garlic, onions and potatoes. Cook until tender.	
3	Add flour and toss to coat flour.	
4	Stir in chicken broth, salt, pepper and milk. Bring to boil.	
5	Reduce heat. Simmer for 20 minutes Add kale just before serving. Serve hot. Top with Parmesan cheese.	Temperature check must reach 165 °F degrees

Time Temperature Sensitive food. *Food safety Standards: hold food for service at an internal temperature above 140° F. Do not mix old product with new. Cool leftover product quickly (within 4 hours) to below 41° F. Follow proper cooling procedures. Store leftovers in a tightly sealed, labeled and dated container. Use leftover within 72 hours if stored in refrigerator or 30 days if stored in the freezer. Reheat leftover product quickly (within 2 hours) to 165 degrees F for 15 seconds. Reheat left over product only once; discard if not used. Cold holding at 41°F or colder or using time alone (less than four hours).*

<u>Texture Modified Diets:</u>
Soft & Bite Size: (aka Bite size) **Food particle size ½ inch (~width of standard fork)** Food must be moist. Cut foods with a knife to a ½" particle size prior to mixing. Moisten with broth as needed. Peel potatoes.
Chopped: **Food particle size ¼ inch (~ ½ width of standard fork)** Food must be moist. Chop foods with a knife to 1/4" particle size prior to mixing. Moisten with broth as needed. Peel potatoes.
Minced and Moist:(aka Minced/Mechanical Soft/Ground) **Food particle size 1/8 inch (fits through prongs of standard fork)** Food must be moist. Use a food processor to grind food particles into 1/8 inch prior to mixing. Moisten with broth as needed. Peel potatoes.
Pureed: Smooth and cohesive. Use a food processor to puree to a smooth consistency. Foods are processed by grinding and then pureeing them. May add broth or sauce to puree. Do not add to much liquid. Puree should still hold its shape. Must not be firm or sticky. Puree foods while still hot. Appearance should be smooth like pudding. Peel potatoes
 Serve ½ cup puree Italian turkey sausage, ½ cup puree potatoes and ½ puree kale separately.
<u>Therapeutic Modified Diets:</u>
Lowfat: no changes
Diabetic/No added Sugar/No Conc. Sweets/Calorie Controlled: No changes needed
Bland/Anti Reflux: Omit pepper, garlic, and onions. Use lean ground turkey instead of sausage
Liberal House Renal: Serve SF 2 oz. ground turkey patty, ½ cup cooked SF kale and ½ c. rice
No Added Salt: No changes needed
2 Gram Sodium: Serve SF 2 oz. ground turkey patty, ½ cup cooked SF kale and ½ c. potato
Gluten Free: Use gluten free flour and chicken broth. Prepare foods separately to prevent cross contamination.
Allergy Alerts: When an "X" is present, this indicates the allergen is present. Always read all food labels to ensure allergens are not present.

Wheat	Milk	Eggs	Fish Shellfish	Soy	Peanuts/Nuts	Other
X	X					

Key: SF= Salt Free D= Diet or Sugarfree LF = Lowfat FF = Fat Free GF = Gluten Free

Copyright 2020 Jacqueline Larson M.S., R.D.N. and Associates.   All Rights Reserved

Recipe Name: Pepperoni and Cheese Pizza
Recipe Category: Lunch Entrée
Portion Size: 1 Slice (1/8 pizza)
Ingredients: Yields: 8 servings

Ingredients	Notes:
½ teaspoon garlic powder	
1 (1 pound) loaf frozen bread dough	Thawed
1 small jar pizza sauce	
8 oz. pepperoni slices	
4 cups shredded lowfat mozzarella cheese	

Directions:

Steps:	Directions:	Critical Control Point / Quality Assurance
1	On a floured surface, roll dough into a 13-inch circle	
2	Press onto the bottom and up the sides of a greased 12-inch pizza pan.	
3	Spread sauce over crust to within 1/2 inch of edge	
4	Top with cheese.	
5	Bake at 350 degrees F for 20-25 minutes or until crust is golden and cheese is melted	

Time Temperature Sensitive food. *Food safety Standards: hold food for service at an internal temperature above 140°F. Do not mix old product with new. Cool leftover product quickly (within 4 hours) to below 41°F. Follow proper cooling procedures. Store leftovers in a tightly sealed, labeled and dated container. Use leftover within 72 hours if stored in refrigerator or 30 days if stored in the freezer. Reheat leftover product quickly (within 2 hours) to 165 degrees F for 15 seconds. Reheat left over product only once; discard if not used. Cold holding at 41°F or colder or using time alone (less than four hours).* **Special Diets:**

Texture Modified Diets:

Soft & Bite Size: (aka Bite size) **Food particle size ½ inch (~width of standard fork)** Food must be moist. Bake crust until soft. If crust is hard, it must be processed to 1/8 inch and moistened before adding the toppings. Cut foods with a knife to a ½" particle size prior to layering. Moisten with broth as needed. Omit pepperoni. May use ground Italian sausage (no skin)

Chopped: Food particle size ¼ inch (~ ½ width of standard fork) Food must be moist. Bake crust until soft. If crust is hard, it must be processed to 1/8 inch and moistened before adding the toppings Chop foods with a knife to 1/4" particle size prior to layering. Moisten with broth as needed. Omit pepperoni. May use ground Italian sausage (no skin)

Minced and Moist: (aka Minced/Mechanical Soft/Ground) **Food particle size 1/8 inch (fits through prongs of standard fork)** Food must be moist. Bake crust until soft. Use a food processor to grind food particles into 1/8 inch prior to layering. Moisten with broth as needed. Omit pepperoni. May use ground Italian sausage (no skin).

Pureed: Smooth and cohesive. Use a food processor to puree to a smooth consistency. Foods are processed by grinding and then pureeing them. May add milk or sauce to puree. Do not add to much liquid. Puree should still hold its shape. Must not be firm or sticky. Puree foods while still hot. Appearance should be smooth like pudding. Omit pepperoni. May use ground Italian sausage (no skin). Serve 1 cup serving. Puree pizza with milk.

Therapeutic Modified Diets:

Lowfat: No pepperoni
Diabetic/No added Sugar/No Conc. Sweets/Calorie Controlled: No changes needed
Bland/Anti Reflux: omit garlic and pizza sauce.
Liberal House Renal: Use alternate menu item
No Added Salt: No pepperoni
2 Gram Sodium: Use alternate menu item
Gluten Free: Use gluten free sauce, pepperoni and gluten free dough. Prepare foods separately to prevent cross contamination.

Allergy Alerts: When an "X" is present, this indicates the allergen is present. Always read all food labels to ensure allergens are not present.

Wheat	Milk	Eggs	Fish Shellfish	Soy	Peanuts/Nuts	Other
X	x					

Key: SF= Salt Free D= Diet or Sugarfree LF = Lowfat FF = Fat Free GF = Gluten Free

Recipe Name: Winter Vegetables Turkey Sausage and Spelt Soup
Recipe Category: Lunch Entrée
Portion Size: 1 ½ cup of soup
Ingredients: Yields: 8 servings

Ingredients	Notes:
2 cups spelt (or other whole grain –barley, Farro, Brown rice, Etc.)	
2 Tablespoons olive oil	
16 oz. lean Italian sausage, casings removed (turkey)	Or Use bulk.
2 cups washed, peeled and cubed butternut squash	Cut into 1 inch pieces
1 ½ cups washed, peeled and slices carrots	Cut into 1 inch pieces
1 ½ cups washed, peeled and sliced parsnips	Cut into 1 inch pieces
1 large onion, diced	Wash, peel and dice
3 gloves garlic, minced	Wash, peel and dice
2 tablespoons thyme	
8 cups low sodium chicken broth	
1 teaspoon salt	
¼ teaspoon black pepper	

Directions:

Steps:	Directions:	Critical Control Point Quality Assurance
1	In a large lidded pot, heat olive oil over medium heat.	
2	Add sausage breaking up with a spoon.	
3	Cook 8 to 10 minutes, until browned. Drain fat.	
4	Stir in butternut squash, carrots, parsnips, onion, garlic and thyme	
5	Cook 5 minutes stirring occasionally.	
6	Add chicken broth, 1 cup water and spelt	
7	Bring to a boil	
8	Reduce heat to a simmer and cook covered, for 60 minutes or until spelt is tender	
9	Stir in salt and pepper.	

Time Temperature Sensitive food. *Food safety Standards: hold food for service at an internal temperature above 140° F. Do not mix old product with new. Cool leftover product quickly (within 4 hours) to below 41° F. Follow proper cooling procedures. Store leftovers in a tightly sealed, labeled and dated container. Use leftover within 72 hours if stored in refrigerator or 30 days if stored in the freezer. Reheat leftover product quickly (within 2 hours) to 165 degrees F for 15 seconds. Reheat left over product only once; discard if not used. Cold holding at 41 °F or colder using time alone (less than four hours).*

<u>**Texture Modified Diets: NO Cassings. Use bulk Italian sausage.**</u>
Soft & Bite Size: (aka Bite size) **Food particle size ½ inch (~width of standard fork)** Food must be moist. Cut foods with a knife to a ½" particle size prior to mixing. Moisten with broth as needed.
Chopped: Food particle size ¼ inch (~ ½ width of standard fork) Food must be moist. Chop foods with a knife to 1/4" particle size prior to mixing. Moisten with broth as needed.
Minced and Moist: (aka Minced/Mechanical Soft/Ground) **Food particle size 1/8 inch (fits through prongs of standard fork)** Food must be moist. Use a food processor to grind food particles into 1/8 inch prior to mixing. Moisten with broth as needed.
Pureed: Smooth and cohesive. Use a food processor to puree to a smooth consistency. Foods are processed by grinding and then pureeing them. May add broth or sauce to puree. Do not add to much liquid. Puree should still hold its shape. Must not be firm or sticky. Puree foods while still hot. Appearance should be smooth like pudding.
(strain broth and puree ingredients) Serve 1 ½ c. serving.
<u>*Therapeutic Modified Diets:*</u>
Low fat: No changes needed
Diabetic/No added Sugar/No Conc. Sweets/Calorie Controlled: No changes needed
Bland/Anti Reflux: Omit onion, garlic, thyme and pepper
Liberal House Renal: Use SF chicken or turkey. Omit salt. Use SF broth or water.
No Added Salt: No changes needed.
2 Gram Sodium: Use SF chicken or turkey. Omit salt. Use SF broth or water.
Gluten Free: Use Brown Rice. (no barley or other grain containing gluten.) Use gluten free broth and turkey sausage. Prepare foods separately to prevent cross contamination.
Allergy Alerts: When an "X" is present, this indicates the allergen is present. Always read all food labels to ensure allergens are not present.

Wheat	Milk	Eggs	Fish Shellfish	Soy	Peanuts/Nuts	Other
X						

Key: SF= Salt Free D= Diet or Sugarfree LF = Lowfat FF = Fat Free GF = Gluten Free

248

Copyright 2020 Jacqueline Larson M.S., R.D.N. and Associates.   All Rights Reserved

SEAFOOD DINNER RECIPES

Copyright 2020- Jacqueline Larson M.S., R.D.N. and Associates. All Rights Reserved

Recipe Name: Baked Codfish with Lemon
Recipe Category: Dinner Entrée
Portion Size: 4 oz.
Ingredients: Yields: 8 servings

Ingredients	Notes:
8 (4 oz.) Codfish fillets	Or other white fish
½ teaspoon salt	
¼ teaspoon pepper	
¼ teaspoon paprika	
3 tablespoons of small capers	Optional
¼ cup olive oil	
¼ cup fresh parsley	Wash, trim and chop fine. Or 2 T. dried parsley
16 lemon slices	
½ cup tartar sauce	

Directions:

Steps:	Directions:	Critical Control Point / Quality Assurance
1	Preheat oven 375 degrees	
2	Spray baking pan with non-stick cooking spray	
3	Place fish in pan. Brush each with olive oil.	
4	Sprinkle with salt, pepper, and paprika	
5	Top each fillet with 2 lemon slices and sprinkle with capers. Transfer to preheated broiler. Heat on top rack for 3-5 minutes.	Bake 8-10 minutes. Broil for 3 minutes or until lemon slightly browned at edges. Cook until internal temperature reaches 145° F for 15 seconds.
6	Sprinkle each with parsley. Serve while hot. Serve tartar sauce on the side as a condiment.	

Time Temperature Sensitive food. *Food safety Standards: hold food for service at an internal temperature above 140° F. Do not mix old product with new. Cool leftover product quickly (within 4 hours) to below 41° F. Follow proper cooling procedures. Reheat leftover product quickly (within 2 hours) to 165 degrees F for 15 seconds. Cold holding at 41°F or colder or using time alone (less than four hours).*

<u>Texture Modified Diets:</u>
Soft & Bite Size: (aka Bite size) **Food particle size ½ inch (~width of standard fork)** Food must be moist. Cut foods with a knife to a ½" particle size prior to mixing. Moisten with tartar sauce as needed. Foods that do not process well should be omitted. Omit: capers and lemon slices. Drizzle with lemon juice.
Chopped: Food particle size ¼ inch (~ ½ width of standard fork) Food must be moist. Chop foods with a knife to 1/4" particle size prior to mixing. Moisten with tartar sauce as needed. Foods that do not process well should be omitted. Omit: capers and lemon slices. Drizzle with lemon juice.
Minced and Moist:(aka Minced/Mechanical Soft/Ground) **Food particle size 1/8 inch (fits through prongs of standard fork)** Food must be moist. Use a food processor to grind food particles into 1/8 inch prior to mixing. Moisten with tartar sauce as needed. Foods that do not process well should be omitted. Omit: capers and lemon slices. Drizzle with lemon juice.
Pureed: Smooth and cohesive. Use a food processor to puree to a smooth consistency. Foods are processed by grinding and then pureeing them. May add tartar sauce to puree. Do not add to much liquid. Puree should still hold its shape. Must not be firm or sticky. Puree foods while still hot. Appearance should be smooth like pudding. Foods that do not process well should be omitted. Omit: capers and lemon slices. Drizzle with lemon juice. Serve ½ c. puree fish serving.

<u>Therapeutic Modified Diets:</u>
Lowfat: No changes needed
Diabetic/No added Sugar/No Conc. Sweets/Calorie Controlled: No changes needed
Bland/Anti Reflux: omit pepper, parsley, lemon and capers
Liberal House Renal: Omit salt, lemon and capers
No Added Salt: Omit capers
2 Gram Sodium: Omit salt and capers
Gluten Free: No changes needed. Prepare foods separately to prevent cross contamination.
Allergy Alerts: When an "X" is present, this indicates the allergen is present.
Always read all food labels to ensure allergens are not present.

Wheat	Milk	Eggs	Fish Shellfish	Soy	Peanuts/Nuts	Other
		X	X			

Key: SF= Salt Free D= Diet or Sugarfree LF = Lowfat FF = Fat Free GF = Gluten Free

Recipe Name: Baked Fish with Cilantro Lime
Recipe Category: Dinner Entrée
Portion Size: 4 oz.
Ingredients: Yields: 8 servings

Ingredients	Notes:
8 Codfish or haddock fillets	4 oz. each or other white fish
½ teaspoon salt	
¼ teaspoon pepper and paprika	
½ cup snipped fresh cilantro	
1 tablespoon olive oil	
1 teaspoon lime zest	
2 tablespoon fresh lime juice	

Directions:

Steps:	Directions:	Critical Control Point / Quality Assurance
1	Preheat oven to 375 degrees	
2	Spray baking pan with non stick cooking spray	
3	Place fish in pan. Brush with olive oil.	
4	Sprinkle with salt, pepper, and paprika	Bake 8 to 10 minutes
5	Transfer to preheated broiler	Broil for 3 minutes until lemon slightly browned at the edges. Cook until internal temperature reaches 145° F for 15 seconds
6	In a small bowl, stir together cilantro, lime zest, and lime juice. Spoon over fish. Serve hot.	

Time Temperature Sensitive food. *Food safety Standards: hold food for service at an internal temperature above 140° F. Do not mix old product with new. Cool leftover product quickly (within 4 hours) to below 41° F. Follow proper cooling procedures. Store leftovers in a tightly sealed, labeled and dated container. Use leftover within 72 hours if stored in refrigerator or 30 days if stored in the freezer. Reheat leftover product quickly (within 2 hours) to 165 degrees F for 15 seconds. Reheat left over product only once; discard if not used. Cold holding at 41°F or colder or using time alone (less than four hours). Always wash hands and wash and sanitize counter tops utensils and containers between steps when working with raw seafood.*

Texture Modified Diets:

Soft & Bite Size: (aka Bite size) **Food particle size ½ inch (~width of standard fork)** Food must be moist. Cut foods with a knife to a ½" particle size prior to mixing. Moisten with tartar sauce as needed.
Chopped: Food particle size ¼ inch (~ ½ width of standard fork) Food must be moist. Chop foods with a knife to 1/4" particle size prior to mixing. Moisten with tartar sauce as needed.
Minced and Moist: (aka Minced/Mechanical Soft/Ground) **Food particle size 1/8 inch (fits through prongs of standard fork)** Food must be moist. Use a food processor to grind food particles into 1/8 inch prior to mixing. Moisten with tartar sauce as needed. **Pureed: Smooth and cohesive.** Use a food processor to puree to a smooth consistency. Foods are processed by grinding and then pureeing them. May add tartar sauce to puree. Do not add to much liquid. Puree should still hold its shape. Must not be firm or sticky. Puree foods while still hot. Appearance should be smooth like pudding. Serve ½ c. puree fish serving.

Therapeutic Modified Diets:

Lowfat: No changes needed
Diabetic/No added Sugar/No Conc. Sweets/Calorie Controlled: No changes needed
Bland/Anti Reflux: omit pepper, paprika, cilantro, lime and lime zest
Liberal House Renal: Omit salt and lime
No Added Salt: No changes needed
2 Gram Sodium: omit salt
Gluten Free: No changes needed. Prepare foods separately to prevent cross contamination.

Allergy Alerts: When an "X" is present, this indicates the allergen is present. Always read all food labels to ensure allergens are not present.

Wheat	Milk	Eggs	Fish Shellfish	Soy	Peanuts/Nuts	Other
			X			

Key: SF= Salt Free D= Diet or Sugarfree LF = Lowfat FF = Fat Free GF = Gluten Free

Copyright 2020 Jacqueline Larson M.S., R.D.N. and Associates.   All Rights Reserved

Recipe Name: Blackened Tilapia Fish
Recipe Category: Dinner Entrée
Portion Size: 4 oz.
Ingredients: Yields: 8 servings

Ingredients	Notes:
8 Tilapia	4 oz. each or other white fish fillets
1 teaspoon salt	
¼ teaspoon pepper	
2 teaspoons paprika	
2 tablespoons light brown sugar	
2 tablespoons olive oil	
1 teaspoon ground cumin	
2 teaspoons garlic powder	
1 teaspoon dried oregano	

Directions:

Steps:	Directions:	Critical Control Point / Quality Assurance
1	Combine paprika, brown sugar, oregano, garlic powder, cumin, pepper, and salt in a deep dish. Mix until well combined	
2	Heat oil over medium high heat in a large pan.	
3	Saute the fillets for 2-3 minutes on each side until reddish brown on the outside and flaky on the inside. Serve immediately.	Saute for 2-3 minutes until slightly browned at the edges. Cook until internal temperature reaches 145° F for 15 seconds

Time Temperature Sensitive food. *Food safety Standards: hold food for service at an internal temperature above 140° F. Do not mix old product with new. Cool leftover product quickly (within 4 hours) to below 41° F. Follow proper cooling procedures. Store leftovers in a tightly sealed, labeled and dated container. Use leftover within 72 hours if stored in refrigerator or 30 days if stored in the freezer. Reheat leftover product quickly (within 2 hours) to 165 degrees F for 15 seconds. Reheat left over product only once; discard if not used. Cold holding at 41°F or colder or using time alone (less than four hours). Always wash hands and wash and sanitize counter tops utensils and containers between steps when working with raw seafood.*

Texture Modified Diets:

Soft & Bite Size: (aka Bite size) **Food particle size ½ inch (~width of standard fork)** Food must be moist. Cut foods with a knife to a ½" particle size prior to mixing. Moisten with tartar sauce as needed.
Chopped: Food particle size ¼ inch (~ ½ width of standard fork) Food must be moist. Chop foods with a knife to 1/4" particle size prior to mixing. Moisten with tartar sauce as needed. **Minced and Moist:**(aka Minced/Mechanical Soft/Ground) **Food particle size 1/8 inch (fits through prongs of standard fork)** Food must be moist. Use a food processor to grind food particles into 1/8 inch prior to mixing. Moisten with tartar sauce as needed..
Pureed: Smooth and cohesive. Use a food processor to puree to a smooth consistency. Foods are processed by grinding and then pureeing them. May add tartar sauce to puree. Do not add to much liquid. Puree should still hold its shape. Must not be firm or sticky. Puree foods while still hot. Appearance should be smooth like pudding. Serve ½ c. puree fish serving.

Therapeutic Modified Diets:

Lowfat: No changes needed
Diabetic/No added Sugar/No Conc. Sweets/Calorie Controlled: No changes needed
Bland/Anti Reflux: omit pepper, oregano, garlic powder, and cumin
Liberal House Renal: Omit salt
No Added Salt: No changes needed
2 Gram Sodium: omit salt
Gluten Free: No changes needed. Prepare foods separately to prevent cross contamination.

Allergy Alerts: When an "X" is present, this indicates the allergen is present. Always read all food labels to ensure allergens are not present.

Wheat	Milk	Eggs	Fish Shellfish	Soy	Peanuts/Nuts	Other
			X			

Key: SF= Salt Free D= Diet or Sugarfree LF = Lowfat FF = Fat Free GF = Gluten Free

Copyright 2020 Jacqueline Larson M.S., R.D.N. and Associates.   All Rights Reserved

Recipe Name: Brazilian Fish Stew
Recipe Category: Dinner Entrée
Portion Size: 1 cup Fish Stew over ½ c. rice
Ingredients: Yields: 8 servings

Ingredients	Notes:
8 boneless fillet of fish and 1 pounds of assorted shellfish, shells removed.	3 oz. of fillet each. (shelled shellfish is optional)
3 garlic cloves, minced	
¼ cup lemon juice	
1 teaspoon lemon zest	Wash lemon before zesting.
½ teaspoon salt	
1/2 teaspoon pepper	
1 large onion, finely sliced	Wash, peel and slice
1 green pepper	Wash, trim and dice
1 red pepper	Wash, trim and dice
2 large fresh tomatoes	Wash, trim and dice
1 teaspoon coriander	
1 (6 oz.) can tomato paste	
¼ cup olive oil	
2 cups light coconut milk	
2 cups cooked brown rice	See recipe in cookbook for brown rice
¼ cup Fresh parsley	Wash, trim and chop

Directions:

Steps:	Directions:	Critical Control Point / Quality Assurance
1	Rinse fish and place in a bowl with garlic, lemon juice, salt and pepper	
2	Marinate in refrigerator for 15 minutes	
3	Place oil in pan and sauté onion, green pepper, red pepper, until tender	
4	Add tomatoes, coriander, and tomato paste	
5	Bring to boil and add fish and shell fish. Add coconut milk and heat through.	Lower heat to medium and cook for 5 to 7 minutes. Cook until internal temperature reaches 165° F for 15 seconds.
6	Serve hot over brown rice.	
7	Garnish with lemon zest and parsley .	

Time Temperature Sensitive food. *Food safety Standards: hold food for service at an internal temperature above 140° F. Do not mix old product with new. Cool leftover product quickly (within 4 hours) to below 41° F. Follow proper cooling procedures. Store leftovers in a tightly sealed, labeled and dated container. Use leftover within 72 hours if stored in refrigerator or 30 days if stored in the freezer. Reheat leftover product quickly (within 2 hours) to 165 degrees F for 15 seconds. Reheat left over product only once; discard if not used. Cold holding at 41°F or colder or using time alone (less than four hours). Always wash hands and wash and sanitize counter tops utensils and containers between steps when working with raw seafood.*

<u>**Texture Modified Diets:**</u>
Soft & Bite Size: (aka Bite size) **Food particle size ½ inch (~width of standard fork)** Food must be moist. Cut foods with a knife to a ½" particle size prior to mixing. Moisten with tartar sauce as needed.
Chopped: Food particle size ¼ inch (~ ½ width of standard fork) Food must be moist. Chop foods with a knife to 1/4" particle size prior to mixing. Moisten with tartar sauce as needed.
Minced and Moist:(aka Minced/Mechanical Soft/Ground) **Food particle size 1/8 inch (fits through prongs of standard fork)** Food must be moist. Use a food processor to grind food particles into 1/8 inch prior to mixing. Moisten with tartar sauce as needed.
Pureed: Smooth and cohesive. Use a food processor to puree to a smooth consistency. Foods are processed by grinding and then pureeing them. May add tartar sauce to puree. Do not add to much liquid. Puree should still hold its shape. Must not be firm or sticky. Puree foods while still hot. Appearance should be smooth like pudding. Serve ½ c. puree fish serving and ½ cup puree brown rice separately.

Copyright 2020 Jacqueline Larson M.S., R.D.N. and Associates.   All Rights Reserved

Therapeutic Modified Diets:
Lowfat: No changes needed
Diabetic/No added Sugar/No Conc. Sweets/Calorie Controlled: No changes needed
Bland/Anti Reflux: Serve plain baked fish and plain brown rice
Liberal House Renal: Omit salt, tomato paste, and tomatoes
No Added Salt: No changes needed
2 Gram Sodium: Omit salt
Gluten Free: No changes needed. Prepare foods separately to prevent cross contamination.
Allergy Alerts: When an "X" is present, this indicates the allergen is present.
Always read all food labels to ensure allergens are not present.

Wheat	Milk	Eggs	Fish Shellfish	Soy	Peanuts/Nuts	Other
			X			X

Key: SF= Salt Free D= Diet or Sugarfree LF = Lowfat FF = Fat Free GF = Gluten Free

Recipe Name: Broiled Fish Parmesan
Recipe Category: Dinner Entrée
Portion Size: 4 oz.

Ingredients: Yields: 8 servings

Ingredients	Notes:
2 ½ pounds fish fillets	May use any white boneless fish (cod, halibut, perch, sole, trout etc.)
2 cups light mayonnaise	
¼ cup grated parmesan cheese	
2 teaspoons grated onion	
¼ teaspoon Tabasco hot pepper sauce (optional)	

Directions:

Steps:	Directions:	Critical Control Point / Quality Assurance
1	Place fillet in a shallow baking tray. Broil for 5 minutes or less.	
2	Combine mayonnaise, cheese, onion, and Tabasco; mix well. Spread mixture on fish. Return to broiler.	
3	Broil until topping is brown, bubbly, and fish flakes easily with a fork. Serve hot.	Cook until internal temperature reaches 145° F for 15 seconds.

Time Temperature Sensitive food. Food safety Standards: hold food for service at an internal temperature above 140° F. Do not mix old product with new. Cool leftover product quickly (within 4 hours) to below 41° F. Follow proper cooling procedures. Store leftovers in a tightly sealed, labeled and dated container. Use leftover within 72 hours if stored in refrigerator or 30 days if stored in the freezer. Reheat leftover product quickly (within 2 hours) to 165 degrees F for 15 seconds. Reheat left over product only once; discard if not used. Cold holding at 41°F or colder or using time alone (less than four hours). Always wash hands and wash and sanitize counter tops utensils and containers between steps when working with raw seafood.

Texture Modified Diets:

Soft & Bite Size: (aka Bite size) **Food particle size ½ inch (~width of standard fork)** Food must be moist. Cut foods with a knife to a ½" particle size prior to mixing. Moisten with tartar sauce as needed. Foods that do not process well should be omitted.

Chopped: Food particle size ¼ inch (~ ½ width of standard fork) Food must be moist. Chop foods with a knife to 1/4" particle size prior to mixing. Moisten with tartar sauce as needed.

Minced and Moist: (aka Minced/Mechanical Soft/Ground) **Food particle size 1/8 inch (fits through prongs of standard fork)** Food must be moist. Use a food processor to grind food particles into 1/8 inch prior to mixing. Moisten with tartar sauce as needed.

Pureed: Smooth and cohesive. Use a food processor to puree to a smooth consistency. Foods are processed by grinding and then pureeing them. May add tartar sauce to puree. Do not add to much liquid. Puree should still hold its shape. Must not be firm or sticky. Puree foods while still hot. Appearance should be smooth like pudding. Serve ½ c. puree fish serving.

Therapeutic Modified Diets:

Lowfat: No changes needed
Diabetic/No added Sugar/No Conc. Sweets/Calorie Controlled: No changes needed
Bland/Anti Reflux: omit Tabasco sauce
Liberal House Renal: Omit mayonnaise and Parmesan cheese. Drizzle with olive oil.
No Added Salt: No changes needed
2 Gram Sodium: Omit mayonnaise and Parmesan cheese. Drizzle with olive oil
Gluten Free: No changes needed. Prepare foods separately to prevent cross contamination.
Allergy Alerts: When an "X" is present, this indicates the allergen is present.
Always read all food labels to ensure allergens are not present.

Wheat	Milk	Eggs	Fish Shellfish	Soy	Peanuts/Nuts	Other
	X	X	X			

Key: SF= Salt Free D= Diet or Sugarfree LF = Lowfat FF = Fat Free GF = Gluten Free

Copyright 2020 Jacqueline Larson M.S., R.D.N. and Associates.   All Rights Reserved

Recipe Name: Crab Cakes with Red Pepper Sauce
Recipe Category: Dinner Entrée
Portion Size: 4 oz.
Ingredients: Yields: 8 servings

Ingredients	Notes:
½ cup light mayonnaise	
¼ cup fresh chives	Wash, trim and chop
2 tablespoons fresh parsley	Wash, trim and mince
1 tablespoon lemon juice	
½ teaspoon paprika	
1 pound lump crabmeat, cartilage removed	Drained
½ cup bread crumbs	
RED PEPPER SAUCE:	
1/2 cup sweet red pepper	Wash, trim and finely chop
1/4 cup green onions	Wash, trim and finely chop (including green tops)
1/4 cup Dijon mustard	
1/4 cup light mayonnaise	
1/4 cup light sour cream	
2 tablespoons red onion	Wash, peeled and minced
2 teaspoons parsley flakes	
1 tablespoon lemon juice	
¼ teaspoon salt	
¼ teaspoon pepper	
3 tablespoons olive oil	
8 Lemon wedges	(optional garnish)

Directions:

Steps:	Directions:	Critical Control Point / Quality Assurance
1	In a large bowl, combine mayonnaise, chives, parsley, lemon juice, paprika, pepper, crabmeat and bread crumbs; mix well.	
2	Shape 1/4 cup of crab mixture into patties.	
3	For sauce, in a blender or food processor, combine the red pepper, onions, mustard, mayonnaise, sour cream, onion, parsley, honey, lemon juice, salt and pepper; cover and process until finely chopped. Chill.	Refrigerate until serving.
4	In a large skillet, heat ½ oil to medium high heat.	
5	Place half of the crab cakes in skillet.	Cook over medium heat for 5 minutes on each side or until lightly browned (carefully turn the delicate cakes over)
6	Repeat with remaining oil and crab cakes. Serve with sauce and lemon wedges.	Cook until internal temperature reaches 145° F for 15 seconds.

Time Temperature Sensitive food. *Food safety Standards: hold food for service at an internal temperature above 140° F. Do not mix old product with new. Cool leftover product quickly (within 4 hours) to below 41° F. Follow proper cooling procedures. Store leftovers in a tightly sealed, labeled and dated container. Use leftover within 72 hours if stored in refrigerator or 30 days if stored in the freezer. Reheat leftover product quickly (within 2 hours) to 165 degrees F for 15 seconds. Reheat left over product only once; discard if not used. Cold holding at 41 °F or colder or using time alone (less than four hours).*

Copyright 2020 Jacqueline Larson M.S., R.D.N. and Associates.   All Rights Reserved

Texture Modified Diets:

Soft & Bite Size: (aka Bite size) **Food particle size ½ inch (~width of standard fork)** Food must be moist. Cut foods with a knife to a ½" particle size prior to mixing. Moisten with sauce as needed. Foods that do not process well should be omitted. Omit: green onions

Chopped: Food particle size ¼ inch (~ ½ width of standard fork) Food must be moist. Chop foods with a knife to 1/4" particle size prior to mixing. Moisten with sauce as needed. Foods that do not process well should be omitted. Omit: green onions.

Minced and Moist: (aka Minced/Mechanical Soft/Ground) **Food particle size 1/8 inch (fits through prongs of standard fork)** Food must be moist. Use a food processor to grind food particles into 1/8 inch prior to mixing. Moisten with sauce as needed. Foods that do not process well should be omitted. Omit: green onions.

Pureed: Smooth and cohesive. Use a food processor to puree to a smooth consistency. Foods are processed by grinding and then pureeing them. May add sauce to puree. Do not add to much liquid. Puree should still hold its shape. Must not be firm or sticky. Puree foods while still hot. Appearance should be smooth like pudding. Foods that do not process well should be omitted. Omit: green onions.
Serve ½ c. puree fish serving. Top with puree sauce.

Therapeutic Modified Diets:

Lowfat: No changes needed
Diabetic/No added Sugar/No Conc. Sweets/Calorie Controlled: No changes needed
Bland/Anti Reflux: omit, parsley, chives, lemon juice, paprika, lemons. For sauce top with mayonnaise and sour cream mixture only.
Liberal House Renal: Omit salt, bread crumbs, mayonnaise and red pepper sauce
No Added Salt: No changes needed
2 Gram Sodium: omit salt, bread crumbs, mayonnaise and red pepper sauce
Gluten Free: Omit bread crumbs and Substitute with GF crushed cornflakes or oatmeal. Prepare foods separately to prevent cross contamination.
Allergy Alerts: When an "X" is present, this indicates the allergen is present.
Always read all food labels to ensure allergens are not present.

Wheat	Milk	Eggs	Fish Shellfish	Soy	Peanuts/Nuts	Other
X	X	X	X			

Key: SF= Salt Free D= Diet or Sugarfree LF = Lowfat FF = Fat Free GF = Gluten Free

Recipe Name: Creamed Salmon
Recipe Category: Dinner Entrée
Portion Size: ½ cup creamed salmon over 1 English muffin half
Ingredients: Yields: 8 servings

Ingredients	Notes:
1/2 cup sliced green onion	Wash, trim and slice. (including green tops)
1/2 teaspoon salt	
1/4 teaspoon pepper	
1/4 cup oil	
1/4 cup flour	
2 1/2 cups nonfat milk	
1 cup light sour cream	
4 cups canned salmon, drained (water packed) or fresh boneless skinless salmon, cut into small pieces	
4 English muffins, split and toasted	May use whole grain muffins
1/4 cup silvered almonds, toasted	(optional)

Directions:

Steps:	Directions:	Critical Control Point / Quality Assurance
1	In a saucepan cook onion in oil till tender.	
2	Stir in flour, salt, and pepper. Add milk all at once.	Cook and stir till thickened and bubbly.
3	Stir about 2 cups of the hot mixture into sour cream; return all to saucepan.	
4	Gently stir in salmon and 1/4 cup milk. Heat through (do not boil). Serve over muffin halves. Sprinkle with almonds.	Cook until internal temperature reaches 165° F for 15 seconds.

Time Temperature Sensitive food. *Food safety Standards: hold food for service at an internal temperature above 140° F. Do not mix old product with new. Cool leftover product quickly (within 4 hours) to below 41° F. Follow proper cooling procedures. Store leftovers in a tightly sealed, labeled and dated container. Use leftover within 72 hours if stored in refrigerator or 30 days if stored in the freezer. Reheat leftover product quickly (within 2 hours) to 165 degrees F for 15 seconds. Reheat left over product only once; discard if not used. Cold holding at 41°F or colder or using time alone (less than four hours). Always wash hands and wash and sanitize counter tops utensils and containers between steps when working with raw seafood.*

Texture Modified Diets:

Soft & Bite Size: (aka Bite size) **Food particle size ½ inch (~width of standard fork)** Food must be moist. Cut foods with a knife to a ½" particle size prior to mixing. Moisten with sauce as needed. Foods that do not process well should be omitted. Omit: green onions and almonds. Serve over soft moist bread.

Chopped: Food particle size ¼ inch (~ ½ width of standard fork) Food must be moist. Chop foods with a knife to 1/4" particle size prior to mixing. Moisten with sauce as needed. Foods that do not process well should be omitted. Omit: green onions and almonds. Serve over soft moist bread.

Minced and Moist: (aka Minced/Mechanical Soft/Ground) **Food particle size 1/8 inch (fits through prongs of standard fork)** Food must be moist. Use a food processor to grind food particles into 1/8 inch prior to mixing. Moisten with sauce as needed. Foods that do not process well should be omitted. Omit: green onions and almonds. Serve over soft moist bread

Pureed: Smooth and cohesive. Use a food processor to puree to a smooth consistency. Foods are processed by grinding and then pureeing them. May add sauce to puree. Do not add to much liquid. Puree should still hold its shape. Must not be firm or sticky. Puree foods while still hot. Appearance should be smooth like pudding. Foods that do not process well should be omitted. Omit: green onions and almonds. Serve ½ c. puree fish serving and ½ c. puree bread separately. Top with puree sauce.

Therapeutic Modified Diets:

Lowfat: Omit nuts
Diabetic/No added Sugar/No Conc. Sweets/Calorie Controlled: No changes needed
Bland/Anti Reflux: omit pepper and almonds
Liberal House Renal: Omit salt, sour cream, almonds and milk. Serve on SF toast (see recipe)
No Added Salt: No changes needed
2 Gram Sodium: omit salt. Serve on SF toast (see recipe)
Gluten Free: Gluten-free flour. Use gluten free English muffins or gluten free bread. Prepare foods separately to prevent cross contamination.

Allergy Alerts: When an "X" is present, this indicates the allergen is present. Always read all food labels to ensure allergens are not present.

Milk	Eggs	Fish Shellfish	Soy	Peanuts/Nuts	Other
X	X	X		X	

Key: SF= Salt Free D= Diet or Sugarfree LF = Lowfat FF = Fat Free GF = Gluten Free

Recipe Name: Creamed Tuna
Recipe Category: Dinner Entrée
Portion Size: ½ cup creamed tuna over 1 English muffin half
Ingredients: Yields: 8 servings

Ingredients	Notes:
1/2 cup sliced green onion	Wash, trim and slice. (including green tops)
1/2 teaspoon salt	
1/4 teaspoon pepper	
1/4 cup oil	
1/4 cup flour	
2 1/2 cups nonfat milk	
1 cup light sour cream	
4 cups tuna, drained (water packed)	
4 English muffins, spilt and toasted	May use whole grain muffins
1/4 cup silvered almonds, toasted	(optional)

Directions:

Steps:	Directions:	Critical Control Point Quality Assurance
1	In a saucepan cook onion in oil till tender.	
2	Stir in flour, salt, and pepper. Add milk all at once.	Cook and stir till thickened and bubbly.
3	Stir about 2 cups of the hot mixture into sour cream; return all to saucepan.	
4	Gently stir in tuna and 1/4 cup milk. Heat through (do not boil). Serve over muffin halves. Sprinkle with almonds.	Cook until internal temperature reaches 165° F for 15 seconds.

Time Temperature Sensitive food. *Food safety Standards: hold food for service at an internal temperature above 140° F. Do not mix old product with new. Cool leftover product quickly (within 4 hours) to below 41° F. Follow proper cooling procedures. Store leftovers in a tightly sealed, labeled and dated container. Use leftover within 72 hours if stored in refrigerator or 30 days if stored in the freezer. Reheat leftover product quickly (within 2 hours) to 165 degrees F for 15 seconds. Reheat left over product only once; discard if not used. Cold holding at 41 °F or colder or using time alone (less than four hours). Always wash hands and wash and sanitize counter tops utensils and containers between steps when working with raw seafood.*

Texture Modified Diets:

Soft & Bite Size: (aka Bite size) **Food particle size ½ inch (~width of standard fork)** Food must be moist. Cut foods with a knife to a ½" particle size prior to mixing. Moisten with sauce as needed. Foods that do not process well should be omitted. Omit: green onions and almonds. Serve over soft moist bread.

Chopped: Food particle size ¼ inch (~ ½ width of standard fork) Food must be moist. Chop foods with a knife to 1/4" particle size prior to mixing. Moisten with sauce as needed. Foods that do not process well should be omitted. Omit: green onions and almonds. Serve over soft moist bread.

Minced and Moist: (aka Minced/Mechanical Soft/Ground) **Food particle size 1/8 inch (fits through prongs of standard fork)** Food must be moist. Use a food processor to grind food particles into 1/8 inch prior to mixing. Moisten with sauce as needed. Foods that do not process well should be omitted. Omit: green onions and almonds. Serve over soft moist bread

Pureed: Smooth and cohesive. Use a food processor to puree to a smooth consistency. Foods are processed by grinding and then pureeing them. May add sauce to puree. Do not add to much liquid. Puree should still hold its shape. Must not be firm or sticky. Puree foods while still hot. Appearance should be smooth like pudding. Foods that do not process well should be omitted. Omit: green onions and almonds. Serve ½ c. puree fish serving and ½ c. puree bread separately. Top with puree sauce.

Therapeutic Modified Diets:
Lowfat: Omit nuts
Diabetic/No added Sugar/No Conc. Sweets/Calorie Controlled: No changes needed
Bland/Anti Reflux: omit pepper and almonds
Liberal House Renal: Omit salt, sour cream, almonds and milk. Serve on SF toast (see recipe)
No Added Salt: No changes needed
2 Gram Sodium: omit salt. Serve on SF toast (see recipe)
Gluten Free: Gluten-free flour. Use gluten free English muffins or gluten free bread. Prepare foods separately to prevent cross contamination.

Allergy Alerts: When an "X" is present, this indicates the allergen is present. Always read all food labels to ensure allergens are not present.

Wheat	Milk	Eggs	Fish Shellfish	Soy	Peanuts/Nuts	Other
X	X	X	X		X	

Key: SF= Salt Free D= Diet or Sugarfree LF = Lowfat FF = Fat Free GF = Gluten Free

Recipe Name: Creamy Pesto Shrimp with Linguine
Recipe Category: Dinner Entrée
Portion Size: 1 cup
Ingredients: Yields: 8 servings

Ingredients	Notes:
1 pound linguine pasta	May use whole grain pasta
2 tablespoons olive oil	
3 cloves garlic, minced	
2 tablespoons all purpose flour	
1 cup low sodium chicken broth	
1 (14 oz.) can fat free evaporated milk	Or half and half
1/2 cup pine nuts	
1/4 cup nonfat milk	
1/2 teaspoon ground black pepper	
1 cup grated Parmesan cheese	
2 cups fresh basil	Wash and trim before processing
2 1/2 pounds large shrimp, peeled and deveined	

Directions:

Steps:	Directions:	Critical Control Point / Quality Assurance
1	Bring a large pot of water to a boil. Add linguine pasta	Cook for 8 to 10 minutes, or until al dente; drain
2	In a large skillet, heat oil over medium heat. Add garlic and stir. Stir in flour, and stir	Cook for 1 minute
3	Over medium high heat add chicken broth and evaporated milk	Cook 6 to 8 minutes, stirring occasionally until thick and bubbly
4	In a small food processor, add pine nuts, nonfat milk, black pepper, Parmesan cheese and fresh basil; Add to sauce	Process until smooth
5	Stir in the shrimp to sauce	Cook until they turn pink ~ 5 minutes. Cook until internal temperature reaches 145° F for 15 seconds.
6	Serve over the hot linguine.	

Time Temperature Sensitive food. *Food safety Standards: hold food for service at an internal temperature above 140° F. Do not mix old product with new. Cool leftover product quickly (within 4 hours) to below 41° F. Follow proper cooling procedures. Store leftovers in a tightly sealed, labeled and dated container. Use leftover within 72 hours if stored in refrigerator or 30 days if stored in the freezer. Reheat leftover product quickly (within 2 hours) to 165 degrees F for 15 seconds. Reheat left over product only once; discard if not used. Cold holding at 41 °F or colder or using time alone (less than four hours). Always wash hands and wash and sanitize counter tops utensils and containers between steps when working with raw seafood.*

<u>**Texture Modified Diets: TIP: use pasta in correct particle size.**</u>
Soft & Bite Size: (aka Bite size) **Food particle size ½ inch (~width of standard fork)** Food must be moist. Cut foods with a knife to a ½" particle size prior to mixing. Moisten with broth as needed. Foods that do not process well should be omitted. Omit: pine nuts.
Chopped: Food particle size ¼ inch (~ ½ width of standard fork) Food must be moist. Chop foods with a knife to 1/4" particle size prior to mixing. Moisten with broth as needed. Foods that do not process well should be omitted. Omit: pine nuts
Minced and Moist: (aka Minced/Mechanical Soft/Ground) **Food particle size 1/8 inch (fits through prongs of standard fork)** Food must be moist. Use a food processor to grind food particles into 1/8 inch prior to mixing. Moisten with broth as needed. Foods that do not process well should be omitted. Omit: pine nuts
Pureed: Smooth and cohesive. Use a food processor to puree to a smooth consistency. Foods are processed by grinding and then pureeing them. May add broth or sauce to puree. Do not add to much liquid. Puree should still

Copyright 2020 Jacqueline Larson M.S., R.D.N. and Associates.   All Rights Reserved

hold its shape. Must not be firm or sticky. Puree foods while still hot. Appearance should be smooth like pudding. Foods that do not process well should be omitted. Omit: pine nuts
Serve ½ c. puree shrimp/sauce serving and ½ c. puree pasta separately.

Therapeutic Modified Diets:
Lowfat: Use evaporated milk, no half and half
Diabetic/No added Sugar/No Conc. Sweets/Calorie Controlled: No changes needed
Bland/Anti Reflux: omit garlic, black pepper, basil, and pine nuts
Liberal House Renal: Serve plain cooked shrimp and pasta. Drizzle with olive oil, basil and garlic.
No Added Salt: No changes needed
2 Gram Sodium: Serve plain cooked shrimp and pasta. Drizzle with olive oil, basil and garlic
Gluten Free: Use Gluten-free broth. Use GF Pasta and GF all purpose flour. Prepare foods separately to prevent cross contamination.
Allergy Alerts: When an "X" is present, this indicates the allergen is present.
Always read all food labels to ensure allergens are not present.

Wheat	Milk	Eggs	Fish Shellfish	Soy	Peanuts/Nuts	Other
X	X	X	X		X	

Key: SF= Salt Free D= Diet or Sugarfree LF = Lowfat FF = Fat Free GF = Gluten Free

Recipe Name: Creamy Salmon and Pasta Salad
Recipe Category: Dinner Entrée
Portion Size: 1 1/2 cup
Ingredients: Yields: 8 servings

Ingredients	Notes:
1 lb. pasta	May use whole grain pasta
4 cups canned salmon water packed, drained, flaked	
1/4 cup light mayonnaise	
1 cup plain nonfat Greek yogurt	
2 tablespoons fresh lemon juice	
1 teaspoon lemon zest	Wash and zest
1 cup celery, diced	Wash, trim and dice.
1 cup frozen peas, thawed	
½ cup red bell pepper, diced	Wash, trim and dice.
1 cup carrot, shredded	Wash peel, trim and shred.
1/2 cup chopped green onion	Wash, trim, and slice. (including green tops)
2 tablespoons chopped parsley, dried	Or ¼ cup fresh chopped

Directions:

Steps:	Directions:	Critical Control Point /Quality Assurance
1	Cook pasta according to package directions.	
2	In a large bowl mix Greek yogurt, mayonnaise, lemon juice and zest, and pepper together.	
3	When pasta is finished cooking, drain, then run under cool water until it's no longer hot.	
4	Add pasta to yogurt dressing, along with celery, red pepper, peas, carrots, onions, and parsley.	
5	Gently mix all the ingredients together until combined.	
6	Refrigerate for 1 hour or overnight before serving.	

Time Temperature Sensitive food. *Food safety Standards: hold food for service at an internal temperature above 140° F. Do not mix old product with new. Cool leftover product quickly (within 4 hours) to below 41° F. Follow proper cooling procedures. Store leftovers in a tightly sealed, labeled and dated container. Use leftover within 72 hours if stored in refrigerator or 30 days if stored in the freezer. Cold holding at 41°F or colder or using time alone (less than four hours).*

<u>Texture Modified Diets: TIP: Use pasta in correct particle size.</u>
Soft & Bite Size: (aka Bite size) **Food particle size ½ inch (~width of standard fork)** Food must be moist. Cut foods with a knife to a ½" particle size prior to mixing. Moisten with broth as needed. Foods that do not process well should be omitted. Omit: green onion
Chopped: Food particle size ¼ inch (~ ½ width of standard fork) Food must be moist. Chop foods with a knife to 1/4" particle size prior to mixing. Moisten with broth as needed. Foods that do not process well should be omitted. Omit: green onion
Minced and Moist:(aka Minced/Mechanical Soft/Ground) **Food particle size 1/8 inch (fits through prongs of standard fork)** Food must be moist. Use a food processor to grind food particles into 1/8 inch prior to mixing. Moisten with broth as needed. Foods that do not process well should be omitted. Omit: green onion
Pureed: Smooth and cohesive. Use a food processor to puree to a smooth consistency. Foods are processed by grinding and then pureeing them. May add broth or sauce to puree. Do not add to much liquid. Puree should still hold its shape. Must not be firm or sticky. Puree foods while still hot. Appearance should be smooth like pudding. Foods that do not process well should be omitted. Omit: green onion. Serve ½ c. puree salmon and ½ c. puree pasta separately.

<u>Therapeutic Modified Diets:</u>
Lowfat: No changes needed
Diabetic/No added Sugar/No Conc. Sweets/Calorie Controlled: No changes needed
Bland/Anti Reflux: omit lemon, celery, green onion and parsley
Liberal House Renal: Omit salt, mayonnaise, and yogurt. Toss with olive oil.
No Added Salt: No changes needed
2 Gram Sodium: omit salt and mayonnaise. Toss with olive oil.
Gluten Free: Gluten-free pasta Prepare foods separately to prevent cross contamination.

Allergy Alerts: When an "X" is present, this indicates the allergen is present. Always read all food labels to ensure allergens are not present.

Wheat	Milk	Eggs	Fish Shellfish	Soy	Peanuts/Nuts	Other
X	X	X	X			

Key: SF= Salt Free D= Diet or Sugarfree LF = Lowfat FF = Fat Free GF = Gluten Free

Recipe Name: Creamy Tuna and Pasta Salad
Recipe Category: Dinner Entrée
Portion Size: 1 1/2 cup
Ingredients: Yields: 8 servings

Ingredients	Notes:
1 lb. pasta	May use whole grain pasta
4 cups canned tuna water packed, drained, flaked	
1/4 cup light mayonnaise	
1 cup plain nonfat Greek yogurt	
2 tablespoons fresh lemon juice	
1 teaspoon lemon zest	Wash and zest
1 cup celery, diced	Wash, trim and dice.
1 cup frozen peas, thawed	
½ cup red bell pepper, diced	Wash, trim and dice.
1 cup carrot, shredded	Wash peel, trim and shred.
1/2 cup chopped green onion	Wash, trim, and slice. (including green tops)
2 tablespoons chopped parsley, dried	Or ¼ cup fresh chopped

Directions:

Steps:	Directions:	Critical Control Point /Quality Assurance
1	Cook pasta according to package directions.	
2	In a large bowl mix Greek yogurt, mayonnaise, lemon juice and zest, and pepper together.	
3	When pasta is finished cooking, drain, then run under cool water until it's no longer hot.	
4	Add pasta to yogurt dressing, along with celery, red pepper, peas, carrots, onions, and parsley.	
5	Gently mix the ingredients together until combined.	
6	Refrigerate for 1 hour or overnight before serving.	

Time Temperature Sensitive food. *Food safety Standards: hold food for service at an internal temperature above 140° F. Do not mix old product with new. Cool leftover product quickly (within 4 hours) to below 41° F. Follow proper cooling procedures. Store leftovers in a tightly sealed, labeled and dated container. Use leftover within 72 hours if stored in refrigerator or 30 days if stored in the freezer. Cold holding at 41°F or colder or using time alone (less than four hours).*

Texture Modified Diets:

Soft & Bite Size: (aka Bite size) **Food particle size ½ inch (~width of standard fork)** Food must be moist. Cut foods with a knife to a ½" particle size prior to mixing. Moisten with broth as needed. Foods that do not process well should be omitted. Omit: green onions.

Chopped: Food particle size ¼ inch (~ ½ width of standard fork) Food must be moist. Chop foods with a knife to 1/4" particle size prior to mixing. Moisten with broth as needed. Foods that do not process well should be omitted. Omit: green onions.

Minced and Moist: (aka Minced/Mechanical Soft/Ground) **Food particle size 1/8 inch (fits through prongs of standard fork)** Food must be moist. Use a food processor to grind food particles into 1/8 inch prior to mixing. Moisten with broth as needed. Foods that do not process well should be omitted. Omit: green onions.

Pureed: Smooth and cohesive. Use a food processor to puree to a smooth consistency. Foods are processed by grinding and then pureeing them. May add broth or sauce to puree. Do not add to much liquid. Puree should still hold its shape. Must not be firm or sticky. Puree foods while still hot. Appearance should be smooth like pudding. Foods that do not process well should be omitted. Omit: green onions.
Serve ½ c. puree tuna serving, ½ puree pasta and ½ cup puree cooked carrots separately.

Therapeutic Modified Diets:

Lowfat: No changes needed
Diabetic/No added Sugar/No Conc. Sweets/Calorie Controlled: No changes needed
Bland/Anti Reflux: omit lemon, celery, green onion and parsley
Liberal House Renal: Omit salt, mayonnaise, and yogurt. Toss with olive oil.
No Added Salt: No changes needed
2 Gram Sodium: omit salt and mayonnaise. Toss with olive oil.
Gluten Free: Gluten-free pasta Prepare foods separately to prevent cross contamination.

Allergy Alerts: When an "X" is present, this indicates the allergen is present. Always read all food labels to ensure allergens are not present.

Wheat	Milk	Eggs	Fish Shellfish	Soy	Peanuts/Nuts	Other
X	X	X	X			

Key: SF= Salt Free D= Diet or Sugarfree LF = Lowfat FF = Fat Free GF = Gluten Free

Recipe Name: Fish Tacos with Corn Salsa
Recipe Category: Dinner Entrée
Portion Size: 3 oz. Fish, 1 tortillas
Ingredients: Yields: 8 servings

Ingredients	Notes:
1 cup frozen corn, thawed	
1/2 cup diced red onion	Wash, peel and dice
1 cup jicama	Wash, peel and finely chop
1/2 cup fresh cilantro leaves,	Wash, trim and finely chop
1/2 cup red bell pepper	Wash, trim and finely chop
1 lime, zested and juiced	Wash, zest and juice
1/4 cup light sour cream	
1/2 teaspoon cayenne pepper	
1/2 teaspoon ground black pepper	
1 teaspoon salt	
8 (4 ounce) fillets tilapia	May use other white fish.
2 tablespoons olive oil	
8 corn tortillas, warmed	

Directions:

Steps:	Directions:	Critical Control Point /Quality Assurance
1	In a medium bowl, mix together corn, red onion, jicama, red bell pepper, sour cream and cilantro	
2	Stir in lime juice and zest	
3	In a small bowl, combine cayenne pepper, ground black pepper, and salt	
4	Brush each fillet with olive oil, and sprinkle with spices.	
5	Preheat oven to 400 degrees F	
6	Arrange fillets on baking sheet. Cook for 7 minutes per side.	Cook until internal temperature reaches 145 degrees F
7	For each fish taco, top corn tortillas with fish, sour cream, and corn salsa	

Time Temperature Sensitive food. Food safety Standards: hold food for service at an internal temperature above 140° F. Do not mix old product with new. Cool leftover product quickly (within 4 hours) to below 41° F. Follow proper cooling procedures. Store leftovers in a tightly sealed, labeled and dated container. Use leftover within 72 hours if stored in refrigerator or 30 days if stored in the freezer. Reheat leftover product quickly (within 2 hours) to 165 degrees F for 15 seconds. Reheat left over product only once; discard if not used. Cold holding at 41°F or colder or using time alone (less than four hours). Always wash hands and wash and sanitize counter tops utensils and containers between steps when working with raw seafood.

<u>**Texture Modified Diets:**</u>
Soft & Bite Size: (aka Bite size) **Food particle size ½ inch (~width of standard fork)** Food must be moist. Cut foods with a knife to a ½" particle size prior to layering. Moisten with broth as needed. Foods that do not process well should be omitted. Omit: corn. Mince red onion, jicama, red bell pepper and cilantro.
Chopped: Food particle size ¼ inch (~ ½ width of standard fork) Food must be moist. Chop foods with a knife to 1/4" particle size prior to layering. Moisten with broth as needed. Foods that do not process well should be omitted. Omit: corn. Mince red onion, jicama, red bell pepper and cilantro.
Minced and Moist: (aka Minced/Mechanical Soft/Ground) **Food particle size 1/8 inch (fits through prongs of standard fork)** Food must be moist. Use a food processor to grind food particles into 1/8 inch prior to layering. Moisten with broth as needed. Foods that do not process well should be omitted. Omit: corn. Mince red onion, jicama, red bell pepper and cilantro.
Pureed: Smooth and cohesive. Use a food processor to puree to a smooth consistency. Foods are processed by grinding and then pureeing them. May add broth or sauce to puree. Do not add to much liquid. Puree should still hold its shape. Must not be firm or sticky. Puree foods while still hot. Appearance should be smooth like pudding. Foods that do not process well should be omitted. Omit: corn. Puree red onion, jicama, red bell pepper and cilantro.
½ c. puree serving, ½ c. puree tortilla, topped with 2 Tablespoons puree salsa.
<u>**Therapeutic Modified Diets:**</u>
Lowfat: No changes needed
Diabetic/No added Sugar/No Conc. Sweets/Calorie Controlled: No changes needed
Bland/Anti Reflux: omit corn salsa, cayenne pepper and black pepper
Liberal House Renal: Omit salt and sour cream. Use low sodium tortillas (see recipe)
No Added Salt: No changes needed
2 Gram Sodium: omit salt and sour cream. Use low sodium tortillas (see recipe)
Gluten Free: No changes needed. Prepare foods separately to prevent cross contamination.
Allergy Alerts: When an "X" is present, this indicates the allergen is present. Always read all food labels to ensure allergens are not present.

Wheat	Milk	Eggs	FishShellfish	Soy	Peanuts/Nuts	Other
	X		X			

Key: SF= Salt Free D= Diet or Sugarfree LF = Lowfat FF = Fat Free GF = Gluten Free

Copyright 2020 Jacqueline Larson M.S., R.D.N. and Associates.   All Rights Reserved

Recipe Name: Fish Tacos with Creamy Cilantro Lime dressing
Recipe Category: Dinner Entrée
Portion Size: 2 small tacos
Ingredients: Yields: 8 servings

Ingredients	Notes:
2 1/2 Pounds white fish, cut into thin strips	Red snapper, tilapia, any mild white fish
1 tablespoon olive oil	
1 tablespoon chili powder	
1/2 teaspoon garlic powder	
1/4 teaspoon onion powder	
1/2 teaspoon paprika	
1 teaspoon ground cumin	
1/2 teaspoon salt	
1/4 teaspoon ground black pepper	
1/2 teaspoon sugar	
1/4 Cup shredded low fat cheddar cheese	
3 Cups shredded cabbage	Wash, trim and chop
16 Flour small tortillas	May use whole grain
Sauce:	
¼ cup thinly sliced green onions	Washed, trimmed and sliced thin.
¼ cup chopped fresh cilantro	
¼ cup light mayonnaise	
1/2 teaspoon zest of lime	
2 tablespoons lime juice	
¼ teaspoon salt	
1 clove garlic, minced	Washed trimmed and minced
½ cup light sour cream	

Directions:

Steps:	Directions:	Critical Control Point /Quality Assurance
1	In a large flat bowl combine chili powder, garlic powder, onion powder, paprika, cumin, salt, black pepper and sugar.	
2	Heat oil in large pan heat oil to medium high heat.	
3	Dredge fish in seasoning and cook in pan.	Cook until internal temperature reaches 145 F degrees for 15 seconds.
4	Prepare sauce in a small bowl by mixing, green onions, cilantro, mayonnaise, lime zest, lime juice, salt, garlic and sour cream .	
5	Wrap tortillas in foil and 350 warm in oven for 20 minutes. In heated tortillas and top with fish, cabbage, cheese and sauce.	

Time Temperature Sensitive food. *Food safety Standards: hold food for service at an internal temperature above 140° F. Do not mix old product with new. Cool leftover product quickly (within 4 hours) to below 41° F. Follow proper cooling procedures. Store leftovers in a tightly sealed, labeled and dated container. Use leftover within 72 hours if stored in refrigerator or 30 days if stored in the freezer. Reheat leftover product quickly (within 2 hours) to 165 degrees F for 15 seconds. Reheat left over product only once; discard if not used. Cold holding at 41°F or colder or using time alone (less than four hours). Always wash hands and wash and sanitize counter tops utensils and containers between steps when working with raw meat.*

Texture Modified Diets:

Soft & Bite Size: (aka Bite size) **Food particle size ½ inch (~width of standard fork)** Food must be moist. Cut foods with a knife to a ½" particle size prior to mixing. Moisten with broth as needed. Foods that do not process well should be omitted. Omit: green onions. Cook cabbage to soften or mince.

Chopped: Food particle size ¼ inch (~ ½ width of standard fork) Food must be moist. Chop foods with a knife to 1/4" particle size prior to mixing. Moisten with broth as needed. Foods that do not process well should be omitted. Omit: green onions. Cook cabbage to soften or mince.

Minced and Moist: (aka Minced/Mechanical Soft/Ground) **Food particle size 1/8 inch (fits through prongs of standard fork)** Food must be moist. Use a food processor to grind food particles into 1/8 inch prior to mixing. Moisten with broth as needed. Foods that do not process well should be omitted. Omit: green onions.

Pureed: Smooth and cohesive. Use a food processor to puree to a smooth consistency. Foods are processed by grinding and then pureeing them. May add broth or sauce to puree. Do not add to much liquid. Puree should still

hold its shape. Must not be firm or sticky. Puree foods while still hot. Appearance should be smooth like pudding. Foods that do not process well should be omitted. Omit: green onions.
Serve ½ c. puree meat on top of ½ c. puree tortillas serving. Melt cheese on top of meat. Top with 1 T. puree tomato and 1 T. puree lettuce and 1 t. sour cream.

Therapeutic Modified Diets:
Lowfat: No changes needed
Diabetic/No added Sugar/No Conc. Sweets/Calorie Controlled: No changes needed
Bland/Anti Reflux: Serve plain fish on tortilla
Liberal House Renal: Omit sauce and cheese. Use SF tortillas.
No Added Salt: No changes needed
2 Gram Sodium: Omit salt and cheese. Use low sodium tortillas. (See recipe)
Gluten Free: Omit flour whole grain tortillas for gluten free corn tortillas. Prepare foods separately to prevent cross contamination.
Allergy Alerts: When an "X" is present, this indicates the allergen is present.
Always read all food labels to ensure allergens are not present.

Wheat	Milk	Eggs	Fish Shellfish	Soy	Peanuts/Nuts	Other
X	X	X	X			

Key: SF= Salt Free D= Diet or Sugarfree LF = Lowfat FF = Fat Free GF = Gluten Free

Recipe Name: Garlic, Ginger and Coconut White Fish
Recipe Category: Dinner Entrée
Portion Size: 4 oz.
Ingredients: **Yields: 8 servings**

Ingredients	Notes:
8 Codfish or haddock fillets	4 oz. each or other white fish
½ teaspoon salt	
2 cloves garlic, minced	Washed, peeled, and minced
2 tablespoons olive oil	
2 tablespoons curry powder	
¼ teaspoon ground ginger	
1 red bell pepper	Washed, trimmed and diced
1 cup reduced fat coconut milk	
½ teaspoon paprika	
1 cup shredded carrots	Washed, peeled and shredded
4 green onions	Washed, trimmed and sliced
¼ teaspoon pepper and paprika	
½ cup snipped fresh basil or 2 tablespoons dried.	
1 teaspoon lime zest	
2 tablespoon fresh lime juice	

Directions:

Steps:	Directions:	Critical Control Point / Quality Assurance
1	Preheat oven to 400 degrees	
2	In a baking dish add the garlic, coconut milk, oil, lime juice, lime zest, curry powder, salt.	
3	Add the bell pepper, carrots and green onions, and season thoroughly with salt. Stir until vegetables are well coated with sauce and evenly distributed through the dish.	
4	Cover the baking dish and cook for 15 minutes.	Bake 8 to 10 minutes
5	Remove dish from oven and carefully remove cover. Season the fish with salt and nestle each piece of fish into the baking dish so that two pieces of fish are overlapping.	Broil for 3 minutes until lemon slightly browned at the edges. Cook until internal temperature reaches 145° F for 15 seconds
6	Cover the baking dish and cook for about 15-18 minutes longer or until fish is flaky, white, and opaque through the center.	
7	Transfer fish to serving plates and add heaping spoonfuls of vegetables and coconut curry sauce. Top with chopped basil. Serve hot over rice.	

Time Temperature Sensitive food. *Food safety Standards: hold food for service at an internal temperature above 140° F. Do not mix old product with new. Cool leftover product quickly (within 4 hours) to below 41° F. Follow proper cooling procedures. Store leftovers in a tightly sealed, labeled and dated container. Use leftover within 72 hours if stored in refrigerator or 30 days if stored in the freezer. Reheat leftover product quickly (within 2 hours) to 165 degrees F for 15 seconds. Reheat left over product only once; discard if not used. Cold holding at 41°F or colder or using time alone (less than four hours). Always wash hands and wash and sanitize counter tops utensils and containers between steps when working with raw seafood.*

Texture Modified Diets:

Soft & Bite Size: (aka Bite size) **Food particle size ½ inch (~width of standard fork)** Food must be moist. Cut foods with a knife to a ½" particle size prior to mixing. Moisten with sauce as needed. Foods that do not process well should be omitted. Omit: green onions.

Chopped: Food particle size ¼ inch (~ ½ width of standard fork) Food must be moist. Chop foods with a knife to 1/4" particle size prior to mixing. Moisten with sauce as needed. Foods that do not process well should be omitted. Omit: green onions.

Copyright 2020 Jacqueline Larson M.S., R.D.N. and Associates.   All Rights Reserved

Minced and Moist: (aka Minced/Mechanical Soft/Ground) **Food particle size 1/8 inch (fits through prongs of standard fork)** Food must be moist. Use a food processor to grind food particles into 1/8 inch prior to mixing. Moisten with sauce as needed. Foods that do not process well should be omitted. Omit: green onions.

Pureed: Smooth and cohesive. Use a food processor to puree to a smooth consistency. Foods are processed by grinding and then pureeing them. May add broth or sauce to puree. Do not add to much liquid. Puree should still hold its shape. Must not be firm or sticky. Puree foods while still hot. Appearance should be smooth like pudding. Foods that do not process well should be omitted. Omit: green onions.

<u>Therapeutic Modified Diets:</u>

Lowfat: No changes needed

Diabetic/No added Sugar/No Conc. Sweets/Calorie Controlled: No changes needed

Bland/Anti Reflux: omit pepper, bell pepper, green onion, paprika, basil, lime and lime zest

Liberal House Renal: Omit salt and lime

No Added Salt: No changes needed

2 Gram Sodium: omit salt

Gluten Free: No changes needed. Prepare foods separately to prevent cross contamination.

Allergy Alerts: When an "X" is present, this indicates the allergen is present.
Always read all food labels to ensure allergens are not present.

Wheat	Milk	Eggs	Fish Shellfish	Soy	Peanuts/Nuts	Other
			X			

Key: SF= Salt Free D= Diet or Sugarfree LF = Lowfat FF = Fat Free GF = Gluten Free

Recipe Name: Glazed Salmon
Recipe Category: Dinner Entrée
Portion Size: 3 oz.
Ingredients: Yields: 8 servings

Ingredients	Notes:
1/2 cup light soy sauce	
1/2 cup honey	
2 tablespoons cornstarch	
2 tablespoons sesame seeds	
½ teaspoon garlic powder	Or 2 cloves fresh garlic, minced
1/2 teaspoon ground ginger	
2 tablespoons oil	
2 ½ lbs. Salmon	May use other white fish.
1/4 cup green onion	Wash, trim and chop. (including green tops)

Directions:

Steps:	Directions:	Critical Control Point / Quality Assurance
1	To make the sauce: In a small bowl; combine soy sauce, honey, sesame seeds, garlic powder, cornstarch, and ginger.; set aside.	
2	Heat the oil in a large skillet	
3	Add salmon and sauté for 8 to 10 minutes or until juices run clear. Pour sauce over Salmon. Cook until thick.	Cook until internal temperature reaches 145° F for 15 seconds.
4	Top with green onions. Serve hot	

Time Temperature Sensitive food. Food safety Standards: hold food for service at an internal temperature above 140° F. Do not mix old product with new. Cool leftover product quickly (within 4 hours) to below 41°F. Follow proper cooling procedures. Store leftovers in a tightly sealed, labeled and dated container. Use leftover within 72 hours if stored in refrigerator or 30 days if stored in the freezer. Reheat leftover product quickly (within 2 hours) to 165 degrees F for 15 seconds. Reheat left over product only once; discard if not used. Cold holding at 41°F or colder or using time alone (less than four hours). Always wash hands and wash and sanitize counter tops utensils and containers between steps when working with raw seafood.

<u>Texture Modified Diets:</u>
Soft & Bite Size: (aka Bite size) **Food particle size ½ inch (~width of standard fork)** Food must be moist. Cut foods with a knife to a ½" particle size after cooking. Moisten with broth as needed. Foods that do not process well should be omitted. Omit: green onions.
Chopped: Food particle size ¼ inch (~ ½ width of standard fork) Food must be moist. Chop foods with a knife to 1/4" particle size after cooking. Moisten with broth as needed. Foods that do not process well should be omitted. Omit: green onions
Minced and Moist:(aka Minced/Mechanical Soft/Ground) **Food particle size 1/8 inch (fits through prongs of standard fork)** Food must be moist. Use a food processor to grind food particles into 1/8 inch prior to after cooking. Moisten with broth as needed. Foods that do not process well should be omitted. Omit: green onions
Pureed: Smooth and cohesive. Use a food processor to puree to a smooth consistency. Foods are processed by grinding and then pureeing them. May add broth or sauce to puree. Do not add to much liquid. Puree should still hold its shape. Must not be firm or sticky. Puree foods while still hot. Appearance should be smooth like pudding. Foods that do not process well should be omitted. Omit: green onions and sesame seeds.

<u>Therapeutic Modified Diets:</u>
Lowfat: No changes needed
Diabetic/No added Sugar/No Conc. Sweets/Calorie Controlled: omit honey
Bland/Anti Reflux: omit sesame seeds, garlic, and green onion
Liberal House Renal: Omit sauce. Top with green onions. Season with sesame seeds, garlic powder and ginger
No Added Salt: Omit sauce. Top with green onions. Season with sesame seeds, garlic powder and ginger
2 Gram Sodium: Omit sauce. Top with green onions. Season with sesame seeds, garlic powder and ginger
Gluten Free: Use gluten free soy sauce. Prepare foods separately to prevent cross contamination.

Allergy Alerts: When an "X" is present, this indicates the allergen is present. Always read all food labels to ensure allergens are not present.

Wheat	Milk	Eggs	Fish Shellfish	Soy	Peanuts/Nuts	Other
X			X	X		

Key: SF= Salt Free D= Diet or Sugarfree LF = Lowfat FF = Fat Free GF = Gluten Free

Recipe Name: Honey Mustard Salmon
Recipe Category: Dinner Entrée
Portion Size: 4 ounces fish with sauce
Ingredients: **Yields: 8 servings**

Ingredients	Notes:
¼ cup honey mustard	(may sub 1 tablespoon honey with 3 tablespoons Dijon mustard
2 teaspoons garlic, minced	Washed, peeled and minced
2 tablespoons lemon juice	
2 tablespoons olive oil	
1 teaspoon dried dill	
¼ teaspoon salt	
8 boneless skinless fresh salmon	Or see recipe for salmon patties

Directions:

Steps:	Directions:	Critical Control Point /Quality Assurance
1	Pre heat oven to 400°F. In a small bowl, whisk together honey, mustard, garlic, olive oil, dill and salt	
2	On a baking sheet, add salmon. Brush with honey mustard sauce. Bake in oven for 8-10 minutes. (do not over cook)	Cook until internal temperature reaches 145 degrees F.

Time Temperature Sensitive food. *Food safety Standards: hold food for service at an internal temperature above 140°F. Do not mix old product with new. Cool leftover product quickly (within 4 hours) to below 41°F. Follow proper cooling procedures. Store leftovers in a tightly sealed, labeled and dated container. Use leftover within 72 hours if stored in refrigerator or 30 days if stored in the freezer. Reheat leftover product quickly (within 2 hours) to 165 degrees F for 15 seconds. Reheat left over product only once; discard if not used. Cold holding at 41°F or colder or using time alone (less than four hours). Always wash hands and wash and sanitize counter tops utensils and containers between steps when working with raw poultry.*

Texture Modified Diets:

Soft & Bite Size: (aka Bite size) **Food particle size ½ inch (~width of standard fork)** Food must be moist. Cut foods with a knife to a ½" particle size after cooking. Moisten with sauce as needed after cutting.
Chopped: Food particle size ¼ inch (~ ½ width of standard fork) Food must be moist. Chop foods with a knife to 1/4" particle size after cooking. Moisten with sauce as needed after chopping.
Minced and Moist: (aka Minced/Mechanical Soft/Ground) **Food particle size 1/8 inch (fits through prongs of standard fork)** Food must be moist. Use a food processor to grind food particles into 1/8 inch after cooking. Moisten with sauce as needed after processing.
Pureed: Smooth and cohesive. Use a food processor to puree to a smooth consistency. Foods are processed by grinding and then pureeing them. May add milk or sauce to puree. Do not add to much liquid. Puree should still hold its shape. Must not be firm or sticky. Puree foods while still hot. Appearance should be smooth like pudding. Serve ½ cup serving with sauce.

Therapeutic Modified Diets:

Lowfat: No changes needed.
Diabetic/No added Sugar/No Conc. Sweets/Calorie Controlled: No changes needed.
Bland/Anti Reflux: Omit mustard, garlic and dill.
Liberal House Renal: Omit salt.
No Added Salt: No changes needed.
2 Gram Sodium: Omit salt
Gluten Free: Use GF Dijon mustard. Prepare foods separately to prevent cross contamination.
Allergy Alerts: When an "X" is present, this indicates the allergen is present.
Always read all food labels to ensure allergens are not present.

Wheat	Milk	Eggs	Fish Shellfish	Soy	Peanuts/Nuts	Other
X			X			

Key: SF= Salt Free D= Diet or Sugarfree LF = Lowfat FF = Fat Free GF = Gluten Free

Recipe Name: Lemon Dijon Baked Fish
Recipe Category: Dinner Entrée
Portion Size: 4 oz.
Ingredients: **Yields: 8 servings**

Ingredients	Notes:
2 1/2 pounds orange roughly fillets (boneless)	May use other white fish.
3 tablespoons Dijon mustard	
3 tablespoons unsalted butter, melted	
2 tablespoon lemon juice	
1 teaspoon Worchester sauce	
1 cup bread crumbs	
½ c. tartar sauce	

Directions:

Steps:	Directions:	Critical Control Point / Quality Assurance
1	Preheat oven to 425 degrees	
2	Cut fillets in half & arrange in lightly greased baking dish	
3	Combine mustard, butter, lemon juice and Worcester sauce in a small bowl.	
4	Dip fillets in mustard mixture and then dip in bread crumbs.	
5	Bake 20-25 minutes or until fish flakes easily with a fork. Serve immediately with tartar sauce on the side.	Cook until internal temperature reaches 145° F for 15 seconds.

Time Temperature Sensitive food. *Food safety Standards: hold food for service at an internal temperature above 140°F. Do not mix old product with new. Cool leftover product quickly (within 4 hours) to below 41°F. Follow proper cooling procedures. Store leftovers in a tightly sealed, labeled and dated container. Use leftover within 72 hours if stored in refrigerator or 30 days if stored in the freezer. Reheat leftover product quickly (within 2 hours) to 165 degrees F for 15 seconds. Reheat left over product only once; discard if not used. Cold holding at 41°F or colder or using time alone (less than four hours). Always wash hands and wash and sanitize counter tops utensils and containers between steps when working with raw seafood.*

Texture Modified Diets:

Soft & Bite Size: (aka Bite size) **Food particle size ½ inch (~width of standard fork)** Food must be moist. Cut foods with a knife to a ½" particle size after cooking. Moisten with tartar sauce as needed after cutting.

Chopped: Food particle size ¼ inch (~ ½ width of standard fork) Food must be moist. Chop foods with a knife to 1/4" particle size after cooking. Moisten with tartar sauce as needed after chopping.

Minced and Moist: (aka Minced/Mechanical Soft/Ground) **Food particle size 1/8 inch (fits through prongs of standard fork)** Food must be moist. Use a food processor to grind food particles into 1/8 inch after cooking. Moisten with tartar sauce as needed after processing.

Pureed: Smooth and cohesive. Use a food processor to puree to a smooth consistency. Foods are processed by grinding and then pureeing them. May add milk or tartar sauce to puree. Do not add to much liquid. Puree should still hold its shape. Must not be firm or sticky. Puree foods while still hot. Appearance should be smooth like pudding. Serve ½ c. puree fish serving.

Therapeutic Modified Diets:

Lowfat: No changes needed
Diabetic/No added Sugar/No Conc. Sweets/Calorie Controlled: No changes needed
Bland/Anti Reflux: omit lemon juice and Worchester sauce
Liberal House Renal: Omit Worchester sauce and bread crumbs
No Added Salt: No changes needed
2 Gram Sodium: omit Worchester sauce and bread crumbs
Gluten Free: Use gluten free bread crumbs or GF crushed cornflakes. Prepare foods separately to prevent cross contamination.

Allergy Alerts: When an "X" is present, this indicates the allergen is present. Always read all food labels to ensure allergens are not present.

Wheat	Milk	Eggs	Fish Shellfish	Soy	Peanuts/Nuts	Other
X	X	X	X			

Key: SF= Salt Free D= Diet or Sugarfree LF = Lowfat FF = Fat Free GF = Gluten Free

Recipe Name: Mediterranean Salmon Orzo Salad
Recipe Category: Dinner Entrée
Portion Size: 2 cups (1 cup salmon/ orzo and 1 cup spinach)
Ingredients: Yields: 8 servings

Ingredients	Notes:
4 cups water packed salmon, drained and flaked	
8 cups baby fresh spinach, washed	Wash and trim
1 red bell pepper, finely chopped	Wash, trim and finely chop
2 medium tomatoes, diced	Wash, trim, and dice
4 green onions with tops, chopped	Wash, trim and chop
1 lb. package orzo	May use whole grain pasta
1 can (15 oz.) garbanzo beans, rinsed and drained	Low-Sodium Canned Garbanzo beans
1/4 Cup olive oil	
½ cup Red Wine vinegar	
2 tablespoons dried parsley	Or ¼ cup fresh parsley finely chopped
2 clove garlic, minced	
2 tablespoons Dijon mustard	
1/2 teaspoon salt	
1/4 teaspoon pepper	
4 oz. low fat feta cheese	

Directions:

Steps:	Directions:	Critical Control Point / Quality Assurance
1	Prepare Orzo according to the directions on the package; Drain	
2	In a small bowl whisk together, olive oil, red wine vinegar, parmesan, parsley, garlic, Dijon mustard, salt and pepper.	
3	In a large bowl, add orzo, salmon flakes, bell pepper, green onion, tomato and garbanzo beans.	
4	Drizzle with dressing and gently toss to coat.	
5	On serving plate add baby spinach and top with salmon mixture. Top with feta cheese. Serve cold.	

Time Temperature Sensitive food. *Food safety Standards: hold food for service at an internal temperature above 140° F. Do not mix old product with new. Cool leftover product quickly (within 4 hours) to below 41° F. Follow proper cooling procedures. Store leftovers in a tightly sealed, labeled and dated container. Use leftover within 72 hours if stored in refrigerator or 30 days if stored in the freezer. Reheat leftover product quickly (within 2 hours) to 165 degrees F for 15 seconds. Reheat left over product only once; discard if not used. Cold holding at 41 °F or colder or using time alone (less than four hours).*

Texture Modified Diets:

Soft & Bite Size: (aka Bite size) **Food particle size ½ inch (~width of standard fork)** Food must be moist. Cut foods with a knife to a ½" particle size prior to mixing. Moisten with broth as needed. Foods that do not process well should be omitted. Omit: green onions. Cook spinach and bell peppers to soften.

Chopped: Food particle size ¼ inch (~ ½ width of standard fork) Food must be moist. Chop foods with a knife to 1/4" particle size prior to mixing. Moisten with broth as needed. Foods that do not process well should be omitted. Omit: green onions. Cook spinach and bell peppers to soften.

Minced and Moist: (aka Minced/Mechanical Soft/Ground) **Food particle size 1/8 inch (fits through prongs of standard fork)** Food must be moist. Use a food processor to grind food particles into 1/8 inch prior to mixing. Moisten with broth as needed. Foods that do not process well should be omitted. Omit: green onions.

Pureed: Smooth and cohesive. Use a food processor to puree to a smooth consistency. Foods are processed by grinding and then pureeing them. May add broth or sauce to puree. Do not add to much liquid. Puree should still hold its shape. Must not be firm or sticky. Puree foods while still hot. Appearance should be smooth like pudding. Foods that do not process well should be omitted. Omit: green onions. Serve ½ c. puree tuna serving and 1/2c. puree orzo mixture separately.

Therapeutic Modified Diets:

Lowfat: No changes needed

Diabetic/No added Sugar/No Conc. Sweets/Calorie Controlled: No changes needed

Bland/Anti Reflux: Serve on ½ c. cooked spinach. Omit: pepper, tomato, onion, garbanzo beans, red wine vinegar, parsley, garlic Dijon must and black pepper

Liberal House Renal: Omit salt, garbanzo beans, and feta cheese
No Added Salt: No changes needed
2 Gram Sodium: omit salt and feta cheese
Gluten Free: Use gluten free pasta in place of orzo. Prepare foods separately to prevent cross contamination.
Allergy Alerts: When an "X" is present, this indicates the allergen is present.
Always read all food labels to ensure allergens are not present.

Wheat	Milk	Eggs	Fish Shellfish	Soy	Peanuts/Nuts	Other
X	X	X	X			

Key: SF= Salt Free D= Diet or Sugarfree LF = Lowfat FF = Fat Free GF = Gluten Free

Recipe Name: Mediterranean Tuna Orzo Salad
Recipe Category: Dinner Entrée
Portion Size: 2 cups (1 cup tuna/ orzo and 1 cup spinach)
Ingredients: Yields: 8 servings

Ingredients	Notes:
4 cups water packed tuna, drained and flaked	
8 cups baby fresh spinach, washed	Wash and trim
1 red bell pepper, finely chopped	Wash, trim and finely chop
2 medium tomatoes, diced	Wash, trim, and dice
4 green onions with tops, chopped	Wash, trim and chop
1 lb. package orzo	May use whole grain pasta
1 can (15 oz.) garbanzo beans, rinsed and drained	Low-Sodium Canned Garbanzo beans
1/4 cup olive oil	
½ cup Red Wine vinegar	
2 tablespoons dried parsley	Or ¼ cup fresh parsley finely chopped
2 clove garlic, minced	
2 tablespoons Dijon mustard	
1/2 teaspoon salt	
1/4 teaspoon pepper	
4 oz. low fat feta cheese	

Directions:

Steps:	Directions:	Critical Control Point /Quality Assurance
1	Prepare Orzo according to the directions on the package; Drain.	
2	In a small bowl whisk together, olive oil, red wine vinegar, parmesan, parsley, garlic, Dijon mustard, salt and pepper.	
3	In a large bowl, add orzo, tuna flakes, bell pepper, green onion, tomato and garbanzo beans.	
4	Drizzle with dressing and gently toss to coat.	
5	On serving plate add baby spinach and top with tuna mixture. Top with feta cheese. Serve cold.	

Time Temperature Sensitive food. *Food safety Standards: hold food for service at an internal temperature above 140°F. Do not mix old product with new. Cool leftover product quickly (within 4 hours) to below 41°F. Follow proper cooling procedures. Store leftovers in a tightly sealed, labeled and dated container. Use leftover within 72 hours if stored in refrigerator or 30 days if stored in the freezer. Reheat leftover product quickly (within 2 hours) to 165 degrees F for 15 seconds. Reheat left over product only once; discard if not used. Cold holding at 41°F or colder or using time alone (less than four hours).*

Texture Modified Diets:

Soft & Bite Size: (aka Bite size) **Food particle size ½ inch (~width of standard fork)** Food must be moist. Cut foods with a knife to a ½" particle size prior to mixing. Moisten with broth as needed. Foods that do not process well should be omitted. Omit: green onions. Cook spinach and bell peppers to soften

Chopped: Food particle size ¼ inch (~ ½ width of standard fork) Food must be moist. Chop foods with a knife to 1/4" particle size prior to mixing. Moisten with broth as needed. Foods that do not process well should be omitted. Omit: green onions. Cook spinach and bell peppers to soften

Minced and Moist: (aka Minced/Mechanical Soft/Ground) **Food particle size 1/8 inch (fits through prongs of standard fork)** Food must be moist. Use a food processor to grind food particles into 1/8 inch prior to mixing. Moisten with broth as needed. Foods that do not process well should be omitted. Omit: green onions.

Pureed: Smooth and cohesive. Use a food processor to puree to a smooth consistency. Foods are processed by grinding and then pureeing them. May add broth or sauce to puree. Do not add to much liquid. Puree should still hold its shape. Must not be firm or sticky. Puree foods while still hot. Appearance should be smooth like pudding. Foods that do not process well should be omitted. Omit: green onions. Serve ½ c. puree tuna serving and 1/2c. puree orzo mixture separately.

Therapeutic Modified Diets:

Lowfat: No changes needed
Diabetic/No added Sugar/No Conc. Sweets/Calorie Controlled: No changes needed
Bland/Anti Reflux: Serve on ½ c. cooked spinach. Omit: pepper, tomato, onion, garbanzo beans, red wine vinegar, parsley, garlic Dijon must and black pepper

Liberal House Renal: Omit salt, garbanzo beans, and feta cheese
No Added Salt: No changes needed
2 Gram Sodium: omit salt and feta cheese
Gluten Free: Use gluten free pasta in place of orzo. Prepare foods separately to prevent cross contamination.
Allergy Alerts: When an "X" is present, this indicates the allergen is present.
Always read all food labels to ensure allergens are not present.

Wheat	Milk	Eggs	Fish Shellfish	Soy	Peanuts/Nuts	Other
X	X	X	X			

Key: SF= Salt Free D= Diet or Sugarfree LF = Lowfat FF = Fat Free GF = Gluten Free

Recipe Name: Salmon and Peas Pasta Salad
Recipe Category: Dinner Entrée
Portion Size: 1 cup
Ingredients: Yields: 8 servings

Ingredients	Notes:
1 lb. pasta	May use whole grain pasta
4 cups canned salmon	water packed, drained, flaked
1 cup frozen peas, thawed	
1/4 cup olive oil	
2 garlic cloves, minced	Washed, peeled and minced
1/2 cup fresh lemon juice	
1 teaspoon lemon zest	
1/2 teaspoon salt	
1/4 teaspoon pepper	
1/4 cup Parmesan Cheese	

Directions:

Steps:	Directions:	Critical Control Point /Quality Assurance
1	Bring a pot of water to a boil. Cook pasta until al dente, about 9 minutes, or as package directs	Reserve 1 cup of cooking water; drain pasta
2	In a large bowl add garlic and salmon. Flake salmon.	
3	Add lemon juice, lemon zest, salt, olive oil and pepper.	
4	Toss to coat. Add pasta and peas. Gently toss. Chill.	
5	Top with Parmesan cheese just before serving	
6	Serve chilled	

Time Temperature Sensitive food. *Food safety Standards: hold food for service at an internal temperature above 140° F. Do not mix old product with new. Cool leftover product quickly (within 4 hours) to below 41° F. Follow proper cooling procedures. Store leftovers in a tightly sealed, labeled and dated container. Use leftover within 72 hours if stored in refrigerator or 30 days if stored in the freezer. Cold holding at 41°F or colder or using time alone (less than four hours).*

Texture Modified Diets: TIP: Use pasta with the correct particle size.

Soft & Bite Size: (aka Bite size) **Food particle size ½ inch (~width of standard fork)** Food must be moist. Cut foods with a knife to a ½" particle size prior to mixing. Moisten with broth as needed.

Chopped: Food particle size ¼ inch (~ ½ width of standard fork) Food must be moist. Chop foods with a knife to 1/4" particle size prior to mixing. Moisten with broth as needed.

Minced and Moist: (aka Minced/Mechanical Soft/Ground) **Food particle size 1/8 inch (fits through prongs of standard fork)** Food must be moist. Use a food processor to grind food particles into 1/8 inch prior to mixing. Moisten with broth as needed.

Pureed: Smooth and cohesive. Use a food processor to puree to a smooth consistency. Foods are processed by grinding and then pureeing them. May add broth or sauce to puree. Do not add to much liquid. Puree should still hold its shape. Must not be firm or sticky. Puree foods while still hot. Appearance should be smooth like pudding. Tip: combine all ingredients except salmon. Puree pasta mixture and salmon s separately.

Therapeutic Modified Diets:

Lowfat: No changes needed
Diabetic/No added Sugar/No Conc. Sweets/Calorie Controlled: No changes needed
Bland/Anti Reflux: omit garlic, lemon juice, lemon zest and pepper
Liberal House Renal: Omit salt, lemon juice, lemon zest and Parmesan cheese
No Added Salt: No changes needed
2 Gram Sodium: omit salt and Parmesan cheese.
Gluten Free: Gluten-free pasta. Prepare foods separately to prevent cross contamination.

Allergy Alerts: When an "X" is present, this indicates the allergen is present. Always read all food labels to ensure allergens are not present.

Wheat	Milk	Eggs	Fish Shellfish	Soy	Peanuts/Nuts	Other
X	X	X	X			

Key: SF= Salt Free D= Diet or Sugarfree LF = Lowfat FF = Fat Free GF = Gluten Free

Copyright 2020 Jacqueline Larson M.S., R.D.N. and Associates. All Rights Reserved

Recipe Name: Salmon Cakes
Recipe Category: Dinner Entrée
Portion Size: 4 oz.
Ingredients: Yields: 8 servings

Ingredients	Notes:
4 cups canned Salmon	Drained and flaked. Or may use fresh boneless skinless salmon diced.
1 cup bread crumbs	
1/2 cup minced onion	Washed, peeled and minced
3 eggs, beaten	
1 teaspoon salt	
1/4 teaspoon paprika	
2 tablespoons Dijon mustard	
2 tablespoons olive oil	

Directions:

Steps:	Directions:	Critical Control Point / Quality Assurance
1	Combine tuna, bread crumbs, onions, eggs, salt, Dijon mustard and paprika.	
2	Form these ingredients into cakes	
3	Sauté in olive oil until brown. Turning once.	Cook until internal temperature reaches 165° F for 15 seconds.

Time Temperature Sensitive food. Food safety Standards: hold food for service at an internal temperature above 140° F. Do not mix old product with new. Cool leftover product quickly (within 4 hours) to below 41° F. Follow proper cooling procedures. Store leftovers in a tightly sealed, labeled and dated container. Use leftover within 72 hours if stored in refrigerator or 30 days if stored in the freezer. Reheat leftover product quickly (within 2 hours) to 165 degrees F for 15 seconds. Reheat left over product only once; discard if not used. Cold holding at 41°F or colder or using time alone (less than four hours). Always wash hands and wash and sanitize counter tops utensils and containers between steps when working with raw seafood.

Texture Modified Diets:

Soft & Bite Size: (aka Bite size) **Food particle size ½ inch (~width of standard fork)** Food must be moist. Cut foods with a knife to a ½" particle size after cooking. Moisten with sauce as needed after cutting.

Chopped: Food particle size ¼ inch (~ ½ width of standard fork) Food must be moist. Chop foods with a knife to 1/4" particle size after cooking. Moisten with sauce as needed after chopping.

Minced and Moist: (aka Minced/Mechanical Soft/Ground) **Food particle size 1/8 inch (fits through prongs of standard fork)** Food must be moist. Use a food processor to grind food particles into 1/8 inch after cooking. Moisten with sauce as needed after processing.

Pureed: Smooth and cohesive. Use a food processor to puree to a smooth consistency. Foods are processed by grinding and then pureeing them. May add milk or sauce to puree. Do not add to much liquid. Puree should still hold its shape. Must not be firm or sticky. Puree foods while still hot. Appearance should be smooth like pudding. Puree with broth or tarter sauce if needed. Serve ½ c. meat serving.

Therapeutic Modified Diets:

Lowfat: No changes needed
Diabetic/No added Sugar/No Conc. Sweets/Calorie Controlled: No changes needed
Bland/Anti Reflux: omit onion, Dijon Mustard and paprika
Liberal House Renal: Omit salt and bread crumbs
No Added Salt: No changes needed
2 Gram Sodium: omit salt and bread crumbs
Gluten Free: Use GF bread crumbs or salt Prepare foods separately to prevent cross contamination.
Allergy Alerts: When an "X" is present, this indicates the allergen is present.
Always read all food labels to ensure allergens are not present.

Wheat	Milk	Eggs	Fish Shellfish	Soy	Peanuts/Nuts	Other
X	X	X	X			

Key: SF= Salt Free D= Diet or Sugarfree LF = Lowfat FF = Fat Free GF = Gluten Free

Recipe Name: Salmon Cakes with Creamy Citrus Sauce
Recipe Category: Dinner Entrée
Portion Size: 3 oz. and 2 tablespoons sauce
Ingredients: Yields: 8 servings

Ingredients	Notes:
4 cups, water packed salmon	drained and flaked
1 1/2 cup seasoned bread crumbs	
1/2 cup minced onions	Wash, peel and mince
1/2 cup red bell pepper	Wash, trim and chop finely
3 eggs	
1 cup nonfat milk	
1 teaspoon salt	
1/4 cup oil	
Sauce: 1/2 cup light mayonnaise 1/4 cup light sour cream 2 tablespoons nonfat milk 1 teaspoon lime zest 1/4 cup fresh lime juice 1/4 teaspoon ground cumin	Or use lemon zest and lemon juice Or use orange zest and orange juice

Directions:

Steps:	Directions:	Critical Control Point /Quality Assurance
1	In a large bowl toss together salmon, bread crumbs, onions, eggs, nonfat milk bread crumbs, salt and red pepper	
2	Shape mixture into 8 patties	
3	In a large nonstick skillet heat oil. Sauté patties, a few at a time, until golden brown on both sides, about 3 minutes per side	Cook until internal temperature reaches 165° F for 15 seconds. Keep warm
4	For sauce, in a small combine mayonnaise, milk, lime juice, lime zest and cumin	
5	For each serving, spoon over sauce.	

Time Temperature Sensitive food. *Food safety Standards: hold food for service at an internal temperature above 140° F. Do not mix old product with new. Cool leftover product quickly (within 4 hours) to below 41° F. Follow proper cooling procedures. Store leftovers in a tightly sealed, labeled and dated container. Use leftover within 72 hours if stored in refrigerator or 30 days if stored in the freezer. Reheat leftover product quickly (within 2 hours) to 165 degrees F for 15 seconds. Reheat left over product only once; discard if not used. Cold holding at 41°F or colder or using time alone (less than four hours). Always wash hands and wash and sanitize counter tops utensils and containers between steps when working with raw seafood.*

<u>*Texture Modified Diets:*</u>
Soft & Bite Size: (aka Bite size) **Food particle size ½ inch (~width of standard fork)** Food must be moist. Cut foods with a knife to a ½" particle size after cooking. Moisten with sauce as needed after cutting.
Chopped: Food particle size ¼ inch (~ ½ width of standard fork) Food must be moist. Chop foods with a knife to 1/4" particle size after cooking. Moisten with sauce as needed after chopping.
Minced and Moist:(aka Minced/Mechanical Soft/Ground) **Food particle size 1/8 inch (fits through prongs of standard fork)** Food must be moist. Use a food processor to grind food particles into 1/8 inch after cooking. Moisten with sauce as needed after processing.
Pureed: Smooth and cohesive. Use a food processor to puree to a smooth consistency. Foods are processed by grinding and then pureeing them. May add milk or sauce to puree. Do not add to much liquid. Puree should still hold its shape. Must not be firm or sticky. Puree foods while still hot. Appearance should be smooth like pudding. Serve ½ c. meat serving topped with sauce.

<u>*Therapeutic Modified Diets:*</u>
Lowfat: No changes needed
Diabetic/No added Sugar/No Conc. Sweets/Calorie Controlled: No changes needed
Bland/Anti Reflux: omit onion, red pepper, zest, juice and cumin.
Liberal House Renal: Omit salt, bread crumbs and sauce.
No Added Salt: No changes needed
2 Gram Sodium: omit salt, bread crumbs and sauce. May sprinkle with citrus juice

Copyright 2020 Jacqueline Larson M.S., R.D.N. and Associates. All Rights Reserved

Gluten Free: Use GF bread crumbs, oats or crushed cornflakes. Prepare foods separately to prevent cross contamination.

Allergy Alerts: When an "X" is present, this indicates the allergen is present. Always read all food labels to ensure allergens are not present.

Wheat	Milk	Eggs	Fish Shellfish	Soy	Peanuts/Nuts	Other
X	X	X	X			

Key: SF= Salt Free D= Diet or Sugarfree LF = Lowfat FF = Fat Free GF = Gluten Free

Recipe Name: Salmon Cakes with Lemon Dill Sauce
Recipe Category: Dinner Entrée
Portion Size: 4 oz. plus 1 tablespoon sauce
Ingredients: Yields: 8 servings

Ingredients	Notes:
4 cups, water packed salmon, drained and flaked	May use fresh boneless skin less salmon
1 1/2 cup seasoned bread crumbs	
1/2 cup green onions	Wash, trim and finely chop (including green tops)
1/4 cup chopped, drained pimiento	
2 eggs	
1 cup nonfat milk	
1 teaspoon grated lemon peel	
2 tablespoons oil	
Lemon slices (optional)	
4 cups, water packed salmon drained and flaked	
Sauce: 2 Tablespoons margarine or butt 2 Tablespoons flour 1/2 Cup low sodium chicken broth 2 Tablespoons lemon juice 1/2 Teaspoon dill weed	

Directions:

Steps:	Directions:	Critical Control Point / Quality Assurance
1	In a large bowl toss together salmon, breadcrumbs, onions and pimiento.	
2	In a small bowl beat together egg and milk; stir in lemon peel. Stir into salmon mixture; toss until moistened.	
3	With lightly flour hands, shape mixture into 16 four-inch patties.	
4	In a large skillet heat oil.	
5	Sauté patties, a few at a time, until golden brown on both sides, about 3 minutes per side	Cook until internal temperature reaches 165° F for 15 seconds. Keep warm.
6	For sauce, in a small saucepan, melt margarine	
7	Add flour and stir Add broth, lemon juice, and dill	
8	Heat to boiling	
9	For each serving, spoon over sauce Top with lemon slices	

Time Temperature Sensitive food. *Food safety Standards: hold food for service at an internal temperature above 140° F. Do not mix old product with new. Cool leftover product quickly (within 4 hours) to below 41° F. Follow proper cooling procedures. Store leftovers in a tightly sealed, labeled and dated container. Use leftover within 72 hours if stored in refrigerator or 30 days if stored in the freezer. Reheat leftover product quickly (within 2 hours) to 165 degrees F for 15 seconds. Reheat left over product only once; discard if not used. Cold holding at 41°F or colder or using time alone (less than four hours). Always wash hands and wash and sanitize counter tops utensils and containers between steps when working with raw seafood.*

<u>**Texture Modified Diets:**</u>

Soft & Bite Size: (aka Bite size) **Food particle size ½ inch (~width of standard fork)** Food must be moist. Cut foods with a knife to a ½" particle size after cooking. Moisten with sauce as needed after cutting. Omit green onions.
Chopped: Food particle size ¼ inch (~ ½ width of standard fork) Food must be moist. Chop foods with a knife to 1/4" particle size after cooking. Moisten with sauce as needed after chopping. Omit green onions.
Minced and Moist: (aka Minced/Mechanical Soft/Ground) **Food particle size 1/8 inch (fits through prongs of standard fork)** Food must be moist. Use a food processor to grind food particles into 1/8 inch after cooking. Moisten with sauce as needed after processing. Omit green onions.
Pureed: Smooth and cohesive. Use a food processor to puree to a smooth consistency. Foods are processed by grinding and then pureeing them. May add milk or sauce to puree. Do not add to much liquid. Puree should still hold its shape. Must not be firm or sticky. Puree foods while still hot. Appearance should be smooth like pudding. Omit green onions.

Copyright 2020 Jacqueline Larson M.S., R.D.N. and Associates.   All Rights Reserved

Serve ½ c. meat serving topped with sauce.

Therapeutic Modified Diets:
Lowfat: No changes needed
Diabetic/No added Sugar/No Conc. Sweets/Calorie Controlled: No changes needed
Bland/Anti Reflux: omit onion, pimento, lemon peel, lemon juice, lemon slices, and dill.
Liberal House Renal: Omit sauce, pimentos and bread crumbs.
No Added Salt: No changes needed
2 Gram Sodium: omit sauce, pimentos and bread crumbs. Drizzle with lemon juice.
Gluten Free: Use gluten-free flour. Use GF bread crumbs, oats or crushed cornflakes. Use GF broth. Prepare foods separately to prevent cross contamination.
Allergy Alerts: When an "X" is present, this indicates the allergen is present.
Always read all food labels to ensure allergens are not present.

Wheat	Milk	Eggs	Fish Shellfish	Soy	Peanuts/Nuts	Other
X	X	X	X	X		

Key: SF= Salt Free D= Diet or Sugarfree LF = Lowfat FF = Fat Free GF = Gluten Free

Recipe Name: Salmon Cakes with Red Pepper Sauce
Recipe Category: Dinner Entrée
Portion Size: 4 oz.
Ingredients: **Yields: 8 servings**

Ingredients	Notes:
½ cup light mayonnaise	
¼ cup fresh chives	Wash, trim and chop
2 tablespoons fresh parsley	Wash, trim and mince
1 tablespoon lemon juice	
½ teaspoon paprika	
2 ½ cups canned salmon or fresh diced	Drained, and measured
½ cup bread crumbs	
RED PEPPER SAUCE:	
1/2 cup sweet red pepper	Wash, trim and finely chop
1/4 cup green onions	Wash, trim and finely chop (including green tops)
1/4 cup Dijon mustard	
1/4 cup light mayonnaise	
1/4 cup light sour cream	
2 tablespoons red onion	Wash, peeled and minced
2 teaspoons parsley flakes	
1 tablespoon lemon juice	
¼ teaspoon salt	
¼ teaspoon pepper	
3 tablespoons olive oil	
8 Lemon wedges	(optional garnish)

Directions:

Steps:	Directions:	Critical Control Point / Quality Assurance
1	In a large bowl, combine mayonnaise, chives, parsley, lemon juice, paprika, pepper, salmon and bread crumbs; mix well.	
2	Shape 1/4 cup full of salmon mixture into patties.	
3	Meanwhile, for sauce, in a blender of food processor, combine the red pepper, onions, mustard, mayonnaise, sour cream, onion, parsley, honey, lemon juice, salt and pepper; cover and process until finely chopped.	Refrigerate until serving.
4	In a large skillet, heat ½ oil to medium high heat.	
5	Place half of the salmon cakes in skillet.	Cook over medium heat for 5 minutes on each side or until lightly browned (carefully turn the delicate cakes over)
6	Repeat with remaining oil and salmon cakes. Serve with sauce and lemon wedges.	Cook until internal temperature reaches 145° F for 15 seconds.

Time Temperature Sensitive food. *Food safety Standards: hold food for service at an internal temperature above 140° F. Do not mix old product with new. Cool leftover product quickly (within 4 hours) to below 41° F. Follow proper cooling procedures. Store leftovers in a tightly sealed, labeled and dated container. Use leftover within 72 hours if stored in refrigerator or 30 days if stored in the freezer. Reheat leftover product quickly (within 2 hours) to 165 degrees F for 15 seconds. Reheat left over product only once; discard if not used. Cold holding at 41°F or colder or using time alone (less than four hours).*

<u>Texture Modified Diets:</u>
Soft & Bite Size: (aka Bite size) **Food particle size ½ inch (~width of standard fork)** Food must be moist. Cut foods with a knife to a ½" particle size after cooking. Moisten with sauce as needed after cutting.

Chopped: Food particle size ¼ inch (~ ½ width of standard fork) Food must be moist. Chop foods with a knife to 1/4" particle size after cooking. Moisten with sauce as needed after chopping.

Minced and Moist: (aka Minced/Mechanical Soft/Ground) **Food particle size 1/8 inch (fits through prongs of standard fork)** Food must be moist. Use a food processor to grind food particles into 1/8 inch after cooking. Moisten with sauce as needed after processing.

Pureed: Smooth and cohesive. Use a food processor to puree to a smooth consistency. Foods are processed by grinding and then pureeing them. May add milk or sauce to puree. Do not add to much liquid. Puree should still hold its shape. Must not be firm or sticky. Puree foods while still hot. Appearance should be smooth like pudding. Serve ½ c. meat serving topped with sauce.

Therapeutic Modified Diets:

Lowfat: No changes needed

Diabetic/No added Sugar/No Conc. Sweets/Calorie Controlled: No changes needed

Bland/Anti Reflux: omit, parsley, chives, lemon juice, paprika, lemons. For sauce top with mayonnaise and sour cream mixture only.

Liberal House Renal: Omit salt, bread crumbs, mayonnaise and red pepper sauce

No Added Salt: No changes needed

2 Gram Sodium: omit salt, bread crumbs, mayonnaise and red pepper sauce

Gluten Free: Omit bread crumbs and Substitute with GF crushed cornflakes or oatmeal. Prepare foods separately to prevent cross contamination.

Allergy Alerts: When an "X" is present, this indicates the allergen is present.
Always read all food labels to ensure allergens are not present.

Wheat	Milk	Eggs	Fish Shellfish	Soy	Peanuts/Nuts	Other
X	X	X	X			

Key: SF= Salt Free D= Diet or Sugarfree LF = Lowfat FF = Fat Free GF = Gluten Free

Recipe Name: Salmon Chowder
Recipe Category: Dinner Entrée
Portion Size: 2 cups
Ingredients: Yields: 8 servings

Ingredients	Notes:
4 Cups canned salmon drained and flaked (water packed)	May use fresh salmon
2 tablespoons olive oil	
1 large onion, chopped	Wash, peel and chop
Dash of cayenne pepper	Optional
1 cup celery, diced	Wash, trim and dice
1 cup carrots	Wash, peel and dice
1/2 teaspoon salt	
2 bay leaves	
3 cloves, garlic minced	Or 1 teaspoon garlic powder
2 (14 oz.) can diced tomatoes	Use Low-sodium canned tomato
4 cups low sodium chicken broth	
3 cups red potatoes	Wash, trim and dice. (may leave on peel)
2 cups frozen corn kernels	
1/4 cup parsley flakes	Wash, trim and chop. Or use 2 tablespoons dried

Directions:

Steps:	Directions:	Critical Control Point /Quality Assurance
1	In a large saucepan, over medium heat, add the oil.	
2	When the oil is hot, stir in the onions, celery, and carrots.	
3	Season the vegetables with salt, cayenne, and bay leaves. Saute for 6 minutes, or until the vegetables are soft and tender. Stir in the chicken broth and tomatoes and bring up to a boil. Add the potatoes and corn.	Simmer for 15 minutes, or until the potatoes are fork tender
4	Add the salmon and simmer the soup for 5 minutes. Remove bay leaf. Stir in the parsley and ladle the soup into serving bowls.	Cook until internal temperature reaches 165° F for 15 seconds.

Time Temperature Sensitive food. *Food safety Standards: hold food for service at an internal temperature above 140° F. Do not mix old product with new. Cool leftover product quickly (within 4 hours) to below 41° F. Follow proper cooling procedures. Store leftovers in a tightly sealed, labeled and dated container. Use leftover within 72 hours if stored in refrigerator or 30 days if stored in the freezer. Reheat leftover product quickly (within 2 hours) to 165 degrees F for 15 seconds. Reheat left over product only once; discard if not used. Cold holding at 41°F or colder or using time alone (less than four hours). Always wash hands and wash and sanitize counter tops utensils and containers between steps when working with raw seafood.*

<u>Texture Modified Diets:</u>
Chopped: Peel potatoes. Omit corn. All food must be cut into pieces no larger than ¼" X ¼ " X ¼ " (Pea size) Food must also be moist. Serve 2 c. chowder serving. Moisten with broth if needed.) Tip: process all foods to correct size before serving.
Mechanical Soft/Ground: Peel potatoes. Omit corn. All food must be cut into pieces no larger than ⅛" X ⅛" X ⅛ " (small curd cottage cheese consistency) Food must also be moist Serve 2 c. chowder serving. Moisten with broth if needed. Tip: process all foods to correct size before cooking.
Puree: Peel potatoes. Omit corn. All foods are prepared to a smooth consistency by grinding and then pureeing them. Appearance is smooth like pudding. Puree with broth if needed. Serve ½ c. puree fish ½ c. puree potatoes (no skin) and ½ c. puree carrots separately.

<u>Therapeutic Modified Diets:</u>
Lowfat: No changes needed
Diabetic/No added Sugar/No Conc. Sweets/Calorie Controlled: No changes needed
Bland/Anti Reflux: omit onion, cayenne pepper, bay leaf, celery, garlic, tomatoes, corn and parsley. Peel potatoes.
Liberal House Renal: Omit salt, tomatoes, and use SF broth or water.
No Added Salt: No changes needed
2 Gram Sodium: omit salt and use SF broth or water. Substitute fresh tomatoes for canned.
Gluten Free: Gluten-free broth. Prepare foods separately to prevent cross contamination.

Allergy Alerts: When an "X" is present, this indicates the allergen is present. Always read all food labels to ensure allergens are not present.

Wheat	Milk	Eggs	Fish Shellfish	Soy	Peanuts/Nuts	Other
X			X			

Key: SF= Salt Free D= Diet or Sugarfree LF = Lowfat FF = Fat Free GF = Gluten Free

Recipe Name: Salmon Leek Casserole
Recipe Category: Dinner Entrée
Portion Size: 1 cup
Ingredients: **Yields: 8 servings**

Ingredients	Notes:
1 lb. Noodles or pasta	May use whole grain noodles or pasta
4 cups canned salmon water packed, drained, flaked	
2 tablespoons olive oil	
2 tablespoons flour	
2 garlic cloves, minced	
4 large leeks	Wash, trim and slice thin
3 cups nonfat milk	
1 (8oz.) light cream cheese softened	
2 tablespoons Dijon mustard	
1/4 cup fresh lemon juice	
1 teaspoon lemon zest	
1 cup grated low fat shredded Monterey jack cheese	
1/4 cup bread crumbs	

Directions:

Steps:	Directions:	Critical Control Point /Quality Assurance
1	Preheat oven to 350 degrees	
2	Cook noodles according to the directions on the package	
3	Heat oil in large skillet over medium heat Add leeks	Cook until leeks are tender
4	Sprinkle with flour	
5	Gradually stir in milk	Cook 5 minutes stirring constantly
6	Stir in cream cheese, and mustard	
7	Remove from heat and stir in noodles, lemon juice, zest, salmon and half of the cheese	
8	Spray baking dish with nonstick cooking spray	
9	Add mixture to baking dish	
10	Top with remaining cheese and bread crumbs	
11	Bake in 350 degree oven uncovered for 20-30 minutes until hot	Cook until internal temperature reaches 165° F for 15 seconds.

Time Temperature Sensitive food. *Food safety Standards: hold food for service at an internal temperature above 140° F. Do not mix old product with new. Cool leftover product quickly (within 4 hours) to below 41° F. Follow proper cooling procedures. Store leftovers in a tightly sealed, labeled and dated container. Use leftover within 72 hours if stored in refrigerator or 30 days if stored in the freezer. Reheat leftover product quickly (within 2 hours) to 165 degrees F for 15 seconds. Reheat left over product only once; discard if not used. Cold holding at 41°F or colder or using time alone (less than four hours). Always wash hands and wash and sanitize counter tops utensils and containers between steps when working with raw seafood.*

Texture Modified Diets: Tip: use pasta that is the correct particle size.
Soft & Bite Size: (aka Bite size) **Food particle size ½ inch (~width of standard fork)** Food must be moist. Cut foods with a knife to a ½" particle size before mixing. Moisten with sauce as needed after cutting. Omit leeks and add white onions.
Chopped: Food particle size ¼ inch (~ ½ width of standard fork) Food must be moist. Chop foods with a knife to 1/4" particle size before mixing. Moisten with sauce as needed after chopping. Omit leeks and add white onions.
Minced and Moist:(aka Minced/Mechanical Soft/Ground) **Food particle size 1/8 inch (fits through prongs of standard fork)** Food must be moist. Use a food processor to grind food particles into 1/8 inch before mixing. Moisten with sauce as needed after processing. Omit leeks and add white onions.
Pureed: Smooth and cohesive. Use a food processor to puree to a smooth consistency. Foods are processed by grinding and then pureeing them. May add milk or sauce to puree. Do not add to much liquid. Puree should still hold its shape. Must not be firm or sticky. Puree foods while still hot. Appearance should be smooth like pudding. Omit leeks and add white onions. Serve ½ cup puree salmon and ½ cup puree pasta with sauce separately.
Therapeutic Modified Diets:

Copyright 2020 Jacqueline Larson M.S., R.D.N. and Associates.   All Rights Reserved

Lowfat: No changes needed
Diabetic/No added Sugar/No Conc. Sweets/Calorie Controlled: No changes needed
Bland/Anti Reflux: omit garlic, leeks, Dijon mustard, lemon zest and lemon juice.
Liberal House Renal: Omit cream cheese, bread crumbs and cheese. Omit lemon juice and lemon zest.
No Added Salt: No changes needed
2 Gram Sodium: omit cream cheese, bread crumbs, and cheese
Gluten Free: Gluten-free flour. Use gluten free pasta. Use GF bread crumbs or sub. With GF cornflakes. Prepare foods separately to prevent cross contamination.
Allergy Alerts: When an "X" is present, this indicates the allergen is present.
Always read all food labels to ensure allergens are not present.

Wheat	Milk	Eggs	Fish Shellfish	Soy	Peanuts/Nuts	Other
X	X	X	X			

Key: SF= Salt Free D= Diet or Sugarfree LF = Lowfat FF = Fat Free GF = Gluten Free

Recipe Name: Salmon Loaf
Recipe Category: Dinner Entrée
Portion Size: 3 oz.
Ingredients: Yields: 8 servings

Ingredients	Notes:
1/2 cup finely chopped onion	Wash, peel and chop
2 teaspoons dried dill weed	
1/4 teaspoon pepper	
2 tablespoons olive oil	
3 eggs, beaten	
1 cup bread crumbs	
½ cup red bell pepper	Washed, trimmed and diced
1/2 cup milk	
4 cups salmon, drained and broken into chunks (water packed)	Canned
8 oz. low fat cheddar cheese	

Directions:

Steps:	Directions:	Critical Control Point / Quality Assurance
1	In a saucepan cook onion, dill weed, and pepper in olive oil till onion is tender.	
2	Combine egg, bread crumbs, milk, and onion mixture.	
3	Add salmon and peppers; mix well.	
4	Shape into a loaf in a greased shallow baking pan.	
5	Bake in a 350 degree oven for 30 to 35 minutes. Top with cheese	Cook until internal temperature reaches 165° F for 15 seconds.

Time Temperature Sensitive food. *Food safety Standards: hold food for service at an internal temperature above 140° F. Do not mix old product with new. Cool leftover product quickly (within 4 hours) to below 41° F. Follow proper cooling procedures. Store leftovers in a tightly sealed, labeled and dated container. Use leftover within 72 hours if stored in refrigerator or 30 days if stored in the freezer. Reheat leftover product quickly (within 2 hours) to 165 degrees F for 15 seconds. Reheat left over product only once; discard if not used. Cold holding at 41 °F or colder or using time alone (less than four hours). Always wash hands and wash and sanitize counter tops utensils and containers between steps when working with raw seafood.*

Texture Modified Diets:

Soft & Bite Size: (aka Bite size) **Food particle size ½ inch (~width of standard fork)** Food must be moist. Cut foods with a knife to a ½" particle size after cooking. Moisten with sauce as needed after cutting.

Chopped: Food particle size ¼ inch (~ ½ width of standard fork) Food must be moist. Chop foods with a knife to 1/4" particle size after cooking. Moisten with sauce as needed after chopping.

Minced and Moist: (aka Minced/Mechanical Soft/Ground) **Food particle size 1/8 inch (fits through prongs of standard fork)** Food must be moist. Use a food processor to grind food particles into 1/8 inch after cooking. Moisten with sauce as needed after processing.

Pureed: Smooth and cohesive. Use a food processor to puree to a smooth consistency. Foods are processed by grinding and then pureeing them. May add milk or sauce to puree. Do not add to much liquid. Puree should still hold its shape. Must not be firm or sticky. Puree foods while still hot. Appearance should be smooth like pudding. Serve ½ c. meat serving topped with sauce.

Therapeutic Modified Diets:

Lowfat: No changes needed
Diabetic/No added Sugar/No Conc. Sweets/Calorie Controlled: No changes needed
Bland/Anti Reflux: omit onion, dill, bell peppers and pepper
Liberal House Renal: Omit cheese and bread crumbs
No Added Salt: No changes needed
2 Gram Sodium: omit cheese and bread crumbs
Gluten Free: Use gluten free bread crumbs or oats. Prepare foods separately to prevent cross contamination.
Allergy Alerts: When an "X" is present, this indicates the allergen is present. Always read all food labels to ensure allergens are not present.

Wheat	Milk	Eggs	Fish Shellfish	Soy	Peanuts/Nuts	Other
X	X	X	X			

Key: SF= Salt Free D= Diet or Sugarfree LF = Lowfat FF = Fat Free GF = Gluten Free

Recipe Name: Salmon Muffin Melt
Recipe Category: Dinner Entrée
Portion Size: 3 oz.
Ingredients: Yields: 8 servings

Ingredients	Notes:
4 cups salmon	(drained water packed)
1/2 cup light mayonnaise	
1 (8 oz.) light cream cheese	softened
1/2 cup celery, diced	Wash, trim and dice
8 green onions	Wash, trim and slice with green tops
8 oz. low fat shredded cheddar cheese	
8 English Muffins	

Directions:

Steps:	Directions:	Critical Control Point /Quality Assurance
1	In a medium sized bowl, combine salmon, mayonnaise, cream cheese and celery.	
2	Spilt muffins in half. Top with salmon salad Spread and flatten.	
3	Top with cheddar cheese and green onions Bake in a 400 degree oven 10 to 12 minutes	Cook until internal temperature reaches 165° F for 15 seconds.

Time Temperature Sensitive food. Food safety Standards: hold food for service at an internal temperature above 140° F. Do not mix old product with new. Cool leftover product quickly (within 4 hours) to below 41° F. Follow proper cooling procedures. Store leftovers in a tightly sealed, labeled and dated container. Use leftover within 72 hours if stored in refrigerator or 30 days if stored in the freezer. Reheat leftover product quickly (within 2 hours) to 165 degrees F for 15 seconds. Reheat left over product only once; discard if not used. Cold holding at 41°F or colder or using time alone (less than four hours).

Texture Modified Diets:
Soft & Bite Size: (aka Bite size) **Food particle size ½ inch (~width of standard fork)** Food must be moist. Cut foods with a knife to a ½" particle size after cooking. Moisten with sauce or milk as needed after cutting. Use soft moist bread. Omit green onions.

Chopped: Food particle size ¼ inch (~ ½ width of standard fork) Food must be moist. Chop foods with a knife to 1/4" particle size after cooking. Moisten with sauce or milk as needed after chopping. Use soft moist bread. Omit green onions.

Minced and Moist: (aka Minced/Mechanical Soft/Ground) **Food particle size 1/8 inch (fits through prongs of standard fork)** Food must be moist. Use a food processor to grind food particles into 1/8 inch after cooking. Moisten with sauce or milk as needed after processing. Use soft moist bread. Omit green onions.

Pureed: Smooth and cohesive. Use a food processor to puree to a smooth consistency. Foods are processed by grinding and then pureeing them. May add milk or sauce to puree. Do not add to much liquid. Puree should still hold its shape. Must not be firm or sticky. Puree foods while still hot. Appearance should be smooth like pudding. Serve ½ c. puree tuna mixture and ½ c. puree muffin separately. Omit green onions.

Therapeutic Modified Diets:
Lowfat: No changes needed
Diabetic/No added Sugar/No Conc. Sweets/Calorie Controlled: No changes needed
Bland/Anti Reflux: omit celery and green onions
Liberal House Renal: Omit mayonnaise, cream cheese, and cheese. Omit English muffins use low sodium toast.
No Added Salt: No changes needed
2 Gram Sodium: omit mayonnaise, cream cheese and cheese. Omit English muffins use low sodium toast
Gluten Free: Gluten-free muffins. Prepare foods separately to prevent cross contamination.

Allergy Alerts: When an "X" is present, this indicates the allergen is present. Always read all food labels to ensure allergens are not present.

Wheat	Milk	Eggs	Fish Shellfish	Soy	Peanuts/Nuts	Other
X	X	X	X			

Key: SF= Salt Free D= Diet or Sugarfree LF = Lowfat FF = Fat Free GF = Gluten Free

Recipe Name: Salmon Noodle Casserole
Recipe Category: Dinner Entrée
Portion Size: 1 cup
Ingredients: Yields: 8 servings

Ingredients	Notes:
1 lb. noodles	May use whole grain noodles or pasta
4 cups canned salmon	Water packed, drained, flaked.
2 tablespoons olive oil	
2 tablespoons flour	
2 garlic cloves, minced	Wash, peel and mince
1 large onion, chopped	Wash, peel and chop
1 cup carrots	Wash, peel, trim and dice.
1 cup celery, diced	Wash, trim and dice
3 cups nonfat milk	
1 (8oz.) light cream cheese	softened
2 tablespoons Dijon mustard	
1 cup frozen peas	
1 cup grated Parmesan Cheese	
1/4 cup bread crumbs	

Directions:

Steps:	Directions:	Critical Control Point /Quality Assurance
1	Preheat oven to 350 degrees.	
2	Cook noodles according to the directions on the package.	
3	Heat oil in large skillet over medium heat. Add garlic, onion, carrots and celery. Cook until carrot is tender Sprinkle with flour.	
4	Gradually stir in milk; Cook 5 minutes stirring constantly.	
5	Stir in cream cheese, and mustard.	
6	Remove from heat and stir in noodles, peas and half of the parmesan. Stir salmon	
7	Spray baking dish with nonstick cooking spray Add mixture to baking dish	
8	Top with remaining cheese and bread crumbs Bake in 350 degree oven uncovered for 20-30 minutes until hot	Cook until internal temperature reaches 165° F for 15 seconds.

Time Temperature Sensitive food. *Food safety Standards: hold food for service at an internal temperature above 140° F. Do not mix old product with new. Cool leftover product quickly (within 4 hours) to below 41° F. Follow proper cooling procedures. Store leftovers in a tightly sealed, labeled and dated container. Use leftover within 72 hours if stored in refrigerator or 30 days if stored in the freezer. Reheat leftover product quickly (within 2 hours) to 165 degrees F for 15 seconds. Reheat left over product only once; discard if not used. Cold holding at 41°F or colder or using time alone (less than four hours). Always wash hands and wash and sanitize counter tops utensils and containers between steps when working with raw seafood.*

<u>**Texture Modified Diets: Tip: use pasta that is the correct particle size.**</u>
Soft & Bite Size: (aka Bite size) **Food particle size ½ inch (~width of standard fork)** Food must be moist. Cut foods with a knife to a ½" particle size before mixing. Moisten with sauce as needed after cutting. Omit leeks and add white onions.
Chopped: Food particle size ¼ inch (~ ½ width of standard fork) Food must be moist. Chop foods with a knife to 1/4" particle size before mixing. Moisten with sauce as needed after chopping. Omit leeks and add white onions.
Minced and Moist:(aka Minced/Mechanical Soft/Ground) **Food particle size 1/8 inch (fits through prongs of standard fork)** Food must be moist. Use a food processor to grind food particles into 1/8 inch before mixing. Moisten with sauce as needed after processing. Omit leeks and add white onions.
Pureed: Smooth and cohesive. Use a food processor to puree to a smooth consistency. Foods are processed by grinding and then pureeing them. May add milk or sauce to puree. Do not add to much liquid. Puree should still hold its shape. Must not be firm or sticky. Puree foods while still hot. Appearance should be smooth like pudding. Omit leeks and add white onions. Serve ½ cup puree salmon and ½ cup puree pasta with sauce separately.
Tip prepare casserole without salmon to puree separately.
<u>**Therapeutic Modified Diets:**</u>

Copyright 2020 Jacqueline Larson M.S., R.D.N. and Associates. All Rights Reserved

Lowfat: No changes needed
Diabetic/No added Sugar/No Conc. Sweets/Calorie Controlled: No changes needed
Bland/Anti Reflux: omit onions, celery, and Dijon mustard
Liberal House Renal: Omit cream cheese, bread crumbs and Parmesan cheese
No Added Salt: No changes needed
2 Gram Sodium: Omit cream cheese, bread crumbs and Parmesan cheese.
Gluten Free: Gluten-free flour and noodles. Use GF bread crumbs or GF crushed cornflakes. Prepare foods separately to prevent cross contamination.
Allergy Alerts: When an "X" is present, this indicates the allergen is present.
Always read all food labels to ensure allergens are not present.

Wheat	Milk	Eggs	Fish Shellfish	Soy	Peanuts/Nuts	Other
X	X	X	X			

Key: SF= Salt Free D= Diet or Sugarfree LF = Lowfat FF = Fat Free GF = Gluten Free

Recipe Name: Salmon Patties with Cheese Sauce
Recipe Category: Dinner Entrée
Portion Size: 4 oz. patty with 2 tablespoons sauce
Ingredients: Yields: 8 servings

Ingredients	Notes:
4 cups canned salmon, drained and flaked	May use fresh boneless skinless salmon
1 cup bread crumbs	May use whole grain bread crumbs
1/2 cup minced onion	Wash, peel and dice
3 Eggs, beaten	
2 tablespoons lemon juice	
3/4 teaspoon salt	
1/4 teaspoon pepper	
1/2 cup nonfat milk	
2 tablespoons Dijon mustard	
Sauce: ¼ c. margarine ¼ c. flour ¼ teaspoon paprika ½ teaspoon dry mustard 2 cups nonfat milk 1 cup shredded low fat Swiss Cheese ½ cup shredded low fat Cheddar Cheese Salt and Pepper to taste	

Directions:

Steps:	Directions:	Critical Control Point / Quality Assurance
1	Preheat oven to 350 degrees	
2	Combine salmon, bread crumbs, onions, eggs, salt, lemon juice, milk, mustard and pepper.	
3	Form these ingredients into 8 patties	
4	Place into baking dish sprayed with nonstick vegetable dish. Bake for about 45 minutes.	Cook until internal temperature reaches 165° F for 15 seconds.
5	For sauce: melt margarine in medium saucepan over low heat.	
6	Stir in flour. Pour in milk. Add paprika, and mustard	
7	Cook stirring constantly until thickened. Stir in cheeses.	
8	Heat until melted and well blended	

Time Temperature Sensitive food. *Food safety Standards: hold food for service at an internal temperature above 140° F. Do not mix old product with new. Cool leftover product quickly (within 4 hours) to below 41° F. Follow proper cooling procedures. Store leftovers in a tightly sealed, labeled and dated container. Use leftover within 72 hours if stored in refrigerator or 30 days if stored in the freezer. Reheat leftover product quickly (within 2 hours) to 165 degrees F for 15 seconds. Reheat left over product only once; discard if not used. Cold holding at 41°F or colder or using time alone (less than four hours). Always wash hands and wash and sanitize counter tops utensils and containers between steps when working with raw seafood.*

Texture Modified Diets:

Soft & Bite Size: (aka Bite size) **Food particle size ½ inch (~width of standard fork)** Food must be moist. Cut foods with a knife to a ½" particle size after cooking. Moisten with sauce or milk as needed after cutting. **Chopped: Food particle size ¼ inch (~ ½ width of standard fork)** Food must be moist. Chop foods with a knife to 1/4" particle size after cooking. Moisten with sauce or milk as needed after chopping.
Minced and Moist:(aka Minced/Mechanical Soft/Ground) **Food particle size 1/8 inch (fits through prongs of standard fork)** Food must be moist. Use a food processor to grind food particles into 1/8 inch after cooking. Moisten with sauce or milk as needed after processing. Use soft moist bread.
Pureed: Smooth and cohesive. Use a food processor to puree to a smooth consistency. Foods are processed by grinding and then pureeing them. May add milk or sauce to puree. Do not add to much liquid. Puree should still hold its shape. Must not be firm or sticky. Puree foods while still hot. Appearance should be smooth like pudding. .

Therapeutic Modified Diets:

Lowfat: No changes needed
Diabetic/No added Sugar/No Conc. Sweets/Calorie Controlled: No changes needed

Bland/Anti Reflux: omit onion, lemon juice, pepper, paprika, dry mustard, and Dijon mustard.
Liberal House Renal: Omit salt, bread crumbs and cheese sauce.
No Added Salt: No changes needed
2 Gram Sodium: omit salt, bread crumbs and cheese sauce.
Gluten Free: Use gluten-free flour and GF bread crumbs or oats. Prepare foods separately to prevent cross contamination.

Allergy Alerts: When an "X" is present, this indicates the allergen is present. Always read all food labels to ensure allergens are not present.

Wheat	Milk	Eggs	Fish Shellfish	Soy	Peanuts/Nuts	Other
X	X	X	X	X		

Key: SF= Salt Free D= Diet or Sugarfree LF = Lowfat FF = Fat Free GF = Gluten Free

Recipe Name: Salmon with Almonds and Herbs
Recipe Category: Dinner Entrée
Portion Size: 4 oz.
Ingredients: **Yields: 8 servings**

Ingredients	Notes:
8 (5oz.) Fresh or Frozen skinless salmon fillets	May use other fresh fish types.
1/2 cup light mayonnaise	
2 Slices Whole Wheat Bread, torn	
½ cup sliced almonds	
¼ cup snipped fresh basil	Or 2 Tablespoons dried basil, crushed
¼ cup onion	Wash, peel and chop fine.
2 tablespoon snipped fresh parsley	or 1 Tablespoon dried parsley
½ teaspoon salt	
2 cloves garlic, minced	
¼ cup lemon Juice	
½ teaspoon black pepper	

Directions:

Steps:	Directions:	Critical Control Point /Quality Assurance
1	Preheat oven to 400 degrees F.	
2	Coat a shallow baking pan with nonstick cooking spray.	
3	Combine bread, almonds, snipped or dried basil, onion, parsley, salt and salt and garlic in a food processor until coarsely chopped.	
4	Place fish in baking dish. Drizzle with lemon juice. Spread mayonnaise on each piece of fish.	
5	Gently pat some of the dry mixture on top of each piece of fish.	
6	Bake uncovered for 10-12 minutes or until fish flakes easily when tested with a fork	Cook until internal temperature reaches 145° F for 15 seconds.

Time Temperature Sensitive food. *Food safety Standards: hold food for service at an internal temperature above 140° F. Do not mix old product with new. Cool leftover product quickly (within 4 hours) to below 41° F. Follow proper cooling procedures. Store leftovers in a tightly sealed, labeled and dated container. Use leftover within 72 hours if stored in refrigerator or 30 days if stored in the freezer. Reheat leftover product quickly (within 2 hours) to 165 degrees F for 15 seconds. Reheat left over product only once; discard if not used. Cold holding at 41°F or colder or using time alone (less than four hours). Always wash hands and wash and sanitize counter tops utensils and containers between steps when working with raw seafood.*

<u>**Texture Modified Diets:**</u>
Soft & Bite Size: (aka Bite size) **Food particle size ½ inch (~width of standard fork)** Food must be moist. Cut foods with a knife to a ½" particle size after cooking. Moisten with sauce or milk as needed after cutting. Omit almonds.
Chopped: Food particle size ¼ inch (~ ½ width of standard fork) Food must be moist. Chop foods with a knife to 1/4" particle size after cooking. Moisten with sauce or milk as needed after chopping. Omit almonds
Minced and Moist:(aka Minced/Mechanical Soft/Ground) **Food particle size 1/8 inch (fits through prongs of standard fork)** Food must be moist. Use a food processor to grind food particles into 1/8 inch after cooking. Moisten with sauce or milk as needed after processing. Use soft moist bread. Omit almonds
Pureed: Smooth and cohesive. Use a food processor to puree to a smooth consistency. Foods are processed by grinding and then pureeing them. May add milk or sauce to puree. Do not add to much liquid. Puree should still hold its shape. Must not be firm or sticky. Puree foods while still hot. Appearance should be smooth like pudding. Omit almonds.
<u>**Therapeutic Modified Diets:**</u>
Lowfat: No changes needed
Diabetic/No added Sugar/No Conc. Sweets/Calorie Controlled: No changes needed
Bland/Anti Reflux: omit almonds, onion, basil, garlic, lemon juice and pepper
Liberal House Renal: Omit salt, bread and lemon juice
No Added Salt: No changes needed
2 Gram Sodium: omit salt and bread
Gluten Free: Use GF bread crumbs or corn flakes. Prepare foods separately to prevent cross contamination.
Allergy Alerts: When an "X" is present, this indicates the allergen is present. Always read all food labels to ensure allergens are not present.

Wheat	Milk	Eggs	Fish Shellfish	Soy	Peanuts/Nuts	Other
X	X	X	X		X	

Key: SF= Salt Free D= Diet or Sugarfree LF = Lowfat FF = Fat Free GF = Gluten Free

Recipe Name: Salmon Pasta with Creamy Linguine
Recipe Category: Dinner Entrée
Portion Size: 1 cup
Ingredients: **Yields: 8 servings**

Ingredients	Notes:
1 lb. linguine	May use whole grain linguine
4 cups canned salmon	water packed, drained, flaked. May use fresh tuna
1/4 cup unsalted butter	
1/4 cup all-purpose flour	
1 tablespoon olive oil	
6 garlic cloves, minced	Wash, peeled and minced
1 1/2 cup fresh sliced mushrooms	Wash, trim and slice
1 cup celery, diced	Wash, trim and dice
1/2 teaspoon salt	
1/4 teaspoon pepper	
2 tablespoons parsley flakes	
1 cup Parmesan cheese	

Directions:

Steps:	Directions:	Critical Control Point / Quality Assurance
1	Bring a pot of water to a boil. Cook linguine until al dente, about 9 minutes, or as package directs. Reserve 1/2 cup of cooking water; drain pasta	
2	Melt butter in a small pan over medium-low heat. Sprinkle in flour and cook, stirring, until thickened but not browned, about 2 minutes. Whisk in milk and continue to whisk until sauce is thick enough to coat the back of a spoon, about 3 minutes. Season with salt and pepper. Remove from heat	
3	Warm oil in a large skillet over medium-high heat. Add garlic and cook, stirring, until golden, about 1 minute. Add mushrooms and sauté until they release their liquid and begin to turn golden, about 5 minutes. Add onion, celery and cook, stirring, until vegetables are tender, about 5 minutes longer	
4	Stir sauce and reserved pasta water into vegetable mixture and cook, stirring, until heated through, about 5 minutes. Reduce heat to medium-low, add salmon, breaking it up, and cook until warmed through, about 2 minutes. Season with salt and pepper. Toss linguine with sauce, sprinkle with parsley and Parmesan cheese, and serve hot	Cook until internal temperature reaches 165° F for 15 seconds.

Time Temperature Sensitive food. *Food safety Standards: hold food for service at an internal temperature above 140° F. Do not mix old product with new. Cool leftover product quickly (within 4 hours) to below 41° F. Follow proper cooling procedures. Store leftovers in a tightly sealed, labeled and dated container. Use leftover within 72 hours if stored in refrigerator or 30 days if stored in the freezer. Reheat leftover product quickly (within 2 hours) to 165 degrees F for 15 seconds. Reheat left over product only once; discard if not used. Cold holding at 41°F or colder or using time alone (less than four hours). Always wash hands and wash and sanitize counter tops utensils and containers between steps when working with raw seafood.*

<u>Texture Modified Diets: Tip: use pasta that is the correct particle size.</u>
Soft & Bite Size: (aka Bite size) **Food particle size ½ inch (~width of standard fork)** Food must be moist. Cut foods with a knife to a ½" particle size before mixing. Moisten with sauce as needed after cutting.
Chopped: Food particle size ¼ inch (~ ½ width of standard fork) Food must be moist. Chop foods with a knife to 1/4" particle size before mixing. Moisten with sauce as needed after chopping.
Minced and Moist: (aka Minced/Mechanical Soft/Ground) **Food particle size 1/8 inch (fits through prongs of standard fork)** Food must be moist. Use a food processor to grind food particles into 1/8 inch before mixing. Moisten with sauce as needed after processing.

Pureed: Smooth and cohesive. Use a food processor to puree to a smooth consistency. Foods are processed by grinding and then pureeing them. May add milk or sauce to puree. Do not add to much liquid. Puree should still hold its shape. Must not be firm or sticky. Puree foods while still hot. Appearance should be smooth like pudding. Serve ½ cup puree salmon and ½ cup puree pasta with sauce separately. Tip prepare casserole without salmon to puree separately.

Therapeutic Modified Diets:
Lowfat: No changes needed
Diabetic/No added Sugar/No Conc. Sweets/Calorie Controlled: No changes needed
Bland/Anti Reflux: omit celery, pepper and parsley.
Liberal House Renal: Omit salt and Parmesan cheese
No Added Salt: No changes needed
2 Gram Sodium: omit salt and Parmesan cheese.
Gluten Free: Gluten-free flour and pasta. Prepare foods separately to prevent cross contamination.
Allergy Alerts: When an "X" is present, this indicates the allergen is present.
Always read all food labels to ensure allergens are not present.

Wheat	Milk	Eggs	Fish Shellfish	Soy	Peanuts/Nuts	Other
X	X	X	X			

Key: SF= Salt Free D= Diet or Sugarfree LF = Lowfat FF = Fat Free GF = Gluten Free

Recipe Name: Salmon with Fettuccini or Tuna with Fettuccini
Recipe Category: Dinner Entrée
Portion Size: 1 cup
Ingredients: Yields: 8 servings

Ingredients	Notes:
4 Cups canned salmon or tuna, drained and flaked	(water packed) May use fresh salmon or tuna
1 lb. package fettuccine	May use spinach fettuccine or whole grain fettucine
1 1/2 cups nonfat milk	
1 (8 oz.) fresh sliced mushrooms	
2 tablespoons olive oil	
2 tablespoon flour	
1/2 cup low sodium chicken broth	
1 cup grated parmesan cheese	
1 tablespoon parsley flakes	
2 teaspoons dried dill weed	(Optional)
1/2 teaspoon salt	
1/8 teaspoon black pepper	

Directions:

Steps:	Directions:	Critical Control Point /Quality Assurance
1	Cook pasta according to the directions on package	
2	Meanwhile, prepare sauce. In a large pan, melt oil over medium heat. Add onion and mushrooms; Cook until onion is tender. Reduce heat to low, and stir in flour. Remove from heat.	
3	Stir into cooked vegetables, the milk mixture and broth.	
4	Return pan to heat, and bring to a boil, stirring frequently.	
5	Reduce heat, and simmer for 2 minutes.	
6	Cut into salmon into chunks; stir into the sauce. Stir in Parmesan cheese, parsley, and dill. Season with salt and pepper to taste, and heat though. Serve over hot pasta. Toss to coat.	Cook until internal temperature reaches 165° F for 15 seconds.

Time Temperature Sensitive food. *Food safety Standards: hold food for service at an internal temperature above 140° F. Do not mix old product with new. Cool leftover product quickly (within 4 hours) to below 41° F. Follow proper cooling procedures. Store leftovers in a tightly sealed, labeled and dated container. Use leftover within 72 hours if stored in refrigerator or 30 days if stored in the freezer. Reheat leftover product quickly (within 2 hours) to 165 degrees F for 15 seconds. Reheat left over product only once; discard if not used. Cold holding at 41 °F or colder or using time alone (less than four hours). Always wash hands and wash and sanitize counter tops utensils and containers between steps when working with raw seafood.*

Texture Modified Diets: Tip: use pasta that is the correct particle size.

Soft & Bite Size: (aka Bite size) **Food particle size ½ inch (~width of standard fork)** Food must be moist. Cut foods with a knife to a ½" particle size before mixing. Moisten with sauce as needed after cutting.

Chopped: Food particle size ¼ inch (~ ½ width of standard fork) Food must be moist. Chop foods with a knife to 1/4" particle size before mixing. Moisten with sauce as needed after chopping.

Minced and Moist: (aka Minced/Mechanical Soft/Ground) **Food particle size 1/8 inch (fits through prongs of standard fork)** Food must be moist. Use a food processor to grind food particles into 1/8 inch before mixing. Moisten with sauce as needed after processing.

Pureed: Smooth and cohesive. Use a food processor to puree to a smooth consistency. Foods are processed by grinding and then pureeing them. May add milk or sauce to puree. Do not add to much liquid. Puree should still hold its shape. Must not be firm or sticky. Puree foods while still hot. Appearance should be smooth like pudding. Serve ½ cup puree salmon and ½ cup puree pasta with sauce separately. Tip prepare casserole without salmon to puree separately.

Therapeutic Modified Diets:

Lowfat: No changes needed
Diabetic/No added Sugar/No Conc. Sweets/Calorie Controlled: No changes needed
Bland/Anti Reflux: omit parsley, dill weed and black pepper.
Liberal House Renal: Omit salt and Parmesan cheese
No Added Salt: No changes needed
2 Gram Sodium: Omit salt and Parmesan cheese
Gluten Free: Use gluten free pasta, broth, and flour. Prepare foods separately to prevent cross contamination.

Allergy Alerts: When an "X" is present, this indicates the allergen is present. Always read all food labels to ensure allergens are not present.

Wheat	Milk	Eggs	FishShellfish	Soy	Peanuts/Nuts	Other
X	X	X	X			

Key: SF= Salt Free D= Diet or Sugarfree LF = Lowfat FF = Fat Free GF = Gluten Free

Copyright 2020 Jacqueline Larson M.S., R.D.N. and Associates.   All Rights Reserved

Recipe Name: Salmon with Mango Salsa
Recipe Category: Dinner Entrée
Portion Size: 4 oz. with 2 tablespoons salsa
Ingredients: **Yields: 8 servings**

Ingredients	Notes:
8 (5oz.) Fresh or Frozen skinless salmon fillets	May use other fresh or frozen fish.
3 tablespoons olive oil	
1 small red onion, diced	Washed, peeled and diced
2 cloves garlic, peeled and minced	Washed, peeled and minced
1 avocado, peeled and diced	Washed, peeled, seed removed and diced
1 tablespoon fresh cilantro, chopped	Washed, trimmed and chopped
2 mangos	Washed, peeled, seeded and diced
1 tablespoon red wine vinegar	

Directions:

Steps:	Directions:	Critical Control Point /Quality Assurance
1	Preheat oven to 400 degrees F.	
2	Coat a shallow baking pan with nonstick cooking spray.	
3	Place fish in baking dish. Brush with olive oil. Bake uncovered for 10-12 minutes or until fish flakes easily when tested with a fork.	Cook until internal temperature reaches 145° F for 15 seconds.
4	For Salsa: In a small bowl, combine red onion, garlic, avocado, cilantro, mango and red wine vinegar. Toss gently. Serve immediately on top of Salmon.	

Time Temperature Sensitive food. *Food safety Standards: hold food for service at an internal temperature above 140° F. Do not mix old product with new. Cool leftover product quickly (within 4 hours) to below 41° F. Follow proper cooling procedures. Store leftovers in a tightly sealed, labeled and dated container. Use leftover within 72 hours if stored in refrigerator or 30 days if stored in the freezer. Reheat leftover product quickly (within 2 hours) to 165 degrees F for 15 seconds. Reheat left over product only once; discard if not used. Cold holding at 41°F or colder or using time alone (less than four hours). Always wash hands and wash and sanitize counter tops utensils and containers between steps when working with raw seafood.*

Texture Modified Diets:

Soft & Bite Size: (aka Bite size) **Food particle size ½ inch (~width of standard fork)** Food must be moist. Cut foods with a knife to a ½" particle size after cooking. Moisten with sauce or milk as needed after cutting.

Chopped: Food particle size ¼ inch (~ ½ width of standard fork) Food must be moist. Chop foods with a knife to 1/4" particle size after cooking. Moisten with sauce or milk as needed after chopping.

Minced and Moist: (aka Minced/Mechanical Soft/Ground) **Food particle size 1/8 inch (fits through prongs of standard fork)** Food must be moist. Use a food processor to grind food particles into 1/8 inch after cooking. Moisten with sauce or milk as needed after processing. Use soft moist bread.

Pureed: Smooth and cohesive. Use a food processor to puree to a smooth consistency. Foods are processed by grinding and then pureeing them. May add milk or sauce to puree. Do not add to much liquid. Puree should still hold its shape. Must not be firm or sticky. Puree foods while still hot. Appearance should be smooth like pudding.

Therapeutic Modified Diets:

Lowfat: No changes needed
Diabetic/No added Sugar/No Conc. Sweets/Calorie Controlled: No changes needed
Bland/Anti Reflux: omit onion, garlic, cilantro and red wine vinegar
Liberal House Renal: no changes needed
No Added Salt: No changes needed
2 Gram Sodium: No changes needed
Gluten Free: No changes needed.
Allergy Alerts: When an "X" is present, this indicates the allergen is present.
Always read all food labels to ensure allergens are not present.

Wheat	Milk	Eggs	Fish Shellfish	Soy	Peanuts/Nuts	Other
			X			

Key: SF= Salt Free D= Diet or Sugarfree LF = Lowfat FF = Fat Free GF = Gluten Free

Recipe Name: Sesame Ginger Salmon
Recipe Category: Dinner Entrée
Portion Size: 4 ounces chicken with sauce
Ingredients: Yields: 8 servings

Ingredients	Notes:
1/2 cup reduced sodium soy sauce	
1/2 cup honey	
2 tablespoons sesame seeds	
2 tablespoons cornstarch	
1/2 teaspoon garlic powder	
1/2 teaspoon ground ginger	
2 tablespoons oil	
8 boneless skinless fresh salmon	
4 green onions	Wash, trim and cut into thin strips including tops.

Directions:

Steps:	Directions:	Critical Control Point /Quality Assurance
1	In a small bowl; combine soy sauce, honey, sesame seeds, cornstarch, garlic powder and ground ginger. Set aside.	
2	Cut the salmon into 8 (3 oz.) pieces. Heat the oil in a large skillet. Add salmon and sauté for 8 to 10 minutes or until juices run clear.	Cook until internal temperature reaches 145 degrees F.
3	Pour sauce over salmon. Heat until thick and bubbly. Garnish with onions.	

Time Temperature Sensitive food. *Food safety Standards: hold food for service at an internal temperature above 140°F. Do not mix old product with new. Cool leftover product quickly (within 4 hours) to below 41°F. Follow proper cooling procedures. Store leftovers in a tightly sealed, labeled and dated container. Use leftover within 72 hours if stored in refrigerator or 30 days if stored in the freezer. Reheat leftover product quickly (within 2 hours) to 165 degrees F for 15 seconds. Reheat left over product only once; discard if not used. Cold holding at 41°F or colder or using time alone (less than four hours). Always wash hands and wash and sanitize counter tops utensils and containers between steps when working with raw seafood.*

Texture Modified Diets:
Soft & Bite Size: (aka Bite size) **Food particle size ½ inch (~width of standard fork)** Food must be moist. Cut foods with a knife to a ½" particle size after cooking. Moisten with sauce as needed after cutting. Omit green onions.
Chopped: Food particle size ¼ inch (~ ½ width of standard fork) Food must be moist. Chop foods with a knife to 1/4" particle size after cooking. Moisten with sauce as needed after chopping. Omit green onions.
Minced and Moist:(aka Minced/Mechanical Soft/Ground) **Food particle size 1/8 inch (fits through prongs of standard fork)** Food must be moist. Use a food processor to grind food particles into 1/8 inch after cooking. Moisten with sauce as needed after processing. Omit green onions.
Pureed: Smooth and cohesive. Use a food processor to puree to a smooth consistency. Foods are processed by grinding and then pureeing them. May add milk or sauce to puree. Do not add to much liquid. Puree should still hold its shape. Must not be firm or sticky. Puree foods while still hot. Appearance should be smooth like pudding. Omit green onions. Serve ½ c. meat serving topped with sauce.

Therapeutic Modified Diets:
Lowfat: No changes needed.
Diabetic/No added Sugar/No Conc. Sweets/Calorie Controlled: No changes needed.
Bland/Anti Reflux: Omit sesame seeds, garlic powder and green onions
Liberal House Renal: Omit honey and soy sauce; season chicken with garlic powder, ground ginger, sesame seeds and green onion
No Added Salt: No changes needed.
2 Gram Sodium: Omit honey and soy sauce; season chicken with garlic powder and ground ginger sesame seeds and green onion.
Gluten Free: Use GF soy sauce Prepare foods separately to prevent cross contamination.

Allergy Alerts: When an "X" is present, this indicates the allergen is present. Always read all food labels to ensure allergens are not present.

Wheat	Milk	Eggs	Fish Shellfish	Soy	Peanuts/Nuts	Other
X			X	X		

Key: SF= Salt Free D= Diet or Sugarfree LF = Lowfat FF = Fat Free GF = Gluten Free

Recipe Name: Shrimp and Gouda in Pastry Shells
Recipe Category: Dinner Entrée
Portion Size: ½ cup over 1 pastry shell
Ingredients: **Yields: 12 servings**

Ingredients	Notes:
1 (10 ounce) package Puff Pastry Shells	Or use toasted English muffins or bread
1 tablespoon olive oil	
1 small onion	Wash, trim and chop
1 teaspoon garlic powder	
2 lbs. fresh shrimp	Peeled, tail removed and deveined
1 cup frozen peas, thawed	
1 can fat free evaporated milk	
2 (8oz.) light cream cheese	
2 eggs, beaten	
8 oz. Smoked Gouda Cheese	Shredded

Directions:

Steps:	Directions:	Critical Control Point / Quality Assurance
1	Bake the pastry shells according to the package directions	Remove from the baking sheet and cool on a wire rack
2	Heat the oil in a 10-inch skillet over medium heat	
3	Add the onion and garlic powder. Stir in shrimp.	Cook for about 5 minutes or until tender
4	In a large bowl whip, cream cheese, evaporated milk, eggs and Gouda Cheese.	
5	In a large skillet over low heat cheese mixture, heat to boil. (Stir frequently). Reduce the heat to low. Add shrimp and cook. Just before serving add peas and heat.	Cook until internal temperature 145 Degree F. for 15 seconds.
6	Spoon about 1/2 cup of the shrimp mixture in each shell	
7	Serve immediately.	

Time Temperature Sensitive food. *Food safety Standards: hold food for service at an internal temperature above 140° F. Do not mix old product with new. Cool leftover product quickly (within 4 hours) to below 41° F. Follow proper cooling procedures. Store leftovers in a tightly sealed, labeled and dated container. Use leftover within 72 hours if stored in refrigerator or 30 days if stored in the freezer. Reheat leftover product quickly (within 2 hours) to 165 degrees F for 15 seconds. Reheat left over product only once; discard if not used. Cold holding at 41 °F or colder or using time alone (less than four hours). Always wash hands and wash and sanitize counter tops utensils and containers between steps when working with raw seafood.*

<u>Texture Modified Diets:</u>
Soft & Bite Size: (aka Bite size) **Food particle size ½ inch (~width of standard fork)** Food must be moist. Cut foods with a knife to a ½" particle size prior to mixing. Moisten with broth as needed. Foods that do not process well should be omitted. Omit: Puff pastry. Serve over soft bread.
Chopped: Food particle size ¼ inch (~ ½ width of standard fork) Food must be moist. Chop foods with a knife to 1/4" particle size prior to mixing. Moisten with broth as needed. Foods that do not process well should be omitted. Omit: puff pastry. Serve over soft bread.
Minced and Moist:(aka Minced/Mechanical Soft/Ground) **Food particle size 1/8 inch (fits through prongs of standard fork)** Food must be moist. Use a food processor to grind food particles into 1/8 inch prior to mixing. Moisten with broth as needed. Foods that do not process well should be omitted. Omit: puff pastry. Serve over soft bread.
Pureed: Smooth and cohesive. Use a food processor to puree to a smooth consistency. Foods are processed by grinding and then pureeing them. May add broth or sauce to puree. Do not add to much liquid. Puree should still hold its shape. Must not be firm or sticky. Puree foods while still hot. Appearance should be smooth like pudding. Foods that do not process well should be omitted. Omit: puff pastry.. Serve ½ c. meat ½ c. puree bread separately.

<u>Therapeutic Modified Diets:</u>

Lowfat: No puff pastry. Use toast or English muffin
Diabetic/No added Sugar/No Conc. Sweets/Calorie Controlled: No changes needed
Bland/Anti Reflux: No puff pastry, use toast or English muffin. Omit garlic and onion. **Liberal House Renal:** Serve 3 oz. plain shrimp sauté with garlic and onion, garlic powder on low sodium toast
No Added Salt: No changes needed
2 Gram Sodium: Serve 3 oz. plain shrimp sauté with garlic and onion, on low sodium toast
Gluten Free: Gluten-free broth. Serve on gluten free toast. Prepare foods separately to prevent cross contamination.
Allergy Alerts: When an "X" is present, this indicates the allergen is present.
Always read all food labels to ensure allergens are not present.

Wheat	Milk	Eggs	Fish Shellfish	Soy	Peanuts/Nuts	Other
X	X	X	X			

Key: SF= Salt Free D= Diet or Sugarfree LF = Lowfat FF = Fat Free GF = Gluten Free

Recipe Name: Shrimp Fajitas
Recipe Category: Dinner Entrée
Portion Size: 2 fajitas with 1 (1 whole grain tortilla) plus 1 1/2 oz. shrimp for a total of 2 tortillas and 3 oz. meat.
Ingredients: **Yields: 8 servings**

Ingredients	Notes:
2 1/2 pounds shrimp (deveined, peeled and tail off)	
16 (6 inch) flour tortillas	May use whole grain
2 teaspoons vegetable oil	
3 green bell peppers	Wash, trim and slice into strips
1 tablespoon cornstarch	
2 teaspoons chili powder	
1 teaspoon salt	
1 teaspoon sugar	
½ teaspoon onion powder	
½ teaspoon garlic powder	
¼ teaspoon cayenne pepper	
½ teaspoon ground cumin	
2/3 cup water	
1 cup tomato, diced	Wash, trim and dice
1 cup shredded low fat cheddar cheese	
½ cup light sour cream	
avocado	(optional)

Directions:

Steps:	Directions:	Critical Control Point / Quality Assurance
1	Sauté onions and peppers in 1 teaspoon oil in a large pan until tender crisp on medium high heat. Remove from pan.	
2	In the same pan on medium high heat, sauté shrimp in 1 teaspoon oil until browned.	
3	In a small bowl combine cornstarch, chili powder, salt, paprika, sugar, onion powder, garlic powder, cayenne pepper, cumin and water.	
4	Combine seasoning mix with cooked shrimp.	
5	Simmer 10 to 15 minutes.	Minimum Temperature 165°F for 15 seconds
6	Heat tortilla according to package directions.	
7	To serve, spoon shrimp mixture evenly down center of each warm tortilla. Top with green peppers and onions.	
8	Sprinkle with cheese and roll up. Serve with s cheddar cheese, sour cream, and tomato	

Time Temperature Sensitive food. *Food safety Standards: hold food for service at an internal temperature above 140° F. Do not mix old product with new. Cool leftover product quickly (within 4 hours) to below 41° F. Follow proper cooling procedures. Store leftovers in a tightly sealed, labeled and dated container. Use leftover within 72 hours if stored in refrigerator or 30 days if stored in the freezer. Reheat leftover product quickly (within 2 hours) to 165 degrees F for 15 seconds. Reheat left over product only once; discard if not used. Cold holding at 41 ºF or colder or using time alone (less than four hours). Always wash hands and wash and sanitize counter tops utensils and containers between steps when working with raw meat.*

Texture Modified Diets:

Soft & Bite Size: (aka Bite size) **Food particle size ½ inch (~width of standard fork)** Food must be moist. Cut foods with a knife to a ½" particle size prior to layering. Moisten with broth as needed.

Chopped: Food particle size ¼ inch (~ ½ width of standard fork) Food must be moist. Chop foods with a knife to 1/4" particle size prior to layering. Moisten with broth as needed.

Minced and Moist: (aka Minced/Mechanical Soft/Ground) **Food particle size 1/8 inch (fits through prongs of standard fork)** Food must be moist. Use a food processor to grind food particles into 1/8 inch prior to layering. Moisten with broth as needed.

Pureed: Smooth and cohesive. Use a food processor to puree to a smooth consistency. Foods are processed by grinding and then pureeing them. May add broth or sauce to puree. Do not add to much liquid. Puree should still hold its shape. Must not be firm or sticky. Puree foods while still hot. Appearance should be smooth like pudding. . Serve ½ c. meat serving and pasta separately. May puree pasta puree with sauce for flavor.
Serve 1/2 c. puree shrimp mixture separately.1 cup puree tortilla separately. May puree tomato and add to sour cream and tomato top of tortilla to moisten. May melt cheese on meat mixture.

Therapeutic Modified Diets:

Lowfat: No changes needed
Diabetic/No added Sugar/No Conc. Sweets/Calorie Controlled: No changes needed
Bland: omit all seasonings except salt
Liberal House Renal: Omit tomato, salt, cheddar cheese, sour cream and bell pepper, Use low sodium tortillas. (see recipe)
No Added Salt: no changes
2 Gram Sodium: Omit salt, cheddar cheese, sour cream. Use low sodium tortillas. (See recipe)
Gluten Free: Use GF corn tortillas. Prepare foods separately to prevent cross contamination.
Allergy Alerts: When an "X" is present, this indicates the allergen is present.
Always read all food labels to ensure allergens are not present.

Wheat	Milk	Eggs	Fish Shellfish	Soy	Peanuts/Nuts	Other
X	X		X			

Key: SF= Salt Free D= Diet or Sugarfree LF = Lowfat FF = Fat Free GF = Gluten Free

Recipe Name: Shrimp Gumbo in Pastry Shells
Recipe Category: Dinner Entrée
Portion Size: ½ cup over 1 pastry shell
Ingredients: Yields: 8 servings

Ingredients	Notes:
1 (10 ounce) package Puff Pastry Shells	Or use toasted English muffins or bread
1 tablespoon olive oil	
1 small green pepper, chopped	Wash, trim and chop
1 small red pepper, chopped	Wash, trim and chop
1 teaspoon garlic powder	
1/4 teaspoon ground red pepper	
1/4 c. all purpose flour	
2 (14 oz.) cans fat free evaporated milk	
1 cup low sodium chicken broth	
½ lb. diced cooked chicken	
1 lb. cooked shrimp	Shelled, deveined and coarsely chopped
1 lb. ounces kielbasa, diced	

Directions:

Steps:	Directions:	Critical Control Point / Quality Assurance
1	Bake the pastry shells according to the package directions	Remove from the baking sheet and cool on a wire rack
2	Heat the oil in a 10-inch skillet over medium heat	
3	Add the green pepper, red pepper, garlic powder and ground red pepper	Cook for about 5 minutes or until tender
4	Stir in flour. Stir the evaporated milk, chicken broth, chicken, shrimp, and kielbasa into the skillet	
5	Heat to a boil. Reduce the heat to low. Cook for 5 minutes.	Cook until internal temperature reaches 165° F for 15 seconds.
6	Spoon about 1/2 cup of the chicken mixture in each shell.	
7	Serve immediately	

Time Temperature Sensitive food. *Food safety Standards: hold food for service at an internal temperature above 140° F. Do not mix old product with new. Cool leftover product quickly (within 4 hours) to below 41° F. Follow proper cooling procedures. Store leftovers in a tightly sealed, labeled and dated container. Use leftover within 72 hours if stored in refrigerator or 30 days if stored in the freezer. Reheat leftover product quickly (within 2 hours) to 165 degrees F for 15 seconds. Reheat left over product only once; discard if not used. Cold holding at 41°F or colder or using time alone (less than four hours). Always wash hands and wash and sanitize counter tops utensils and containers between steps when working with raw seafood.*

Texture Modified Diets:

Soft & Bite Size: (aka Bite size) **Food particle size ½ inch (~width of standard fork)** Food must be moist. Cut foods with a knife to a ½" particle size prior to mixing. Moisten with broth as needed. Foods that do not process well should be omitted. Omit: Puff pastry. Serve over soft bread.

Chopped: Food particle size ¼ inch (~ ½ width of standard fork) Food must be moist. Chop foods with a knife to 1/4" particle size prior to mixing. Moisten with broth as needed. Foods that do not process well should be omitted. Omit: puff pastry. Serve over soft bread.

Minced and Moist: (aka Minced/Mechanical Soft/Ground) **Food particle size 1/8 inch (fits through prongs of standard fork)** Food must be moist. Use a food processor to grind food particles into 1/8 inch prior to mixing. Moisten with broth as needed. Foods that do not process well should be omitted. Omit: puff pastry. Serve over soft bread.

Pureed: Smooth and cohesive. Use a food processor to puree to a smooth consistency. Foods are processed by grinding and then pureeing them. May add broth or sauce to puree. Do not add to much liquid. Puree should still hold its shape. Must not be firm or sticky. Puree foods while still hot. Appearance should be smooth like pudding. Foods that do not process well should be omitted. Omit: puff pastry.. Serve ½ c. meat ½ c. puree bread separately.

Therapeutic Modified Diets:

Lowfat: No puff pastry. Use toast or English muffin
Diabetic/No added Sugar/No Conc. Sweets/Calorie Controlled: No changes needed
Bland/Anti Reflux: No puff pastry, use toast or English muffin. Omit green pepper, red pepper, and kielbasa
Liberal House Renal: Serve 3 oz. plain shrimp sauté with green and red pepper, garlic powder on low sodium toast
No Added Salt: No changes needed
2 Gram Sodium: Serve 3 oz. plain shrimp sauté with green and red pepper, powder on on low sodium toast
Gluten Free: Gluten-free broth and kielbasa. Serve on gluten free toast. Prepare foods separately to prevent cross contamination.
Allergy Alerts: When an "X" is present, this indicates the allergen is present.
Always read all food labels to ensure allergens are not present.

Wheat	Milk	Eggs	Fish Shellfish	Soy	Peanuts/Nuts	Other
X	X	X	X			

Key: SF= Salt Free D= Diet or Sugarfree LF = Lowfat FF = Fat Free GF = Gluten Free©

Recipe Name: Shrimp Lo Mein
Recipe Category: Dinner Entrée
Portion Size: 3 oz. boneless meat, ½ cup pasta, ½ cup vegetables (approx. 1 ½ cups)
Ingredients: **Yields: 8 servings**

Ingredients	Notes:
2 ½ pounds shrimp	Deveined and tail removed
1 lb. spaghetti	May use whole grain
1/2 cup reduced-sodium soy sauce	
1 tablespoon sesame oil	
¼ cup hot water	
1 tablespoon chicken bouillon	
¼ cup brown sugar	
2 teaspoons garlic powder or garlic cloves minced	
2 tablespoon oil	
2 cups carrots	Wash thoroughly, peeled, and sliced thin
2 cups broccoli	Wash thoroughly, cut into bite size pieces
1 large onion	Wash thoroughly before cutting, sliced
2 tablespoons sesame seeds, toasted	

Directions:

Steps:	Directions:	Critical Control Point /Quality Assurance
1	In a small bowl, dissolve bouillon in hot water. Add soy sauce, brown sugar, sesame oil and garlic in the small bowl. Stir.	
2	Prepare pasta according to directions on package. Drain reserving 1 cup water	
3	In a medium high heated skillet, add oil. Add shrimp and until no longer translucent.	
4	Add sauce mixture, cook all together for about 2 minutes and remove from pan.	Minimum Temperature 145°F for 15 seconds for shrimp
5	In the same pan, sauté onions until golden brown. Remove from heat.	
6	In a separate skillet, stir fry carrot until just tender. Add broccoli and cook until just tender.	
7	In a large pot combine reserved water, pasta, vegetables and shrimp. Toss to coat.	
8	Top with sesame seeds. Serve hot.	

Time Temperature Sensitive food. *Food safety Standards: hold food for service at an internal temperature above 140°F. Do not mix old product with new. Cool leftover product quickly (within 4 hours) to below 41°F. Follow proper cooling procedures. Store leftovers in a tightly sealed, labeled and dated container. Use leftover within 72 hours if stored in refrigerator or 30 days if stored in the freezer. Reheat leftover product quickly (within 2 hours) to 165 degrees F for 15 seconds. Reheat left over product only once; discard if not used. Cold holding at 41°F or colder or using time alone (less than four hours). Always wash hands and wash and sanitize counter tops utensils and containers between steps when working with raw meat.*

Texture Modified Diets: Tip: Use pasta that is the correct particle size.
Soft & Bite Size: (aka Bite size) **Food particle size ½ inch (~width of standard fork)** Food must be moist. Cut foods with a knife to a ½" particle size prior to mixing. Moisten with broth as needed.
Chopped: Food particle size ¼ inch (~ ½ width of standard fork) Food must be moist. Chop foods with a knife to 1/4" particle size prior to mixing. Moisten with broth as needed.
Minced and Moist:(aka Minced/Mechanical Soft/Ground) **Food particle size 1/8 inch (fits through prongs of standard fork)** Food must be moist. Use a food processor to grind food particles into 1/8 inch prior to mixing. Moisten with broth as needed.
Pureed: Smooth and cohesive. Use a food processor to puree to a smooth consistency. Foods are processed by grinding and then pureeing them. May add broth or sauce to puree. Do not add to much liquid. Puree should still hold its shape. Must not be firm or sticky. Puree foods while still hot. Appearance should be smooth like pudding. Serve ½ c. puree meat serving, ½ cup puree pasta and ½ cup puree vegetables separately. Omit sesame seeds.
Therapeutic Modified Diets:
Lowfat: No changes needed

Copyright 2020 Jacqueline Larson M.S., R.D.N. and Associates. All Rights Reserved

Diabetic/No added Sugar/No Conc. Sweets/Calorie Controlled: No changes needed
Bland: omit sesame seeds, garlic powder, broccoli and onion
Liberal House Renal: Omit sauce, season with no salt herbs
No Added Salt: Omit sauce
2 Gram Sodium: omit sauce, season with no salt herbs
Gluten Free: Use GF soy sauce. Use gluten free pasta. Prepare foods separately to prevent cross contamination.
Allergy Alerts: When an "X" is present, this indicates the allergen is present.
Always read all food labels to ensure allergens are not present.

Wheat	Milk	Eggs	Fish Shellfish	Soy	Peanuts/Nuts	Other
X		X	x	X		

Key: SF= Salt Free D= Diet or Sugarfree LF = Lowfat FF = Fat Free GF = Gluten Free

Recipe Name: Shrimp Marinated in Chili Garlic Sauce
Recipe Category: Dinner Entrée
Portion Size: 3 oz.
Ingredients: Yields: 8 servings

Ingredients	Notes:
3 1/2 lbs. of fresh shrimp, peeled, deveined and tails removed	
2 tablespoon chili garlic sauce	
1/2 cup light soy sauce	
3 garlic cloves, minced	Wash, peel and mince
3 teaspoons honey	
2 tablespoons oil	

Directions:

Steps:	Directions:	Critical Control Point / Quality Assurance
1	Combine chili garlic sauce, soy sauce, garlic and honey in a bowl; Stir	
2	Add shrimp and marinate for 15 minutes.	
3	In a large skillet, heat oil on high until hot.	
4	Drain excess liquid from shrimp.	
5	Carefully add to the hot oil.	
6	Stir fry until cooked.	About 5-7 minutes. Cook until internal temperature reaches 145° F for 15 seconds.

Time Temperature Sensitive food. *Food safety Standards: hold food for service at an internal temperature above 140° F. Do not mix old product with new. Cool leftover product quickly (within 4 hours) to below 41° F. Follow proper cooling procedures. Store leftovers in a tightly sealed, labeled and dated container. Use leftover within 72 hours if stored in refrigerator or 30 days if stored in the freezer. Reheat leftover product quickly (within 2 hours) to 165 degrees F for 15 seconds. Reheat left over product only once; discard if not used. Cold holding at 41 °F or colder or using time alone (less than four hours). Always wash hands and wash and sanitize counter tops utensils and containers between steps when working with raw seafood.*

Texture Modified Diets:

Soft & Bite Size: (aka Bite size) **Food particle size ½ inch (~width of standard fork)** Food must be moist. Cut foods with a knife to a ½" particle size after cooking. Moisten with sauce as needed after cutting.

Chopped: Food particle size ¼ inch (~ ½ width of standard fork) Food must be moist. Chop foods with a knife to 1/4" particle size after cooking. Moisten with sauce as needed after chopping.

Minced and Moist: (aka Minced/Mechanical Soft/Ground) **Food particle size 1/8 inch (fits through prongs of standard fork)** Food must be moist. Use a food processor to grind food particles into 1/8 inch after cooking. Moisten with sauce as needed after processing.

Pureed: Smooth and cohesive. Use a food processor to puree to a smooth consistency. Foods are processed by grinding and then pureeing them. May add milk or sauce to puree. Do not add to much liquid. Puree should still hold its shape. Must not be firm or sticky. Puree foods while still hot. Appearance should be smooth like pudding. Serve ½ c. meat serving.

Therapeutic Modified Diets:

Lowfat: No changes needed
Diabetic/No added Sugar/No Conc. Sweets/Calorie Controlled: No changes needed
Bland/Anti Reflux: omit chili garlic sauce,
Liberal House Renal: Omit soy sauce and chili garlic sauce
No Added Salt: Omit soy sauce
2 Gram Sodium: Omit soy sauce and chili garlic sauce
Gluten Free: Use gluten free soy sauce. Prepare foods separately to prevent cross contamination.
**Allergy Alerts: When an "X" is present, this indicates the allergen is present.
Always read all food labels to ensure allergens are not present.**

Wheat	Milk	Eggs	Fish Shellfish	Soy	Peanuts/Nuts	Other
			X	X		

Key: SF= Salt Free D= Diet or Sugarfree LF = Lowfat FF = Fat Free GF = Gluten Free

Recipe Name: Shrimp Salad with Creamy Tarragon Dressing
Recipe Category: Dinner Entrée
Portion Size: ½ c. shrimp salad on ½ c. watercress leaves
Ingredients: Yields: 8 servings

Ingredients	Notes:
4 cups cooked small shrimp	Deveined, peeled and tail removed.
1/2 cup light mayonnaise	
1 teaspoon fresh lemon zest	
1/2 cup fresh lemon juice	
1/4 cup fresh Tarragon	
1 teaspoon Dijon mustard	
1/4 teaspoon salt	
1/4 teaspoon pepper	
4 cups chopped watercress leaves	Or other green leafy vegetable. Remove any tough stems or membranes.
2 tablespoons drained capers	
1 large avocado	Wash, peel, seed and dice. (optional)

Directions:

Steps:	Directions:	Critical Control Point /Quality Assurance
1	In a small bowl, combine mayonnaise, lemon zest, lemon juice, tarragon, mustard, salt, shrimp, cappers and pepper.	
2	On individual serving plates. Place ½ cup watercress leaves. Top with ½ cup shrimp.	
3	Just before serving top with avocado. Serve chilled.	

Time Temperature Sensitive food. *Food safety Standards: hold food for service at an internal temperature above 140° F. Do not mix old product with new. Cool leftover product quickly (within 4 hours) to below 41° F. Follow proper cooling procedures. Store leftovers in a tightly sealed, labeled and dated container. Use leftover within 72 hours if stored in refrigerator or 30 days if stored in the freezer. Cold holding at 41°F or colder or using time alone (less than four hours). Always wash hands and wash and sanitize counter tops utensils and containers between steps when working with raw seafood.*

<u>Texture Modified Diets:</u>

Soft & Bite Size: (aka Bite size) **Food particle size ½ inch (~width of standard fork)** Food must be moist. Cut foods with a knife to a ½" particle size prior to mixing. Moisten with broth as needed. Foods that do not process well should be omitted. Omit: capers

Chopped: Food particle size ¼ inch (~ ½ width of standard fork) Food must be moist. Chop foods with a knife to 1/4" particle size prior to mixing. Moisten with broth as needed. Foods that do not process well should be omitted. Omit: capers

Minced and Moist: (aka Minced/Mechanical Soft/Ground) **Food particle size 1/8 inch (fits through prongs of standard fork)** Food must be moist. Use a food processor to grind food particles into 1/8 inch prior to mixing. Moisten with broth as needed. Foods that do not process well should be omitted. Omit: capers

Pureed: Smooth and cohesive. Use a food processor to puree to a smooth consistency. Foods are processed by grinding and then pureeing them. May add broth or sauce to puree. Do not add to much liquid. Puree should still hold its shape. Must not be firm or sticky. Puree foods while still hot. Appearance should be smooth like pudding. Foods that do not process well should be omitted. Omit: capers Puree with broth if needed. Serve ½ c. puree shrimp salad and ½. Puree greens separately. May process greens with bread to thicken.

<u>Therapeutic Modified Diets:</u>

Lowfat: No changes needed
Diabetic/No added Sugar/No Conc. Sweets/Calorie Controlled: No changes needed
Bland/Anti Reflux: omit lemon zest, lemon juice, Dijon mustard, capers and Tarragon. Finely shred greens
Liberal House Renal: Omit salt, capers and substitute olive oil for mayonnaise
No Added Salt: No changes needed
2 Gram Sodium: omit salt, capers and substitute olive oil for mayonnaise
Gluten Free: No changes needed. Prepare foods separately to prevent cross contamination.

Allergy Alerts: When an "X" is present, this indicates the allergen is present. Always read all food labels to ensure allergens are not present.

Wheat	Milk	Eggs	Fish Shellfish	Soy	Peanuts/Nuts	Other
		X	X			

Key: SF= Salt Free D= Diet or Sugarfree LF = Lowfat FF = Fat Free GF = Gluten Free©

Copyright 2020 Jacqueline Larson M.S., R.D.N. and Associates.   All Rights Reserved

Recipe Name: Shrimp Tacos with Creamy Cilantro Lime dressing
Recipe Category: Dinner Entrée
Portion Size: 2 small tacos
Ingredients: Yields: 8 servings

Ingredients	Notes:
2 1/2 Pounds shrimp	Peeled, deveined and tail removed
1 tablespoon olive oil	
1 tablespoon chili powder	
1/2 teaspoon garlic powder	
1/4 teaspoon onion powder	
1/2 teaspoon paprika	
1 teaspoon ground cumin	
1/2 teaspoon salt	
1/4 teaspoon ground black pepper	
1/2 teaspoon sugar	
1/4 Cup shredded low fat cheddar cheese	
3 Cups shredded cabbage	Wash, trim and chop
16 Flour small tortillas	May use whole grain
Sauce:	
¼ cup thinly sliced green onions	Washed, trimmed and sliced thin.
¼ cup chopped fresh cilantro	
¼ cup light mayonnaise	
1/2 teaspoon zest of lime	
2 tablespoons lime juice	
¼ teaspoon salt	
1 clove garlic, minced	Washed trimmed and minced
½ cup light sour cream	

Directions:

Steps:	Directions:	Critical Control Point /Quality Assurance
1	In a large flat bowl combine chili powder, garlic powder, onion powder, paprika, cumin, salt, black pepper and sugar.	
2	Heat oil in large pan heat oil to medium high heat.	
3	Dredge shrimp in seasoning and cook in pan.	Cook until internal temperature reaches 145 F degrees for 15 seconds.
4	Prepare sauce in a small bowl by mixing, green onions, cilantro, mayonnaise, lime zest, lime juice, salt, garlic and sour cream .	
5	Wrap tortillas in foil and 350 warm in oven for 20 minutes. In heated tortillas and top with shrimp, cabbage, cheese and sauce..	

Time Temperature Sensitive food. *Food safety Standards: hold food for service at an internal temperature above 140° F. Do not mix old product with new. Cool leftover product quickly (within 4 hours) to below 41° F. Follow proper cooling procedures. Store leftovers in a tightly sealed, labeled and dated container. Use leftover within 72 hours if stored in refrigerator or 30 days if stored in the freezer. Reheat leftover product quickly (within 2 hours) to 165 degrees F for 15 seconds. Reheat left over product only once; discard if not used. Cold holding at 41°F or colder or using time alone (less than four hours). Always wash hands and wash and sanitize counter tops utensils and containers between steps when working with raw meat.*

Texture Modified Diets: Serve chopped meat mixture, tomatoes, lettuce, cheese and sour cream on top of chopped/ minced tortillas. Do not mix

Soft & Bite Size: (aka Bite size) **Food particle size ½ inch (~width of standard fork)** Food must be moist. Cut foods with a knife to a ½" particle size prior to mixing. Moisten with broth as needed. Foods that do not process well should be omitted. Omit: green onions.

Chopped: Food particle size ¼ inch (~ ½ width of standard fork) Food must be moist. Chop foods with a knife to 1/4" particle size prior to mixing. Moisten with broth as needed. Foods that do not process well should be omitted. Omit: green onions.

Minced and Moist:(aka Minced/Mechanical Soft/Ground) **Food particle size 1/8 inch (fits through prongs of standard fork)** Food must be moist. Use a food processor to grind food particles into 1/8 inch prior to mixing. Moisten with broth as needed. Foods that do not process well should be omitted. Omit: green onions.

Pureed: Smooth and cohesive. Use a food processor to puree to a smooth consistency. Foods are processed by grinding and then pureeing them. May add broth or sauce to puree. Do not add to much liquid. Puree should still hold its shape. Must not be firm or sticky. Puree foods while still hot. Appearance should be smooth like pudding.

Foods that do not process well should be omitted. Omit: green onions. . Serve ½ c. puree meat on top of ½ c. puree tortillas serving. Melt cheese on top of meat. Top with1 T. puree tomato and 1 T. puree lettuce and 1 t. sour cream.

Therapeutic Modified Diets:
Lowfat: No changes needed
Diabetic/No added Sugar/No Conc. Sweets/Calorie Controlled: No changes needed
Bland/Anti Reflux: Serve plain shrimp on tortilla
Liberal House Renal: Omit sauce and cheese. Use SF tortillas.
No Added Salt: No changes needed
2 Gram Sodium: Omit salt and cheese. Use low sodium tortillas. (See recipe)
Gluten Free: Omit flour whole grain tortillas for gluten free corn tortillas. Prepare foods separately to prevent cross contamination.
Allergy Alerts: When an "X" is present, this indicates the allergen is present.
Always read all food labels to ensure allergens are not present.

Wheat	Milk	Eggs	Fish Shellfish	Soy	Peanuts/Nuts	Other
X	X	X	X			

Key: SF= Salt Free D= Diet or Sugarfree LF = Lowfat FF = Fat Free GF = Gluten Free

Recipe Name: Southwest Style Salmon Casserole
Recipe Category: Dinner Entrée
Portion Size: 1 cup
Ingredients: **Yields: 8 servings**

Ingredients	Notes:
8 flour tortillas	May use whole wheat tortillas
4 cups canned salmon, in water, drained	
1 (15 oz.) can no added salt black beans	drained and rinsed
1 cup frozen whole kernel corn, thawed	
1 (10 oz.) can enchilada sauce	
1 small onion, finely chopped	Wash, peel and chop
2 teaspoons chili powder	
2 teaspoons cumin	
8 oz. low fat cheddar or Monterey Jack cheese	
1/2 cup light sour cream	
1/2 cup salsa	
1 Avocado, peeled (optional)	Wash, seed, peel and dice

Directions:

Steps:	Directions:	Critical Control Point /Quality Assurance
1	Preheat oven to 350 degrees F	
2	Spray baking pan with cooking spray; Line pan with 4 flour tortillas	
3	Mix together the salmon, corn and beans	or Salmon
4	Spread 1/3 mixture over tortillas	
5	Sprinkle with 1/3 of cheese	
6	Layer with 4 tortillas. Spread the remaining salmon mixture over the top. Add the remaining cheese.	
7	Cover with foil and bake for 25 minutes until hot throughout	
8	Sprinkle with remaining cheese	
9	Return to top shelf under broiler for 1-2 minutes until cheese is just browned.	Cook until internal temperature reaches 165° F for 15 seconds.
10	Serve with sour cream, avocado and salsa as desired	

Time Temperature Sensitive food. *Food safety Standards: hold food for service at an internal temperature above 140° F. Do not mix old product with new. Cool leftover product quickly (within 4 hours) to below 41° F. Follow proper cooling procedures. Store leftovers in a tightly sealed, labeled and dated container. Use leftover within 72 hours if stored in refrigerator or 30 days if stored in the freezer. Reheat leftover product quickly (within 2 hours) to 165 degrees F for 15 seconds. Reheat left over product only once; discard if not used. Cold holding at 41°F or colder or using time alone (less than four hours).*

Texture Modified Diets:
Soft & Bite Size: (aka Bite size) **Food particle size ½ inch (~width of standard fork)** Food must be moist. Cut foods with a knife to a ½" particle size prior to mixing. Moisten with broth as needed. Foods that do not process well should be omitted. Omit: corn.

Chopped: Food particle size ¼ inch (~ ½ width of standard fork) Food must be moist. Chop foods with a knife to 1/4" particle size prior to mixing. Moisten with broth as needed. Foods that do not process well should be omitted. Omit: corn.

Minced and Moist: (aka Minced/Mechanical Soft/Ground) **Food particle size 1/8 inch (fits through prongs of standard fork)** Food must be moist. Use a food processor to grind food particles into 1/8 inch prior to mixing. Moisten with broth as needed. Foods that do not process well should be omitted. Omit: corn.

Pureed: Smooth and cohesive. Use a food processor to puree to a smooth consistency. Foods are processed by grinding and then pureeing them. May add broth or sauce to puree. Do not add to much liquid. Puree should still hold its shape. Must not be firm or sticky. Puree foods while still hot. Appearance should be smooth like pudding. Foods that do not process well should be omitted. Omit: corn.
Puree with broth if needed. Serve ½ c. puree salmon (season with cumin and chili) topped with puree salsa/sour cream and ½ cup puree beans with cheese separately.

Therapeutic Modified Diets:
Lowfat: No changes needed

Diabetic/No added Sugar/No Conc. Sweets/Calorie Controlled: No changes needed
Bland/Anti Reflux: Serve ½ c. plain salmon on tortilla. (heated). Top with cheese and sour cream
Liberal House Renal: Omit enchilada sauce, cheese, sour cream and salsa. Use low sodium tortillas
No Added Salt: No changes needed
2 Gram Sodium: omit enchilada sauce, cheese and sour cream. Use low sodium tortillas
Gluten Free: Use corn tortillas. Prepare foods separately to prevent cross contamination.
Allergy Alerts: When an "X" is present, this indicates the allergen is present.
Always read all food labels to ensure allergens are not present.

Wheat	Milk	Eggs	Fish Shellfish	Soy	Peanuts/Nuts	Other
X	X		X			

Key: SF= Salt Free D= Diet or Sugarfree LF = Lowfat FF = Fat Free GF = Gluten Free

Recipe Name: Southwest Style Tuna Casserole
Recipe Category: Dinner Entrée
Portion Size: 1 cup
Ingredients: **Yields: 8 servings**

Ingredients	Notes:
8 flour tortillas	May use whole wheat tortillas
4 cups light tuna in water, drained	
1 (15 oz.) can no added salt black beans	drained and rinsed
1 cup frozen whole kernel corn, thawed	
1 (10 oz.) can enchilada sauce	
1 small onion, finely chopped	Wash, peel and chop
2 teaspoons chili powder	
2 teaspoons cumin	
8 oz. low fat cheddar or Monterey Jack cheese	
1/2 cup light sour cream	
1/2 cup salsa	
1 Avocado, peeled (optional)	Wash, seed, peel and dice

Directions:

Steps:	Directions:	Critical Control Point /Quality Assurance
1	Preheat oven to 350 degrees F	
2	Spray baking pan with cooking spray; Line pan with 4 flour tortillas	
3	Mix together the tuna, corn and beans	or Salmon
4	Spread 1/3 mixture over tortillas	
5	Sprinkle with 1/3 of cheese	
6	Layer with 4 tortillas. Spread the remaining tuna mixture over the top. Add the remaining cheese.	
7	Cover with foil and bake for 25 minutes until hot throughout	
8	Sprinkle with remaining cheese	
9	Return to top shelf under broiler for 1-2 minutes until cheese is just browned.	Cook until internal temperature reaches 165° F for 15 seconds.
10	Serve with sour cream, avocado and salsa as desired	

Time Temperature Sensitive food. Food safety Standards: hold food for service at an internal temperature above 140° F. Do not mix old product with new. Cool leftover product quickly (within 4 hours) to below 41° F. Follow proper cooling procedures. Store leftovers in a tightly sealed, labeled and dated container. Use leftover within 72 hours if stored in refrigerator or 30 days if stored in the freezer. Reheat leftover product quickly (within 2 hours) to 165 degrees F for 15 seconds. Reheat left over product only once; discard if not used. Cold holding at 41°F or colder or using time alone (less than four hours).

Texture Modified Diets:

Soft & Bite Size: (aka Bite size) **Food particle size ½ inch (~width of standard fork)** Food must be moist. Cut foods with a knife to a ½" particle size prior to mixing. Moisten with broth as needed. Foods that do not process well should be omitted. Omit: corn.

Chopped: Food particle size ¼ inch (~ ½ width of standard fork) Food must be moist. Chop foods with a knife to 1/4" particle size prior to mixing. Moisten with broth as needed. Foods that do not process well should be omitted. Omit: corn.

Minced and Moist: (aka Minced/Mechanical Soft/Ground) **Food particle size 1/8 inch (fits through prongs of standard fork)** Food must be moist. Use a food processor to grind food particles into 1/8 inch prior to mixing. Moisten with broth as needed. Foods that do not process well should be omitted. Omit: corn.

Pureed: Smooth and cohesive. Use a food processor to puree to a smooth consistency. Foods are processed by grinding and then pureeing them. May add broth or sauce to puree. Do not add to much liquid. Puree should still hold its shape. Must not be firm or sticky. Puree foods while still hot. Appearance should be smooth like pudding. Foods that do not process well should be omitted. Omit: corn.

Puree with broth if needed. Serve ½ c. puree salmon (season with cumin and chili) topped with puree salsa/sour cream and ½ cup puree beans with cheese separately.

Therapeutic Modified Diets:

Lowfat: No changes needed
Diabetic/No added Sugar/No Conc. Sweets/Calorie Controlled: No changes needed
Bland/Anti Reflux: Serve ½ c. plain tuna on tortilla. (heated). Top with cheese and sour cream
Liberal House Renal: Omit enchilada sauce, cheese, sour cream and salsa. Use low sodium tortillas
No Added Salt: No changes needed
2 Gram Sodium: omit enchilada sauce, cheese and sour cream. Use low sodium tortilas
Gluten Free: Use corn tortillas. Prepare foods separately to prevent cross contamination.
Allergy Alerts: When an "X" is present, this indicates the allergen is present.
Always read all food labels to ensure allergens are not present.

Wheat	Milk	Eggs	Fish Shellfish	Soy	Peanuts/Nuts	Other
X	X		X			

Key: SF= Salt Free D= Diet or Sugarfree LF = Lowfat FF = Fat Free GF = Gluten Free

Recipe Name: Sweet and Sour Shrimp
Recipe Category: Dinner Entrée
Portion Size: 3 oz. pork, 1 c. serving size with sauce and vegetables
Ingredients: **Yields: 8 servings**

Ingredients	Notes:
2 ½ lb. shrimp	Deveined, peeled and tail removed
1 16 ounce can pineapple chunks (juice packed)	
2/3 cup sugar	
½ cup vinegar	
¼ cup cornstarch	
2 teaspoons instant chicken bouillon granules	
¼ cup lite soy sauce	
2 eggs, beaten	
½ cup cornstarch	
½ cup flour	
½ cup water	
¼ teaspoon black pepper	
2 Tablespoon oil	
4 medium carrots	Wash, Peel, and thinly sliced at an angle
4 cloves garlic, minced	
2 Large Bell peppers Green or Red	Wash, remove stem and seeds, and cut into ½ inch pieces
4 Cups, hot cooked rice	May use brown or white enriched rice

Directions:

Steps:	Directions:	Critical Control Point / Quality Assurance
1	For sauce, drain pineapple, reserving juice. Cut pineapple into ½ inch pieces.	
2	Add water to reserved juice to equal 1 ½ cups	
3	Stir in sugar, vinegar, the 2 Tablespoons cornstarch, soy sauce and bouillon and set aside	
4	For batter: In a small bowl, combine egg the ¼ cup cornstarch, flour, water and pepper.	
5	Whisk thoroughly, until smooth.	
6	Dip shrimp into batter. In small amount of oil, sauté about 1/3 of the shrimp. Cook pieces for 4-5 minutes on medium high heat. Batter Should be golden brown. Repeat until all chicken is cooked. Drain any excess oil on paper towels.	Cook 165° F degrees for chicken
7	In a large skillet or wok, Add 1 Tablespoon oil, and heat over medium high heat.	
8	Stir fry carrots and garlic for 1 minute.	
9	Add sweet peppers and stir fry for 1 to 2 minutes, or till tender crisp	
10	Push from center of pan. Stir in sauce into center of pan or wok. Cook until thick and bubbly	
11	Stir in all pineapple and shrimp. Stir together all ingredients to coat with sauce. Heat through.	Cook until temperature reaches 165°F. Serve.

Time Temperature Sensitive food. *Food safety Standards: hold food for service at an internal temperature above 140° F. Do not mix old product with new. Cool leftover product quickly (within 4 hours) to below 41° F. Follow proper cooling procedures. Store leftovers in a tightly sealed, labeled and dated container. Use leftover within 72 hours if stored in refrigerator or 30 days if stored in the freezer. Reheat leftover product quickly (within 2 hours) to 165 degrees F for 15 seconds. Reheat left over product only once; discard if not used. Cold holding at 41°F or colder or using time alone (less than four hours). Always wash hands and wash and sanitize counter tops utensils and containers between steps when working with raw seafood.*

Copyright 2020 Jacqueline Larson M.S., R.D.N. and Associates.   All Rights Reserved

Texture Modified Diets:

Soft & Bite Size: (aka Bite size) **Food particle size ½ inch (~width of standard fork)** Food must be moist. Cut foods with a knife to a ½" particle size prior to mixing. Moisten with broth as needed. Foods that do not process well should be omitted. Omit: pineapple

Chopped: Food particle size ¼ inch (~ ½ width of standard fork) Food must be moist. Chop foods with a knife to 1/4" particle size prior to mixing. Moisten with broth as needed. Foods that do not process well should be omitted. Omit: pineapple

Minced and Moist: (aka Minced/Mechanical Soft/Ground) **Food particle size 1/8 inch (fits through prongs of standard fork)** Food must be moist. Use a food processor to grind food particles into 1/8 inch prior to mixing. Moisten with broth as needed. Foods that do not process well should be omitted. Omit: pineapple

Pureed: Smooth and cohesive. Use a food processor to puree to a smooth consistency. Foods are processed by grinding and then pureeing them. May add broth or sauce to puree. Do not add to much liquid. Puree should still hold its shape. Must not be firm or sticky. Puree foods while still hot. Appearance should be smooth like pudding. Foods that do not process well should be omitted. Omit: pineapple

Therapeutic Modified Diets:

Lowfat: No changes needed
Diabetic/No added Sugar/No Conc. Sweets/Calorie Controlled: No changes needed
Bland/Anti Reflux: omit pepper and garlic
Liberal House Renal: omit chicken granules and soy sauce
No Added Salt: omit chicken granules and soy sauce
2 Gram Sodium: omit chicken granules and soy sauce
Gluten Free: Use gluten free soy sauce. Use gluten free flour. Omit chicken granules and use gluten free chicken broth in place of water. Prepare foods separately to prevent cross contamination.

Allergy Alerts: When an "X" is present, this indicates the allergen is present.
Always read all food labels to ensure allergens are not present.

Wheat	Milk	Eggs	Fish Shellfish	Soy	Peanuts/Nuts	Other
X		X	X	X		

Key: SF= Salt Free D= Diet or Sugarfree LF = Lowfat FF = Fat Free GF = Gluten Free

Recipe Name: Tuna and Peas Pasta Salad
Recipe Category: Dinner Entrée
Portion Size: 1 cup
Ingredients: **Yields: 8 servings**

Ingredients	Notes:
1 lb. pasta	May use whole grain pasta
4 cups canned tuna	water packed, drained, flaked
1 cup frozen peas, thawed	
1/4 cup olive oil	
2 garlic cloves, minced	Washed, peeled and minced
1/2 cup fresh lemon juice	
1 teaspoon lemon zest	
1/2 teaspoon salt	
1/4 teaspoon pepper	
1/4 cup Parmesan Cheese	

Directions:

Steps:	Directions:	Critical Control Point /Quality Assurance
1	Bring a pot of water to a boil. Cook pasta until al dente, about 9 minutes, or as package directs	Reserve 1 cup of cooking water; drain pasta
2	In a large bowl add garlic and tuna. Flake tuna.	
3	Add lemon juice, lemon zest, salt, olive oil and pepper.	
4	Toss to coat. Add pasta and peas. Gently toss. Chill.	
5	Top with Parmesan cheese just before serving.	
6	Serve chilled	

Time Temperature Sensitive food. *Food safety Standards: hold food for service at an internal temperature above 140° F. Do not mix old product with new. Cool leftover product quickly (within 4 hours) to below 41° F. Follow proper cooling procedures. Store leftovers in a tightly sealed, labeled and dated container. Use leftover within 72 hours if stored in refrigerator or 30 days if stored in the freezer. Cold holding at 41°F or colder or using time alone (less than four hours).*

Texture Modified Diets: TIP: Use pasta with the correct particle size.
Soft & Bite Size: (aka Bite size) **Food particle size ½ inch (~width of standard fork)** Food must be moist. Cut foods with a knife to a ½" particle size prior to mixing. Moisten with broth as needed.
Chopped: Food particle size ¼ inch (~ ½ width of standard fork) Food must be moist. Chop foods with a knife to 1/4" particle size prior to mixing. Moisten with broth as needed.
Minced and Moist: (aka Minced/Mechanical Soft/Ground) **Food particle size 1/8 inch (fits through prongs of standard fork)** Food must be moist. Use a food processor to grind food particles into 1/8 inch prior to mixing. Moisten with broth as needed.
Pureed: Smooth and cohesive. Use a food processor to puree to a smooth consistency. Foods are processed by grinding and then pureeing them. May add broth or sauce to puree. Do not add to much liquid. Puree should still hold its shape. Must not be firm or sticky. Puree foods while still hot. Appearance should be smooth like pudding. Serve ½ cup puree tuna and ½ puree pasta with pea separately.

Therapeutic Modified Diets:
Lowfat: No changes needed
Diabetic/No added Sugar/No Conc. Sweets/Calorie Controlled: No changes needed
Bland/Anti Reflux: omit garlic, lemon juice, lemon zest and pepper
Liberal House Renal: Omit salt, lemon juice, lemon zest and Parmesan cheese
No Added Salt: No changes needed
2 Gram Sodium: omit salt and Parmesan cheese.
Gluten Free: Gluten-free pasta. Prepare foods separately to prevent cross contamination.
Allergy Alerts: When an "X" is present, this indicates the allergen is present.
Always read all food labels to ensure allergens are not present.

Wheat	Milk	Eggs	Fish Shellfish	Soy	Peanuts/Nuts	Other
X	X	X	X			

Key: SF= Salt Free D= Diet or Sugarfree LF = Lowfat FF = Fat Free GF = Gluten Free

Recipe Name: Tuna Baked Spaghetti
Recipe Category: Dinner Entrée
Portion Size: 1 cup
Ingredients: Yields: 8 servings

Ingredients	Notes:
1 lb. spaghetti	May use whole grain noodles or pasta
4 cups canned tuna	Water packed, drained, flaked.
2 tablespoons olive oil	
2 garlic cloves, minced	Wash, peel and mince
6 eggs, beaten	
1 cup nonfat milk	
1 large onion, chopped	Wash, peel and chop
1 cup grated Parmesan Cheese	
1/4 cup bread crumbs	

Directions:

Steps:	Directions:	Critical Control Point /Quality Assurance
1	Preheat oven to 350 degrees.	
2	Cook spaghetti according to the directions on the package. Drain	
3	Heat oil in large skillet over medium heat. Add garlic and onion. Cook until tender.	
4	In a large bowl combine, spaghetti, milk, onion, garlic, tuna, and eggs.	
5	Pour mixture in sprayed baking dish.	
6	Top with cheese and bread crumb.	
7	Top with remaining cheese and bread crumbs Bake in 350 degree oven uncovered for 20-30 minutes until hot.	Cook until internal temperature reaches 165° F for 15 seconds.
8	Place under preheated broil and cook until fully set and starting to brown.	

Time Temperature Sensitive food. *Food safety Standards: hold food for service at an internal temperature above 140° F. Do not mix old product with new. Cool leftover product quickly (within 4 hours) to below 41° F. Follow proper cooling procedures. Store leftovers in a tightly sealed, labeled and dated container. Use leftover within 72 hours if stored in refrigerator or 30 days if stored in the freezer. Reheat leftover product quickly (within 2 hours) to 165 degrees F for 15 seconds. Reheat left over product only once; discard if not used. Cold holding at 41 °F or colder or using time alone (less than four hours). Always wash hands and wash and sanitize counter tops utensils and containers between steps when working with raw seafood.*

Texture Modified Diets: TIP: use pasta with correct particle size.
Soft & Bite Size: (aka Bite size) **Food particle size ½ inch (~width of standard fork)** Food must be moist. Cut foods with a knife to a ½" particle size prior to mixing. Moisten with broth as needed.
Chopped: Food particle size ¼ inch (~ ½ width of standard fork) Food must be moist. Chop foods with a knife to 1/4" particle size prior to mixing. Moisten with broth as needed.
Minced and Moist:(aka Minced/Mechanical Soft/Ground) **Food particle size 1/8 inch (fits through prongs of standard fork)** Food must be moist. Use a food processor to grind food particles into 1/8 inch prior to mixing. Moisten with broth as needed.
Pureed: Smooth and cohesive. Use a food processor to puree to a smooth consistency. Foods are processed by grinding and then pureeing them. May add broth or sauce to puree. Do not add to much liquid. Puree should still hold its shape. Must not be firm or sticky. Puree foods while still hot. Appearance should be smooth like pudding. Tip prepare casserole without tuna to puree separately.

Therapeutic Modified Diets:
Lowfat: No changes needed
Diabetic/No added Sugar/No Conc. Sweets/Calorie Controlled: No changes needed
Bland/Anti Reflux: omit onions and garlic.
Liberal House Renal: Omit bread crumbs, milk and cheese
No Added Salt: No changes needed
2 Gram Sodium: Omit bread crumbs and cheese.
Gluten Free: Gluten-free spaghetti. Use GF bread crumbs. Prepare foods separately to prevent cross contamination.
Allergy Alerts: When an "X" is present, this indicates the allergen is present. Always read all food labels to ensure allergens are not present.

Wheat	Milk	Eggs	Fish Shellfish	Soy	Peanuts/Nuts	Other
X	X	X	X			

Key: SF= Salt Free D= Diet or Sugarfree LF = Lowfat FF = Fat Free GF = Gluten Free

Recipe Name: Tuna Cakes
Recipe Category: Dinner Entrée
Portion Size: 4 oz.
Ingredients: Yields: 8 servings

Ingredients	Notes:
4 cups canned tuna	Drained and flaked.
1 cup bread crumbs	
1/2 cup minced onion	Washed, peeled and minced
3 eggs, beaten	
1 teaspoon salt	
1/4 teaspoon paprika	
2 tablespoons Dijon mustard	
2 tablespoons olive oil	

Directions:

Steps:	Directions:	Critical Control Point /Quality Assurance
1	Combine tuna, bread crumbs, onions, eggs, salt, Dijon mustard and paprika.	
2	Form these ingredients into cakes	
3	Sauté in olive oil until brown	Cook until internal temperature reaches 165° F for 15 seconds.

Time Temperature Sensitive food. Food safety Standards: hold food for service at an internal temperature above 140°F. Do not mix old product with new. Cool leftover product quickly (within 4 hours) to below 41°F. Follow proper cooling procedures. Store leftovers in a tightly sealed, labeled and dated container. Use leftover within 72 hours if stored in refrigerator or 30 days if stored in the freezer. Reheat leftover product quickly (within 2 hours) to 165 degrees F for 15 seconds. Reheat left over product only once; discard if not used. Cold holding at 41 °F or colder or using time alone (less than four hours). Always wash hands and wash and sanitize counter tops utensils and containers between steps when working with raw seafood.

Texture Modified Diets:

Soft & Bite Size: (aka Bite size) **Food particle size ½ inch (~width of standard fork)** Food must be moist. Cut foods with a knife to a ½" particle size after cooking. Moisten with sauce as needed after cutting.
Chopped: Food particle size ¼ inch (~ ½ width of standard fork) Food must be moist. Chop foods with a knife to 1/4" particle size after cooking. Moisten with sauce as needed after chopping.
Minced and Moist: (aka Minced/Mechanical Soft/Ground) **Food particle size 1/8 inch (fits through prongs of standard fork)** Food must be moist. Use a food processor to grind food particles into 1/8 inch after cooking. Moisten with sauce as needed after processing.
Pureed: Smooth and cohesive. Use a food processor to puree to a smooth consistency. Foods are processed by grinding and then pureeing them. May add milk or sauce to puree. Do not add to much liquid. Puree should still hold its shape. Must not be firm or sticky. Puree foods while still hot. Appearance should be smooth like pudding. Serve ½ c. meat serving topped with sauce.

Therapeutic Modified Diets:

Lowfat: No changes needed
Diabetic/No added Sugar/No Conc. Sweets/Calorie Controlled: No changes needed
Bland/Anti Reflux: omit onion, Dijon Mustard and paprika
Liberal House Renal: Omit salt and bread crumbs
No Added Salt: No changes needed
2 Gram Sodium: omit salt and bread crumbs
Gluten Free: Use GF bread crumbs or salt Prepare foods separately to prevent cross contamination.
**Allergy Alerts: When an "X" is present, this indicates the allergen is present.
Always read all food labels to ensure allergens are not present.**

Wheat	Milk	Eggs	Fish Shellfish	Soy	Peanuts/Nuts	Other
X	X	X	X			

Key: SF= Salt Free D= Diet or Sugarfree LF = Lowfat FF = Fat Free GF = Gluten Free

Recipe Name: Tuna Cakes with Creamy Citrus Sauce
Recipe Category: Dinner Entrée
Portion Size: 3 oz. and 2 tablespoons sauce
Ingredients: Yields: 8 servings

Ingredients	Notes:
4 cups, water packed tuna	drained and flaked
1 1/2 cup seasoned bread crumbs	
1/2 cup minced onions	Wash, peel and mince
1/2 cup red bell pepper	Wash, trim and chop finely
3 eggs	
1 cup nonfat milk	
1 teaspoon salt	
1/4 cup oil	
Sauce: 1/2 cup light mayonnaise 1/4 cup light sour cream 2 tablespoons nonfat milk 1 teaspoon lime zest 1/4 cup fresh lime juice 1/4 teaspoon ground cumin	Or use lemon zest and lemon juice Or use orange zest and orange juice

Directions:

Steps:	Directions:	Critical Control Point /Quality Assurance
1	In a large bowl toss together tuna, bread crumbs, onions, eggs, nonfat milk bread crumbs, salt and red pepper. Shape mixture into 8 patties	
2	In a large nonstick skillet heat oil. Sauté patties, a few at a time, until golden brown on both sides, about 3 minutes per side	Cook until internal temperature reaches 165° F for 15 seconds. Keep warm.
3	For each serving, spoon over sauce tuna cakes.	

Time Temperature Sensitive food. *Food safety Standards: hold food for service at an internal temperature above 140° F. Do not mix old product with new. Cool leftover product quickly (within 4 hours) to below 41° F. Follow proper cooling procedures. Store leftovers in a tightly sealed, labeled and dated container. Use leftover within 72 hours if stored in refrigerator or 30 days if stored in the freezer. Reheat leftover product quickly (within 2 hours) to 165 degrees F for 15 seconds. Reheat left over product only once; discard if not used. Cold holding at 41°F or colder or using time alone (less than four hours). Always wash hands and wash and sanitize counter tops utensils and containers between steps when working with raw seafood.*

Texture Modified Diets:

Soft & Bite Size: (aka Bite size) **Food particle size ½ inch (~width of standard fork)** Food must be moist. Cut foods with a knife to a ½" particle size after cooking. Moisten with sauce as needed after cutting.
Chopped: Food particle size ¼ inch (~ ½ width of standard fork) Food must be moist. Chop foods with a knife to 1/4" particle size after cooking. Moisten with sauce as needed after chopping.
Minced and Moist:(aka Minced/Mechanical Soft/Ground) **Food particle size 1/8 inch (fits through prongs of standard fork)** Food must be moist. Use a food processor to grind food particles into 1/8 inch after cooking. Moisten with sauce as needed after processing.
Pureed: Smooth and cohesive. Use a food processor to puree to a smooth consistency. Foods are processed by grinding and then pureeing them. May add milk or sauce to puree. Do not add to much liquid. Puree should still hold its shape. Must not be firm or sticky. Puree foods while still hot. Appearance should be smooth like pudding. Serve ½ c. meat serving topped with sauce.

Therapeutic Modified Diets:

Lowfat: No changes needed
Diabetic/No added Sugar/No Conc. Sweets/Calorie Controlled: No changes needed
Bland/Anti Reflux: omit onion, red pepper, zest, juice and cumin.
Liberal House Renal: Omit salt, bread crumbs and sauce.
No Added Salt: No changes needed
2 Gram Sodium: omit salt, bread crumbs and sauce. May sprinkle with citrus juice
Gluten Free: Use GF bread crumbs, oats or crushed cornflakes. Prepare foods separately to prevent cross contamination.

Allergy Alerts: When an "X" is present, this indicates the allergen is present. Always read all food labels to ensure allergens are not present.

Wheat	Milk	Eggs	Fish Shellfish	Soy	Peanuts/Nuts	Other
X	X	X	X			

Key: SF= Salt Free D= Diet or Sugarfree LF = Lowfat FF = Fat Free GF = Gluten Free

Copyright 2020 Jacqueline Larson M.S., R.D.N. and Associates.   All Rights Reserved

Recipe Name: Tuna Cakes with Lemon Dill Sauce
Recipe Category: Dinner Entrée
Portion Size: 4 oz. plus 1 tablespoon sauce
Ingredients: **Yields: 8 servings**

Ingredients	Notes:
4 cups, water packed tuna, drained and flaked	
1 1/2 cup seasoned bread crumbs	
1/2 cup green onions	Wash, trim and finely chop (including green tops)
1/4 cup Dijon mustard	
2 Eggs	
½ cup nonfat milk	
1 teaspoon grated lemon peel	(optional)
2 tablespoons lemon juice	
2 tablespoons oil	
Lemon slices (optional)	
Sauce: 2 Tablespoons margarine or butt 2 Tablespoons flour 1/2 Cup low sodium chicken broth 2 Tablespoons lemon juice 1/2 Teaspoon dill weed	

Directions:

Steps:	Directions:	Critical Control Point / Quality Assurance
1	In a large bowl toss together tuna, breadcrumbs, onions and Dijon mustard.	
2	In a small bowl beat together egg and milk; stir in lemon peel and lemon juice. Stir into tuna mixture; toss until moistened.	
3	With lightly flour hands, shape mixture into 16 two-inch patties.	
4	In a large nonstick skillet, heat oil to medium high heat.	
5	Sauté patties, a few at a time, until golden brown on both sides, about 3 minutes per side	Cook until internal temperature reaches 165° F for 15 seconds. Keep warm.
6	For sauce, in a small saucepan, melt margarine	
7	Add flour and stir. Add broth, lemon juice, and dill.	
8	Heat to boiling. Reduce heat and simmer until thick	
9	For each serving, spoon over sauce tuna cakes. Top with lemon slices	

Time Temperature Sensitive food. *Food safety Standards: hold food for service at an internal temperature above 140° F. Do not mix old product with new. Cool leftover product quickly (within 4 hours) to below 41° F. Follow proper cooling procedures. Store leftovers in a tightly sealed, labeled and dated container. Use leftover within 72 hours if stored in refrigerator or 30 days if stored in the freezer. Reheat leftover product quickly (within 2 hours) to 165 degrees F for 15 seconds. Reheat left over product only once; discard if not used. Cold holding at 41°F or colder or using time alone (less than four hours). Always wash hands and wash and sanitize counter tops utensils and containers between steps when working with raw seafood.*

<u>**Texture Modified Diets:**</u>

Soft & Bite Size: (aka Bite size) **Food particle size ½ inch (~width of standard fork)** Food must be moist. Cut foods with a knife to a ½" particle size after cooking. Moisten with sauce as needed after cutting.

Chopped: Food particle size ¼ inch (~ ½ width of standard fork) Food must be moist. Chop foods with a knife to 1/4" particle size after cooking. Moisten with sauce as needed after chopping.

Minced and Moist:(aka Minced/Mechanical Soft/Ground) **Food particle size 1/8 inch (fits through prongs of standard fork)** Food must be moist. Use a food processor to grind food particles into 1/8 inch after cooking. Moisten with sauce as needed after processing.

Pureed: Smooth and cohesive. Use a food processor to puree to a smooth consistency. Foods are processed by grinding and then pureeing them. May add milk or sauce to puree. Do not add to much liquid. Puree should still hold its shape. Must not be firm or sticky. Puree foods while still hot. Appearance should be smooth like pudding. Serve ½ c. meat serving topped with sauce.

<u>**Therapeutic Modified Diets:**</u>

Lowfat: No changes needed
Diabetic/No added Sugar/No Conc. Sweets/Calorie Controlled: No changes needed
Bland/Anti Reflux: omit onion, pimento, lemon peel, lemon juice, lemon slices, and dill.
Liberal House Renal: Omit sauce, pimentos and bread crumbs.
No Added Salt: No changes needed
2 Gram Sodium: omit sauce, pimentos and bread crumbs. Drizzle with lemon juice.
Gluten Free: Use gluten-free flour. Use GF bread crumbs, oats or crushed cornflakes. Use GF broth. Prepare foods separately to prevent cross contamination.
Allergy Alerts: When an "X" is present, this indicates the allergen is present.
Always read all food labels to ensure allergens are not present.

Wheat	Milk	Eggs	Fish Shellfish	Soy	Peanuts/Nuts	Other
X	X	X	X	X		

Key: SF= Salt Free D= Diet or Sugarfree LF = Lowfat FF = Fat Free GF = Gluten Free

Recipe Name: Tuna Cakes with Red Pepper Sauce
Recipe Category: Dinner Entrée
Portion Size: 4 oz.
Ingredients: Yields: 8 servings

Ingredients	Notes:
½ cup light mayonnaise	
¼ cup fresh chives	Wash, trim and chop
2 tablespoons fresh parsley	Wash, trim and mince
1 tablespoon lemon juice	
½ teaspoon paprika	
2 ½ cups canned tuna	Drained, and measured
½ cup bread crumbs	
RED PEPPER SAUCE:	
1/2 cup sweet red pepper	Wash, trim and finely chop
1/4 cup green onions	Wash, trim and finely chop (including green tops)
1/4 cup Dijon mustard	
1/4 cup light mayonnaise	
1/4 cup light sour cream	
2 tablespoons red onion	Wash, peeled and minced
2 teaspoons parsley flakes	
1 tablespoon lemon juice	
¼ teaspoon salt	
¼ teaspoon pepper	
3 tablespoons olive oil	
8 Lemon wedges	(optional garnish)

Directions:

Steps:	Directions:	Critical Control Point / Quality Assurance
1	In a large bowl, combine mayonnaise, chives, parsley, lemon juice, paprika, pepper, tuna and bread crumbs; mix well.	
2	Shape 1/4 cup full of tuna mixture into patties.	
3	Meanwhile, for sauce, in a blender of food processor, combine the red pepper, onions, mustard, mayonnaise, sour cream, onion, parsley, honey, lemon juice, salt and pepper; cover and process until finely chopped.	Refrigerate until serving.
4	In a large skillet, heat ½ oil to medium high heat.	
5	Place half of the tuna cakes in skillet.	Cook over medium heat for 5 minutes on each side or until lightly browned (carefully turn the delicate cakes over)
6	Repeat with remaining oil and tuna cakes. Serve with sauce and lemon wedges.	Cook until internal temperature reaches 145° F for 15 seconds.

Time Temperature Sensitive food. Food safety Standards: hold food for service at an internal temperature above 140° F. Do not mix old product with new. Cool leftover product quickly (within 4 hours) to below 41° F. Follow proper cooling procedures. Store leftovers in a tightly sealed, labeled and dated container. Use leftover within 72 hours if stored in refrigerator or 30 days if stored in the freezer. Reheat leftover product quickly (within 2 hours) to 165 degrees F for 15 seconds. Reheat left over product only once; discard if not used. Cold holding at 41°F or colder or using time alone (less than four hours).

Texture Modified Diets:

Soft & Bite Size: (aka Bite size) **Food particle size ½ inch (~width of standard fork)** Food must be moist. Cut foods with a knife to a ½" particle size after cooking. Moisten with sauce as needed after cutting. Omit green onions.
Chopped: Food particle size ¼ inch (~ ½ width of standard fork) Food must be moist. Chop foods with a knife to 1/4" particle size after cooking. Moisten with sauce as needed after chopping. Omit green onions.

Minced and Moist: (aka Minced/Mechanical Soft/Ground) **Food particle size 1/8 inch (fits through prongs of standard fork)** Food must be moist. Use a food processor to grind food particles into 1/8 inch after cooking. Moisten with sauce as needed after processing. Omit green onions.

Pureed: Smooth and cohesive. Use a food processor to puree to a smooth consistency. Foods are processed by grinding and then pureeing them. May add milk or sauce to puree. Do not add to much liquid. Puree should still hold its shape. Must not be firm or sticky. Puree foods while still hot. Appearance should be smooth like pudding. Omit green onions.

Serve ½ c. meat serving topped with sauce.

Therapeutic Modified Diets:

Lowfat: No changes needed

Diabetic/No added Sugar/No Conc. Sweets/Calorie Controlled: No changes needed

Bland/Anti Reflux: omit, parsley, chives, lemon juice, paprika, lemons. For sauce top with mayonnaise and sour cream mixture only.

Liberal House Renal: Omit salt, bread crumbs, mayonnaise and red pepper sauce

No Added Salt: No changes needed

2 Gram Sodium: omit salt, bread crumbs, mayonnaise and red pepper sauce

Gluten Free: Omit bread crumbs and Substitute with GF crushed cornflakes or oatmeal. Prepare foods separately to prevent cross contamination.

Allergy Alerts: When an "X" is present, this indicates the allergen is present.
Always read all food labels to ensure allergens are not present.

Wheat	Milk	Eggs	Fish Shellfish	Soy	Peanuts/Nuts	Other
X	X	X	X			

Key: SF= Salt Free D= Diet or Sugarfree LF = Lowfat FF = Fat Free GF = Gluten Free

Recipe Name: Tuna Leek Casserole
Recipe Category: Dinner Entrée
Portion Size: 1 cup
Ingredients: **Yields: 8 servings**

Ingredients	Notes:
1 lb. Noodles or pasta	May use whole grain noodles or pasta
4 cups canned tuna water packed, drained, flaked	
2 tablespoons olive oil	
2 tablespoons flour	
2 garlic cloves, minced	
4 large leeks	Wash, trim and slice thin
2 cups nonfat milk	
1 8oz. light cream cheese softened	
2 tablespoons Dijon mustard	
1/4 cup fresh lemon juice	
1 teaspoon lemon zest	
1 cup grated low fat shredded Monterey jack cheese	
1/4 cup bread crumbs	

Directions:

Steps:	Directions:	Critical Control Point / Quality Assurance
1	Preheat oven to 350 degrees	
2	Cook noodles according to the directions on the package.	
3	Heat oil in large skillet over medium heat Add leeks. Sprinkle with flour. Gradually stir in milk	Cook until leeks are tender
4	Stir in cream cheese, and mustard.	Cook 5 minutes stirring constantly
5	Remove from heat and stir in noodles, lemon juice, zest, tuna and half of the cheese.	
6	Spray baking dish with nonstick cooking spray.	
7	Add mixture to baking dish.	
8	Top with remaining cheese and bread crumbs.	
9	Bake in 350 degree oven uncovered for 20-30 minutes until hot	Cook until internal temperature reaches 165° F for 15 seconds.

Time Temperature Sensitive food. *Food safety Standards: hold food for service at an internal temperature above 140° F. Do not mix old product with new. Cool leftover product quickly (within 4 hours) to below 41° F. Follow proper cooling procedures. Store leftovers in a tightly sealed, labeled and dated container. Use leftover within 72 hours if stored in refrigerator or 30 days if stored in the freezer. Reheat leftover product quickly (within 2 hours) to 165 degrees F for 15 seconds. Reheat left over product only once; discard if not used. Cold holding at 41°F or colder or using time alone (less than four hours). Always wash hands and wash and sanitize counter tops utensils and containers between steps when working with raw seafood.*

Texture Modified Diets: TIP: Use pasta with the correct particle size.
Soft & Bite Size: (aka Bite size) **Food particle size ½ inch (~width of standard fork)** Food must be moist. Cut foods with a knife to a ½" particle size prior to mixing. Moisten with broth as needed. Omit leeks. Use onions in place of leeks.
Chopped: Food particle size ¼ inch (~ ½ width of standard fork) Food must be moist. Chop foods with a knife to 1/4" particle size prior to mixing. Moisten with broth as needed. Omit leeks. Use onions in place of leeks.
Minced and Moist:(aka Minced/Mechanical Soft/Ground) **Food particle size 1/8 inch (fits through prongs of standard fork)** Food must be moist. Use a food processor to grind food particles into 1/8 inch prior to mixing. Moisten with broth as needed. Omit leeks. Use onions in place of leeks.
Pureed: Smooth and cohesive. Use a food processor to puree to a smooth consistency. Foods are processed by grinding and then pureeing them. May add broth or sauce to puree. Do not add to much liquid. Puree should still hold its shape. Must not be firm or sticky. Puree foods while still hot. Appearance should be smooth like pudding. Omit leeks. Use onions in place of leeks. Serve ½ c. puree tuna (or salmon) and ½ c. pasta mixture separately. Tip: prepare casserole without tuna to puree separately.

Therapeutic Modified Diets:
Lowfat: No changes needed
Diabetic/No added Sugar/No Conc. Sweets/Calorie Controlled: No changes needed
Bland/Anti Reflux: omit garlic, leeks, Dijon mustard, lemon zest and lemon juice.
Liberal House Renal: Omit cream cheese, bread crumbs and cheese. Omit lemon juice and lemon zest.
No Added Salt: No changes needed
2 Gram Sodium: omit cream cheese, bread crumbs, and cheese
Gluten Free: Gluten-free flour. Use gluten free pasta. Use GF bread crumbs or sub. With GF cornflakes. Prepare foods separately to prevent cross contamination.
Allergy Alerts: When an "X" is present, this indicates the allergen is present.
Always read all food labels to ensure allergens are not present.

Wheat	Milk	Eggs	Fish Shellfish	Soy	Peanuts/Nuts	Other
X	X	X	X			

Key: SF= Salt Free D= Diet or Sugarfree LF = Lowfat FF = Fat Free GF = Gluten Free

Recipe Name: Tuna Loaf
Recipe Category: Dinner Entrée
Portion Size: 4 oz.
Ingredients: Yields: 8 servings

Ingredients	Notes:
1/2 cup finely chopped onion	Wash, peel and chop
2 teaspoons dried dill weed	
1/4 teaspoon pepper	
2 tablespoons Dijon mustard	
2 tablespoons olive oil	
3 eggs, beaten	
1 cup bread crumbs	
1/2 cup milk	
4 cups tuna, drained and broken into chunks (water packed)	
8 oz. low fat cheddar cheese	

Directions:

Steps:	Directions:	Critical Control Point / Quality Assurance
1	In a saucepan cook onion, dill weed, and pepper in olive oil till onion is tender.	
2	Combine egg, bread crumbs, Dijon Mustard. milk, and onion mixture. Add tuna; mix well	
3	Shape into a loaf in a greased shallow baking pan.	
4	Bake in a 350 degree oven for 30 to 35 minutes.	Cook until internal temperature reaches 165° F for 15 seconds.
5	Top with cheese .	

Time Temperature Sensitive food. *Food safety Standards: hold food for service at an internal temperature above 140° F. Do not mix old product with new. Cool leftover product quickly (within 4 hours) to below 41° F. Follow proper cooling procedures. Store leftovers in a tightly sealed, labeled and dated container. Use leftover within 72 hours if stored in refrigerator or 30 days if stored in the freezer. Reheat leftover product quickly (within 2 hours) to 165 degrees F for 15 seconds. Reheat left over product only once; discard if not used. Cold holding at 41°F or colder or using time alone (less than four hours). Always wash hands and wash and sanitize counter tops utensils and containers between steps when working with raw seafood.*

Texture Modified Diets:

Soft & Bite Size: (aka Bite size) **Food particle size ½ inch (~width of standard fork)** Food must be moist. Cut foods with a knife to a ½" particle size after cooking. Moisten with sauce as needed after cutting.
Chopped: Food particle size ¼ inch (~ ½ width of standard fork) Food must be moist. Chop foods with a knife to 1/4" particle size after cooking. Moisten with sauce as needed after chopping.
Minced and Moist:(aka Minced/Mechanical Soft/Ground) **Food particle size 1/8 inch (fits through prongs of standard fork)** Food must be moist. Use a food processor to grind food particles into 1/8 inch after cooking. Moisten with sauce as needed after processing.
Pureed: Smooth and cohesive. Use a food processor to puree to a smooth consistency. Foods are processed by grinding and then pureeing them. May add milk or sauce to puree. Do not add to much liquid. Puree should still hold its shape. Must not be firm or sticky. Puree foods while still hot. Appearance should be smooth like pudding.
Serve ½ c. meat serving topped with sauce.

Therapeutic Modified Diets:

Lowfat: No changes needed
Diabetic/No added Sugar/No Conc. Sweets/Calorie Controlled: No changes needed
Bland/Anti Reflux: omit onion, dill, Dijon mustard, and pepper
Liberal House Renal: Omit cheese and bread crumbs
No Added Salt: No changes needed
2 Gram Sodium: omit cheese and bread crumbs
Gluten Free: Use gluten free bread crumbs or oats. Prepare foods separately to prevent cross contamination.

Allergy Alerts: When an "X" is present, this indicates the allergen is present. Always read all food labels to ensure allergens are not present.

Wheat	Milk	Eggs	Fish Shellfish	Soy	Peanuts/Nuts	Other
X	X	X	X			

Key: SF= Salt Free D= Diet or Sugarfree LF = Lowfat FF = Fat Free GF = Gluten Free

Copyright 2020 Jacqueline Larson M.S., R.D.N. and Associates.   All Rights Reserved

Recipe Name: Tuna Muffin Melt
Recipe Category: Dinner Entrée
Portion Size: 3 oz.
Ingredients: Yields: 8 servings

Ingredients	Notes:
4 cups tuna	(drained water packed)
1/2 cup light mayonnaise	
2 tablespoons Dijon mustard	
1 8 oz. light cream cheese	softened
1/2 cup celery, diced	Wash, trim and dice
8 green onions	Wash, trim and slice with green tops
8 oz. low fat shredded cheddar cheese	
8 English Muffins	

Directions:

Steps:	Directions:	Critical Control Point / Quality Assurance
1	In a medium sized bowl, combine tuna mayonnaise, cream cheese, Dijon mustard, and celery	
2	Spilt muffins in half. Top with tuna salad. Spread and flatten.	
3	Top with cheddar cheese and green onions Bake in a 400 degree oven 10 to 12 minutes	Cook until internal temperature reaches 165° F for 15 seconds.

Time Temperature Sensitive food. Food safety Standards: hold food for service at an internal temperature above 140° F. Do not mix old product with new. Cool leftover product quickly (within 4 hours) to below 41° F. Follow proper cooling procedures. Store leftovers in a tightly sealed, labeled and dated container. Use leftover within 72 hours if stored in refrigerator or 30 days if stored in the freezer. Reheat leftover product quickly (within 2 hours) to 165 degrees F for 15 seconds. Reheat left over product only once; discard if not used. Cold holding at 41°F or colder or using time alone (less than four hours).

<u>Texture Modified Diets:</u>

Soft & Bite Size: (aka Bite size) **Food particle size ½ inch (~width of standard fork)** Food must be moist. Cut foods with a knife to a ½" particle size after cooking. Moisten with sauce or milk as needed after cutting. Use soft moist bread. Omit green onions.

Chopped: Food particle size ¼ inch (~ ½ width of standard fork) Food must be moist. Chop foods with a knife to 1/4" particle size after cooking. Moisten with sauce or milk as needed after chopping. Use soft moist bread. Omit green onions.

Minced and Moist: (aka Minced/Mechanical Soft/Ground) **Food particle size 1/8 inch (fits through prongs of standard fork)** Food must be moist. Use a food processor to grind food particles into 1/8 inch after cooking. Moisten with sauce or milk as needed after processing. Use soft moist bread. Omit green onions.

Pureed: Smooth and cohesive. Use a food processor to puree to a smooth consistency. Foods are processed by grinding and then pureeing them. May add milk or sauce to puree. Do not add to much liquid. Puree should still hold its shape. Must not be firm or sticky. Puree foods while still hot. Appearance should be smooth like pudding. Serve ½ c. puree tuna mixture and ½ c. puree muffin separately. Omit green onions.

<u>Therapeutic Modified Diets:</u>

Lowfat: No changes needed
Diabetic/No added Sugar/No Conc. Sweets/Calorie Controlled: No changes needed
Bland/Anti Reflux: omit celery and green onions
Liberal House Renal: Omit mayonnaise, cream cheese, and cheese. Omit English muffins use low sodium toast.
No Added Salt: No changes needed
2 Gram Sodium: omit mayonnaise, cream cheese and cheese. Omit English muffins use low sodium toast
Gluten Free: Gluten-free muffins. Prepare foods separately to prevent cross contamination.

Allergy Alerts: When an "X" is present, this indicates the allergen is present. Always read all food labels to ensure allergens are not present.

Wheat	Milk	Eggs	Fish Shellfish	Soy	Peanuts/Nuts	Other
X	X	X	X			

Key: SF= Salt Free D= Diet or Sugarfree LF = Lowfat FF = Fat Free GF = Gluten Free

Recipe Name: Tuna Noodle Casserole
Recipe Category: Dinner Entrée
Portion Size: 1 cup
Ingredients: **Yields:** 8 servings

Ingredients	Notes:
1 lb. noodles	May use whole grain noodles or pasta
4 cups canned tuna	Water packed, drained, flaked.
2 tablespoons olive oil	
2 tablespoons flour	
2 garlic cloves, minced	Wash, peel and mince
1 large onion, chopped	Wash, peel and chop
1 cup carrots	Wash, peel, trim and dice.
1 cup celery, diced	Wash, trim and dice
3 cups nonfat milk	
1 (8oz.) light cream cheese	softened
2 tablespoons Dijon mustard	
1 cup frozen peas	
1 cup grated Parmesan Cheese	
1/4 cup bread crumbs	

Directions:

Steps:	Directions:	Critical Control Point /Quality Assurance
1	Preheat oven to 350 degrees.	
2	Cook noodles according to the directions on the package.	
3	Heat oil in large skillet over medium heat. Add garlic, onion, carrots and celery. Cook until carrot is tender. Sprinkle with flour	
4	Gradually stir in milk; Cook 5 minutes stirring constantly.	
5	Stir in cream cheese, and mustard	
6	Remove from heat and stir in noodles, peas and half of the parmesan. Stir in tuna.	
7	Spray baking dish with nonstick cooking spray. Add mixture to baking dish	
8	Top with remaining cheese and bread crumbs Bake in 350 degree oven uncovered for 20-30 minutes until hot	Cook until internal temperature reaches 165° F for 15 seconds.

Time Temperature Sensitive food. *Food safety Standards: hold food for service at an internal temperature above 140° F. Do not mix old product with new. Cool leftover product quickly (within 4 hours) to below 41° F. Follow proper cooling procedures. Store leftovers in a tightly sealed, labeled and dated container. Use leftover within 72 hours if stored in refrigerator or 30 days if stored in the freezer. Reheat leftover product quickly (within 2 hours) to 165 degrees F for 15 seconds. Reheat left over product only once; discard if not used. Cold holding at 41°F or colder or using time alone (less than four hours). Always wash hands and wash and sanitize counter tops utensils and containers between steps when working with raw seafood.*

Texture Modified Diets: TIP: use pasta that is the correct particle size.

Soft & Bite Size: (aka Bite size) **Food particle size ½ inch (~width of standard fork)** Food must be moist. Cut foods with a knife to a ½" particle size prior to mixing. Moisten with broth as needed.

Chopped: Food particle size ¼ inch (~ ½ width of standard fork) Food must be moist. Chop foods with a knife to 1/4" particle size prior to mixing. Moisten with broth as needed.

Minced and Moist:(aka Minced/Mechanical Soft/Ground) **Food particle size 1/8 inch (fits through prongs of standard fork)** Food must be moist. Use a food processor to grind food particles into 1/8 inch prior to mixing. Moisten with broth as needed.

Pureed: Smooth and cohesive. Use a food processor to puree to a smooth consistency. Foods are processed by grinding and then pureeing them. May add broth or sauce to puree. Do not add to much liquid. Puree should still hold its shape. Must not be firm or sticky. Puree foods while still hot. Appearance should be smooth like pudding. Serve ½ c. puree tuna or salmon and ½ c. puree pasta mixture separately. Tip prepare casserole without tuna to puree separately.

Therapeutic Modified Diets:

Lowfat: No changes needed
Diabetic/No added Sugar/No Conc. Sweets/Calorie Controlled: No changes needed
Bland/Anti Reflux: omit onions, celery, and Dijon mustard
Liberal House Renal: Omit cream cheese, bread crumbs and Parmesan cheese
No Added Salt: No changes needed
2 Gram Sodium: Omit cream cheese, bread crumbs and Parmesan cheese.
Gluten Free: Gluten-free flour and noodles. Use GF bread crumbs or GF crushed cornflakes. Prepare foods separately to prevent cross contamination.
Allergy Alerts: When an "X" is present, this indicates the allergen is present.
Always read all food labels to ensure allergens are not present.

Wheat	Milk	Eggs	Fish Shellfish	Soy	Peanuts/Nuts	Other
X	X	X	X			

Key: SF= Salt Free D= Diet or Sugarfree LF = Lowfat FF = Fat Free GF = Gluten Free

Recipe Name: Tuna (or Salmon) Pasta with Lemon Garlic Sauce
Recipe Category: Dinner Entrée
Portion Size: 1 cup
Ingredients: Yields: 8 servings

Ingredients	Notes:
1 lb. pasta	May use whole grain pasta
4 cups canned tuna (or salmon)	Water packed, drained, flaked
1/4 cup olive oil	
6 garlic cloves, minced	Washed, peeled and minced
1/2 cup fresh lemon juice	
1 teaspoon lemon zest	
1/2 teaspoon salt	
1/4 teaspoon pepper	
2 tablespoons parsley flakes	

Directions:

Steps:	Directions:	Critical Control Point /Quality Assurance
1	Bring a pot of water to a boil.	
2	Cook pasta until al dente, about 9 minutes, or as package directs.	
3	Reserve 1 cup of cooking water; drain pasta.	
4	Heat in a large pan over medium-low heat.	
5	Add garlic and sauté 1 minute; Stir in flaked tuna.	
6	Add lemon juice, lemon zest, salt and pepper.	
7	Add pasta and remaining water; toss pasta with sauce, sprinkle with parsley . Serve hot	

Time Temperature Sensitive food. *Food safety Standards: hold food for service at an internal temperature above 140° F. Do not mix old product with new. Cool leftover product quickly (within 4 hours) to below 41° F. Follow proper cooling procedures. Store leftovers in a tightly sealed, labeled and dated container. Use leftover within 72 hours if stored in refrigerator or 30 days if stored in the freezer. Reheat leftover product quickly (within 2 hours) to 165 degrees F for 15 seconds. Reheat left over product only once; discard if not used. Cold holding at 41°F or colder or using time alone (less than four hours).*

<u>**Texture Modified Diets: Tip: Use pasta that is the correct particle size.**</u>
Soft & Bite Size: (aka Bite size) **Food particle size ½ inch (~width of standard fork)** Food must be moist. Cut foods with a knife to a ½" particle size after cooking. Moisten with sauce as needed after cutting.
Chopped: Food particle size ¼ inch (~ ½ width of standard fork) Food must be moist. Chop foods with a knife to 1/4" particle size after cooking. Moisten with sauce as needed after chopping.
Minced and Moist:(aka Minced/Mechanical Soft/Ground) **Food particle size 1/8 inch (fits through prongs of standard fork)** Food must be moist. Use a food processor to grind food particles into 1/8 inch after cooking. Moisten with sauce as needed after processing.
Pureed: Smooth and cohesive. Use a food processor to puree to a smooth consistency. Foods are processed by grinding and then pureeing them. May add milk or sauce to puree. Do not add to much liquid. Puree should still hold its shape. Must not be firm or sticky. Puree foods while still hot. Appearance should be smooth like pudding. Serve ½ c. puree tuna or salmon and ½ c. puree pasta separately. Tip: puree tuna or salmon mixture separate before add to pasta in step 7.
<u>**Therapeutic Modified Diets:**</u>
Lowfat: No changes needed
Diabetic/No added Sugar/No Conc. Sweets/Calorie Controlled: No changes needed
Bland/Anti Reflux: omit garlic, lemon zest, parsley flakes and pepper.
Liberal House Renal: Omit salt
No Added Salt: No changes needed
2 Gram Sodium: omit salt
Gluten Free: Use gluten free pasta . Prepare foods separately to prevent cross contamination.
Allergy Alerts: When an "X" is present, this indicates the allergen is present. Always read all food labels to ensure allergens are not present.

Wheat	Milk	Eggs	Fish Shellfish	Soy	Peanuts/Nuts	Other
X		X	X			

Key: SF= Salt Free D= Diet or Sugarfree LF = Lowfat FF = Fat Free GF = Gluten Free

Recipe Name: Tuna and Pasta Salad with Lemon
Recipe Category: Dinner Entrée
Portion Size: 1 cup
Ingredients: Yields: 8 servings

Ingredients	Notes:
1 lb. pasta	May use whole grain pasta
4 cups canned tuna	water packed, drained, flaked
1 cup frozen peas, thawed	
1/4 cup olive oil	
2 garlic cloves, minced	Washed, peeled and minced
1/2 cup fresh lemon juice	
1 teaspoon lemon zest	
1/2 teaspoon salt	
1/4 teaspoon pepper	
1/4 cup Parmesan Cheese	

Directions:

Steps:	Directions:	Critical Control Point /Quality Assurance
1	Bring a pot of water to a boil. Cook pasta until al dente, about 9 minutes, or as package directs	Reserve 1 cup of cooking water; drain pasta
2	In a large bowl add garlic and tuna. Flake tuna.	
3	Add lemon juice, lemon zest, salt, olive oil and pepper.	
4	Toss to coat. Add pasta and peas. Gently toss. Chill.	
5	Top with Parmesan cheese just before serving.	
6	Serve chilled	

Time Temperature Sensitive food. *Food safety Standards: hold food for service at an internal temperature above 140° F. Do not mix old product with new. Cool leftover product quickly (within 4 hours) to below 41° F. Follow proper cooling procedures. Store leftovers in a tightly sealed, labeled and dated container. Use leftover within 72 hours if stored in refrigerator or 30 days if stored in the freezer. Cold holding at 41°F or colder or using time alone (less than four hours).*

<u>*Texture Modified Diets: Tip: Use pasta that is the correct particle size.*</u>
Soft & Bite Size: (aka Bite size) **Food particle size ½ inch (~width of standard fork)** Food must be moist. Cut foods with a knife to a ½" particle size after cooking. Moisten with sauce as needed after cutting.
Chopped: Food particle size ¼ inch (~ ½ width of standard fork) Food must be moist. Chop foods with a knife to 1/4" particle size after cooking. Moisten with sauce as needed after chopping.
Minced and Moist: (aka Minced/Mechanical Soft/Ground) **Food particle size 1/8 inch (fits through prongs of standard fork)** Food must be moist. Use a food processor to grind food particles into 1/8 inch after cooking. Moisten with sauce as needed after processing.
Pureed: Smooth and cohesive. Use a food processor to puree to a smooth consistency. Foods are processed by grinding and then pureeing them. May add milk or sauce to puree. Do not add to much liquid. Puree should still hold its shape. Must not be firm or sticky. Puree foods while still hot. Appearance should be smooth like pudding.
Serve ½ c. puree tuna or salmon and ½ c. puree pasta separately. Tip: combine all ingredients except tuna Puree pasta mixture and tuna s separately.
<u>*Therapeutic Modified Diets:*</u>
Lowfat: No changes needed
Diabetic/No added Sugar/No Conc. Sweets/Calorie Controlled: No changes needed
Bland/Anti Reflux: omit garlic, lemon juice, lemon zest and pepper
Liberal House Renal: Omit salt, lemon juice, lemon zest and Parmesan cheese
No Added Salt: No changes needed
2 Gram Sodium: omit salt and Parmesan cheese.
Gluten Free: Gluten-free pasta. Prepare foods separately to prevent cross contamination.
Allergy Alerts: When an "X" is present, this indicates the allergen is present. Always read all food labels to ensure allergens are not present.

Wheat	Milk	Eggs	Fish Shellfish	Soy	Peanuts/Nuts	Other
X	X	X	X			

Key: SF= Salt Free D= Diet or Sugarfree LF = Lowfat FF = Fat Free GF = Gluten Free

Recipe Name: Tuna Patties with Cheese Sauce
Recipe Category: Dinner Entrée
Portion Size: 4 oz. patty with 2 tablespoons sauce
Ingredients: **Yields: 8 servings**

Ingredients	Notes:
4 cups canned tuna, drained and flaked	
1 cup bread crumbs	May use whole grain bread crumbs
1/2 cup minced onion	Wash, peel and dice
3 Eggs, beaten	
2 tablespoons lemon juice	
3/4 teaspoon salt	
1/4 teaspoon pepper	
1/2 cup nonfat milk	
2 tablespoons Dijon mustard	
¼ cup green onions with tops.	Wash, trim and slice thin.
Sauce: ¼ c. margarine ¼ c. flour ¼ teaspoon paprika ½ teaspoon dry mustard 2 cups nonfat milk 1 cup shredded low fat Swiss Cheese ½ cup shredded low fat Cheddar Cheese Salt and Pepper to taste	

Directions:

Steps:	Directions:	Critical Control Point / Quality Assurance
1	Preheat oven to 350 degrees	
2	Combine tuna, bread crumbs, onions, eggs, salt, lemon juice, milk, mustard and pepper.	
3	Form these ingredients into patties	
4	Place into baking dish sprayed with nonstick vegetable dish. Bake for about 45 minutes.	Cook until internal temperature reaches 165° F for 15 seconds.
5	For sauce: melt margarine in medium saucepan over low heat	
6	Stir in flour. Pour in milk. Add paprika, and mustard	
7	Cook stirring constantly until thickened. Stir in cheeses.	
8	Heat until melted and well blended. To serve top patty topped with cheese sauce and garnished with green onions.	

Time Temperature Sensitive food. *Food safety Standards: hold food for service at an internal temperature above 140°F. Do not mix old product with new. Cool leftover product quickly (within 4 hours) to below 41°F. Follow proper cooling procedures. Store leftovers in a tightly sealed, labeled and dated container. Use leftover within 72 hours if stored in refrigerator or 30 days if stored in the freezer. Reheat leftover product quickly (within 2 hours) to 165 degrees F for 15 seconds. Reheat left over product only once; discard if not used. Cold holding at 41°F or colder or using time alone (less than four hours). Always wash hands and wash and sanitize counter tops utensils and containers between steps when working with raw seafood.*

<u>**Texture Modified Diets:**</u>

Soft & Bite Size: (aka Bite size) **Food particle size ½ inch (~width of standard fork)** Food must be moist. Cut foods with a knife to a ½" particle size after cooking. Moisten with sauce as needed after cutting. Omit green onions.
Chopped: Food particle size ¼ inch (~ ½ width of standard fork) Food must be moist. Chop foods with a knife to 1/4" particle size after cooking. Moisten with sauce as needed after chopping. Omit green onions.
Minced and Moist:(aka Minced/Mechanical Soft/Ground) **Food particle size 1/8 inch (fits through prongs of standard fork)** Food must be moist. Use a food processor to grind food particles into 1/8 inch after cooking. Moisten with sauce as needed after processing. Omit green onions.
Pureed: Smooth and cohesive. Use a food processor to puree to a smooth consistency. Foods are processed by grinding and then pureeing them. May add milk or sauce to puree. Do not add to much liquid. Puree should still hold

its shape. Must not be firm or sticky. Puree foods while still hot. Appearance should be smooth like pudding. Omit green onions.

Serve ½ c. meat serving topped with sauce.

Therapeutic Modified Diets:

Lowfat: No changes needed

Diabetic/No added Sugar/No Conc. Sweets/Calorie Controlled: No changes needed

Bland/Anti Reflux: omit onion, lemon juice, pepper, paprika, dry mustard, green onions, and Dijon mustard.

Liberal House Renal: Omit salt, bread crumbs and cheese sauce.

No Added Salt: No changes needed

2 Gram Sodium: omit salt, bread crumbs and cheese sauce.

Gluten Free: Use gluten-free flour and GF bread crumbs or oats. Prepare foods separately to prevent cross contamination.

Allergy Alerts: When an "X" is present, this indicates the allergen is present.

Always read all food labels to ensure allergens are not present.

Wheat	Milk	Eggs	Fish Shellfish	Soy	Peanuts/Nuts	Other
X	X	X	X	X		

Key: SF= Salt Free D= Diet or Sugarfree LF = Lowfat FF = Fat Free GF = Gluten Free

Recipe Name: Tuna Pea Pasta Salad
Recipe Category: Dinner Entrée
Portion Size: 1 cup
Ingredients: Yields: 8 servings

Ingredients	Notes:
1 (16 ounce) package pasta	
4 cups peas, frozen	Thaw
3 cups canned tuna	
¼ cup olive oil	
1/4 cup sliced unsalted almonds	Toasted
2 teaspoons parsley flakes	
2/3 cup lemon juice	
1/2 teaspoon grated lemon zest	(optional)
1 clove garlic	Washed, peeled and minced
1/4 cup red onion	Washed, peeled and finely chopped
1 teaspoon salt	
1 pinch ground black pepper	
2 Tablespoons capers	(optional)

Directions:

Steps:	Directions:	Critical Control Point /Quality Assurance
1	In a large pot of salted boiling water, cook pasta until al dente, rinse under cold water and drain.	
2	In a large bowl, combine the olive oil, parsley flakes, lemon juice, lemon zest, garlic salt and peppers. Whisk to combine.	
3	Add pasta, tuna, red onion and peas. Toss to coat. Refrigerate for 1 hour. Top with almonds just before serving.	

Time Temperature Sensitive food. *Food safety Standards: Do not mix old product with new. Cool leftover product quickly (within 4 hours) to below 41°F. Follow proper cooling procedures. Store leftovers in a tightly sealed, labeled and dated container. Use leftover within 72 hours if stored in refrigerator or 30 days if stored in the freezer. Cold holding at 41°F or colder or using time alone (less than four hours).*

Texture Modified Diets: TiP: Use pasta that is the correct particle size.

Soft & Bite Size: (aka Bite size) **Food particle size ½ inch (~width of standard fork)** Food must be moist. Cut foods with a knife to a ½" particle size prior to mixing. Moisten with broth as needed. Foods that do not process well should be omitted. Omit: capers and almonds.

Chopped: Food particle size ¼ inch (~ ½ width of standard fork) Food must be moist. Chop foods with a knife to 1/4" particle size prior to mixing. Moisten with broth as needed. Foods that do not process well should be omitted. Omit: capers and almonds.

Minced and Moist: (aka Minced/Mechanical Soft/Ground) **Food particle size 1/8 inch (fits through prongs of standard fork)** Food must be moist. Use a food processor to grind food particles into 1/8 inch prior to mixing. Moisten with broth as needed. Foods that do not process well should be omitted. Omit: capers and almonds.

Pureed: Smooth and cohesive. Use a food processor to puree to a smooth consistency. Foods are processed by grinding and then pureeing them. May add broth or sauce to puree. Do not add to much liquid. Puree should still hold its shape. Must not be firm or sticky. Puree foods while still hot. Appearance should be smooth like pudding. Foods that do not process well should be omitted. Omit: capers and almonds. Serve ½ cup puree pasta, ½ cup puree green beans and 1/3 cup tuna mixture separately.

Therapeutic Modified Diets:

Lowfat: Omit almonds
Diabetic/No added Sugar/No Conc. Sweets/Calorie Controlled: No changes needed
Bland/Anti Reflux: Omit red onion, almonds, black pepper and garlic
Liberal House Renal: Omit almonds, salt and capers
No Added Salt: Omit capers
2 Gram Sodium: Omit salt and capers
Gluten Free: Use gluten free pasta. Prepare foods separately to prevent cross contamination.

Allergy Alerts: When an "X" is present, this indicates the allergen is present. Always read all food labels to ensure allergens are not present.

Wheat	Milk	Eggs	Fish Shellfish	Soy	Peanuts/Nuts	Other
X		X	x		x	

Key: SF= Salt Free D= Diet or Sugarfree LF = Lowfat FF = Fat Free GF = Gluten Free

Recipe Name: Tuna Salad with Creamy Tarragon Dressing
Recipe Category: Dinner Entrée
Portion Size: ½ c. tuna salad on ½ c. watercress leaves
Ingredients: Yields: 8 servings

Ingredients	Notes:
4 cups canned water packed tuna, drained	
1/2 cup light mayonnaise	
1 teaspoon fresh lemon zest	
1/2 cup fresh lemon juice	
1/4 cup fresh Tarragon	
1 teaspoon Dijon mustard	
1/4 teaspoon salt	
1/4 teaspoon pepper	
4 cups chopped watercress leaves	Or other green leafy vegetable.
2 tablespoons drained capers	
1 large avocado	Wash, peel, seed and dice. (optional)

Directions:

Steps:	Directions:	Critical Control Point / Quality Assurance
1	In a small bowl, combine mayonnaise, lemon zest, lemon juice, tarragon, mustard, salt, tuna, cappers and pepper.	
2	On individual serving plates. Place ½ cup watercress leaves. Top with ½ cup tuna.	
3	Just before serving top with avocado. serve chilled.	

Time Temperature Sensitive food. *Food safety Standards: hold food for service at an internal temperature above 140° F. Do not mix old product with new. Cool leftover product quickly (within 4 hours) to below 41° F. Follow proper cooling procedures. Store leftovers in a tightly sealed, labeled and dated container. Use leftover within 72 hours if stored in refrigerator or 30 days if stored in the freezer. Cold holding at 41°F or colder or using time alone (less than four hours).*

Texture Modified Diets:

Soft & Bite Size: (aka Bite size) **Food particle size ½ inch (~width of standard fork)** Food must be moist. Cut foods with a knife to a ½" particle size prior to mixing. Moisten with broth as needed. Foods that do not process well should be omitted. Omit:capers

Chopped: Food particle size ¼ inch (~ ½ width of standard fork) Food must be moist. Chop foods with a knife to 1/4" particle size prior to mixing. Moisten with broth as needed. Foods that do not process well should be omitted. Omit:capers

Minced and Moist: (aka Minced/Mechanical Soft/Ground) **Food particle size 1/8 inch (fits through prongs of standard fork)** Food must be moist. Use a food processor to grind food particles into 1/8 inch prior to mixing. Moisten with broth as needed. Foods that do not process well should be omitted. Omit: capers

Pureed: Smooth and cohesive. Use a food processor to puree to a smooth consistency. Foods are processed by grinding and then pureeing them. May add broth or sauce to puree. Do not add to much liquid. Puree should still hold its shape. Must not be firm or sticky. Puree foods while still hot. Appearance should be smooth like pudding. Foods that do not process well should be omitted. Omit: capers
Serve ½ c. puree tuna salad and ½. Puree greens separately. May process greens with bread to thicken.

Therapeutic Modified Diets:

Lowfat: No changes needed
Diabetic/No added Sugar/No Conc. Sweets/Calorie Controlled: No changes needed
Bland/Anti Reflux: omit lemon zest, lemon juice, Dijon mustard, capers and Tarragon. Finely shred greens
Liberal House Renal: Omit salt, capers and substitute olive oil for mayonnaise
No Added Salt: No changes needed
2 Gram Sodium: omit salt, capers and substitute olive oil for mayonnaise
Gluten Free: No changes needed. Prepare foods separately to prevent cross contamination.

Allergy Alerts: When an "X" is present, this indicates the allergen is present. Always read all food labels to ensure allergens are not present.

Wheat	Milk	Eggs	Fish Shellfish	Soy	Peanuts/Nuts	Other
		X	X			

Key: SF= Salt Free D= Diet or Sugarfree LF = Lowfat FF = Fat Free GF = Gluten Free

Recipe Name: Tuna Tortilla Roll Ups
Recipe Category: Dinner Entrée
Portion Size: ½ cup tuna mixture on 1 tortilla
Ingredients: Yields: 8 servings

Ingredients	Notes:
4 cups water packed tuna, drained and flaked	
8 lettuce leaves	Wash and trim
1/2 cup celery, finely chopped	Wash, trim and finely chop
1 cup, diced green apple	Wash, core and dice.
1/2 cup light mayonnaise	
8 (8-inch) whole grain flour or corn tortillas	

Directions:

Steps:	Directions:	Critical Control Point / Quality Assurance
1	In a medium bowl, combine tuna, celery, apple and mayonnaise.	
2	Top tortilla with lettuce leaf and tuna salad.	
3	Roll up tightly. Serve cold.	

Time Temperature Sensitive food. *Food safety Standards: hold food for service at an internal temperature above 140° F. Do not mix old product with new. Cool leftover product quickly (within 4 hours) to below 41° F. Follow proper cooling procedures. Store leftovers in a tightly sealed, labeled and dated container. Use leftover within 72 hours and store in refrigerator. Cold holding at 41°F or colder or using time alone (less than four hours*

Texture Modified Diets:

Soft & Bite Size: (aka Bite size) **Food particle size ½ inch (~width of standard fork)** Food must be moist. Cut foods with a knife to a ½" particle size prior to layering. Moisten with broth as needed. Peel apple

Chopped: Food particle size ¼ inch (~ ½ width of standard fork) Food must be moist. Chop foods with a knife to 1/4" particle size prior to layering. Moisten with broth as needed. Peel apple

Minced and Moist: (aka Minced/Mechanical Soft/Ground) **Food particle size 1/8 inch (fits through prongs of standard fork)** Food must be moist. Use a food processor to grind food particles into 1/8 inch prior to layering. Moisten with broth as needed. Peel apple

Pureed: Smooth and cohesive. Use a food processor to puree to a smooth consistency. Foods are processed by grinding and then pureeing them. May add broth or sauce to puree. Do not add to much liquid. Puree should still hold its shape. Must not be firm or sticky. Puree foods while still hot. Appearance should be smooth like pudding. Peel apple. Serve ½ c. puree tuna salad and ½ c puree tortilla separately.

Therapeutic Modified Diets:

Lowfat: No changes needed
Diabetic/No added Sugar/No Conc. Sweets/Calorie Controlled: No changes needed
Bland/Anti Reflux: omit celery and finely chop lettuce. Peel apple
Liberal House Renal: Omit mayonnaise. Use low sodium tortillas. (see recipe in cookbook)
No Added Salt: No changes needed
2 Gram Sodium: omit mayonnaise. Use low sodium tortillas. (see recipe in cookbook)
Gluten Free: Use corn tortillas. Prepare foods separately to prevent cross contamination.
Allergy Alerts: When an "X" is present, this indicates the allergen is present.
Always read all food labels to ensure allergens are not present.

Wheat	Milk	Eggs	Fish Shellfish	Soy	Peanuts/Nuts	Other
X		X	X			

Key: SF= Salt Free D= Diet or Sugarfree LF = Lowfat FF = Fat Free GF = Gluten Free

Recipe Name: Tuna Pasta with Creamy Linguine
Recipe Category: Dinner Entrée
Portion Size: 1 cup
Ingredients: Yields: 8 servings

Ingredients	Notes:
1 lb. linguine	May use whole grain linguine
4 cups canned tuna	water packed, drained, flaked. May use fresh tuna
1/4 cup unsalted butter	
1/4 cup all-purpose flour	
1 tablespoon olive oil	
6 garlic cloves, minced	Wash, peeled and minced
1 1/2 cup fresh sliced mushrooms	Wash, trim and slice
1 cup celery, diced	Wash, trim and dice
1/2 teaspoon salt	
1/4 teaspoon pepper	
2 tablespoons parsley flakes	
1 cup Parmesan cheese	

Directions:

Steps:	Directions:	Critical Control Point / Quality Assurance
1	Bring a pot of water to a boil Cook linguine until al dente, about 9 minutes, or as package directs Reserve 1/2 cup of cooking water; drain pasta	
2	Melt butter in a small pan over medium-low heat Sprinkle in flour and cook, stirring, until thickened but not browned, about 2 minutes Whisk in milk and continue to cook until sauce is thick enough to coat the back of a spoon, about 3 minutes Season with salt and pepper Remove from heat	
3	Warm oil in a large skillet over medium-high heat Add garlic and cook, stirring, until golden, about 1 minute Add mushrooms and sauté until they release their liquid and begin to turn golden, about 5 minutes Add onion, celery and cook, stirring, until vegetables are tender, about 5 minutes longer	
4	Stir sauce and reserved pasta water into vegetable mixture and cook, stirring, until heated through, about 5 minutes Reduce heat to medium-low, add tuna, breaking it up, and cook until warmed through, about 2 minutes Season with salt and pepper Toss linguine with sauce, sprinkle with parsley and Parmesan cheese, and serve hot	Cook until internal temperature reaches 165° F for 15 seconds.

Time Temperature Sensitive food. Food safety Standards: hold food for service at an internal temperature above 140° F. Do not mix old product with new. Cool leftover product quickly (within 4 hours) to below 41° F. Follow proper cooling procedures. Store leftovers in a tightly sealed, labeled and dated container. Use leftover within 72 hours if stored in refrigerator or 30 days if stored in the freezer. Reheat leftover product quickly (within 2 hours) to 165 degrees F for 15 seconds. Reheat left over product only once; discard if not used. Cold holding at 41°F or colder or using time alone (less than four hours). Always wash hands and wash and sanitize counter tops utensils and containers between steps when working with raw seafood.

Texture Modified Diets: TIP: Use pasta that is the correct particle size.
Soft & Bite Size: (aka Bite size) **Food particle size ½ inch (~width of standard fork)** Food must be moist. Cut foods with a knife to a ½" particle size prior to mixing. Moisten with broth as needed.
Chopped: Food particle size ¼ inch (~ ½ width of standard fork) Food must be moist. Chop foods with a knife to 1/4" particle size prior to mixing. Moisten with broth as needed.

Minced and Moist: (aka Minced/Mechanical Soft/Ground) **Food particle size 1/8 inch (fits through prongs of standard fork)** Food must be moist. Use a food processor to grind food particles into 1/8 inch prior to mixing. Moisten with broth as needed.

Pureed: Smooth and cohesive. Use a food processor to puree to a smooth consistency. Foods are processed by grinding and then pureeing them. May add broth or sauce to puree. Do not add to much liquid. Puree should still hold its shape. Must not be firm or sticky. Puree foods while still hot. Appearance should be smooth like pudding. Serve ½ cup puree tuna and puree pasta separately.

Tip: Puree linguine mixture before adding tuna to keep separate.

<u>Therapeutic Modified Diets:</u>

Lowfat: No changes needed

Diabetic/No added Sugar/No Conc. Sweets/Calorie Controlled: No changes needed

Bland/Anti Reflux: omit celery, pepper and parsley.

Liberal House Renal: Omit salt and Parmesan cheese

No Added Salt: No changes needed

2 Gram Sodium: omit salt and Parmesan cheese.

Gluten Free: Gluten-free flour and pasta. Prepare foods separately to prevent cross contamination.

Allergy Alerts: When an "X" is present, this indicates the allergen is present.

Always read all food labels to ensure allergens are not present.

Wheat	Milk	Eggs	Fish Shellfish	Soy	Peanuts/Nuts	Other
X	X	X	X			

Key: SF= Salt Free D= Diet or Sugarfree LF = Lowfat FF = Fat Free GF = Gluten Free

Recipe Name: White Fish with Coconut Curry Sauce
Recipe Category: Dinner Entrée
Portion Size: 4 oz. fish and ½ c. rice
Ingredients: Yields: 8 servings

Ingredients	Notes:
1 teaspoon dark sesame oil, divided	Or may use olive oil
2 teaspoons minced peeled fresh ginger	Or 1 teaspoon ground ginger
2 garlic cloves, minced	Wash, peel and mince
1 cup finely chopped red bell pepper	Wash, core and chop
1 cup chopped green onions	Wash, trim and chop (including green tops)
1 teaspoon curry powder	
1/4 cup red curry paste	(optional)
1 teaspoon ground cumin	
1/3 cup low-sodium soy sauce	
1 tablespoon brown sugar	
1/2 teaspoon salt, divided	
2 (14-ounce) cans light coconut milk	
2 tablespoons chopped fresh cilantro	or 2 teaspoon dried cilantro
8 (4-ounce) white fish fillets	
Cooking spray	
4 cups hot cooked brown rice	
8 lime wedges (optional)	

Directions:

Steps:	Directions:	Critical Control Point / Quality Assurance
1	Preheat broiler	
2	Heat 1/2 teaspoon oil in a large nonstick skillet over medium heat	
3	Add ginger and garlic; cook 1 minute. Add pepper and onions; cook 1 minute	
4	Stir in curry powder, curry paste, and cumin; cook 1 minute	
5	Add soy sauce, sugar, 1/4-teaspoon salt, and coconut milk; bring to a simmer (do not boil) Remove from heat; stir in cilantro	
6	Brush fish with 1/2 teaspoon oil; sprinkle with 1/4 teaspoon salt	
7	Place fish on a baking sheet coated with cooking spray	
8	Broil 7 minutes or until fish flakes easily when tested with a fork	Cook until internal temperature reaches 145° F for 15 seconds.
9	Serve fish with sauce, rice, and lime wedges	

Time Temperature Sensitive food. *Food safety Standards: hold food for service at an internal temperature above 140° F. Do not mix old product with new. Cool leftover product quickly (within 4 hours) to below 41° F. Follow proper cooling procedures. Store leftovers in a tightly sealed, labeled and dated container. Use leftover within 72 hours if stored in refrigerator or 30 days if stored in the freezer. Reheat leftover product quickly (within 2 hours) to 165 degrees F for 15 seconds. Reheat left over product only once; discard if not used. Cold holding at 41°F or colder or using time alone (less than four hours). Always wash hands and wash and sanitize counter tops utensils and containers between steps when working with raw seafood.*

<u>Texture Modified Diets:</u>
Soft & Bite Size: (aka Bite size) **Food particle size ½ inch (~width of standard fork)** Food must be moist. Cut foods with a knife to a ½" particle size after cooking. Moisten with sauce as needed after cutting.
Chopped: Food particle size ¼ inch (~ ½ width of standard fork) Food must be moist. Chop foods with a knife to 1/4" particle size after cooking. Moisten with sauce as needed after chopping.
Minced and Moist:(aka Minced/Mechanical Soft/Ground) **Food particle size 1/8 inch (fits through prongs of standard fork)** Food must be moist. Use a food processor to grind food particles into 1/8 inch after cooking. Moisten with sauce as needed after processing.

Pureed: Smooth and cohesive. Use a food processor to puree to a smooth consistency. Foods are processed by grinding and then pureeing them. May add milk or sauce to puree. Do not add to much liquid. Puree should still hold its shape. Must not be firm or sticky. Puree foods while still hot. Appearance should be smooth like pudding. Serve ½ c. meat serving topped with sauce.

Therapeutic Modified Diets:
Lowfat: No changes needed
Diabetic/No added Sugar/No Conc. Sweets/Calorie Controlled: No changes needed
Bland/Anti Reflux: omit garlic, red pepper, green onion, curry, curry paste, lime and cilantro
Liberal House Renal: Omit soy sauce, salt red curry paste and lime
No Added Salt: Omit soy sauce
2 Gram Sodium: Omit soy sauce, salt and red curry paste
Gluten Free: Use GF soy sauce. Prepare foods separately to prevent cross contamination.
Allergy Alerts: When an "X" is present, this indicates the allergen is present.
Always read all food labels to ensure allergens are not present.

Wheat	Milk	Eggs	Fish Shellfish	Soy	Peanuts/Nuts	Other
X			X	X		

Key: SF= Salt Free D= Diet or Sugarfree LF = Lowfat FF = Fat Free GF = Gluten Free

SEAFOOD LUNCH

Recipe Name: Crab and Pea Pasta Salad
Recipe Category: Lunch Entrée
Portion Size: 1 cup
Ingredients: Yields: 8 servings

Ingredients	Notes:
1 lb. pasta	May use whole grain
2 cups frozen peas	Thawed
½ cup light mayonnaise	
½ cup light sour cream	
1 teaspoon salt	
1 pinch ground back pepper	
3 cups imitation crab meat	Chopped

Directions:

Steps:	Directions:	Critical Control Point / Quality Assurance
1	Prepared pasta according to the directions on package. Drain/	
2	In a large bowl combine mayonnaise, sour cream, salt, pepper and crab meat. Stir to combine. Add pasta and peas. Gently toss to coat.	Keep chilled until ready to toss with salad
3	Chill for at least 1 hour. Serve Chilled	

Time Temperature Sensitive food. *Food safety Standards: Do not mix old product with new. Cool leftover product quickly (within 4 hours) to below 41°F. Follow proper cooling procedures. Store leftovers in a tightly sealed, labeled and dated container. Use leftover within 72 hours if stored in refrigerator or 30 days if stored in the freezer. Cold holding at 41°F or colder or using time alone (less than four hours).*

Texture Modified Diets:

Soft & Bite Size: (aka Bite size) **Food particle size ½ inch (~width of standard fork)** Food must be moist. Cut foods with a knife to a ½" particle size prior to mixing. Moisten with milk as needed.

Chopped: Food particle size ¼ inch (~ ½ width of standard fork) Food must be moist. Chop foods with a knife to 1/4" particle size prior to mixing. Moisten with milk as needed.

Minced and Moist: (aka Minced/Mechanical Soft/Ground) **Food particle size 1/8 inch (fits through prongs of standard fork)** Food must be moist. Use a food processor to grind food particles into 1/8 inch prior to mixing. Moisten with milk as needed.

Pureed: Smooth and cohesive. Use a food processor to puree to a smooth consistency. Foods are processed by grinding and then pureeing them. May add milk or sauce to puree. Do not add to much liquid. Puree should still hold its shape. Must not be firm or sticky. Puree foods while still hot. Appearance should be smooth like pudding. Serve ½ c. puree meat and ½ c. puree noodles and peas separately.

Therapeutic Modified Diets:

Lowfat: No changes needed.
Diabetic/No added Sugar/No Conc. Sweets/Calorie Controlled: No changes needed
Bland/Anti Reflux: Omit pepper.
Liberal House Renal: Omit mayonnaise, salt and imitation crab. Substitute tuna for crab.
No Added Salt: No changes needed.
2 Gram Sodium: Omit mayonnaise, salt and imitation crab. Substitute tuna for crab.
Gluten Free: Use gluten free pasta. Prepare foods separately to prevent cross contamination.
Allergy Alerts: When an "X" is present, this indicates the allergen is present.
Always read all food labels to ensure allergens are not present.

Wheat	Milk	Eggs	Fish Shellfish	Soy	Peanuts/Nuts	Other
X	X	X	X			

Key: SF= Salt Free D= Diet or Sugarfree LF = Lowfat FF = Fat Free GF = Gluten Free

Recipe Name: Crab and Spinach Quiche
Recipe Category: Lunch Entrée
Portion Size: ½ cup
Ingredients: **Yields: 8 servings**

Ingredients	Notes:
1 tablespoon olive oil	
1 large onion	Washed, peeled and diced
1 (14 oz.) package fresh baby spinach	Washed, trimmed and Chopped
8 eggs	May use 2 cups egg substitute
1/2 cup nonfat milk	
8 oz. low fat shredded sharp cheddar cheese or mozzarella cheese	
1/2 cup grated parmesan cheese	
1 teaspoon salt	
1 pinch ground black pepper	
3 cups imitation crab meat, chopped	

Directions:

Steps:	Directions:	Critical Control Point / Quality Assurance
1	Preheat oven to 375 degrees F (190 degrees C). Spray baking dish with cooking spray.	
2	Heat olive oil in a large skillet over medium heat and cook onion until softened, about 2 minutes.	
3	Stir spinach into onion and cook, stirring often, until spinach is wilted and onions are translucent, about 3 more minutes. Drain juice.	
4	Beat eggs with milk in a large bowl until thoroughly combined; beat in Cheese, and 1/2 Parmesan cheeses and season with salt and black pepper. Drain juice.	
5	Pour spinach mixture into the baking pan and top spinach with imitation crabmeat. Slowly and carefully pour egg-cheese mixture over the imitation crab.	
6	Bake in the preheated oven until the egg is set, 25 to 30 minutes.	Internal temperature should reach 160 degrees

Time Temperature Sensitive food. *Food safety Standards: hold food for service at an internal temperature above 140° F. Do not mix old product with new. Cool leftover product quickly (within 4 hours) to below 41° F. Follow proper cooling procedures. Store leftovers in a tightly sealed, labeled and dated container. Use leftover within 72 hours if stored in refrigerator or 30 days if stored in the freezer. Reheat leftover product quickly (within 2 hours) to 165 degrees F for 15 seconds. Reheat left over product only once; discard if not used. Cold holding at 41°F or colder or using time alone (less than four hours).*

Texture Modified Diets:

Soft & Bite Size: (aka Bite size) **Food particle size ½ inch (~width of standard fork)** Food must be moist. Cut foods with a knife to a ½" particle size prior to mixing. Moisten with milk as needed.

Chopped: Food particle size ¼ inch (~ ½ width of standard fork) Food must be moist. Chop foods with a knife to 1/4" particle size prior to mixing. Moisten with milk as needed.

Minced and Moist: (aka Minced/Mechanical Soft/Ground) **Food particle size 1/8 inch (fits through prongs of standard fork)** Food must be moist. Use a food processor to grind food particles into 1/8 inch prior to mixing. Moisten with milk as needed.

Pureed: Smooth and cohesive. Use a food processor to puree to a smooth consistency. Foods are processed by grinding and then pureeing them. May add milk or sauce to puree. Do not add to much liquid. Puree should still hold its shape. Must not be firm or sticky. Puree foods while still hot. Appearance should be smooth like pudding. Puree with broth if needed.

Therapeutic Modified Diets:

Lowfat: Use egg substitute.
Diabetic/No added Sugar/No Conc. Sweets/Calorie Controlled: No changes needed.
Bland/Anti Reflux: Omit onion and pepper. Use egg substitute.
Liberal House Renal: Omit cheese, Parmesan cheese and imitation crab. May add SF fish or chicken in place of crab.
No Added Salt: Omit Salt.

2 Gram Sodium: Omit cheese, Parmesan cheese and imitation crab. May add SF fish or chicken in place of crab.
Gluten Free: No changes needed
**Allergy Alerts: When an "X" is present, this indicates the allergen is present.
Always read all food labels to ensure allergens are not present.**

Wheat	Milk	Eggs	Fish Shellfish	Soy	Peanuts/Nuts	Other
	x	X	X			

Key: SF= Salt Free D= Diet or Sugarfree LF = Lowfat FF = Fat Free GF = Gluten Free

Recipe Name: Crab Enchiladas
Recipe Category: Lunch Entrée
Portion Size: 1 Enchilada
Ingredients: Yields: 8 servings

Ingredients	Notes:
3 cups imitation crab	chopped
1 yellow onion	Washed, peeled and diced
3 cloves garlic	Washed, peeled and minced
1 (14 oz.) package fresh spinach	Washed and stems removed
8 oz. low fat shredded Monterey Jack Cheese	
1 cup low fat ricotta cheese	
1 cup light sour cream	
1 teaspoon salt	
½ teaspoon ground black pepper	
8 flour tortillas	May use whole grain
8 oz. low fat mozzarella cheese	

Directions:

Steps:	Directions:	Critical Control Point / Quality Assurance
1	Preheat oven to 350 degrees F (175 degrees C).	
2	Heat olive oil in a saucepan over medium heat; cook and stir onion and garlic until softened, about 2 minutes.	
3	Fold spinach into mixture and cook until wilted, 3 to 5 minutes.	
4	Mix Monterey Jack cheese, ricotta cheese, sour cream, salt, crab and black pepper into spinach mixture.	
5	Heat a skillet over medium heat; warm tortillas, 1 at a time, in the hot skillet until flexible, about 30 seconds per side.	
6	Spoon spinach mixture down the center of each warmed tortilla.	
7	Roll tortilla around filling; place filled tortillas seam sides down into a 9x13-inch casserole dish. Top with mozzarella cheese.	
8	Bake in the preheated oven until sauce is bubbling and cheese topping is slightly browned, 20 to 25 minutes.	Cook until internal temperature reaches 165°F for 15 seconds.

Time Temperature Sensitive food. *Food safety Standards: hold food for service at an internal temperature above 140°F. Do not mix old product with new. Cool leftover product quickly (within 4 hours) to below 41°F. Follow proper cooling procedures. Store leftovers in a tightly sealed, labeled and dated container. Use leftover within 72 hours if stored in refrigerator or 30 days if stored in the freezer. Reheat leftover product quickly (within 2 hours) to 165 degrees F for 15 seconds. Reheat left over product only once; discard if not used. Cold holding at 41°F or colder or using time alone (less than four hours).*

Special Diets:
Texture Modified Diets:
Soft & Bite Size: (aka Bite size) **Food particle size ½ inch (~width of standard fork)** Food must be moist. Cut foods with a knife to a ½" particle size prior to layering. Moisten with broth as needed.
Chopped: Food particle size ¼ inch (~ ½ width of standard fork) Food must be moist. Chop foods with a knife to 1/4" particle size prior to layering. Moisten with broth as needed.
Minced and Moist: (aka Minced/Mechanical Soft/Ground) **Food particle size 1/8 inch (fits through prongs of standard fork)** Food must be moist. Use a food processor to grind food particles into 1/8 inch prior to layering. Moisten with broth as needed.
Pureed: Smooth and cohesive. Use a food processor to puree to a smooth consistency. Foods are processed by grinding and then pureeing them. May add broth or sauce to puree. Do not add to much liquid. Puree should still hold its shape. Must not be firm or sticky. Puree foods while still hot. Appearance should be smooth like pudding. Serve ½ cup mixture, 1 tortilla separately.
Therapeutic Modified Diets:
Lowfat: No changes needed

Diabetic/No added Sugar/No Conc. Sweets/Calorie Controlled: No changes needed
Bland/Anti Reflux: omit onion, garlic, and black pepper.
Liberal House Renal: Serve 2 oz. SF seasoned fish and ½ c. SF rice, SF pasta or SF tortillas
No Added Salt: no changes needed
2 Gram Sodium: Serve 2 oz. SF seasoned fish and ½ c. SF rice, SF pasta or SF tortillas.
Gluten Free: Use gluten free corn tortilla. Prepare foods separately to prevent cross contamination.
Allergy Alerts: When an "X" is present, this indicates the allergen is present.
Always read all food labels to ensure allergens are not present.

Wheat	Milk	Eggs	Fish Shellfish	Soy	Peanuts/Nuts	Other
X	x		x			

Key: SF= Salt Free D= Diet or Sugarfree LF = Lowfat FF = Fat Free GF = Gluten Free

Recipe Name: Crab Salad
Recipe Category: Lunch Entrée
Portion Size: 1/3 cup
Ingredients: Yields: 8 servings

Ingredients	Notes:
3 cups imitation crab	
1 cup diced celery	Washed, trimmed and diced
1/4 cup onion	Washed, peeled and minced
2 teaspoons lemon juice	
1/2 cup light mayonnaise	
8 Large lettuce leaves	Washed and separated
2 large tomatoes	Washed, trimmed and cut into wedges
4 Hard cooked eggs	Optional

Directions:

Steps:	Directions:	Critical Control Point / Quality Assurance
1	Combine crabmeat and celery	
2	Add lemon juice and Worcestershire sauce to the mayonnaise. Mix well. Fold mayonnaise mixture into crab.	Keep chilled until time to serve.
3	Serve on lettuce leaves and garnish with sections of tomato and hard cooked eggs	

Time Temperature Sensitive food. *Food safety Standards: Do not mix old product with new. Cool leftover product quickly (within 4 hours) to below 41°F. Follow proper cooling procedures. Store leftovers in a tightly sealed, labeled and dated container. Use leftover within 72 hours if stored in refrigerator or 30 days if stored in the freezer. Cold holding at 41°F or colder or using time alone (less than four hours).*

Texture Modified Diets:

Soft & Bite Size: (aka Bite size) **Food particle size ½ inch (~width of standard fork)** Food must be moist. Cut foods with a knife to a ½" particle size prior to mixing. Moisten with milk as needed. Cook onion and celery to soften.
Chopped: Food particle size ¼ inch (~ ½ width of standard fork) Food must be moist. Chop foods with a knife to 1/4" particle size prior to mixing. Moisten with milk as needed. Cook onion and celery to soften.
Minced and Moist: (aka Minced/Mechanical Soft/Ground) **Food particle size 1/8 inch (fits through prongs of standard fork)** Food must be moist. Use a food processor to grind food particles into 1/8 inch prior to mixing. Moisten with milk as needed. Cook onion and celery to soften.
Pureed: Smooth and cohesive. Use a food processor to puree to a smooth consistency. Foods are processed by grinding and then pureeing them. May add broth or sauce to puree. Do not add to much liquid. Puree should still hold its shape. Must not be firm or sticky. Puree foods while still hot. Appearance should be smooth like pudding. Serve 1/3 cup of crab mixture.

Therapeutic Modified Diets:

Lowfat: Omit eggs.
Diabetic/No added Sugar/No Conc. Sweets/Calorie Controlled: No changes needed
Bland/Anti Reflux: omit onion, celery, lemon juice, tomato and egg.
Liberal House Renal: omit tomato, imitation crab and mayonnaise. Serve 2 oz. SF seasoned fish or chicken
No Added Salt: no changes needed
2 Gram Sodium: Omit imitation crab and mayonnaise. Serve 2oz. SF seasoned fish or chicken.
Gluten Free: no changes needed
Allergy Alerts: When an "X" is present, this indicates the allergen is present.
Always read all food labels to ensure allergens are not present.

Wheat	Milk	Eggs	Fish Shellfish	Soy	Peanuts/Nuts	Other
		X	X			

Key: SF= Salt Free D= Diet or Sugarfree LF = Lowfat FF = Fat Free GF = Gluten Free

Recipe Name: Crab Salad with Thousand Island dressing
Recipe Category: Lunch Entrée
Portion Size: 1 cup lettuce and ½ cup crab mixture
Ingredients: **Yields: 8 servings**

Ingredients	Notes:
3 cups imitation crab	Chopped
8 Cups of lettuce	Separated, washed and torn into bite size pieces
1/4 Cup onion	Washed, peeled and minced
1 Medium avocado	(optional) Washed, peeled and diced
1/2 Cup lowfat Thousand Island dressing	* See recipe in cook book
3 Tomatoes	Washed, deseed and diced
1/4 Cup slivered unsalted almonds	Optional

Directions:

Steps:	Directions:	Critical Control Point / Quality Assurance
1	Wash lettuce and tear into bite size pieces	
2	In a large bowl combine crabmeat, onion, dressing and avocado.	
3	Serve on 1 cup lettuce. Garnish with tomato slices and almonds. Serve chilled	

Time Temperature Sensitive food. *Food safety Standards: Do not mix old product with new. Cool leftover product quickly (within 4 hours) to below 41°F. Follow proper cooling procedures. Store leftovers in a tightly sealed, labeled and dated container. Use leftover within 72 hours if stored in refrigerator or 30 days if stored in the freezer. Cold holding at 41°F or colder or using time alone (less than four hours).*

Texture Modified Diets:

Soft & Bite Size: (aka Bite size) **Food particle size ½ inch (~width of standard fork)** Food must be moist. Cut foods with a knife to a ½" particle size prior to mixing. Moisten with broth as needed. Foods that do not process well should be omitted. Omit: almonds

Chopped: Food particle size ¼ inch (~ ½ width of standard fork) Food must be moist. Chop foods with a knife to 1/4" particle size prior to mixing. Moisten with broth as needed. Foods that do not process well should be omitted. Omit: almonds

Minced and Moist: (aka Minced/Mechanical Soft/Ground) **Food particle size 1/8 inch (fits through prongs of standard fork)** Food must be moist. Use a food processor to grind food particles into 1/8 inch prior to mixing. Moisten with broth as needed. Foods that do not process well should be omitted. Omit: almonds

Pureed: Smooth and cohesive. Use a food processor to puree to a smooth consistency. Foods are processed by grinding and then pureeing them. May add broth or sauce to puree. Do not add to much liquid. Puree should still hold its shape. Must not be firm or sticky. Puree foods while still hot. Appearance should be smooth like pudding. Foods that do not process well should be omitted. Omit: almonds.

Therapeutic Modified Diets:

Lowfat: omit avocado and almonds
Diabetic/No added Sugar/No Conc. Sweets/Calorie Controlled: No changes needed
Bland/Anti Reflux: omit onion, avocado and almonds
Liberal House Renal: omit dressing, almonds, avacado and tomatoes. Substitute Renal dressing recipe in cookbook. Substitute SF 2 oz. fish for imitation crab.
No Added Salt: Substitute low sodium dressing recipe in cookbook.
2 Gram Sodium: Omit dressing. Substitute low sodium dressing recipe in cookbook. SF 2 oz. fish for imitation crab.
Gluten Free: Use gluten free dressing. Prepare separately to prevent cross contamination.
Allergy Alerts: When an "X" is present, this indicates the allergen is present.
Always read all food labels to ensure allergens are not present.

Wheat	Milk	Eggs	Fish Shellfish	Soy	Peanuts/Nuts	Other
X	X	X	x		X	

Key: SF= Salt Free D= Diet or Sugarfree LF = Lowfat FF = Fat Free GF = Gluten Free

Recipe Name: Garden Salmon Pasta Salad
Recipe Category: Lunch Entrée
Portion Size: 1 1/2 cup
Ingredients: **Yields: 8 servings**

Ingredients	Notes:
1 (16 ounce) package pasta	May use whole grain pasta
1 cup tomatoes	Washed, peeled, seeded and diced
1 cup cucumber	Washed, seeded and chopped
1 red pepper	Washed, trimmed and diced
1/4 cup red onion	Washed, peeled and diced
1 tablespoon dill	
3 cups salmon	Use water packed canned
1 cup light mayonnaise	
1 teaspoon salt	
1 pinch ground black pepper	

Directions:

Steps:	Directions:	Critical Control Point /Quality Assurance
1	In a large pot of salted boiling water, cook pasta until al dente, rinse under cold water and drain.	
2	In a large bowl, combine the pasta, tomatoes, cucumbers, red pepper, red onion, dill, salt, pepper, mayonnaise, and salmon. Refrigerate for 1 hour.	

Time Temperature Sensitive food. *Food safety Standards: Do not mix old product with new. Cool leftover product quickly (within 4 hours) to below 41°F. Follow proper cooling procedures. Store leftovers in a tightly sealed, labeled and dated container. Use leftover within 72 hours if stored in refrigerator or 30 days if stored in the freezer. Cold holding at 41°F or colder or using time alone (less than four hours).*

Texture Modified Diets:

Soft & Bite Size: (aka Bite size) **Food particle size ½ inch (~width of standard fork)** Food must be moist. Cut foods with a knife to a ½" particle size prior to mixing. Moisten with broth as needed. Foods that do not process well should be omitted. Omit: cucumber peel. Cook peppers and onions to soften.

Chopped: Food particle size ¼ inch (~ ½ width of standard fork) Food must be moist. Chop foods with a knife to 1/4" particle size prior to mixing. Moisten with broth as needed. Foods that do not process well should be omitted. Omit: cucumber peel. Cook peppers and onions to soften.

Minced and Moist:(aka Minced/Mechanical Soft/Ground) **Food particle size 1/8 inch (fits through prongs of standard fork)** Food must be moist. Use a food processor to grind food particles into 1/8 inch prior to mixing. Moisten with broth as needed. Foods that do not process well should be omitted. Omit: cucumber peel.

Pureed: Smooth and cohesive. Use a food processor to puree to a smooth consistency. Foods are processed by grinding and then pureeing them. May add broth or sauce to puree. Do not add to much liquid. Puree should still hold its shape. Must not be firm or sticky. Puree foods while still hot. Appearance should be smooth like pudding. Foods that do not process well should be omitted. Omit: cucumber peel. Serve ½ c. fish, ½ c. puree noodles and ½ c. puree vegetables separately.

Therapeutic Modified Diets:

Lowfat: No changes needed
Diabetic/No added Sugar/No Conc. Sweets/Calorie Controlled: no changes needed
Bland/Anti Reflux: Omit red onion, red pepper, tomatoes and black pepper
Liberal House Renal: Omit salt and mayonnaise. Toss with SF dressing of choice in cookbook.
No Added Salt: Omit salt
2 Gram Sodium: Omit salt and mayonnaise. Toss with SF dressing of choice in cookbook.
Gluten Free: Use gluten free pasta. Prepare foods separately to prevent cross contamination.
Allergy Alerts: When an "X" is present, this indicates the allergen is present.
Always read all food labels to ensure allergens are not present.

Wheat	Milk	Eggs	Fish Shellfish	Soy	Peanuts/Nuts	Other
X		X	x			

Key: SF= Salt Free D= Diet or Sugarfree LF = Lowfat FF = Fat Free GF = Gluten Free

Recipe Name: Garden Tuna Pasta Salad **or** Garden Salmon Pasta Salad
Recipe Category: Lunch Entrée
Portion Size: 1 1/2 cup
Ingredients: Yields: 8 servings

Ingredients	Notes:
1 (16 ounce) package pasta	May use whole grain pasta
1 cup tomatoes	Washed, peeled, seeded and diced
1 cup cucumber	Washed, seeded and chopped
1 red pepper	Washed, trimmed and diced
1/4 cup red onion	Washed, peeled and diced
1 tablespoon dill	
3 cups tuna or salmon	Use water packed canned
1 cup light mayonnaise	
1 teaspoon salt	
1 pinch ground black pepper	

Directions:

Steps:	Directions:	Critical Control Point /Quality Assurance
1	In a large pot of salted boiling water, cook pasta until al dente, rinse under cold water and drain.	
2	In a large bowl, combine the pasta, tomatoes, cucumbers, red pepper, red onion, dill, salt, pepper, mayonnaise, and tuna. Refrigerate for 1 hour.	

Time Temperature Sensitive food. *Food safety Standards: Do not mix old product with new. Cool leftover product quickly (within 4 hours) to below 41°F. Follow proper cooling procedures. Store leftovers in a tightly sealed, labeled and dated container. Use leftover within 72 hours if stored in refrigerator or 30 days if stored in the freezer. Cold holding at 41°F or colder or using time alone (less than four hours).*

Texture Modified Diets:

Soft & Bite Size: (aka Bite size) **Food particle size ½ inch (~width of standard fork)** Food must be moist. Cut foods with a knife to a ½" particle size prior to mixing. Moisten with broth as needed. Foods that do not process well should be omitted. Omit: cucumber peel. Cook peppers and onions to soften.

Chopped: Food particle size ¼ inch (~ ½ width of standard fork) Food must be moist. Chop foods with a knife to 1/4" particle size prior to mixing. Moisten with broth as needed. Foods that do not process well should be omitted. Omit: cucumber peel. Cook peppers and onions to soften.

Minced and Moist: (aka Minced/Mechanical Soft/Ground) **Food particle size 1/8 inch (fits through prongs of standard fork)** Food must be moist. Use a food processor to grind food particles into 1/8 inch prior to mixing. Moisten with broth as needed. Foods that do not process well should be omitted. Omit: cucumber peel.

Pureed: Smooth and cohesive. Use a food processor to puree to a smooth consistency. Foods are processed by grinding and then pureeing them. May add broth or sauce to puree. Do not add to much liquid. Puree should still hold its shape. Must not be firm or sticky. Puree foods while still hot. Appearance should be smooth like pudding. Foods that do not process well should be omitted. Omit: cucumber peel Serve ½ c. fish, ½ c. puree noodles and ½ c. puree vegetables separately.

Therapeutic Modified Diets:

Lowfat: No changes needed
Diabetic/No added Sugar/No Conc. Sweets/Calorie Controlled: no changes needed
Bland/Anti Reflux: Omit red onion, red pepper, tomatoes and black pepper
Liberal House Renal: Omit salt and mayonnaise. Toss with SF dressing of choice in cookbook.
No Added Salt: Omit salt
2 Gram Sodium: Omit salt and mayonnaise. Toss with SF dressing of choice in cookbook.
Gluten Free: Use gluten free pasta. Prepare foods separately to prevent cross contamination.
Allergy Alerts: When an "X" is present, this indicates the allergen is present.
Always read all food labels to ensure allergens are not present.

Wheat	Milk	Eggs	Fish Shellfish	Soy	Peanuts/Nuts	Other
X		X	x			

Key: SF= Salt Free D= Diet or Sugarfree LF = Lowfat FF = Fat Free GF = Gluten Free

Copyright 2020 Jacqueline Larson M.S., R.D.N. and Associates.   All Rights Reserved

Recipe Name: Salmon Pasta Salad with Peas, Red Bell Peppers and Red Onion
Recipe Category: Lunch Entrée
Portion Size: 1 cup
Ingredients: Yields: 8 servings

Ingredients	Notes:
1 (16 ounce) package pasta	
1 cups peas, frozen	
1 red bell pepper	
3 cups canned salmon	Drained
2 tablespoons olive oil	
1 teaspoon dried dill	
1/3 cup lemon juice	
1/2 teaspoon grated lemon zest	(optional)
1 clove garlic	Washed, peeled and minced
1/4 cup red onion	Washed, peeled and finely chopped
1 teaspoon salt	
1 pinch ground black pepper	

Directions:

Steps:	Directions:	Critical Control Point / Quality Assurance
1	In a large pot of salted boiling water, cook pasta until al dente, rinse under cold water and drain.	
2	In a large bowl, combine the olive oil, dill, lemon juice, lemon zest, garlic salt and peppers. Whisk to combine.	
3	Add pasta, salmon, red onion and toss to coat.	
4	Refrigerate for 1 hour.	

Time Temperature Sensitive food. Food safety Standards: Do not mix old product with new. Cool leftover product quickly (within 4 hours) to below 41°F. Follow proper cooling procedures. Store leftovers in a tightly sealed, labeled and dated container. Use leftover within 72 hours if stored in refrigerator or 30 days if stored in the freezer. Cold holding at 41°F or colder or using time alone (less than four hours).

Texture Modified Diets:
Soft & Bite Size: (aka Bite size) **Food particle size ½ inch (~width of standard fork)** Food must be moist. Cut foods with a knife to a ½" particle size prior to mixing. Moisten with broth as needed. May cook bell pepper to soften.
Chopped: Food particle size ¼ inch (~ ½ width of standard fork) Food must be moist. Chop foods with a knife to 1/4" particle size prior to mixing. Moisten with broth as needed. May cook bell pepper to soften.
Minced and Moist:(aka Minced/Mechanical Soft/Ground) **Food particle size 1/8 inch (fits through prongs of standard fork)** Food must be moist. Use a food processor to grind food particles into 1/8 inch prior to mixing. Moisten with broth as needed.
Pureed: Smooth and cohesive. Use a food processor to puree to a smooth consistency. Foods are processed by grinding and then pureeing them. May add broth or sauce to puree. Do not add to much liquid. Puree should still hold its shape. Must not be firm or sticky. Puree foods while still hot. Appearance should be smooth like pudding. Serve ½ cup puree pasta, ½ cup puree peas/pepper and 1/3 cup tuna mixture separately. Mix in the dressing with the tuna.

Therapeutic Modified Diets:
Lowfat: No changes
Diabetic/No added Sugar/No Conc. Sweets/Calorie Controlled: No changes needed
Bland/Anti Reflux: Omit red onion, bell pepper, black pepper, lemon, dill and garlic
Liberal House Renal: Omit salt
No Added Salt: No changes needed
2 Gram Sodium: Omit salt
Gluten Free: Use gluten free pasta. Prepare foods separately to prevent cross contamination.

Allergy Alerts: When an "X" is present, this indicates the allergen is present. Always read all food labels to ensure allergens are not present.

Wheat	Milk	Eggs	Fish Shellfish	Soy	Peanuts/Nuts	Other
X		X	x			

Key: SF= Salt Free D= Diet or Sugarfree LF = Lowfat FF = Fat Free GF = Gluten Free

Recipe Name: Salmon Quesadillas **or** Tuna Quesadillas
Recipe Category: Lunch Entrée
Portion Size: 1 Quesadilla
Ingredients: **Yields: 8 servings**

Ingredients	Notes:
3 Cups drained water packed, canned tuna or salmon	
16 oz. low fat cheddar cheese	
8 whole grain flour tortillas (burrito size)	May use whole grain
1/2 cup diced bell peppers	Washed, trimmed and diced
1/2 cup light sour cream	
1/4 cup sliced green onions	Washed, trimmed and sliced thin
1/2 cup salsa	
1 avocado (optional)	Washed, peeled and diced

Directions:

Steps:	Directions:	Critical Control Point /Quality Assurance
1	Place tortilla on a flat surface and layer with cheese, diced peppers, and salmon or tuna. Fold in half.	
2	Heat a non stick pan coated with vegetable oil over medium heat.	
3	Place quesadilla carefully into heated pan. Heat both sides in pan until golden brown. Turning once.	
4	Cut into 3 pieces. Garnish with sour cream, salsa, green onion and avocado.	

Time Temperature Sensitive food. *Food safety Standards: hold food for service at an internal temperature above 140° F. Do not mix old product with new. Cool leftover product quickly (within 4 hours) to below 41° F. Follow proper cooling procedures. Store leftovers in a tightly sealed, labeled and dated container. Use leftover within 72 hours if stored in refrigerator or 30 days if stored in the freezer. Reheat leftover product quickly (within 2 hours) to 165 degrees F for 15 seconds. Reheat left over product only once; discard if not used. Cold holding at 41°F or colder or using time alone (less than four hours).*

Texture Modified Diets:
Soft & Bite Size: (aka Bite size) **Food particle size ½ inch (~width of standard fork)** Food must be moist. Cut foods with a knife to a ½" particle size after cooking. Moisten with milk as needed. Foods that do not process well should be omitted. Omit: green onions.
Chopped: Food particle size ¼ inch (~ ½ width of standard fork) Food must be moist. Chop foods with a knife to 1/4" particle after cooking. Moisten with milk as needed. Foods that do not process well should be omitted. Omit: green onion.
Minced and Moist: (aka Minced/Mechanical Soft/Ground) **Food particle size 1/8 inch (fits through prongs of standard fork)** Food must be moist. Use a food processor to grind food particles into 1/8 inch after cooking. Moisten with milk as needed. Foods that do not process well should be omitted. Omit: green onions.
Pureed: Smooth and cohesive. Use a food processor to puree to a smooth consistency. Foods are processed by grinding and then pureeing them. May add broth or sauce to puree. Do not add to much liquid. Puree should still hold its shape. Must not be firm or sticky. Puree foods while still hot. Appearance should be smooth like pudding. Foods that do not process well should be omitted. Omit: green onions.

Therapeutic Modified Diets:
Lowfat: No changes needed.
Diabetic/No added Sugar/No Conc. Sweets/Calorie Controlled: No changes needed
Bland/Anti Reflux: Omit green onion, bell pepper and salsa
Liberal House Renal: Serve SF tortilla or ½ c. pasta and 2 oz. SF tuna or salmon.
No Added Salt: No changes needed
2 Gram Sodium: Serve SF tortilla or ½ c. pasta and 2 oz. SF tuna or salmon
Gluten Free: Use gluten free corn tortilla. Prepare foods separately to prevent cross contamination.
Allergy Alerts: When an "X" is present, this indicates the allergen is present.
Always read all food labels to ensure allergens are not present.

Wheat	Milk	Eggs	Fish Shellfish	Soy	Peanuts/Nuts	Other
X	x		x			

Key: SF= Salt Free D= Diet or Sugarfree LF = Lowfat FF = Fat Free GF = Gluten Free

Copyright 2020 Jacqueline Larson M.S., R.D.N. and Associates. All Rights Reserved

Recipe Name: Salmon Salad
Recipe Category: Lunch Entrée
Portion Size: 1/3 cup
Ingredients: Yields: 8 servings

Ingredients	Notes:
3 cups canned salmon	Drained, water packed
2 cups diced celery or cucumber	Washed, trimmed and diced
1/4 cup onion	Washed, peeled and chopped
1 tablespoon chives or parsley	May use dried or fresh.
1/2 cup light mayonnaise	
1 tablespoon lemon juice	
Lettuce and tomato (optional)	Washed, trimmed and sliced

Directions:

Steps:	Directions:	Critical Control Point / Quality Assurance
1	Mix ingredients in a large bowl. Scoop 1/3 cup on plate.	Keep chilled until ready to serve
2	Garnish with lettuce and tomatoes	

Time Temperature Sensitive food. *Food safety Standards: Do not mix old product with new. Cool leftover product quickly (within 4 hours) to below 41°F. Follow proper cooling procedures. Store leftovers in a tightly sealed, labeled and dated container. Use leftover within 72 hours if stored in refrigerator or 30 days if stored in the freezer. Cold holding at 41°F or colder or using time alone (less than four hours).*

Texture Modified Diets:

Soft & Bite Size: (aka Bite size) **Food particle size ½ inch (~width of standard fork)** Food must be moist. Cut foods with a knife to a ½" particle size prior to mixing. Moisten with milk as needed. Foods that do not process well should be omitted. Omit: cucumber peeling. Cook onion and celery to soften.

Chopped: Food particle size ¼ inch (~ ½ width of standard fork) Food must be moist. Chop foods with a knife to 1/4" particle size prior to mixing. Moisten with milk as needed. Foods that do not process well should be omitted. Omit: cucumber peel. Cook celery and onion to soften.

Minced and Moist: (aka Minced/Mechanical Soft/Ground) **Food particle size 1/8 inch (fits through prongs of standard fork)** Food must be moist. Use a food processor to grind food particles into 1/8 inch prior to mixing. Moisten with broth as needed. Foods that do not process well should be omitted. Omit: cucumber peeling.

Pureed: Smooth and cohesive. Use a food processor to puree to a smooth consistency. Foods are processed by grinding and then pureeing them. May add broth or sauce to puree. Do not add to much liquid. Puree should still hold its shape. Must not be firm or sticky. Puree foods while still hot. Appearance should be smooth like pudding. Foods that do not process well should be omitted. Omit: cucumber peeling Serve1/3 cup puree tuna mixture..

Therapeutic Modified Diets:

Lowfat: No changes needed
Diabetic/No added Sugar/No Conc. Sweets/Calorie Controlled: No changes needed.
Bland/Anti Reflux: omit onion, celery, cucumber, chives or parsley, and tomato.
Liberal House Renal: omit tomato and mayonnaise.
No Added Salt: no changes needed
2 Gram Sodium: Omit mayonnaise.
Gluten Free: No changes needed.
Allergy Alerts: When an "X" is present, this indicates the allergen is present.
Always read all food labels to ensure allergens are not present.

Wheat	Milk	Eggs	Fish Shellfish	Soy	Peanuts/Nuts	Other
X		X	X			

Key: SF= Salt Free D= Diet or Sugarfree LF = Lowfat FF = Fat Free GF = Gluten Free

Recipe Name: Salmon Salad Sandwich
Recipe Category: Lunch Entrée
Portion Size: 1 sandwich
Ingredients: Yields: 8 servings

Ingredients	Notes:
3 cups canned salmon	Drained, water packed
2 cups diced celery or cucumber	Washed, trimmed and diced
1/4 cup onion	Washed, peeled and minced
1 tablespoon chives or parsley	May use dried or fresh.
1/2 cup light mayonnaise	
1 tablespoon lemon juice	
1 teaspoon Dijon mustard	
16 slices bread	May use whole wheat bread.
Lettuce and tomato (optional)	Washed, trimmed and sliced

Directions:

Steps:	Directions:	Critical Control Point /Quality Assurance
1	Mix Salmon, celery or cucumber, onion, chives or parsley, mayonnaise, lemon juice and Dijon mustard Spread 1/3 cup mixture on 1 slice bread.	Keep chilled until ready to serve
2	Garnish with lettuce and tomatoes.	
3.	Top with 1 slice of bread.	

Time Temperature Sensitive food. *Food safety Standards: Do not mix old product with new. Cool leftover product quickly (within 4 hours) to below 41°F. Follow proper cooling procedures. Store leftovers in a tightly sealed, labeled and dated container. Use leftover within 72 hours if stored in refrigerator or 30 days if stored in the freezer. Cold holding at 41°F or colder or using time alone (less than four hours).*

Texture Modified Diets:

Soft & Bite Size: (aka Bite size) **Food particle size ½ inch (~width of standard fork)** Food must be moist. Cut foods with a knife to a ½" particle size prior to mixing/layering. Moisten with broth as needed. Foods that do not process well should be omitted. Omit: cucumber peel and chives.

Chopped: Food particle size ¼ inch (~ ½ width of standard fork) Food must be moist. Chop foods with a knife to 1/4" particle size prior to mixing/layering. Moisten with broth as needed. Foods that do not process well should be omitted. Omit: cucumber peel and chives.

Minced and Moist:(aka Minced/Mechanical Soft/Ground) **Food particle size 1/8 inch (fits through prongs of standard fork)** Food must be moist. Use a food processor to grind food particles into 1/8 inch prior to mixing/layering. Moisten with broth as needed. Foods that do not process well should be omitted. Omit: cucumber peel and chives.

Pureed: Smooth and cohesive. Use a food processor to puree to a smooth consistency. Foods are processed by grinding and then pureeing them. May add broth or sauce to puree. Do not add to much liquid. Puree should still hold its shape. Must not be firm or sticky. Puree foods while still hot. Appearance should be smooth like pudding. Foods that do not process well should be omitted. Omit: cucumber peel and chives.
Serve 1/3 cup puree tuna mixture and bread separately. .

Therapeutic Modified Diets:
Lowfat: No changes needed
Diabetic/No added Sugar/No Conc. Sweets/Calorie Controlled: No changes needed.
Bland/Anti Reflux: omit onion, celery, cucumber, chives or parsley, and tomato.
Liberal House Renal: omit tomato and mayonnaise.
No Added Salt: no changes needed
2 Gram Sodium: Omit mayonnaise.
Gluten Free: Use gluten free bread. Prepare separately to prevent cross contamination.

Allergy Alerts: When an "X" is present, this indicates the allergen is present. Always read all food labels to ensure allergens are not present.

Wheat	Milk	Eggs	Fish Shellfish	Soy	Peanuts/Nuts	Other
X		X	X			

Key: SF= Salt Free D= Diet or Sugarfree LF = Lowfat FF = Fat Free GF = Gluten Free

Recipe Name: Seared Ahi Tuna
Recipe Category: Lunch Entrée
Portion Size: 4 oz. boneless
Ingredients: **Yields: 8 servings**

Ingredients	Notes:
8 (4oz.) boneless Tuna steaks	Store frozen or packed on ice (not more than 24 hours)
1 teaspoon salt	May use kosher salt
½ teaspoon cayenne pepper	
½ teaspoon fresh ground pepper	
¼ cup olive oil	
¼ cup butter	

Directions:

Steps:	Directions:	Critical Control Point / Quality Assurance
1	Season steaks with salt, cayenne and pepper.	
2	Melt butter and oil in pan over medium high heat	
3	Gently place seasoned tuna in the skillet and cook until desired doneness or until temperature reaches 145°F	Cook until internal temperature reaches 145° F for 15 seconds. Serve immediately

Time Temperature Sensitive food. Food safety Standards: hold food for service at an internal temperature above 140° F. Do not mix old product with new. Cool leftover product quickly (within 4 hours) to below 41°F. Follow proper cooling procedures. Reheat leftover product quickly (within 2 hours) to 165 degrees F for 15 seconds. Cold holding at 38°F or colder or using time alone (less than four hours). Packed on ice. No more than 24 hours.

<u>Texture Modified Diets:</u>

Soft & Bite Size: (aka Bite size) **Food particle size ½ inch (~width of standard fork)** Food must be moist. Cut foods with a knife to a ½" particle size after cooking. Moisten with sauce as needed after cutting.

Chopped: Food particle size ¼ inch (~ ½ width of standard fork) Food must be moist. Chop foods with a knife to 1/4" particle size after cooking. Moisten with sauce as needed after chopping.

Minced and Moist: (aka Minced/Mechanical Soft/Ground) **Food particle size 1/8 inch (fits through prongs of standard fork)** Food must be moist. Use a food processor to grind food particles into 1/8 inch after cooking. Moisten with sauce as needed after processing.

Pureed: Smooth and cohesive. Use a food processor to puree to a smooth consistency. Foods are processed by grinding and then pureeing them. May add milk or sauce to puree. Do not add to much liquid. Puree should still hold its shape. Must not be firm or sticky. Puree foods while still hot. Appearance should be smooth like pudding.

<u>Therapeutic Modified Diets:</u>

Lowfat: No changes needed
Diabetic/No added Sugar/No Conc. Sweets/Calorie Controlled: No changes needed
Bland/Anti Reflux: omit cayenne pepper and black pepper
Liberal House Renal: Omit salt
No Added Salt: No changes needed
2 Gram Sodium: omit salt
Gluten Free: No changes needed. Prepare foods separately to prevent cross contamination.
Allergy Alerts: When an "X" is present, this indicates the allergen is present.
Always read all food labels to ensure allergens are not present.

Wheat	Milk	Eggs	Fish Shellfish	Soy	Peanuts/Nuts	Other
	X		X			

Key: SF= Salt Free D= Diet or Sugarfree LF = Lowfat FF = Fat Free GF = Gluten Free

Recipe Name: Tuna and Macaroni Salad or Salmon and Macaroni Salad
Recipe Category: Lunch Entrée
Portion Size: 1 ½ cup
Ingredients: **Yields: 8 servings**

Ingredients	Notes:
1 (16 ounce) package macaroni	May use whole grain
3 tomatoes	Washed, seeded and diced
3 stalks celery, chopped	Washed, trimmed and chopped
3 cups canned tuna (or salmon)	Use water packed.
1 cup light mayonnaise	
1 teaspoon salt	
1 pinch ground black pepper	

Directions:

Steps:	Directions:	Critical Control Point / Quality Assurance
1	In a large pot of salted boiling water, cook pasta until al dente, rinse under cold water and drain	
2	In a large bowl, combine the macaroni, tomatoes, salt, pepper, mayonnaise, celery and tuna.	
3	Refrigerate for 1 hour	Keep chilled until ready to serve

Time Temperature Sensitive food. *Food safety Standards: Do not mix old product with new. Cool leftover product quickly (within 4 hours) to below 41°F. Follow proper cooling procedures. Store leftovers in a tightly sealed, labeled and dated container. Use leftover within 72 hours if stored in refrigerator or 30 days if stored in the freezer. Cold holding at 41°F or colder or using time alone (less than four hours).*

Texture Modified Diets: TIP: use pasta with the correct particle size.
Soft & Bite Size: (aka Bite size) **Food particle size ½ inch (~width of standard fork)** Food must be moist. Cut foods with a knife to a ½" particle size prior to mixing. Moisten with broth as needed. Cook celery to soften.
Chopped: Food particle size ¼ inch (~ ½ width of standard fork) Food must be moist. Chop foods with a knife to 1/4" particle size prior to mixing. Moisten with broth as needed. Cook celery to soften.
Minced and Moist: (aka Minced/Mechanical Soft/Ground) **Food particle size 1/8 inch (fits through prongs of standard fork)** Food must be moist. Use a food processor to grind food particles into 1/8 inch prior to mixing. Moisten with broth as needed.
Pureed: Smooth and cohesive. Use a food processor to puree to a smooth consistency. Foods are processed by grinding and then pureeing them. May add broth or sauce to puree. Do not add to much liquid. Puree should still hold its shape. Must not be firm or sticky. Puree foods while still hot. Appearance should be smooth like pudding. Serve ½ cups per serving, puree pasta and ½ cup tuna mixture separately.

Therapeutic Modified Diets:
Lowfat: No changes needed
Diabetic/No added Sugar/No Conc. Sweets/Calorie Controlled: No changes
Bland/Anti Reflux: Omit tomatoes, celery and black pepper
Liberal House Renal: Omit salt, tomatoes and mayonnaise. Toss with olive oil.
No Added Salt: No changes needed
2 Gram Sodium: Omit salt and mayonnaise. Toss with olive oil
Gluten Free: Use gluten free pasta. Prepare foods separately to prevent cross contamination.
Allergy Alerts: When an "X" is present, this indicates the allergen is present.
Always read all food labels to ensure allergens are not present.

Wheat	Milk	Eggs	Fish Shellfish	Soy	Peanuts/Nuts	Other
X		x	x			

Key: SF= Salt Free D= Diet or Sugarfree LF = Lowfat FF = Fat Free GF = Gluten Free

Recipe Name: Tuna and Tomato Open Faced Melts
Salmon and Tomato Open Face Melts or Turkey and Tomato Open Face Melts or Chicken and Tomato Open Face Melts or Roast Beef and Tomato Open Face Melts
Recipe Category: Lunch Entrée
Portion Size: 1 open faced sandwich
Ingredients: **Yields: 8 servings**

Ingredients	Notes:
3 cups Tuna, (or other cooked diced/sliced meat)	water packed drained
1/4 cup red onion	Washed, peeled and finely chopped
2 tablespoon capers	
1 tablespoon fresh lemon juice	
1/2 teaspoon salt	
1/2 teaspoon dried oregano	
8 large slices tomato (or 16 if they are small)	Washed and sliced
1/2 cup light mayonnaise	
8 slices Provolone cheese	
8 slices crusty bread	

Directions:

Steps:	Directions:	Critical Control Point/Quality Assurance
1	Mix together tuna, capers, lemon, oregano, salt, onion, and mayonnaise in a small bowl	
2	Heat broiler, with rack in highest position.	
3	Arrange bread on baking sheet. Divide tuna salad evenly among slices. Top with tomatoes and then cheese. Broil until cheese is golden brown and bubbly. (About 3-4 minutes).	

Time Temperature Sensitive food. Food safety Standards: hold food for service at an internal temperature above 140° F. Do not mix old product with new. Cool leftover product quickly (within 4 hours) to below 41° F. Follow proper cooling procedures. Reheat leftover product quickly (within 2 hours) to 165 degrees F for 15 seconds. Cold holding at 41°F or colder or using time alone (less than four hours).

Texture Modified Diets:

Soft & Bite Size: (aka Bite size) **Food particle size ½ inch (~width of standard fork)** Food must be moist. Cut foods with a knife to a ½" particle size prior to mixing. Moisten with broth as needed. Foods that do not process well should be omitted. Omit: capers. Use soft moist bread.

Chopped: Food particle size ¼ inch (~ ½ width of standard fork) Food must be moist. Chop foods with a knife to 1/4" particle size prior to mixing. Moisten with broth as needed. Foods that do not process well should be omitted. Omit: capers. Use soft moist bread.

Minced and Moist: (aka Minced/Mechanical Soft/Ground) **Food particle size 1/8 inch (fits through prongs of standard fork)** Food must be moist. Use a food processor to grind food particles into 1/8 inch prior to mixing. Moisten with broth as needed. Foods that do not process well should be omitted. Omit: capers. Use soft moist bread.

Pureed: Smooth and cohesive. Use a food processor to puree to a smooth consistency. Foods are processed by grinding and then pureeing them. May add broth or sauce to puree. Do not add to much liquid. Puree should still hold its shape. Must not be firm or sticky. Puree foods while still hot. Appearance should be smooth like pudding. Foods that do not process well should be omitted. Omit: capers. Puree provolone and bread together. Puree tuna mixture separately. ½ cup serving of each.

Therapeutic Modified Diets:

Lowfat: Omit cheese
Diabetic/No added Sugar/No Conc. Sweets/Calorie Controlled: no changes needed
Bland/Anti Reflux: Omit red onion, omit capers, lemon juice, tomatoes and omit oregano
Liberal House Renal: Omit salt, capers, cheese and mayonnaise. Use low sodium bread or serve with pasta
No Added Salt: Omit capers
2 Gram Sodium: Omit salt, capers, cheese and mayonnaise. Use low sodium bread or serve with pasta.
Gluten Free: Use gluten free bread. Prepare foods separately to prevent cross contamination.

Allergy Alerts: When an "X" is present, this indicates the allergen is present. Always read all food labels to ensure allergens are not present.

Wheat	Milk	Eggs	Fish Shellfish	Soy	Peanuts/Nuts	Other
X	x	x	x			

Key: SF= Salt Free D= Diet or Sugarfree LF = Lowfat FF = Fat Free GF = Gluten Free

Recipe Name: Tuna and White Bean Salad **or** Salmon and White Bean Salad
Recipe Category: Lunch Entrée
Portion Size: 1 ½ cup
Ingredients: Yields: 8 servings

Ingredients	Notes:
3 tomatoes	Washed, peeled, seeded and diced
1 yellow bell pepper	Washed, seeded and diced
1/4 cup red onion	Washed, peeled and diced
3 cups tuna (or salmon)	Use water packed, drained
2 cup white beans	Drained and rinsed
8 cups butter lettuce	Washed and chopped
2 tablespoons capers	Drained
1 tablespoon parsley flakes	
1/4 cup white wine vinegar	
1/4 cup fresh lemon juice	
1 teaspoon salt	
1 pinch ground black pepper	

Directions:

Steps:	Directions:	Critical Control Point / Quality Assurance
1	In a small bowl combine, capers, parsley, white wine vinegar, lemon juice, salt and pepper	
2	In a large bowl combine tomatoes, yellow pepper, red onion, tuna, and white beans	
3	Drizzle with dressing and toss to coat. Serve on bed of lettuce	Keep chilled until ready to serve

Time Temperature Sensitive food. *Food safety Standards: Do not mix old product with new. Cool leftover product quickly (within 4 hours) to below 41° F. Follow proper cooling procedures. Store leftovers in a tightly sealed, labeled and dated container. Use leftover within 72 hours if stored in refrigerator or 30 days if stored in the freezer. Cold holding at 41°F or colder or using time alone (less than four hours).*

Texture Modified Diets:
Soft & Bite Size: (aka Bite size) **Food particle size ½ inch (~width of standard fork)** Food must be moist. Cut foods with a knife to a ½" particle size prior to mixing. Moisten with broth as needed. Foods that do not process well should be omitted. Omit: capers Cook onion and yellow pepper to soften.
Chopped: Food particle size ¼ inch (~ ½ width of standard fork) Food must be moist. Chop foods with a knife to 1/4" particle size prior to mixing. Moisten with broth as needed. Foods that do not process well should be omitted. Omit: capers. Cook onion and yellow pepper to soften.
Minced and Moist: (aka Minced/Mechanical Soft/Ground) **Food particle size 1/8 inch (fits through prongs of standard fork)** Food must be moist. Use a food processor to grind food particles into 1/8 inch prior to mixing. Moisten with broth as needed. Foods that do not process well should be omitted. Omit: capers
Pureed: Smooth and cohesive. Use a food processor to puree to a smooth consistency. Foods are processed by grinding and then pureeing them. May add broth or sauce to puree. Do not add to much liquid. Puree should still hold its shape. Must not be firm or sticky. Puree foods while still hot. Appearance should be smooth like pudding. Foods that do not process well should be omitted. Omit: capers Puree beans with vegetables, lettuce and tuna mixture separately. ½ cup serving of each (beans/ vegetable mixture), (lettuce,) and (tuna mixture).

Therapeutic Modified Diets:
Lowfat: No changes needed
Diabetic/No added Sugar/No Conc. Sweets/Calorie Controlled: No changes needed
Bland/Anti Reflux: Serve ½ cup tuna mixed with mayonnaise and ½ cup plain pasta.
Liberal House Renal: Serve ½ cup plain tuna seasoned with olive oil and lemon juice and ½ cup SF pasta
No Added Salt: Omit capers
2 Gram Sodium: Serve ½ cup plain tuna seasoned with olive oil and lemon juice and 1/3 cup no added salt beans.
Gluten Free: No changes needed
Allergy Alerts: When an "X" is present, this indicates the allergen is present. Always read all food labels to ensure allergens are not present.

Wheat	Milk	Eggs	Fish Shellfish	Soy	Peanuts/Nuts	Other
			X			

Key: SF= Salt Free D= Diet or Sugarfree LF = Lowfat FF = Fat Free GF = Gluten Free

Copyright 2020 Jacqueline Larson M.S., R.D.N. and Associates.   All Rights Reserved

Recipe Name: Tuna or Salmon Burger
Recipe Category: Lunch Entrée
Portion Size: 1 Hamburger
Ingredients: Yields: 8 servings

Ingredients	Notes:
3 cups tuna, (or canned Salmon)	Water packed drained
1 cup chopped celery	Washed, trimmed and chopped
1 small onion	Washed, peeled and minced
½ cup chopped ripe olives	
½ cup light mayonnaise	
8 oz. low fat Cheddar or Swiss cheese	
8 whole hamburger buns	May use whole wheat

Directions:

Steps:	Directions:	Critical Control Point / Quality Assurance
1	Mix together tuna, celery, onion, olives, and mayonnaise	
2	Top each bun with tuna mixture and shredded cheese	
3	Wrap in foil; bake in a 275 degree oven for 30 minutes	

Time Temperature Sensitive food. *Food safety Standards: hold food for service at an internal temperature above 140° F. Do not mix old product with new. Cool leftover product quickly (within 4 hours) to below 41° F. Follow proper cooling procedures. Store leftovers in a tightly sealed, labeled and dated container. Use leftover within 72 hours if stored in refrigerator or 30 days if stored in the freezer. Reheat leftover product quickly (within 2 hours) to 165 degrees F for 15 seconds. Reheat left over product only once; discard if not used. Cold holding at 41 °F or colder or using time alone (less than four hours).*

<u>**Texture Modified Diets:**</u>

Soft & Bite Size: (aka Bite size) **Food particle size ½ inch (~width of standard fork)** Food must be moist. Cut foods with a knife to a ½" particle size after cooking. Moisten with milk as needed after cutting.

Chopped: Food particle size ¼ inch (~ ½ width of standard fork) Food must be moist. Chop foods with a knife to 1/4" particle size after cooking. Moisten with milk as needed after chopping.

Minced and Moist:(aka Minced/Mechanical Soft/Ground) **Food particle size 1/8 inch (fits through prongs of standard fork)** Food must be moist. Use a food processor to grind food particles into 1/8 inch after cooking. Moisten with milk as needed after processing.

Pureed: Smooth and cohesive. Use a food processor to puree to a smooth consistency. Foods are processed by grinding and then pureeing them. May add milk or sauce to puree. Do not add to much liquid. Puree should still hold its shape. Must not be firm or sticky. Puree foods while still hot. Appearance should be smooth like pudding. Puree cheese with bun. Serve ½ cup puree tuna mixture and 1 cup puree bread/cheese mixture separately

<u>**Therapeutic Modified Diets:**</u>

Lowfat: Omit olives and cheese
Diabetic/No added Sugar/No Conc. Sweets/Calorie Controlled: No changes needed
Bland/Anti Reflux: Omit onion, celery and olives.
Liberal House Renal: Omit olives, mayonnaise and cheese. Use SF bun or SF bread.
No Added Salt: Omit olives
2 Gram Sodium: Omit olives, mayonnaise and cheese. Use SF bun or SF bread.
Gluten Free: Use gluten free hamburger bun. Prepare foods separately to prevent cross contamination.
Allergy Alerts: When an "X" is present, this indicates the allergen is present.
Always read all food labels to ensure allergens are not present.

Wheat	Milk	Eggs	Fish Shellfish	Soy	Peanuts/Nuts	Other
X	X	X	X			

Key: SF= Salt Free D= Diet or Sugarfree LF = Lowfat FF = Fat Free GF = Gluten Free

Copyright 2020 Jacqueline Larson M.S., R.D.N. and Associates.   All Rights Reserved

Recipe Name: Tuna Melt (or Salmon Melt or Turkey Melt or Chicken Melt or Roast Beef Melt)
Recipe Category: Lunch Entrée
Portion Size: 1 sandwich
Ingredients: **Yields: 8 servings**

Ingredients	Notes:
3 cups tuna, water packed	Drained . (or sub diced cooked meat)
1/2 cup finely chopped celery	Washed, trimmed and minced
1 /2 cup onion	Washed, peeled and minced
½ cup margarine	
½ cup light mayonnaise	
8 oz. low fat Cheddar or Swiss cheese	
16 slices bread	May use whole grain

Directions:

Steps:	Directions:	Critical Control Point / Quality Assurance
1	Mix together tuna, celery, onion and mayonnaise in a small bowl	
2	Spread margarine on each slice of bread.	
	Heat non stick pan to medium high heat. Carefully, place bread margarine side down onto heated pan. Top with 1/3 cup tuna mixture and flatten with a spoon. Top with 1 slice cheese. Top with 1 slice of bread with the margarine side out. Cook until golden brown. Turnover and cook until golden brown.	
3	Repeat until all sandwiches are made. Cut in half.	

Time Temperature Sensitive food. *Food safety Standards: hold food for service at an internal temperature above 140° F. Do not mix old product with new. Cool leftover product quickly (within 4 hours) to below 41° F. Follow proper cooling procedures. Store leftovers in a tightly sealed, labeled and dated container. Use leftover within 72 hours if stored in refrigerator or 30 days if stored in the freezer. Reheat leftover product quickly (within 2 hours) to 165 degrees F for 15 seconds. Reheat left over product only once; discard if not used. Cold holding at 41°F or colder or using time alone (less than four hours).*

Texture Modified Diets:
Soft & Bite Size: (aka Bite size) **Food particle size ½ inch (~width of standard fork)** Food must be moist. Cut foods with a knife to a ½" particle size after cooking. Moisten with milk as needed after cutting.
Chopped: Food particle size ¼ inch (~ ½ width of standard fork) Food must be moist. Chop foods with a knife to 1/4" particle size after cooking. Moisten with milk as needed after chopping.
Minced and Moist:(aka Minced/Mechanical Soft/Ground) **Food particle size 1/8 inch (fits through prongs of standard fork)** Food must be moist. Use a food processor to grind food particles into 1/8 inch after cooking. Moisten with milk as needed after processing.
Pureed: Smooth and cohesive. Use a food processor to puree to a smooth consistency. Foods are processed by grinding and then pureeing them. May add milk or sauce to puree. Do not add to much liquid. Puree should still hold its shape. Must not be firm or sticky. Puree foods while still hot. Appearance should be smooth like pudding. Puree bread with cheese. Serve ½ c. puree tuna mixture and 1 c. bread/cheese mixture separately.

Therapeutic Modified Diets:
Lowfat: No changes needed
Diabetic/No added Sugar/No Conc. Sweets/Calorie Controlled: No changes needed.
Bland/Anti Reflux: Omit onion and celery
Liberal House Renal: Use SF margarine or brush with olive oil. Omit cheese and mayonnaise. Use SF bread. (use only low sodium meat less than 140 mg per serving)
No Added Salt: no changes needed
2 Gram Sodium: Use SF margarine or brush with olive oil. Omit cheese and mayonnaise. Use SF bread. (use only low sodium meat less than 140 mg. per serving)
Gluten Free: Use gluten free bread. Prepare foods separately to prevent cross contamination.

Allergy Alerts: When an "X" is present, this indicates the allergen is present. Always read all food labels to ensure allergens are not present.

Wheat	Milk	Eggs	Fish Shellfish	Soy	Peanuts/Nuts	Other
X	x	x	x	X		

Key: SF= Salt Free D= Diet or Sugarfree LF = Lowfat FF = Fat Free GF = Gluten Free

Copyright 2020 Jacqueline Larson M.S., R.D.N. and Associates.   All Rights Reserved

Recipe Name: Tuna Pasta Salad with Green Beans or Salmon Pasta Salad with Green Beans
Recipe Category: Lunch Entrée
Portion Size: 1 cup
Ingredients: Yields: 8 servings

Ingredients	Notes:
1 (16 ounce) package pasta	
4 cups green beans	Washed, trimmed and halved
3 cups canned tuna or salmon	
2 tablespoons olive oil	
1/4 cup sliced unsalted almonds	Toasted
2 teaspoons parsley flakes	
1/3 cup lemon juice	
1/2 teaspoon grated lemon zest	(optional)
1 clove garlic	Washed, peeled and minced
1/4 cup red onion	Washed, peeled and finely chopped
1 teaspoon salt	
1 pinch ground black pepper	
2 Tablespoons capers	(optional)

Directions:

Steps:	Directions:	Critical Control Point /Quality Assurance
1	In a large pot of salted boiling water, cook pasta until al dente, rinse under cold water and drain.	
2	In a large bowl, combine the olive oil, parsley flakes, lemon juice, lemon zest, garlic salt and peppers. Whisk to combine.	
3	Add pasta, tuna or salmon, red onion and toss to coat.	
4	Refrigerate for 1 hour. Top with almonds just before serving.	

Time Temperature Sensitive food. *Food safety Standards: Do not mix old product with new. Cool leftover product quickly (within 4 hours) to below 41° F. Follow proper cooling procedures. Store leftovers in a tightly sealed, labeled and dated container. Use leftover within 72 hours if stored in refrigerator or 30 days if stored in the freezer. Cold holding at 41 °F or colder or using time alone (less than four hours).*

Texture Modified Diets: TIP : use pasta that is the correct particle size.
Soft & Bite Size: (aka Bite size) **Food particle size ½ inch (~width of standard fork)** Food must be moist. Cut foods with a knife to a ½" particle size prior to mixing. Moisten with broth as needed. Foods that do not process well should be omitted. Omit: almonds and capers.
Chopped: Food particle size ¼ inch (~ ½ width of standard fork) Food must be moist. Chop foods with a knife to 1/4" particle size prior to mixing. Moisten with broth as needed. Foods that do not process well should be omitted. Omit: almonds and capers.
Minced and Moist:(aka Minced/Mechanical Soft/Ground) **Food particle size 1/8 inch (fits through prongs of standard fork)** Food must be moist. Use a food processor to grind food particles into 1/8 inch prior to mixing. Moisten with broth as needed. Foods that do not process well should be omitted. Omit: almonds and capers.
Pureed: Smooth and cohesive. Use a food processor to puree to a smooth consistency. Foods are processed by grinding and then pureeing them. May add broth or sauce to puree. Do not add to much liquid. Puree should still hold its shape. Must not be firm or sticky. Puree foods while still hot. Appearance should be smooth like pudding. Foods that do not process well should be omitted. Omit: almonds and capers. Serve ½ cup puree pasta, ½ cup puree green beans and 1/3 cup tuna mixture separately.
Therapeutic Modified Diets:
Lowfat: Omit almonds
Diabetic/No added Sugar/No Conc. Sweets/Calorie Controlled: No changes needed
Bland/Anti Reflux: Omit red onion, almonds, black pepper and garlic
Liberal House Renal: Omit almonds, salt and capers
No Added Salt: Omit capers
2 Gram Sodium: Omit salt and capers
Gluten Free: Use gluten free pasta. Prepare foods separately to prevent cross contamination.
Allergy Alerts: When an "X" is present, this indicates the allergen is present. Always read all food labels to ensure allergens are not present.

Wheat	Milk	Eggs	Fish Shellfish	Soy	Peanuts/Nuts	Other
X		X	x		x	

Key: SF= Salt Free D= Diet or Sugarfree LF = Lowfat FF = Fat Free GF = Gluten Free

Recipe Name: Tuna Pasta Salad with Peas, Red Bell Peppers and Red Onion
Recipe Category: Lunch Entrée
Portion Size: 1 cup
Ingredients: **Yields: 8 servings**

Ingredients	Notes:
1 (16 ounce) package pasta	
1 cups peas, frozen	
1 red bell pepper	
3 cups canned tuna	
2 tablespoons olive oil	
2 teaspoons parsley flakes	
1/3 cup lemon juice	
1/2 teaspoon grated lemon zest	(optional)
1 clove garlic	Washed, peeled and minced
1/4 cup red onion	Washed, peeled and finely chopped
1 teaspoon salt	
1 pinch ground black pepper	

Directions:

Steps:	Directions:	Critical Control Point /Quality Assurance
1	In a large pot of salted boiling water, cook pasta until al dente, rinse under cold water and drain.	
2	In a large bowl, combine the olive oil, parsley flakes, lemon juice, lemon zest, garlic salt and peppers. Whisk to combine.	
3	Add pasta, tuna, red onion, bell pepper and toss to coat.	
4	Refrigerate for 1 hour.	

Time Temperature Sensitive food. *Food safety Standards: Do not mix old product with new. Cool leftover product quickly (within 4 hours) to below 41°F. Follow proper cooling procedures. Store leftovers in a tightly sealed, labeled and dated container. Use leftover within 72 hours if stored in refrigerator or 30 days if stored in the freezer. Cold holding at 41°F or colder or using time alone (less than four hours).*

Texture Modified Diets: TIP: Use pasta that is the correct particle size.
Soft & Bite Size: (aka Bite size) **Food particle size ½ inch (~width of standard fork)** Food must be moist. Cut foods with a knife to a ½" particle size prior to mixing. Moisten with broth as needed. Cook bell pepper to soften.
Chopped: Food particle size ¼ inch (~ ½ width of standard fork) Food must be moist. Chop foods with a knife to 1/4" particle size prior to mixing. Moisten with broth as needed. Cook bell pepper to soften.
Minced and Moist:(aka Minced/Mechanical Soft/Ground) **Food particle size 1/8 inch (fits through prongs of standard fork)** Food must be moist. Use a food processor to grind food particles into 1/8 inch prior to mixing. Moisten with broth as needed.
Pureed: Smooth and cohesive. Use a food processor to puree to a smooth consistency. Foods are processed by grinding and then pureeing them. May add broth or sauce to puree. Do not add to much liquid. Puree should still hold its shape. Must not be firm or sticky. Puree foods while still hot. Appearance should be smooth like pudding. Serve ½ cup puree pasta, ½ cup puree peas/pepper and 1/3 cup tuna mixture separately. Mix in the dressing with the tuna.

Therapeutic Modified Diets:
Lowfat: No changes
Diabetic/No added Sugar/No Conc. Sweets/Calorie Controlled: No changes needed
Bland/Anti Reflux: Omit red onion, bell pepper, black pepper, lemon, parsley and garlic
Liberal House Renal: Omit salt
No Added Salt: No changes needed
2 Gram Sodium: Omit salt
Gluten Free: Use gluten free pasta. Prepare foods separately to prevent cross contamination.
Allergy Alerts: When an "X" is present, this indicates the allergen is present. Always read all food labels to ensure allergens are not present.

Wheat	Milk	Eggs	Fish Shellfish	Soy	Peanuts/Nuts	Other
X		X	x			

Key: SF= Salt Free D= Diet or Sugarfree LF = Lowfat FF = Fat Free GF = Gluten Free

Recipe Name: Tuna Pasta Salad with White Beans and Olives
Recipe Category: Lunch Entrée
Portion Size: 1 cup
Ingredients: Yields: 8 servings

Ingredients	Notes:
1 (16 ounce) package pasta (medium shells)	
1 can (14 oz.) canned white beans	Drained and rinsed
1 red bell pepper	
2 cups canned tuna	
¼ cup black olive, pitted and sliced	
½ cup light mayonnaise	
1 tablespoon lemon juice	
1/2 teaspoon grated lemon zest	(optional)
1 clove garlic	Washed, peeled and minced
¼ cup light sour cream	
1/4 cup red onion	Washed, peeled and finely chopped
1 teaspoon salt	
1 pinch ground black pepper	

Directions:

Steps:	Directions:	Critical Control Point /Quality Assurance
1	In a large pot of salted boiling water, cook pasta until al dente, rinse under cold water and drain.	
2	In a large bowl, combine the mayonnaise, lemon juice, lemon zest, garlic, sour cream, salt and pepper. Whisk to combine.	
3	Add pasta, tuna, red onion, beans, bell pepper and Toss to coat. Refrigerate for 1 hour.	

Time Temperature Sensitive food. Food safety Standards: Do not mix old product with new. Cool leftover product quickly (within 4 hours) to below 41° F. Follow proper cooling procedures. Store leftovers in a tightly sealed, labeled and dated container. Use leftover within 72 hours if stored in refrigerator or 30 days if stored in the freezer. Cold holding at 41°F or colder or using time alone (less than four hours).

Texture Modified Diets: TIP: use pasta that is the correct particle size.
Soft & Bite Size: (aka Bite size) **Food particle size ½ inch (~width of standard fork)** Food must be moist. Cut foods with a knife to a ½" particle size prior to mixing. Moisten with broth as needed. Cook bell pepper to soften.
Chopped: Food particle size ¼ inch (~ ½ width of standard fork) Food must be moist. Chop foods with a knife to 1/4" particle size prior to mixing. Moisten with broth as needed. Cook bell pepper to soften.
Minced and Moist: (aka Minced/Mechanical Soft/Ground) **Food particle size 1/8 inch (fits through prongs of standard fork)** Food must be moist. Use a food processor to grind food particles into 1/8 inch prior to mixing. Moisten with broth as needed.
Pureed: Smooth and cohesive. Use a food processor to puree to a smooth consistency. Foods are processed by grinding and then pureeing them. May add broth or sauce to puree. Do not add to much liquid. Puree should still hold its shape. Must not be firm or sticky. Puree foods while still hot. Appearance should be smooth like pudding. Serve ½ cup puree pasta, ½ cup puree pasta 1/3 cup tuna mixture separately. Mix in the dressing with the tuna.

Therapeutic Modified Diets:
Lowfat: No changes
Diabetic/No added Sugar/No Conc. Sweets/Calorie Controlled: No changes needed
Bland/Anti Reflux: Omit red onion, bell pepper, black pepper, lemon, parsley and garlic
Liberal House Renal: Omit salt, mayonnaise, white beans and olives
No Added Salt: Omit olives
2 Gram Sodium: Omit salt and olives
Gluten Free: Use gluten free pasta. Prepare foods separately to prevent cross contamination.
Allergy Alerts: When an "X" is present, this indicates the allergen is present. Always read all food labels to ensure allergens are not present.

Wheat	Milk	Eggs	Fish Shellfish	Soy	Peanuts/Nuts	Other
X	X	X	x			

Key: SF= Salt Free D= Diet or Sugarfree LF = Lowfat FF = Fat Free GF = Gluten Free

Copyright 2020 Jacqueline Larson M.S., R.D.N. and Associates.   All Rights Reserved

Recipe Name: Tuna Pesto Pasta Salad with Sun Dried Tomatoes (or Sub. Salmon, Chicken, or Turkey)
Recipe Category: Lunch Entrée
Portion Size: 1 cup
Ingredients: Yields: 8 servings

Ingredients	Notes:
1 (16 ounce) package pasta	May use whole grain
1 cup sun dried tomatoes	Finely chopped
2 tablespoons olive oil	
3 cups tuna*, cooked diced chicken, cooked diced turkey or cooked or canned salmon	*Use water packed tuna
1/2 cup prepared pesto sauce	Use recipe in cookbook for pesto sauce.
2 tablespoons lemon juice	

Directions:

Steps:	Directions:	Critical Control Point /Quality Assurance
1	In a large pot of salted boiling water, cook pasta until al dente, rinse under cold water and drain	
2	In a large bowl, combine the olive oil, lemon juice, sun dried tomatoes, pesto sauce. Add pasta and toss. Gently toss in tuna, salmon, chicken or turkey.	
3	Refrigerate for 1 hour	Keep chilled until ready to serve

Time Temperature Sensitive food. *Food safety Standards: Do not mix old product with new. Cool leftover product quickly (within 4 hours) to below 41° F. Follow proper cooling procedures. Store leftovers in a tightly sealed, labeled and dated container. Use leftover within 72 hours if stored in refrigerator or 30 days if stored in the freezer. Cold holding at 41°F or colder or using time alone (less than four hours).*

<u>Texture Modified Diets: Tip: use pasta that the correct particle size.</u>
Soft & Bite Size: (aka Bite size) **Food particle size ½ inch (~width of standard fork)** Food must be moist. Cut foods with a knife to a ½" particle size prior to mixing. Moisten with broth as needed. Foods that do not process well should be omitted. Omit: Sun dried tomatoes. Sub. fresh tomatoes.
Chopped: Food particle size ¼ inch (~ ½ width of standard fork) Food must be moist. Chop foods with a knife to 1/4" particle size prior to mixing. Moisten with broth as needed. Foods that do not process well should be omitted. Omit: Sun dried tomatoes. Sub. fresh tomatoes.
Minced and Moist: (aka Minced/Mechanical Soft/Ground) **Food particle size 1/8 inch (fits through prongs of standard fork)** Food must be moist. Use a food processor to grind food particles into 1/8 inch prior to mixing. Moisten with broth as needed. Foods that do not process well should be omitted. Omit: Sun dried tomatoes. Sub. fresh tomatoes.
Pureed: Smooth and cohesive. Use a food processor to puree to a smooth consistency. Foods are processed by grinding and then pureeing them. May add broth or sauce to puree. Do not add to much liquid. Puree should still hold its shape. Must not be firm or sticky. Puree foods while still hot. Appearance should be smooth like pudding. Foods that do not process well should be omitted. Omit: Sun dried tomatoes. Sub. fresh tomatoes. Serve ½ cup pasta and ½ cup of tuna mixture. Puree pasta and tuna mixture separately.

<u>Therapeutic Modified Diets:</u>
Lowfat: No changes needed
Diabetic/No added Sugar/No Conc. Sweets/Calorie Controlled: no changes needed
Bland/Anti Reflux: Omit lemon juice, sun dried tomatoes and pesto sauce
Liberal House Renal: Omit sun dried tomatoes and pesto sauce
No Added Salt: No changed needed
2 Gram Sodium: Omit sun dried tomatoes and pesto sauce. May add fresh tomatoes and basil.
Gluten Free: Use gluten free pasta, pesto sauce and sun dried tomatoes. Prepare foods separately to prevent cross contamination.

Allergy Alerts: When an "X" is present, this indicates the allergen is present. Always read all food labels to ensure allergens are not present.

Wheat	Milk	Eggs	Fish Shellfish	Soy	Peanuts/Nuts	Other
X	X	X	X		X	

Key: SF= Salt Free D= Diet or Sugarfree LF = Lowfat FF = Fat Free GF = Gluten Free

Recipe Name: Tuna Salad
Recipe Category: Lunch Entrée
Portion Size: 1/3 cup
Ingredients: Yields: 8 servings

Ingredients	Notes:
3 cups canned tuna	Drained, water packed
1 cup diced celery or cucumber	Washed, trimmed and minced
1/4 cup onion	Washed, peeled and minced
1 tablespoon chives or parsley	May use dried or fresh.
1/2 cup light mayonnaise	
Lettuce and tomato (optional)	Washed, trimmed and sliced

Directions:

Steps:	Directions:	Critical Control Point /Quality Assurance
1	Mix ingredients.	Keep chilled until ready to serve
2	Serve 1/3 cup portion.	
3	Garnish with lettuce and tomatoes.	

Time Temperature Sensitive food. *Food safety Standards: Do not mix old product with new. Cool leftover product quickly (within 4 hours) to below 41°F. Follow proper cooling procedures. Store leftovers in a tightly sealed, labeled and dated container. Use leftover within 72 hours if stored in refrigerator or 30 days if stored in the freezer. Cold holding at 41°F or colder or using time alone (less than four hours).*

<u>Texture Modified Diets:</u>

Soft & Bite Size: (aka Bite size) **Food particle size ½ inch (~width of standard fork)** Food must be moist. Cut foods with a knife to a ½" particle size prior to mixing. Moisten with broth as needed. Foods that do not process well should be omitted. Omit: chives and cucumber peel.

Chopped: Food particle size ¼ inch (~ ½ width of standard fork) Food must be moist. Chop foods with a knife to 1/4" particle size prior to mixing. Moisten with broth as needed. Foods that do not process well should be omitted. Omit: chives and cucumber peel.

Minced and Moist: (aka Minced/Mechanical Soft/Ground) **Food particle size 1/8 inch (fits through prongs of standard fork)** Food must be moist. Use a food processor to grind food particles into 1/8 inch prior to mixing. Moisten with broth as needed. Foods that do not process well should be omitted. Omit: chives. and cucumber peel.

Pureed: Smooth and cohesive. Use a food processor to puree to a smooth consistency. Foods are processed by grinding and then pureeing them. May add broth or sauce to puree. Do not add to much liquid. Puree should still hold its shape. Must not be firm or sticky. Puree foods while still hot. Appearance should be smooth like pudding. Foods that do not process well should be omitted. Omit: chives and cucumber peel.. Serve1/3 cup puree tuna mixture

<u>Therapeutic Modified Diets:</u>

Lowfat: No changes needed
Diabetic/No added Sugar/No Conc. Sweets/Calorie Controlled: no changes
Bland/Anti Reflux: omit onion, celery, cucumber, chives or parsley, and tomato.
Liberal House Renal: omit tomato and mayonnaise.
No Added Salt: no changes needed
2 Gram Sodium: Omit mayonnaise.
Gluten Free: No changes needed
Allergy Alerts: When an "X" is present, this indicates the allergen is present.
Always read all food labels to ensure allergens are not present.

Wheat	Milk	Eggs	Fish Shellfish	Soy	Peanuts/Nuts	Other
		X	X			

Key: SF= Salt Free D= Diet or Sugarfree LF = Lowfat FF = Fat Free GF = Gluten Free

Recipe Name: Tuna Salad Sandwiches
Recipe Category: Lunch Entrée
Portion Size: 1 Sandwich
Ingredients: Yields: 8 servings

Ingredients	Notes:
3 Cups canned tuna	Drained, water packed
2 Cups diced celery or cucumber	Washed, trimmed and diced
1/4 Cup onion	Washed, peeled and chopped
1 Tablespoon chives or parsley	May use dried or fresh.
1/2 Cup light mayonnaise	
16 slices of bread	May use whole grain
Lettuce and tomato (optional)	Washed, trimmed and sliced

Directions:

Steps:	Directions:	Critical Control Point /Quality Assurance
1	Mix ingredients (except bread)	Keep chilled until ready to serve
2	Divide evenly on eight sandwiches.	
3	Garnish sandwiches with lettuce and tomatoes	

Time Temperature Sensitive food. Food safety Standards: Do not mix old product with new. Cool leftover product quickly (within 4 hours) to below 41°F. Follow proper cooling procedures. Store leftovers in a tightly sealed, labeled and dated container. Use leftover within 72 hours if stored in refrigerator or 30 days if stored in the freezer. Cold holding at 41°F or colder or using time alone (less than four hours).

Texture Modified Diets:

Soft & Bite Size: (aka Bite size) **Food particle size ½ inch (~width of standard fork)** Food must be moist. Cut foods with a knife to a ½" particle size prior to mixing. Moisten with milk as needed. Foods that do not process well should be omitted. Omit: chives and cucumber peel.

Chopped: Food particle size ¼ inch (~ ½ width of standard fork) Food must be moist. Chop foods with a knife to 1/4" particle size prior to mixing. Moisten with milk as needed. Foods that do not process well should be omitted. Omit: chives and cucumber peel.

Minced and Moist: (aka Minced/Mechanical Soft/Ground) **Food particle size 1/8 inch (fits through prongs of standard fork)** Food must be moist. Use a food processor to grind food particles into 1/8 inch prior to mixing. Moisten with milk as needed. Foods that do not process well should be omitted. Omit: chives. and cucumber peel.

Pureed: Smooth and cohesive. Use a food processor to puree to a smooth consistency. Foods are processed by grinding and then pureeing them. May add broth or sauce to puree. Do not add to much liquid. Puree should still hold its shape. Must not be firm or sticky. Puree foods while still hot. Appearance should be smooth like pudding. Foods that do not process well should be omitted. Omit: chives and cucumber peel.. Serve1/3 cup puree tuna mixture
Serve1/3 cup puree tuna mixture and 2 slices puree bread separately. Puree bread and tuna separately

Therapeutic Modified Diets:

Lowfat: No changes needed
Diabetic/No added Sugar/No Conc. Sweets/Calorie Controlled: no changes needed
Bland/Anti Reflux: omit onion, celery, cucumber, chives or parsley, and tomato.
Liberal House Renal: omit tomato and mayonnaise. Use low sodium bread.
No Added Salt: no changes needed
2 Gram Sodium: Omit mayonnaise. Use low sodium bread.
Gluten Free: Use gluten free bread. Prepare separately to prevent cross contamination.
Allergy Alerts: When an "X" is present, this indicates the allergen is present.
Always read all food labels to ensure allergens are not present.

Wheat	Milk	Eggs	Fish Shellfish	Soy	Peanuts/Nuts	Other
X		X	X			

Key: SF= Salt Free D= Diet or Sugarfree LF = Lowfat FF = Fat Free GF = Gluten Free

Recipe Name: Tuna Tortilla Wrap
Recipe Category: Lunch Entrée
Portion Size: 1/3 cup
Ingredients: **Yields: 8 servings**

Ingredients	Notes:
3 cups canned tuna	Drained, water packed
½ cup celery	Washed, trimmed and minced
1/4 cup onion	Washed, peeled and minced
1 tablespoon pickle relish	
1/2 cup light mayonnaise	
1 cup spinach leaves	Washed, trimmed and shredded
½ cup diced tomatoes	Washed, trimmed and diced
1 cup low fat sharp cheddar cheese	
8 tortillas	

Directions:

Steps:	Directions:	Critical Control Point /Quality Assurance
1	Combine tuna, celery, onion, pickle relish and mayonnaise in a small bowl.	
2	Spread each tortilla tuna mixture.	
3	Top with spinach, tomato and cheese.	
4	Roll up tight and cover each with plastic wrap. Refrigerate for 1 hour before serving	

Time Temperature Sensitive food. *Food safety Standards: Do not mix old product with new. Cool leftover product quickly (within 4 hours) to below 41°F. Follow proper cooling procedures. Store leftovers in a tightly sealed, labeled and dated container. Use leftover within 72 hours if stored in refrigerator or 30 days if stored in the freezer. Cold holding at 41°F or colder or using time alone (less than four hours).*

Texture Modified Diets:

Soft & Bite Size: (aka Bite size) **Food particle size ½ inch (~width of standard fork)** Food must be moist. Cut foods with a knife to a ½" particle size prior to layering. Moisten with milk as needed. . Arrange on plate separately: Tortilla, tuna salad mixture, cheese, and vegetables. Moisten with milk if needed.

Chopped: Food particle size ¼ inch (~ ½ width of standard fork) Food must be moist. Chop foods with a knife to 1/4" particle size prior to layering. Moisten with milk as needed. . Arrange on plate separately: Tortilla, tuna salad mixture, cheese, and vegetables. Moisten with milk if needed.

Minced and Moist:(aka Minced/Mechanical Soft/Ground) **Food particle size 1/8 inch (fits through prongs of standard fork)** Food must be moist. Use a food processor to grind food particles into 1/8 inch prior to layering. Moisten with broth as needed. . Arrange on plate separately: Tortilla, tuna salad mixture, cheese, and vegetables. Moisten with milk if needed.

Pureed: Smooth and cohesive. Use a food processor to puree to a smooth consistency. Foods are processed by grinding and then pureeing them. May add broth or sauce to puree. Do not add to much liquid. Puree should still hold its shape. Must not be firm or sticky. Puree foods while still hot. Appearance should be smooth like pudding. Use 1/3 cup puree meat. 1 tortilla puree with milk and cheese, and ½ c. per serving. Puree with milk if needed. Spinach, tomato and onion may be puree with tortilla.

Therapeutic Modified Diets:

Lowfat: No changes needed
Diabetic/No added Sugar/No Conc. Sweets/Calorie Controlled: no changes
Bland/Anti Reflux: omit onion, pickle relish, and tomato.
Liberal House Renal: omit tomato, pickle relish, cheese and mayonnaise.
No Added Salt: Omit pickle relish.
2 Gram Sodium: Omit mayonnaise, pickle relish and cheese
Gluten Free: Use gluten free corn tortilla. Prepare foods separately to prevent cross contamination.

Allergy Alerts: When an "X" is present, this indicates the allergen is present. Always read all food labels to ensure allergens are not present.

Wheat	Milk	Eggs	Fish Shellfish	Soy	Peanuts/Nuts	Other
X	X	X	X			

Key: SF= Salt Free D= Diet or Sugarfree LF = Lowfat FF = Fat Free GF = Gluten Free

Copyright 2020 Jacqueline Larson M.S., R.D.N. and Associates. All Rights Reserved

Recipe Name: Tuna or Salmon with Angel Hair Pasta (or Chicken with Angel Hair Pasta Or Turkey with Angel Hair Pasta)
Recipe Category: Lunch Entrée
Portion Size: 1 cup
Ingredients: **Yields: 8 servings**

Ingredients	Notes:
1 lb. angel hair pasta	May use whole grain
3 cups drained water packed, canned tuna, canned salmon, cooked diced chicken or cooked diced turkey	
3 cups of cherry tomatoes	Washed and halved
8 oz. low fat shredded Mozzarella Cheese	
1/2 cup chopped green onions	Washed, trimmed and chopped
1/4 cup grated Parmesan cheese	
1/2 cup lemon juice	
2 tablespoons olive oil	
1 teaspoon minced garlic	Washed, peeled and minced.
1/2 teaspoon salt	
1/4 teaspoon ground black pepper	

Directions:

Steps:	Directions:	Critical Control Point / Quality Assurance
1	Prepare pasta according to the directions on the package. Drain.	
2	In a small bowl combine lemon juice, olive oil, garlic, salt and pepper.	Keep chilled until ready to serve.
3	In a large bowl combine pasta, tuna (or other meat), tomatoes, mozzarella, and green onions.	
4	Drizzle with dressing and toss to coat. Top with Parmesan cheese.	Serve hot or keep chilled until ready to serve chilled.

Time Temperature Sensitive food. *Food safety Standards: Do not mix old product with new. Cool leftover product quickly (within 4 hours) to below 41°F. Follow proper cooling procedures. Store leftovers in a tightly sealed, labeled and dated container. Use leftover within 72 hours if stored in refrigerator or 30 days if stored in the freezer. Cold holding at 41°F or colder or using time alone (less than four hours).*

<u>Texture Modified Diets: TIP: use pasta that is the correct particle size.</u>
Soft & Bite Size: (aka Bite size) **Food particle size ½ inch (~width of standard fork)** Food must be moist. Cut foods with a knife to a ½" particle size prior to mixing. Moisten with broth as needed. Foods that do not process well should be omitted. Omit: green onions.
Chopped: Food particle size ¼ inch (~ ½ width of standard fork) Food must be moist. Chop foods with a knife to 1/4" particle size prior to mixing. Moisten with broth as needed. Foods that do not process well should be omitted. Omit: green onions.
Minced and Moist: (aka Minced/Mechanical Soft/Ground) **Food particle size 1/8 inch (fits through prongs of standard fork)** Food must be moist. Use a food processor to grind food particles into 1/8 inch prior to mixing. Moisten with broth as needed. Foods that do not process well should be omitted. Omit: green onions.
Pureed: Smooth and cohesive. Use a food processor to puree to a smooth consistency. Foods are processed by grinding and then pureeing them. May add broth or sauce to puree. Do not add to much liquid. Puree should still hold its shape. Must not be firm or sticky. Puree foods while still hot. Appearance should be smooth like pudding. Foods that do not process well should be omitted. Omit: green onions.
Serve ½ cup pasta and 1/3 cup of tuna mixture. Puree pasta and tuna mixture separately.
<u>Therapeutic Modified Diets:</u>
Lowfat: no changes needed
Diabetic/No added Sugar/No Conc. Sweets/Calorie Controlled: No changes needed.
Bland/Anti Reflux: Omit lemon juice, green onions, cherry tomatoes and pepper
Liberal House Renal: Omit cherry tomatoes, Mozzarella cheese, Parmesan cheese, and salt
No Added Salt: No changes needed
2 Gram Sodium: Omit Mozzarella cheese, Parmesan cheese and salt.
Gluten Free: Use gluten free pasta. Prepare foods separately to prevent cross contamination.
Allergy Alerts: When an "X" is present, this indicates the allergen is present. Always read all food labels to ensure allergens are not present.

Wheat	Milk	Eggs	Fish Shellfish	Soy	Peanuts/Nuts	Other
X	X	X	X			

Key: SF= Salt Free D= Diet or Sugarfree LF = Lowfat FF = Fat Free GF = Gluten Free

Meats Recipe Index
Beef Dinner Recipes Index
Asian Skirt Steak 10
Baked Rigatoni with Beef 11
Beef and Broccoli 12
Beef and Brown Rice Casserole 14
Beef and Brown Rice Salad 15
Beef and Tatar Casserole 17
Beef Barley Skillet 18
Beef Barley Soup 19
Beef Carnitas 21
Beef Cubes with Peppers 22
Beef Fajitas 23
Beef Goulash 25
Beef Lo Mein 26
Beef Pepper Steak 28
Beef Pizza 29
Beef Pot Roast 30
Beef Sesame Stir Fry 31
Beef Stew 32
Beef Stroganoff 33
Beef Tacos 34
Beef Tenderloin 36
Beef Tenderloin Medallions 37
Beef Tips and Noodles 38
Beef Tostada 39
Broiled steak 40
Cabbage Roll Casserole 41
Cheese Hamburger Casserole 42
Chili 43
Chili and Macaroni 44
Corn Beef And Cabbage 45
Cornbread Tamale Bake 46
Cornbread Tamale Pie 48
Curried Beef 50
Curried Beef Couscous 51
English Muffin Pizzas 52
Greek Salad with Steak 53
Hamburgers 54
Korean Beef 55
Lasagna 56
Lasagna with Italian Sausage 57
Meat and Pasta Bake 59
Meatballs in Dijon Gravy 60
Meatballs in Tomato Sauce 61
Meatballs in Cheese Sauce 62
Meatloaf 63
Mexican spaghetti 64
Mongolian Beef 65
Open Faced Roast Beef Sandwich with Gravy 66

Pasta with Creamy Tomato Basil Meat Sauce 68
Pasta with Tomato Meat Sauce 69
Patty Melt 70
Penne Pasta with Meat Sauce 71
Pizza Casserole 72
Porcupine Meatballs 73
Pot Roast in Foil 74
Pot Roast with Potatoes and Carrots 75
Roast Beef with Gravy 76
Salisbury Steak 77
Sauerbraten 78
Sauté Beef Liver and Onions 79
Shephard's Pie 80
Sloppy Joes on a Bun 81
Spaghetti and Meat Sauce 82
Steak with Barley Kale Salad 83
Stuffed Peppers 84
Stuffed Potato with Chili 85
Stuffing Hamburger Casserole 86
Swedish Meatballs 87
Swiss Steak 88
Taco Beef Pizza 89
Taco Pasta 90
Taco Supreme 91
Teriyaki Beef 92
Vegetable Beef Soup 93
Beef Lunch Recipes Index
Asian Pasta Salad with Beef and Broccoli 95
Beef Gyros 97
Beef Pizzas 99
Beef Salad 100
Corn Beef Hash 101
French Dip Sandwich 102
French Onion Sandwich 103
Grilled Roast Beef and Cheese Sandwich 104
Meatball Sandwich 105
Pita Pocket Sandwich 106
Reuben Sandwiches 107
Roast Beef Sandwich 108
Roast Beef Tortilla Wraps 109
Sesame Lime Steak Wraps 110
Taco Salad 112
Ham Dinner Entrees Recipes Index
Apricot Glazed Ham 115
Baked Ham 116
Boneless Baked Ham 118
Cheese Ham and Pasta Bake 119

Cheese Ham and Red Potato Bake 121
Cheese Ham Broccoli Bake 123
Florentine Ham Casserole 124
Glazed Ham Loaf 125
Grilled Ham Steak with Pineapple 126
Ground Ham on Pineapple Slices or Peach Halves 127
Ham and Bean Skillet 128
Ham and Dijon Pineapple Sauce 129
Ham Fettuccini 130
Ham and Macaroni Twists 131
Ham and Pasta Salad 133
Ham and Tortellini Alfredo 135
Ham Hocks and Beans 136
Ham Jambalaya 137
Ham Noodle Casserole 138
Honey Dijon Ham 140
Ham Lunch Entrees Recipes Index
Chef Salad 142
Ham and Cheese Sandwich 143
Ham and Linguini Primavera 144
Ham Salad 145
Lima Beans and Ham Salad 146
Submarine Sandwich 147
Lamb Dinner Entrees Recipes Index
Acorn Squash with Lamb 149
Lamb Chops with Mint Jelly 150
Spicy Apricot Lamb Chops 151
Pork Dinner Entrees Recipes Index
Asian Pork Tenderloin 153
Baked Pork Chop 154
BBQ Pork Sandwich 155
Breaded Pork Chop 156
Lemon Garlic Pork Tenderloin 157
Oriental Pork Tortillas 158
Pork Carnitas 160
Pork Chop Adobo 162
Pork Chop and Rice 163
Pork Chop and Stuffing 164
Pork Chop Dijon 165
Pork Chop O' Brien 166
Pork Chop Sauté 167
Pork Chops in Sour Cream 168
Pork Chops in Spiced Peaches 169
Pork Chops in Tangy Sauce 170
Pork Chops in Apple Curry 171
Pork Chops with Apple Mustard Glaze 172
Pork chop with Apple Raisin Sauce 173

Copyright 2020- Jacqueline Larson M.S., R.D.N. and Associates.   All Rights Reserved

Pork Chop with Apricot Ginger Teriyaki Sauce 174
Pork Chop with Cheesy Rice Casserole 175
Pork Chop with Chili Rub and Pineapple Salsa 176
Pork Chops with Coriander 177
Pork Chop with Cranberry Applesauce 178
Pork Chop with Creamy Herb Sauce 179
Pork Chop with Curry Mango Sauce 180
Pork Chop with Fresh Plum Sauce 181
Pork Chop with Honey Garlic Glaze 183
Pork Chop with Honey Orange Glaze 184
Pork Chop with Lemon Sauce 185
Pork Chop with Mexicali Sauce 186
Pork Chop with Mexican Marinade 187
Pork Chops with Mushrooms 188
Pork Chops with Orange Mustard Sauce 189
Pork Chop with Quinoa Salad 190
Pork Chop with Ratatouille 192
Pork Chow Mein 194
Pork Fajitas 195
Pork Lettuce Wraps 197
Pork Low Mein 199
Pork Mediterranean 201
Pork Roast with Sauerkraut 202
Pork Stir Fry with Vegetables 203
Pork Tenderloin Brown Rice Salad 204
Pork Tenderloin Medallions 206
Pork Tenderloin Piccata 207
Pork Tenderloin with Cranberry Glaze 208
Pork Tetrazzini 209
Spicy Apricot Pork Chops 210
Sweet and Sour Pork 211
Pork Lunch Entrees Recipes Index
Asian Pork Noodle Soup 214
Bacon Lettuce Tomato Sandwich 215
Bacon Lettuce Tomato Wrap 216
Grilled Ham and Cheese Sandwich 217
Pork and Corn Salad 218

Pork Tenderloin and Couscous Salad with Raisins and Walnuts 219
Sausage Dinner Recipes Index
Brats Sandwich 222
Cheese Sausage Quiche 223
Hawaiian Pineapple with Sweet and Sour Turkey Sausage 224
Italian Sausage Minestrone Soup 225
Italian Sausage Sandwich 227
Italian Sausage Soup with Tortellini 228
Italian Sausage with Sweet Pepper and Pasta 230
Jambalaya 231
Kielbasa Potato Bake 233
Kielbasa, Sauerkraut and Red Potato Stew 234
Pasta and Italian Sausage in a Creamy Basil Tomato Sauce 235
Pepperoni Stromboli 236
Rigatoni with Cream Basil Tomato Sauce and Italian Sausage 237
Turkey Sausage and Pasta with Alfredo Sauce 238
Turkey Sausage and Pasta with Sun Dried Tomatoes 239
Turkey Sausage Skillet 240
Zucchini Stuffed with Italian Sausage 241
Sausage Lunch Recipes Index
Hot Dogs on a Bun 244
Hot Dogs with Chili 245
Kale and Sausage Soup 246
Pepperoni Pizza 247
Winter Vegetable Turkey Sausage and Spelt Soup 248
Seafood Dinner Recipes Index
Baked Cod with Lemon 250
Baked Fish Cilantro Lime 251
Blackened Tilapia Fish 252
Brazilian Fish Stew 253
Broiled Parmesan Fish 255
Crab Cakes with Red Pepper Sauce 256
Cream Salmon 258
Cream Tuna 259
Creamy Pesto Shrimp with Linguine 260
Creamy Salmon and Pasta Salad 262
Creamy Tuna and Pasta Salad 263
Fish Tacos with Corn Salsa 264

Fish Tacos with Creamy Cilantro Lime Dressing 265
Garlic Ginger and Coconut White Fish 267
Glazed Salmon 269
Homey Mustard Salmon 270
Lemon Dijon Baked Fish 271
Mediterranean Salmon Orzo Salad 272
Mediterranean Tuna Orzo Salad 274
Salmon and Peas Pasta Salad 276
Salmon Cakes 277
Salmon Cakes with Creamy Citrus Sauce 278
Salmon Cakes with Lemon Dill Sauce 280
Salmon Cakes with Red Pepper Sauce 282
Salmon Chowder 284
Salmon Leek Casserole 285
Salmon Loaf 287
Salmon Muffin Melt 288
Salmon Noodle Casserole 289
Salmon Patties with Cheese Sauce 291
Salmon with Almonds and Herbs 293
Salmon with Creamy Linguini 294
Salmon with Fettuccini 296
Salmon with Mango Salsa 297
Sesame Ginger Salmon 298
Shrimp and Gouda in Pastry Shells 299
Shrimp Fajitas 301
Shrimp Gumbo in Pastry Shells 303
Shrimp Lo Mein 305
Shrimp Marinated in Chili Garlic Sauce 307
Shrimp Salad with Creamy Tarragon Dressing 308
Shrimp Taco with Cilantro Lime Dressing 309
Southwestern Style Salmon Casserole 311
Southwestern Style Tuna Casserole 313
Sweet and Sour Shrimp 315
Tuna and Pea Pasta Salad 317
Tuna Baked Spaghetti 318
Tuna Cakes 319
Tuna Cakes with Citrus Sauce 320

Tuna Cakes with Lemon Dill Sauce 321
Tuna Cakes with Red Pepper Sauce 323
Tuna Leek Casserole 325
Tuna Loaf 327
Tuna Muffin Melt 328
Tuna Noodle Casserole 329
Tuna or Salmon Pasta with Lemon Garlic Sauce 331
Tuna and Pasta Salad with Lemon 332
Tuna Patties with Cheese Sauce 333
Tuna Pea Pasta Salad 335
Tuna Salad with Creamy Tarragon Dressing 336
Tuna Tortilla Roll Ups 337
Tuna Pasta with Creamy Linguine 338

White Fish with Coconut Curry Sauce 340

Seafood Lunch Recipes Index
Crab and Pea Pasta Salad 343
Crab and Spinach Quiche 344
Crab Enchilada 346
Crab Salad 348
Crab Salad with Thousand Island Dressing 349
Garden Salmon Pasta Salad 350
Garden Tuna Pasta Salad 351
Salmon Pasta Salad with Peas, Red Bell Peppers and Red Onion 352
Salmon Quesadillas 353
Salmon Salad 354
Salmon Salad Sandwich 355
Seared Ahi Tuna 356
Tuna and Macaroni Salad 357

Tuna and Tomato Open Faced Melts 358
Tuna and White Bean Salad 359
Tuna Burger 360
Tuna Melt 361
Tuna Pasta Salad with Green Beans 362
Tuna Pasta Salad with Peas, Red Bell Peppers and Red Onion 363
Tuna Pasta Salad with White Beans and Olives 364
Tuna Pesto Pasta Salad with Sun Dried Tomatoes 365
Tuna Salad 366
Tuna Salad Sandwiches 367
Tuna Tortilla Wrap 368
Tuna with Angel Hair Pasta 369

NOTES

Made in the USA
Las Vegas, NV
19 October 2023